New Developments in Diagnosing, Assessing, and Treating ADHD

Rejani Thudalikunnil Gopalan
Mahatma Gandhi Medical College and Hospital, India

IGI Global
PUBLISHER of TIMELY KNOWLEDGE

A volume in the Advances in Medical Diagnosis, Treatment, and Care (AMDTC) Book Series

Published in the United States of America by
IGI Global
Medical Information Science Reference (an imprint of IGI Global)
701 E. Chocolate Avenue
Hershey PA, USA 17033
Tel: 717-533-8845
Fax: 717-533-8661
E-mail: cust@igi-global.com
Web site: http://www.igi-global.com

Library of Congress Cataloging-in-Publication Data

Names: Gopalan, Rejani Thudalikunnil, 1974- editor.
Title: New developments in diagnosing, assessing, and treating ADHD / Rejani Thudalikunnil Gopalan, editor.
Description: Hershey, PA : Medical Information Science Reference, [2021] | Includes bibliographical references and index. | Summary: "This book explores issues and updated knowledge on the diagnosis, epidemiology, causes, risk factors, assessments, and management of ADHD"-- Provided by publisher.
Identifiers: LCCN 2020007228 (print) | LCCN 2020007229 (ebook) | ISBN 9781799854951 (hardcover) | ISBN 9781799854968 (ebook)
Subjects: MESH: Attention Deficit Disorder with Hyperactivity
Classification: LCC RC394.A85 (print) | LCC RC394.A85 (ebook) | NLM WS 350.8.A8 | DDC 616.85/89--dc23
LC record available at https://lccn.loc.gov/2020007228
LC ebook record available at https://lccn.loc.gov/2020007229

This book is published in the IGI Global book series Advances in Medical Diagnosis, Treatment, and Care (AMDTC) (ISSN: 2475-6628; eISSN: 2475-6636)

British Cataloguing in Publication Data
A Cataloguing in Publication record for this book is available from the British Library.

Advances in Medical Diagnosis, Treatment, and Care (AMDTC) Book Series

ISSN:2475-6628
EISSN:2475-6636

Mission

Advancements in medicine have prolonged the life expectancy of individuals all over the world. Once life-threatening conditions have become significantly easier to treat and even cure in many cases. Continued research in the medical field will further improve the quality of life, longevity, and wellbeing of individuals.

The **Advances in Medical Diagnosis, Treatment, and Care (AMDTC)** book series seeks to highlight publications on innovative treatment methodologies, diagnosis tools and techniques, and best practices for patient care. Comprised of comprehensive resources aimed to assist professionals in the medical field apply the latest innovations in the identification and management of medical conditions as well as patient care and interaction, the books within the AMDTC series are relevant to the research and practical needs of medical practitioners, researchers, students, and hospital administrators.

Coverage

- Patient Interaction
- Medical Testing
- Alternative Medicine
- Patient-Centered Care
- Medical Procedures
- Internal Medicine
- Emergency Medicine
- Chronic Conditions
- Experimental Medicine
- Disease Prevention

IGI Global is currently accepting manuscripts for publication within this series. To submit a proposal for a volume in this series, please contact our Acquisition Editors at Acquisitions@igi-global.com or visit: http://www.igi-global.com/publish/.

The Advances in Medical Diagnosis, Treatment, and Care (AMDTC) Book Series (ISSN 2475-6628) is published by IGI Global, 701 E. Chocolate Avenue, Hershey, PA 17033-1240, USA, www.igi-global.com. This series is composed of titles available for purchase individually; each title is edited to be contextually exclusive from any other title within the series. For pricing and ordering information please visit http://www.igi-global.com/book-series/advances-medical-diagnosis-treatment-care/129618. Postmaster: Send all address changes to above address.

Titles in this Series

For a list of additional titles in this series, please visit: www.igi-global.com/book-series

Noninvasive Ventilation Technologies and Healthcare for Geriatric Patients
César Fonseca (Universidade de Évora, Portugal) Manuel José Lopes (Universidade de Évora, Portugal) David Mendes (Universidade de Évora, Portugal) Jose Garcia-Alonso (University of Extremadura, Spain) and Felismina Mendes (Universidade de Évora,Portugal)
Medical Information Science Reference • ©2020 • 252pp • H/C (ISBN: 9781799835318) • US $245.00

Diagnostic and Treatment Methods for Ulcerative Colitis and Colitis-Associated Cancer
Ashok Kumar Pandurangan (B.S. Abdur Rahman Crescent Institute of Science and Technology, India)
Medical Information Science Reference • ©2020 • 300pp • H/C (ISBN: 9781799835806) • US $295.00

Biopsychosocial Perspectives and Practices for Addressing Communicable and Non-Communicable Diseases
Simon George Taukeni (University of Namibia, Namibia)
Medical Information Science Reference • ©2020 • 368pp • H/C (ISBN: 9781799821397) • US $265.00

Role of Nutrition in Providing Pro-/Anti-Inflammatory Balance Emerging Research and Opportunities
Uğur Günşen (Bandırma Onyedi Eylül University, Turkey) and Ramazan Mert Atan (Bandırma Onyedi Eylül University, Turkey)
Medical Information Science Reference • ©2020 • 214pp • H/C (ISBN: 9781799835943) • US $235.00

Handbook of Research on Prenatal, Postnatal, and Early Childhood Development
Neriman Aral (Ankara University, Turkey)
Medical Information Science Reference • ©2020 • 470pp • H/C (ISBN: 9781799829522) • US $365.00

Ethnomedicinal Plant Use and Practice in Traditional Medicine
Akash (Gurukul Kangri University, India) Navneet (Gurukul Kangri University, India) and B.S. Bhandari (Garhwal University, India)
Medical Information Science Reference • ©2020 • 380pp • H/C (ISBN: 9781799813200) • US $295.00

Interdisciplinary Approaches to Altering Neurodevelopmental Disorders
Tanu Wadhera (Dr. B. R. Ambedkar National Institute of Technology, Jalandhar, India) and Deepti Kakkar (Dr. B. R. Ambedkar National Institute of Technology, Jalandhar, India)
Medical Information Science Reference • ©2020 • 386pp • H/C (ISBN: 9781799830696) • US $295.00

IGI Global
PUBLISHER of TIMELY KNOWLEDGE

701 East Chocolate Avenue, Hershey, PA 17033, USA
Tel: 717-533-8845 x100 • Fax: 717-533-8661
E-Mail: cust@igi-global.com • www.igi-global.com

The book is dedicated to those who lost their lives, those who suffered and still suffering with COVID 19 health pandemic.

Editorial Advisory Board

Table of Contents

Detailed Table of Contents

Attention Deficit Hyperactivity Disorder (ADHD) is one of the most common neurodevelopmental disorders of the childhood which is characterized by inattention, hyperactivity and impulsivity. Diagnostic and Statistical Manual of Mental Disorders (DSM) and International Classification of Diseases (ICD) have established and revised the guidelines defining the diagnostic criteria for ADHD. This chapter focused on the diagnostic criteria for ADHD given by the ICD and DSM, and also compared the two. Children are mostly very energetic and active and hence it becomes difficult to decide if the level of activity is to be considered normal or should be taken as an indication of an ADHD symptom. Hence even when the symptoms of ADHD are observable, they require a proper assessment to reach to a diagnostic conclusion and hence diagnostic tools for assessing ADHD were also discussed in the chapter. A brief account of the disorders associated with ADHD was mentioned with an emphasis on how these symptoms would affect the academic, emotional and social areas of lives of the children. Different etiological factors including biological factors, brain anatomy, environmental factors, food /diet were discussed along with the pharmacological as well as non-pharmacological management of ADHD. Pharmacological management included brief discussion about stimulant as well as non-stimulant drugs. On the other hand, non-pharmacological treatment included behavioral interventions, neurofeedback, exercise, family therapy, social skill training and parent training.

Attention deficit hyperactivity disorder (ADHD) is the most common psychiatric condition in children. It comprises three core characteristics, namely inattention, hyperactivity, and impulsivity. The current chapter highlighted the comorbidity of ADHD with other psychiatric conditions like autism spectrum, learning disorders, bipolar disorder, externalizing problems, and sleep difficulties along with familial and academic difficulties. It also focused on the behavioral manifestation of ADHD including mental health issues like anxiety, depression, poor self-esteem, suicide, substance use, and sensory processing

This chapter focuses on ADHD in the adult population. The authors of this chapter incorporate new developments in existing understanding of the disorder. This chapter includes journey of 'ADHD diagnosis in adults' to current practice. Understanding of newer aspect of etiological research and its application in identification of adult ADHD is given utmost importance in this chapter. Core parts of the disorder like clinical features, diagnosis, comorbidity, and management are discussed in detail, keeping in mind disease progression from childhood to adulthood. Finally, the authors discussed a lacunae in current scenario and possible future interventions that can improve overall outcome of functional impairments in adults.

The chapter highlights the role of comprehensive assessment and its meaningful elements to construe ADHD in terms of diagnosis and management. The cognitive, affective, and behavioral symptoms must not be attributed to emotional or mood disturbance or psycho-social adjustments. The chapter explains an assessment pyramid explaining of multi-level assessment and domains with an acronym of CTP depicting cognitive, temperament, and psychopathology. Assessment may be more precise when a professional has knowledge of developmental theories. Attention hyperactivity disorder (ADHD) entails a detailed assessment, involving varied social agents, to understand the dynamic manifestation of different ages as well as the dysfunction caused by it. The current chapter emphasizes psycho-social factors, comorbidities, and dual-diagnosis issues that may exacerbate or mask the presentation of ADHD in children, adolescents, and adults.

The pharmacological treatment for ADHD has been researched well and we have efficacious drugs. Drugs are the mainstay of treatment particularly for over 6 years of age. There are two broad classes of drugs that are used in the treatment, psychostimulants and non-stimulants. Transcranial current stimulation and neurofeedback are other mechanisms that have been tried. There are various formulations and doses available for each and only certain drugs are available in India. The various guidelines broadly put stimulant Methylphenidate as the first choice and recommend early shift to a longer acting formulation. Treatment, various comorbidities, and side-effects of these drugs have to be kept in mind and dealt accordingly. Further psychosocial treatments should be used concurrently to improve the outcome.

Children with attention deficit/hyperactivity disorder (ADHD) are drawn against a number of challenges including staying on task or taking extended time to complete, having trouble listening attentively, or difficulty sitting still. In the past, it was thought that children with ADHD would eventually outgrow the symptoms of the disorder. However, children generally continue to show symptoms of the disorder well into adulthood. The presence of ADHD transforms over the course of a person's lifespan, and the way in which the disorder affects children also changes dramatically when they are older. In adults, one of the core difficulties is executive functioning, which results in restlessness, disorganisation, deviating attention, procrastination, impulsive decision making, and more. In order to prevent the development and escalation of more deviant behaviours, early assessment and treatment program for ADHD should be considered from young age. A highly effective treatment practice for ADHD is a multi-modal approach that combines both pharmacological and behavioural interventions.

The prevalence of ADHD is estimated at 5–7% worldwide, which makes it one of the most common psychiatric disorders in children and adolescents. Children with Attention deficit hyperactivity disorder can become difficult if the child is not monitored using correct strategies and techniques. Parents play an integral role in shaping a child. Parenting involves biological as well as the legal aspects and other equally if not more important dimensions of care, protection, nurturance, understanding, guidance, mutual interaction, and partnership occurring within the protective environment of a family. Parenting a differently abled child is very demanding and challenging and the role of family and parents in caring for a child is very crucial, especially development, socializing, and protecting the child.

This chapter is an attempt to discuss the interpersonal difficulties encountered by adults with ADHD. ADHD is one of the most common psychiatric disorders, while adult ADHD still remains the most undiagnosed one due to its comorbidity with other psychiatric disorders. It was until recently that the importance of adult ADHD was recognized to have an impact on the interpersonal difficulties faced by them. The core symptoms of ADHD in the form of behavioral and cognitive impairments along with social skill deficits are associated with maladjustments in their social and personal relationships that often lead to marital discord, problems with peers, family dysfunction, and parent-child conflicts.

Attention-deficit/hyperactivity disorder (ADHD) is one of the most common behavioral disorders of childhood. Children with ADHD exhibit developmentally inappropriate levels of inattention, impulsivity, and/or motor activity. Attention-deficit/hyperactivity disorder (ADHD) is one of the most frequent mental disorders affecting children. ADHD also affects many adults. Symptoms of ADHD include inattention, hyperactivity, and impulsivity. ADHD may also negatively affect the learning environment in children's homes. This chapter talks about social functioning, social deficits, interpersonal difficulties, and social skills training in ADHD. Individuals with ADHD have problems in the areas of peer interaction, emotional regulation, and pro-social behaviours. These social problems are associated with a greater risk for developing problems later in life.

Attention deficit hyperactivity disorder (ADHD) is one of the widely prevalent externalizing disorders from the category of neurodevelopmental disorders. With the constant rise in the diagnosis of a number of cases presenting ADHD or ADHD-like symptoms, the need to understand issues as experienced by the student requires the right interventions for effective management. The core challenges in the area of academics and overall presentation lie with the executive function deficits that the child has. Hence, addressing those and working on skills like attention, working memory, response inhibition, goal setting, planning, problem solving, and organization has to be considered as part of the management plan. The current chapter explores evidence-based issues and strategies to be targeted in the classroom set up for students with ADHD. It also highlights some classroom-specific strategies, which can be focused by the teachers and remedial therapists.

Children and adolescents with ADHD are at an increased risk for various substance use disorders and developing early-onset substance abuse. Both ADHD and substance abuse are said to be disorders of disinhibition, which suggests that both share an underlying vulnerability and have more chances to co-occur. The substance abuse in children and adolescents with ADHD is growing, and many factors accumulate to heighten the risk for such problem. The symptoms of ADHD and their secondary problems, availability of drugs, poor coping mechanisms, and the need for adventure and excitement lead them into substance abuse easily. Once they are trapped into substance abuse, it becomes difficult for them to quit, and the tolerance for drugs and risk taking behaviours makes them experiment with new drugs with more quantity. This in turn results in severe consequences and affects them physically, psychologically, and socially, as well as their overall quality of life.

ADHD or attention deficit hyperactivity disorder has gained immense importance both among the clinicians and researchers because of its early onset, variable clinical presentations, and prominent heritability. Along with the established symptom clusters of attention deficit and hyperactivity, a load of comorbidities have been found hugely prevalent for this population, increasing the morbidity and distress level and turning the management more complex. The early childhood and adolescent onset of this externalizing behavior-based disorder also makes the individual more prone to other externalizing behavioral problems, like addiction to variable psychoactive substances. Adolescent, being a natural age towards risk taking and novelty seeking, addiction proneness itself is a major individual and public health challenge to which ADHD works as potential fuel. In recent times, the upsurge of various behavioral addictions has also been seen prominently in the ADHD population increasing the morbidity and complexity. Treatment options need to be researched in detail.

Methylphenidate (MPH) is the most commonly used drug to treat attention deficit/hyperactivity disorder (ADHD) in children effectively and safely. However, in spite of its widespread application throughout what is considered one of the most plastic and sensitive phases of brain development in children, very little is known to date about its long-term effects on brain structure and function leading well into later adolescence and adulthood. Additionally, there is scant information available to parents, clinicians, and clients with ADD/ADHD about the influence of MPH on brain development. More importantly, recent human and animal studies suggest that MPH alters the dopaminergic system with long-term effects beyond the termination of treatment. As such, a multimodal treatment with psychodynamic therapies can assist the treatment team to support the development of the client's pro-social skills in addition to medication treatment, thus reducing full reliance on MPH as the primary treatment for ADD/ADHD.

Attention deficit hyperactivity (ADHD) manifests with symptoms of inattention, hyperactivity, and impulsivity. The long term consequences of ADHD have been explored on different dimensions such as physical growth, cognitive functions, and other mental health problems. The link between ADHD and criminal activities in adolescents and adulthood were also studied cross sectional and longitudinal methods and many found a relation with criminal activities. But it is important to explore how the disorder, its symptoms, co morbidities including addiction, social and familial adversities affects the relation. This chapter attempted to find the link on these dimensions. Studies have pointed out that ADHD diagnosis poses the increased risk for committing offenses and repetition of acts as well as prone for bullying and victimization, and it is not the symptoms but other environmental and familial factors are also need to be looked in to understand the link between ADHD and crime. Though many studies have shown an association of ADHD with co morbid Addictive disorders to crime, more studies are required to establish exact nature of the relationship.

Many studies have proven that parental stress was associated with childhood mental disorders and disabilities, and in recent years, studies have shown that parents of children with neurodevelopmental disorders (NDDs) experience more parenting stress than parents of typically developing children. Parents living with a child with ADHD experienced stress as they struggled to cope with the child's symptoms amidst the stigmatizing attitudes from family and community members. The chapter tried to explore various factors related with parental stress and ADHD such as quality of life, parental rating of ADHD symptoms and related issues, treatment outcome, marital life, and mental health. One of the important factors contributing to stress is stigma, and the chapter also attempted to explore the link between parental stress and stigma, especially related to ADHD and its interventions. The chapter emphasized the role of mindfulness training for treating ADHD and parental stress while pointing out the methodological limitations.

Attention deficit hyperactivity disorder (ADHD) is a neurodevelopmental disorder that commonly occurs among children between the age ranges of 3-10 years. Though pharmacotherapy in combination of play therapy and behavior therapy has been proved to be effective for the treatment of ADHD, but the results derived from them does not seem to sustain for a longer period of time. There are other alternative therapies too, which can help in management of the symptoms of ADHD. This chapter talks about the different aspects of yoga and effect of different asanas, pranayama, and meditation on ADHD. As medication has its own negative side effects, practitioners have started to research other techniques to be helpful for managing ADHD, and Yoga is proved to be one of the effective ways to reduce the symptoms of ADHD. Yoga is not only limited to the physical exercise; it also includes breathing exercises, meditation, and relaxation exercises, which help to have a balance between mind and body. Through regular practice of yoga, one can attain peace of mind and can lead a happy and healthy life.

ADHD is a neurodevelopmental disorder affecting a significant number of people. It is characterized by inattention and/or hyperactivity and/or impulsivity. It impacts various aspects of an individual's life. Rehabilitation is a holistic process, aiming at restoring and training an individual to improve their quality of life, increase independence, increase social participation and social inclusion. A combination of various rehabilitation strategies are used depending on the individual's needs, severity of the disorder, and developmental phase. Apart from the client, involving parents, caregivers, teachers, schools, and employers and co-workers ensure a consistent and effective rehabilitation process. This chapter focuses on the rehabilitation strategies like medication, behavioral training, psychoeducation, psychotherapy, social skills training, remediation methods, classroom management, parent training, coaching, support groups, lifestyle changes, and career and vocational guidance. Using timely intervention strategies and training enhances the rehabilitation process.

Preface

First of all, I would like to mention that the final editing of this book has been done in the midst of lockdown due to COVID 19 health pandemic. In a way it is a historical attempt as entire world was standstill with fear and ambiguities and saddened with news of death of millions. Many of the authors, reviewers and editorial members were directly and indirectly involved in the management of COVID 19, especially related to the mental health aspects of public, suspected patients, quarantine clients and health workers. Lots of struggles were encountered but everyone put their heart and soul and worked with commitments to complete this book.

With immense gratitude towards those who put hard work to write and review the chapters, I would briefly introduce this book. Our understanding about the clinical symptoms, causes and management of Attention Deficit and Hyperactivity disorder has gone through remarkable changes in past few decades though ambiguity still continues on many dimensions. My interest in ADHD intensified while doing PhD and I am thankful to Late Professor Anna Oommen, National Institute of Mental Health and Neuro Sciences (NIMHANS), India for introducing this area to me and guiding me for my PhD work. I am glad that I could get in touch with thousands many children, adolescents, and adults with ADHD and their families throughout my career which helped me to understand them better way and motivated to explore more innovative ways to help them. The confession of many parents, disappointments and frustrations of clients always made me to feel that our current understanding about ADHD is not adequate enough to address their concerns and issues and we have a long way to go. Two decades back, researchers were more focused on children with ADHD and their families, and then started to focus on adolescents and now focusing on adults with ADHD and their interpersonal, marital and parenting skills too. The management was also evolved on different dimensions. This book is an attempt to explore and combine recent development in the area of ADHD on different dimensions with an objective of imparting knowledge mainly for students, researchers, clinicians and academicians.

The book focused on history, diagnostic classifications, etiology, specific focus on clinical features, assessment and management of children, adolescents and adults with ADHD, co morbidities, Pharmacological, Psychosocial and multimodal managements, classroom issues and remediation, parenting and parental stress, and legal issues.

The first chapter deals with the diagnostic criteria for ADHD given by the ICD and DSM, and also compares the two. Diagnostic tools for assessing ADHD, brief account of the disorders associated with ADHD, etiological factors including biological factors, brain anatomy, environmental factors, food /diet are discussed along with the pharmacological as well as non-pharmacological management of ADHD. Pharmacological management includes brief discussion about stimulant as well as non-stimulant drugs. On the other hand, non-pharmacological treatment includes behavioral interventions, neurofeedback, exercise, family therapy, social skill training, and parent training.

Chapter 2 discusses about the co morbidity of ADHD with other psychiatric conditions like autism spectrum disorders, learning disorders, bipolar affective disorders, externalizing problems, and sleep difficulties along with familial and academic difficulties. It also focused on the behavioral manifestation of ADHD including mental health issues like anxiety, depression, poor self-esteem, suicide, substance use, and sensory processing deficits. Non Pharmacological treatments like behavioral methods, Parent and teacher's training methods, cognitive behavioral therapy and physical activity training are mentioned as treatment strategies.

Chapter 3 explores on pre, peri and post natal risk factors in ADHD. With heritability accounting for 75% to 80% of the variability seen in ADHD, the remaining is explained through environmental risk factors that are exposed during critical period of pre-, peri- and postnatal development. The chapter discusses about prenatal stressors mainly maternal substance use during pregnancy, cigarette smoking, and abuse of illicit drugs, environmental toxins, maternal stress, and maternal characteristics during pregnancy. The chapter also discuss about perinatal Stressors such as hypoxia, low birth weight (LBW) and pre-term baby and postnatal Stressors as quality of parent-child relationship, socioeconomic factors and adverse childhood experiences, respiratory disorders and infections. The author concluded that though literature on the risk factors has been mostly controversial, certain associations have been made with regards to ADHD pathophysiology.

Chapter 4 deals with children and ADHD. It explores classification, assessment and psychological management of ADHD in children and factor related to better outcomes in children. The psychological management focuses on the intervention for better educational outcomes, attention enhancement strategies, improving motivation through internal and external modifications.

Chapter 5 attempts to individually understand the concept of adolescence and ADHD before it combines to the understanding of the progression of ADHD as a neurodevelopmental and behavioural disorder moving through the lifespan in different formats/symptoms. This understanding would provide the clinicians and academicians to develop clarity and be able to follow the golden rule of 'early diagnosis early intervention' by identifying the progressive nature in terms of genetic, biochemistry, psycho-social and personality aspects maintaining the disorder. This chapter would provide overview about the possible interventions and treatment plans available and briefly discuss the recent issues and trends.

Chapter 6 focuses on ADHD in adult population. Recent acceptance of ADHD as a disorder of lifespan has increased research on the subject which leads to tremendous knowledge expansion in this field. Authors of this chapter are making an effort to incorporate new developments in to existing understanding of the disorder. This chapter includes journey of 'ADHD diagnosis in adult' to current practice. Understanding of newer aspect of etiological research and its application in identification of adult ADHD has been emphasized in this chapter. Core part of disorder like clinical features, diagnosis, co morbidity and management are discussed in details keeping in mind about disease progression from childhood to adulthood. Finally, authors discussed about lacunae in current scenario and possible future interventions which can improve overall outcome of functional impairments in adults.

Chapter 7 deals with assessment of ADHD among children, adolescents and adults. Authors attempts to explain the assessment process at different levels such as individual, family, Academic/Occupational/Interpersonal relationship and listed the tools for assessment and observation. They emphasized that one should always be observant while eliciting family or marital history if a family member of the index case shows the manifestation of 'never identified' ADHD and contributes to family psychopathology or disturbed family functioning.

Chapter 8 covers pharmacological management for ADHD. It discusses about management under two broad classes: Psychostimulants and Non-stimulants which included Methylphenidate, Amphetamines, and Clonidine. There are various formulations and doses available for each drug. Guidelines broadly put Stimulant, Methylphenidate as the first choice and recommend early shift to a longer acting formulation. While treatment, various comorbidities like tics, anxiety symptoms, mood symptoms along with side-effects of these drugs have to be kept in mind and dealt accordingly to improve the outcome and also to ensure adherence. Further certain salient points for administration of these drugs are highlighted in the chapter.

Chapter 9 draws attention to the integrated understanding of individual Children with attention deficit/ hyperactivity disorder (ADHD). A highly effective treatment practice for ADHD is multi-modal approach that combines both pharmacological and behavioral interventions. The chapter mainly focuses on the behavioral management and its techniques for different age groups. Authors attempt to explain various techniques like token economy, contingency management, modeling, extinction, and tips for parents in addition to mentioning about CBT, mindfulness, social skill training and exercises.

Parents play an integral role in shaping a child and chapter ten concentrates on parenting with children diagnosed to have ADHD. Parenting a differently abled child is very demanding and challenging and the role of family and parents in caring for a child is very crucial especially development, socializing and protecting the child. The chapter delves into different aspects of parenting and describes parenting styles, parenting challenges, and also discusses the impact of parent-child interactions. Stress and coping of parents are also mentioned. A detailed description of parent training programs and its techniques are highlighted in the chapter.

Chapter 11 covers issues related to ADHD and its impact on interpersonal relationships. The core symptoms of ADHD in the form of behavioral and cognitive impairments, along with social skill deficits are associated with maladjustments in their social and personal relationships that often lead to peers issues, sexual problems, marital discords, and parental capabilities. The chapter focuses on issues and challenges in friendship and with peer groups, dating and romance, and sexual behavior. It also explores difficulties face at marriage and parenting. The residue of the marital complications, along with ADHD symptoms, can be seen in the parental capabilities of these individuals.

Chapter 12 aimed to draw attention to the social functioning, interpersonal difficulties, and social deficits associated with ADHD. Individuals with ADHD have problems in the areas of peer interaction, emotional regulation, and pro-social behaviours. These social problems are associated with a greater risk for developing problems later in life. This chapter talks about all these issues and it also mention about social skills training for individuals with ADHD.

Chapter 13 focuses on executive function deficits among ADHD Students in classroom learning. The core challenges in the area of academics and overall presentation lie with the executive function deficits that the child has. Hence addressing those and working on skills like attention, working memory, response inhibition, goal setting, planning, problem solving and organization has to be considered as part of the management plan. The current chapter explores evidence based issues and strategies to be targeted in the classroom set up for the students with ADHD. It also highlights some classroom specific strategies which can be focused by the teachers and remedial therapists.

Chapter 14 explores about Substance Abuse in Children and Adolescents with ADHD. Both ADHD and substance abuse are said to be disorders of disinhibition, which suggests that both share an underlying vulnerability and has more chances to co-occur. In the present chapter the link between ADHD and substance abuse is discussed. The risk factors for the occurrence of substance abuse in individuals with ADHD along the consequences of it on one's body and mind, and treatment options are also highlighted in the chapter.

Chapter 15 deals with ADHD and addiction. Adolescent, being a natural age towards risk taking and novelty seeking, addiction proneness itself is a major individual and public health challenge, to which ADHD works as potential fuel. In the recent times, the upsurge of various behavioral addictions has also been seen prominently in the ADHD population increasing the morbidity and complexity. The chapter deals with Adult ADHD and Addiction and its pharmacological and psychosocial treatment strategies.

Chapter 16 explores ADHD and comorbidity with Substance Abuse & Brain Development and the long term impact of Methylphenidate on adolescents. Methylphenidate (MPH) is the most commonly used drug to treat attention deficit/hyperactivity disorder (ADHD) in children effectively and safely. However, in spite of its widespread application throughout what is considered one of the most plastic and sensitive phases of brain development in children very little is known to date about its long-term effects on brain structure and function leading well into later adolescence and adulthood. Additionally, there is scant information available to parents, clinicians clients with an ADD/ADHD about the influence of MPH on brain development. The chapter discuses various issues related to it.

Chapter 17 deals with ADHD and offences. The link between ADHD and criminal activities in adolescents and adulthood were studied cross sectional and longitudinal methods and many found a relation with criminal activities. But it is important to explore how the disorder, its symptoms, co morbidities including addiction, social and familial adversities affects the relation. This chapter attempted to find the link on these dimensions. Studies have pointed out that ADHD diagnosis poses the increased risk for committing offenses and repetition of acts as well as prone for bullying and victimization, and it is not the symptoms but other environmental and familial factors are also need to be looked in to understand the link between ADHD and crime. The author concluded that though many studies have shown an association of ADHD with co morbid Addictive disorders to crime, more studies are required to establish exact nature of the relationship.

Chapter 18 covers parental stress, coping, and stigma related to ADHD. Parents living with a child with ADHD experienced stress as they struggle to cope with the child's symptoms amidst the stigmatizing attitudes from family and community members. The chapter tried to explore various factors related with parental stress and ADHD such as quality of life, parental rating of ADHD symptoms and related issues, treatment outcome, marital life and mental health. One of the important factors contributing to stress is stigma and the chapter also attempted to explore the link between parental stress and stigma, especially related to ADHD and its interventions. The chapter emphasized role of mindfulness training for treating ADHD and parental stress while pointing out the methodological limitations.

Chapter 19 focuses on yoga and ADHD. As medication has its own negative side effects, practitioners have started to research on other techniques to be helpful for managing ADHD and Yoga is proved to be one of the effective ways to reduce the symptoms of ADHD. Yoga is not only limited to the physical exercise but it also includes breathing exercises, meditation and relaxation exercises which helps to have a balance between mind and body. This chapter talks about the different aspects of yoga and effect of different asanas, pranayama and meditation on ADHD.

Finally, Chapter 20 deals with rehabilitation strategies for individuals suffering with ADHD. Rehabilitation is a holistic process, aiming at restoring and training an individual to improve their quality of life, increase independence, increase social participation and social inclusion. A combination of various rehabilitation strategies are used depending on the individual's needs, severity of the disorder and developmental phase. This chapter focuses on the rehabilitation strategies like medication, behavioral training, psychoeducation, psychotherapy, social skills training, remediation methods, classroom management, parent training, coaching, support groups, lifestyle changes and career and vocational guidance.

This book was aimed to provide the latest empirical research findings in the area of Attention Deficit/Hyperactivity Disorder (ADHD) focusing on epidemiology, assessment, causes, and comorbidities, ADHD at various stages (childhood, adolescence, and adulthood), educational issues, sexuality, marriage and parenting issues, forensic issues, stigma, and mental health problems among family members. It would also provide a fresh approach and comprehensive knowledge on ADHD and its various aspects and I think the chapters have done justice to the objective of the book.

I am hopeful that the target audience of this book (composed of professionals and researchers working in the mental health area such as clinicians (especially Psychiatrists, Clinical Psychologists,Pediatricians), academicians, special educators, social workers, Psychiatric nurses, rehabilitation centres, and students in the area of mental health) would be benefited from this book. This book is useful for Universities, hospitals, and the public. Moreover, it would provide a deep knowledge on ADHD and its various issues from a developmental approach and it is valuable as it deals with their sexual issues, marriage, parenting skills and issues faced by the family members such as stigma, stress and mental health problems. It will further enrich our current knowledge of ADHD. I hope this book will be another stepping stone to understand ADHD in a more comprehensive way especially in understanding the various psychosocial issues related to the condition.

The research works cited in this book is referenced according to APA guidelines.

Acknowledgment

I express my gratitude towards all who have contributed and joined with me in the process of writing this book. I would like to thank my son Harikrishnan for his patience, family members for their encouragements and support. Special thanks to all authors, reviewers and editorial members for their constant support and enthusiasm. My heartfelt thanks to the publisher for their continuous support and suggestions.

Special thanks authors, reviewers, editorial members who were involved in mental health aid for people affected with COVID 19.

Chapter 1
Attention Deficit Hyperactivity Disorder (ADHD):
An Overview

Girija Shirish Patwardhan
https://orcid.org/0000-0002-8893-6852
Dhruv Educational and Research Foundation, India

ABSTRACT

Attention Deficit Hyperactivity Disorder (ADHD) is one of the most common neurodevelopmental disorders of the childhood which is characterized by inattention, hyperactivity and impulsivity. Diagnostic and Statistical Manual of Mental Disorders (DSM) and International Classification of Diseases (ICD) have established and revised the guidelines defining the diagnostic criteria for ADHD. This chapter focused on the diagnostic criteria for ADHD given by the ICD and DSM, and also compared the two. Children are mostly very energetic and active and hence it becomes difficult to decide if the level of activity is to be considered normal or should be taken as an indication of an ADHD symptom. Hence even when the symptoms of ADHD are observable, they require a proper assessment to reach to a diagnostic conclusion and hence diagnostic tools for assessing ADHD were also discussed in the chapter. A brief account of the disorders associated with ADHD was mentioned with an emphasis on how these symptoms would affect the academic, emotional and social areas of lives of the children. Different etiological factors including biological factors, brain anatomy, environmental factors, food /diet were discussed along with the pharmacological as well as non-pharmacological management of ADHD. Pharmacological management included brief discussion about stimulant as well as non-stimulant drugs. On the other hand, non-pharmacological treatment included behavioral interventions, neurofeedback, exercise, family therapy, social skill training and parent training.

WHAT IS ADHD

ADHD stands for Attention Deficit Hyperactivity Disorder. A paediatrician, George Still, from UK first described a syndrome called as hyperkinetic disorder, in 1902.ADHD is one of the most common

DOI: 10.4018/978-1-7998-5495-1.ch001

neurodevelopmental disorders of the childhood and is characterized by, impulsivity, excessive or exaggerated motor behaviour and difficulty in sustaining attention. It is characterized by developmentally inappropriate functioning in the domains of inattention, hyperactivity and impulsivity. Due to their overactivity and impulsivity, children with ADHD struggle to fit into the school structure (Lange, Reichl, Lange, Tucha, & Tucha, 2010).

As mentioned above, this disorder is marked by inattention, impulsiveness, low tolerance for frustration, and a great deal of in appropriate activity. All children show such traits at times, but for ADHD children, such behaviour is common, interfering with their home and school functioning (Nigg, 2001). It is often difficult to distinguish between children who are highly active and those with ADHD (Feldman, 2010). Hence indicates that it's a matter of degree in terms of the level of activity, but children with ADHD show a variety of other behaviours which makes them difficult to deal with. Even when it seems difficult to draw the line, significant people who tend to be around the child for a longer period of time, like parents and specifically teachers, can observe these children in comparison with other children of the same chronological age.

According to Thomas Brown in his article, ADD/ADHD is seen as a cognitive disorder, according to him it is a developmental impairment of executive functions, the self- management system of the brain. This impairment results in chronic difficulties in executive wide variety of daily tasks (Brown, 2009).

In a study to understand executive function deficits in Attention Deficit/ Hyperactivity Disorder; the researchers compared children's performance on both neuropsychological and real life measures of executive function and processing speed. They used Stroop and Wisconsin Card Sorting Task as neuropsychological measures and videogame and zoo task as real life measures. There was no difference in two groups in executive performance on Stroop effect or zoo task but ADHD group showed deficits in set-shifting assessed by WCST (Perseverative errors and responses). Also, ADHD group showed slowed processing speed on the task of Stroop (slower in colour naming). It was clear from the study, that children with ADHD exhibit impairments in executive function and processing speed in real life activities as well as in neuropsychological testing. Cognitive deficits detected by standardized neuropsychological tests are related to performance difficulties in real world activities (Lawrence, Houghton, Douglas, Durkin, & Whiting, 2004).

In an analysis, ADHD symptoms as mentioned in DSM-5, were found to be strongly correlated with and predictive deficits in executive functioning (Silverstein, et al., 2018).

Clinical Picture of ADHD

As mentioned above, this disorder is marked by inattention, impulsivity and hyperactivity. Some people with ADHD seem to exhibit motor hyperactivity. Children with ADHD are often fidgety, unable to sit still for a longer period of time. Due to this they may disturb the entire class. People also tend to complain about their actions without thinking. Children exhibiting hyperactivity are most frequent referrals to mental health and paediatric faculties.

ADHD is associated with a broad range of cognitive deficits, including inhibition, memory, temporal discounting, decision making, timing and Reaction Time Variability (Coghill, Seth, & Matthews, 2014).

A study exploring the mechanism of verbal working memory deficit of attention deficit hyperactive disorder showed that the children with ADHD show deficits in advanced process of verbal working memory when they were engaged in memory updating (Zhang, Fan, & Jiang, 2016).

To find the relation between IQ score and attention deficits in children with ADHD, studies of various methodologies were reviewed. The review showed a weak correlation between IQ score and attention deficits. The meta-analysis indicated that the associations between I.Q are modest with attention deficit, affecting the I.Q by 2 to 5 Points (Jepsen, Fagerlund, & Mortensen, 2009). It is difficult to understand though, if the performance is poor due to the lower levels of intelligence or due to their symptoms like distractibility, inattention, inability to pay attention to details, or impulsivity etc.

Children with ADHD experience a wide range of challenges with daily life and their education, compromising the expectations from parents and teachers according to the skills performed by other children of their age (Ayuso, Maestu, Gonzalez, RomoBarrientos, & Andrade, 2006).

ADHD adversely affects long term academic outcomes (Arnold, Hodgkins, Kahle, Madhoo, & Kewley, 2020). Children with ADHD achieve academically at a lower level as compared to their given level of intellectual abilities. Having average levels of intellectual abilities, they perform significantly below the prediction in reading, writing and mathematics skills as compared to the children with similar level of intellectual abilities but no ADHD. Research has indicated that the severity of ADHD symptoms based on parent reports, significantly predicted academic underachievement in reading, writing and maths. More severe behavioural symptoms of children with ADHD is, more negatively impacted is the school performance (Barry, Lyman, & Klinger, 2002).

Reading difficulties and academic problems associated with ADHD are also common. Langer (2015), studied how the disorders interact and to what extent can they be differentiated. Structural and functional magnetic resonance techniques were combined with comprehensive behavioural tests, in order to characterize behaviour, brain structure, and neural correlates of executive function, phonological processing and reading fluency in children with diagnosis of ADHD, RD, Comorbidity and controls. The neuroimaging results demonstrated structural and functional atypicalities for comorbidity regions that are frequently associated with deficits in children who have ADHD or RD (Langer, Benjamin, Becker, & Gaab, 2015).

Children with ADHD achieve academically at a lower level as compared to their given level of intellectual abilities. A study examined whether the students identified as gifted underachievers were more likely to manifest symptoms of ADHD, as measured by ADHD-IV. Over half of these gifted underachievers met the screening criteria for ADHD based on the teacher reports, and almost 30% of them met screening criteria for ADHD based on the parent reports. Most of these students had elevated scores on inattention. The results of the study suggested that a substantial percentage of gifted underachievers exhibit attentional problems at home, and these attentional problems are severe enough to merit further examination (McCoach, Siegle, & Rubenstein, 2020).

It is difficult to pin point the exact reason behind poor academic performance exhibited by children diagnosed with ADHD. Different studies have been carried out by researchers to understand different aspects of cognitive functions along with the anatomical differences in the brain among children diagnosed with ADHD. The studies that focus on brain anatomy of the children with ADHD have used scanning techniques like fMRI etc; whereas studies conducted in order to evaluate the cognitive functioning base their research on different psychological test batteries or rating scales; usually the group of children with ADHD is compared with the control group.

It might be a result of different factors like basic differences in brain anatomy, difficulties in emotion regulation etc. different studies have been conducted based on the academic performances of children with ADHD. A study based on academic achievements in children with Autism and ADHD, showed underachievement in ADHD children (Mayes, Waschbusch, Calhoun, & Mattison, 2019).

Along with difficulties in academic performance, children with ADHD also have difficulties with peers, disturbing their social lives. A study examined process involved in peer problems among the children with a diagnosis of ADHD. Measures of social skills, aggression, positive illusory bias in social and behavioural domains, and peer rejection were taken. It was found that peer rejection was related to impaired social skills, which in turn predict later peer rejection. And in this way it turns into a viscous cycle (Murray-Close, et al., 2010). Children with ADHD also experience emotional problems. Children with ADHD have been found to face difficulties with emotion regulation. DSM-III noted emotional disturbance as associated features of ADHD and not a diagnostic criterion. In a study, the authors found that emotion dysregulation is prevalent in ADHD, they also reported that emotion dysregulation in ADHD may arise as a result of deficits in orienting towards, recognizing and/or allotting attention to emotional stimuli; these are related to the dysfunction within straito-amygdalo-medial prefrontal cortical network (Shaw, Stringaris, Nigg, & Leinbenluft, 2014). Secondary complications include low self-esteem and antisocial behaviour.

Emotional symptoms are very common in attention deficit hyperactivity disorder patients and associated with much morbidity, some consider it to be a core feature rather than an associated trait. Emotional symptoms in ADHD cause clinically significant impairments. Even when emotional symptoms are common in other psychiatric disorders, emotional impulsivity and deficient emotional self- regulation, may be specifically for ADHD as a diagnostic criteria (Faraone, et al., 2019).

Emotion Dysregulation is associated with ADHD among young adolescents, and is associated with social impairment. Emotion dysregulation includes behavioural dyscontrol in the presence of strong emotions and inflexibility or slow return to emotional baseline (Bunford, Evans, & Langberg, 2014).

If we try to look at the issues they face, the issues seem to be related to each other. Cognitive symptoms, along with the emotional symptom might lead to poor performance in academics. That might lead to rise in emotional symptoms and social issues. Social issues again leading to the emotional disturbances and the cycle continues.

Prevalence

The prevalence of ADHD is about 5.2% of the child population across all regions of the world (Polanczyk, Lima, Horta, Biederman, & Rohde, 2007).

Sometimes children who are very active are misdiagnosed as suffering with ADHD. The appropriateness or inappropriateness of a behaviour differs from culture to culture. This very fact can also affect the number of cases being labelled as ADHD. Generally for better diagnosis, the appropriateness of the behaviour is looked at from the chronological age and IQ of the children.

As mentioned in ICD-10, ADHD is several times more frequent in boys than in girls. The reason behind the gender difference is not known yet. A meta-analysis of relevant research including 18 studies was conducted. Compared to ADHD boys, ADHD girls displayed greater intellectual impairment, lower level of hyperactivity, and lower rates of other externalizing behaviours (Gaub & Carlson, 1997).

Diagnosis

There are two systems that provide the guidelines for the diagnostic criteria of different disorders, namely Diagnostic and Statistical Manual of Mental Disorders (DSM) and the International Statistical Classification of Diseases and Related Health Problems (ICD).

The International Classification of Disease (Version 10), i.e ICD-10, uses the term Hyperkinetic disorder, whereas, the Statistical and Diagnostic Manual of Mental Disorders (Version 5), i.e. DSM 5, has adopted the term Attention Deficit Hyperactivity disorder. Both of the systems have similar yet not identical criteria for the same.

ADHD is never diagnosed based on a single symptom, but a group of symptoms, broadly divided as Inattention, Hyperactivity and Impulsivity. From the time, ADHD was included in DSM, it has undergone many changes in the criteria for its diagnosis. The diagnostic classification has undergone several revisions.

The Diagnostic Criteria for ADHD

Diagnostic and Statistical Manual for Mental Disorders- IV-TR (DSM-IV-TR)

According to the DSM-IV-TR, the diagnostic criteria for ADHD include six or more symptoms of inattention, persisted for at least a period of 6 months which are maladaptive for the child's development. Or six or more symptoms of Hyperactivity-impulsivity, to a maladaptive degree, present over the period of at least 6 months (American Psychiatric Association, 2000).

A major shift was made in the overall DSM-5 was in terms of its multi-axial system. The multi-axial system was eliminated in the fifth edition of DSM. Another major change was made by creating a new chapter called " Neurodevelopmental Disorders". ADHD was removed from the "Disorders of Childhood and Adolescence" and was included in this new category of "Neurodevelopmental disorders". The diagnostic criteria for ADHD underwent some revisions in DSM-5.

Diagnostic and Statistical Manual for Mental Disorders-5 (DSM 5)

According to DSM-5, two categories of symptoms are specified. One is Inattention and the other is Hyperactivity and Impulsivity. Symptoms like not listening to others while they talk, not being able to pay attention to details, inability to follow through the instructions given, getting distracted easily due to some external stimulus, avoidance of doing a task which demands mental effort etc. comprise the first category of symptoms, which are named as Inattention. On the other hand inability to sit at one place when expected, inappropriate climbing, fidgeting, excessive talking etc are symptoms that indicate Hyperactivity and, intruding others, not being able to wait for their turn indicate Impulsivity.

It is also necessary to specify, if the presentation of the symptoms is a combination of Inattention and Hyperactive- Impulsive symptoms, or if it is predominantly inattentive or predominantly Hyperactive-Impulsive presentation.

It is also needed to specify the severity 'mild', 'moderate' or 'severe', depending on the symptoms and the degree to which the impairment in functioning are seen (American Psychiatric Association, 2013).

As mentioned in their review, Doernberg & Hollander (2016), the changes in the diagnostic criteria for ADHD made from DSM-IV-TR to DSM-5 include following:

1. Same symptom criteria were continued in DSM-5, but specific examples were added under each criterion, to facilitate easier classification of the disorder.
2. Another change made was regarding the age of onset. The age of onset was changed from 7 years to 12 years. Hence now, according to DSM-5 the symptoms must occur before the age of 12 years.

3. Inclusion of specifiers in order to designating either predominantly inattentive or predominantly hyperactive/impulsive presentation of ADHD was another feature in the diagnostic criteria for ADHD according to DSM-5.
4. A change in threshold of symptoms has been made for adults. The cut-off for the diagnosis of adults has been changed to 5 symptoms of inattention or hyperactivity instead of 6 (Doernberg & Hollander, 2016).

Epstein and Loren (2013) mention that in DSM-IV, ADHD was described in different types. In the recent criteria for ADHD, according to DSM-5, the modifiers are added to specify the severity of the disorder, as 'mild', 'moderate', or 'severe'. ADHD can now also be coded as 'in partial remission'.

As they mention in their review, the modifications in DSM-5 have a potential to make the diagnosis of ADHD more reliable. The change from the subtypes to the presentation of the disorder in DSM-5 reflects the increase in evidence that the symptoms are more fluid within the individuals across the lifespan. The switch from requirement of the evidence from impairment to the evidence of the presence of symptoms for both the pervasiveness and age onset criteria is likely to improve the reliability. Also, by not changing the core symptoms, but changing how these symptoms affect in different areas of a person's life, like academic, interpersonal, occupational etc. DSM-5 leads to a much reliable diagnosis (Epstein & Loren, 2013).

In a study, parent ratings were collected and compared, as the changes in the diagnostic criteria for ADHD were expanded to include new descriptors referred to adolescent and adult symptom manifestations in DSM-5. It was observed that in a sample of already diagnosed DSM-IV-TR ADHD, parents led to endorse slightly more symptoms of inattention (Sibley & Yeguez, 2018).

Diagnostic Criteria by ICD-10

According to ICD-10, the Hyperkinetic disorder is classified under Behavioural and Emotional Disorders with Onset Usually Occurring in Childhood and Adolescence, and is coded as F90 (World Health Organization, 1992).

The diagnostic criteria by ICD-10 are more strict as compared to the criteria given by DSM-5. According to ICD-10, hyperkinetic disorders is a group of disorders that is characterized by early onset, a combination of overactive, poorly modulated behaviour with marked inattention and lack of persistence in involvement of the task. Hyperkinetic disorder always arise early in development, usually during the first 5 years of life.

While doing the tasks that require cognitive involvement, these children tend to show lack of persistence. Usually they tend to move into the next task leaving behind the task at hand incomplete; along with excessive activity, disorganization and ill regulated activity is often observed in these children. As mentioned in ICD-10, they also find themselves in trouble with disciplinary activities. Their relationship with the adults is often socially disinhibited, they are unpopular with other children and may also become isolated.

As per the diagnostic guidelines given by ICD-10, the cardinal features of Hyperkinetic disorder are impaired attention and overactivity, and both of these features are required to be evident in more than one situation like at home as well as in school.

1. Impaired attention is manifested by breaking off from task prematurely and leaving the activities unfinished. Children seem to lose interest from one activity as they are diverted to another. It is diagnosed only if the behaviours are excessive for the child's age and IQ.
2. Overactivity implies excessive restlessness, specially in situations where calmness is expected, child running and jumping around, getting up from the seat when s/he is expected to be seated, excess talkativeness, fidgeting and wriggling. The activity should be excessive in the context of the given situation, and compared to the other children of the same age and IQ.
3. The behaviour problems should be of early onset (before age 6 years) and a longer duration (World Health Organization, 1992).

Comparing the DSM-5 and ICD-10 Criteria for ADHD

- If we compare the two diagnostic systems i.e DSM-5 and ICD-10, in terms of diagnostic criteria for ADHD, we can see that in contrast to DSM-5, ICD-10 does not outline the different sub-types of Hyperkinetic disorder.

For DSM-5, six or more symptoms of Inattention and/ or six or more symptoms of Hyperactivity/Impulsion are required to fulfil the criteria for diagnosing ADHD. On the other hand, according to ICD-10, impaired attention and overactivity, both are necessary for the diagnosis and should be evident in more than one settings like school, home etc.

- In both the systems there are two similarities. One, it needs the symptoms to have been present for at least 6 months to a degree that it is inconsistent with the developmental level corresponding to that age and second, the symptoms need to be present across more than one setting like in school, at home, on the ground etc.

A study was conducted with an objective to see the extent to which ICD-10 hyperkinetic disorder and DSM-IV ADHD identify the same children with same difficulties. The children those were referred for symptoms of overactivity, inattention and impulsivity and also a normal control group was the sample. ICD-10 and DSM-IV criteria were applied and four groups were identified as Hyperkinetic disorder & ADHD, ADHD only, Clinic control and normal control. The groups were then compared on the measure reflecting the central characteristics of ADHD, neurodevelopmental functioning, academic and cognitive functioning and presence of conduct problems. DSM-IV criteria identify a broader group of children than those identified by ICD-10. However a significant overlap was observed between these groups formed with these basic criteria (Tripp, Luk, Schaughency, & Singh, 1999).

In another study the predictive validity of the two main diagnostic schemata for childhood hyperactivity-attention deficit hyperactivity disorder DSM-IV and ICD-10 was studied. It was found that ICD-10 and DSM-IV continue to delineate diagnostic entities with substantially different prevalence in clinical samples (Lee, et al., 2008).

The diagnostic guidelines differ between DSM Attention Deficit Hyperactivity Disorder (ADHD) and ICD Hyperkinetic Disorder (HKD). Only 145 out of 597 children from the age range 7 years to 9 years in a multimodal treatment study of ADHD with combined types as given by DSM-IV ADHD met the criteria for ICD-10 HKD. This happened due to major internalizing comorbidities and more stringent symptom count requirements excluded the most (Arnold, et al., 2019).

ASSOCIATED DISORDERS

Children diagnosed with ADHD are sometimes also found to have another condition occurring along with ADHD. We can see that the common conditions that occur along with ADHD include Conduct Disorder, Tourette's Syndrome, Learning Disabilities. Oppositional Defiant Disorder, Substance Use disorder (Timothy, 1997), Epilepsy (Gonzalez, et al., 2007), Anxiety, Sleep Disorders etc.

Tourette syndrome is a neurodevelopmental disorder, found frequently comorbid with Attention Deficit/ Hyperactivity Disorder (ADHD). Using a TIC database of 6805 cases, and the clinical differences were ascertained between subjects with and without ADHD. The reported prevalence of ADHD in Tourette syndrome was 55%. Subjects with Tourette Syndrome have high rates of ADHD and complex associations with other disorders (Freeman, 2007).

In a group of 2861 subjects evaluated, 67% met criteria for ADHD, 34% had only ADHD, but 66% had at-least one comorbid psychiatric condition, Learning disability being the most often, followed by sleep disorder, ODD and by anxiety (Reale, et al., 2017).

Another study examined prevalence of ODD, Anxiety and Depression among children with ADHD. When the self- report measures were given to the children for internalizing symptoms, and parents were given the measures for externalizing symptoms, it was found that 42% of them showed prevalence of Anxiety, 23% showed prevalence for Depression and 19% for ODD (Mitchison & Njardvik, 2019).

Children with ADHD often have comorbid oppositional defiant disorder (ODD) and conduct disorder in addition to having developmental and social problems (Barkley, 2002).

A study was conducted to evaluate the association between ADHD and cigarette smoking in children and adolescents. 128 boys with DSM-III-R ADHD and 109 non ADHD aged 6 to 17 years were followed for 4 years. The socioeconomic status, IQ and psychiatric comorbidity were controlled. They were evaluated. Information on cigarette smoking was obtained. It was found that ADHD was a significant predictor of cigarette smoking. The findings also revealed that ADHD was associated with an early initiation of cigarette smoking. The study indicated that ADHD, particularly the comorbid subtype was a significant risk factor for early initiation of cigarette smoking in children and adolescents (Milberger, Biederman, Faraone, Chen, & Jones, 1997).

Diagnosis of ADHD is associated with increase in classroom disruption and decreased resistance to provocation by the peers . Social skill programs should target social deficits associated with ODD and ADHD (Frankel & Feinberg, 2002).

DIAGNOSTIC TOOLS

There is no medical test for diagnosing ADHD. It is a childhood disorder that cannot be diagnosed using some physiological test. There are different psychological tests or scales which guide the professionals in reaching to the correct diagnosis of ADHD.

Even when the symptoms of ADHD are quite clear and easily observable, professionals conduct the assessment of ADHD using different checklists or rating scales in order to see the severity of the symptom. The parents or the teachers of these children are asked to respond to the given statements in these scales.

These tests are designed based on the diagnostic criteria given by different classification systems like DSM or ICD.

Very commonly used scales for diagnosing ADHD include Child Behaviour Checklist (CBCL), Conner's Comprehensive Behaviour Rating Scale (CBRS), Conner-Well's Adolescent Self Report test for adolescents. A research findings supported Conners' 3 Parent short form and CBCL as good instruments in identifying ADHD among children (Gomez, Vance, Watson, & Stavropoulos, 2019).

Conners Adult ADHD Rating Scales (CAARS)

Earlier ADHD was thought to be a disorder of childhood, but research has shown that it also affects individuals through adolescence and adulthood. We can also see the changes made in the diagnostic criteria for the disorder accordingly. The Conners' Adult Rating scale was designed specially to assess ADHD in adults. It is designed for individuals aged through 18 years up to 50 years. The scale consists of items based on the symptoms as described in the DSM in its fourth edition. Overall the scale is used in various forms including short (with 26 items), long (with 66 items) and screening (with 30 items). The scale consists of statements which are to be rated on a four point Likert scale. 0 being "not at all" or "Never", 1 being "just a little or Once in a while", 2 for "pretty much often" and 3 for "very much or very frequently". CAARS has moderate to high level of Reliability and Validity. And the standardized norms are established. (Macey, 2003).

Another scale called The Strength and Difficulties Questionnaire has been evaluated and tested by different researchers in order to check, how well does it help in screening the children with ADHD. This scale was developed by Robert Goodman. The scale is constructed for children from age 2 to 17 years. It was compared against the Rutter questionnaires to parents and teachers. The findings indicated that SDQ functioned as well as the Rutter questionnaires, while offering additional advantages like focus on strengths along with the difficulties, better coverage of inattention, peer relationships, and prosocial behaviour (Goodman, 1997).

A study was conducted in Indonesia, where the teachers of 222 elementary school children aged 7 to 14 years old participated. The Strength and Difficulties questionnaire teacher report was administered on them with the aim to find its validity to screen hyperkinetic disorder in children in Indonesia. The scores were compared with the clinical diagnostic classification from the clinical psychologists. After undergoing the statistical analysis, it was found that Strength and Difficulties Questionnaire Teacher Report, SDQ-TR was a valid instrument for screening hyperkinetic disorder in Indonesian school aged children (Siregar & Wimbarti, 2018). Hence along with the other tools, this scale can also be considered as one of the tools for screening children with ADHD.

AETIOLOGY/ CAUSES OF ATTENTION DEFICIT HYPERACTIVITY DISORDER

The causal factors behind ADHD has been a topic of research for a very long time. It still remains unclear, to what extent do the biological factors dominate the picture and to what extent do the environmental factors. Research indicates both genetic (Naddar, Silberg, Eaves, Maes, & Meyer, 1998) and social factors. Few researches have also been conducted that suggest the interaction between the biological as well as environmental factors to play a role.

Biological Factors: Majority of the studies performed to find the causes of ADHD are performed to assess genetic risk factors of ADHD. Twin studies have shown that in 74% of cases the inheritance from the parents has played a strong role in the child getting diagnosed with ADHD.

It is believed that it's a number of different genes that are responsible in ADHD (Elia & Devoto, 2007). Many amongst these genes affect the neurotransmission of Dopamine in the brain. Some research has also shown that adrenergic genes play a greater role in ADHD than either dopaminergic or serotonergic genes combined (Comings, et al., 2000).

Brain Anatomy: Certain studies have reported that the prefrontal cortex is often the most affected region in ADHD. The prefrontal cortex as we all know is essential for executive functioning. A study indicate that there is a reduction in total as well as specific brain structure volume in prefrontal cortex, caudate nucleus, corpus collosum and cerebellar vermis. The reduction is also seen in Ventral striatum (Tripp & Wickens, 2009).

Caudate Nucleus and Globus Pallidus are found to be smaller in ADHD. These areas contain high density of Dopamine receptors. This supports the dopamine deficit theory of ADHD (Swanson, et al., 2007).

Neuroimaging studies have shown structural alterations in several brain regions in children and adults with ADHD. In a study, 1713 participants with ADHD were compared with 1529 controls with a median age of 14 years on MRI brain scans. The findings of the study reveal that volumes of the accumbens, amygdala, caudate, hippocampus, putamen and intracranial volume were smaller in individuals with ADHD. No difference in the volume size was found in pallidum and thalamus between the two groups (Hoogman, et al., 2017).

Environmental Factors: Several biological and environmental factors have also been proposed as a risk factors for ADHD. These factors include food additives/diet, lead contamination, cigarette and alcohol exposure, maternal smoking during pregnancy, and low birth weight. Based on the reviewed studies, it is clear that, although a substantial part of aetiology is hereditary factors, the interaction between the genes and environmental factors also increase the risk factor for developing ADHD (Banerjee, Middleton, & Faraone, 2007).

In a review, the relationship between prenatal exposure to nicotine, alcohol, caffeine, and psychosocial stress during pregnancy to the risk of developing behavioural problems related to attention deficit hyperactivity disorder (ADHD) in childhood. 24 studies on Nicotine, 9 on alcohol, 1 on Caffeine and 5 on psychosocial stress, all of which were published between 1973 to 2002 were identified. The studies indicated greater risk of ADHD related disorders among children whose mothers smoked during pregnancy. The studies based on psychosocial stress during pregnancy were inconsistent but indicated modest contribution to ADHD in the child (Linnet, et al., 2003).

A review aimed to analyse the relationship between Attention Deficit Hyperactivity Disorder, Oppositional Defiant Disorder and Conduct Disorder, particularly regarding the importance of genetic and environmental factors in development of these disorders. It was found that the causes of development of these disorders are more related to the genetic factors, but role of the environmental factors is also recognized. The results also indicate that children with ADHD have a predisposition to manifest the behaviours that are common to ODD as well as CD, including the antisocial behaviours (Azeredo, Moreira, & Barbosa, 2018).

The role of psychological causes of hyperactivity are not well known yet. It is highly possible that a child is diagnosed with ADHD, but the assessed symptoms are manifestations of some different underlying causes like a dysfunctional families, constant comparison with other classmates who are performing well academically.

In a study, 100 non-referred children and adolescents with ADHD-I i.e the inattentive type ADHD according to DSM-IV along with 100 non-ADHD controls were assessed. The aim was to find if the family environment risk factors are associated with ADHD of Inattentive type. Different aspects of family environment were assessed through structured diagnostic interviews. These included marital discord, low social class, large family size, paternal criminality, maternal mental disorder as measured under Family Adversity Index; family cohesion, expressiveness and conflict under Family Environmental Scale and the family relationship index. The findings of this study indicated that low family cohesion, family adversity in general and specifically the low family relationship index were associated with an increase in the risk for ADHD-I (Pheula, Rohde, & Schmitz, 2011).

Hence as mentioned already it is very difficult to draw the line and labelling a child with a diagnosis. A very careful and thorough investigation and assessment is important for correct diagnosis.

Food/Diet: Researches are being conducted to observe different types of factors that may be contributing to the development of ADHD in children. Food or diet is one of such factors which is being researched quite frequently in recent times.

Along with the important role in immune function, growth and reproduction, Zinc plays an important role in the development of brain. A review given by Arnold(2005) includes reports of different studies conducted across the world, all of which found the lower levels of Zinc present in children with ADHD; and also the correlation between the lower levels of zinc and severity of the ADHD symptoms (Arnold & DiSilvestro, 2005).

A study was conducted on 20 patients with ADHD to estimate the levels of Magnesium, zinc and copper levels in the sera and hair of children diagnosed with ADHD. Magnesium, zinc and copper deficiencies were found in children with ADHD. Also magnesium and zinc deficiencies were found to be correlated with hyperactivity, inattention and impulsivity; this correlation was not observed in the copper deficient ADHD cases (Elbaz, Zahra, & Hanafy, 2017).

In a review, the authors have noted the food elimination diets and history of their investigation in relation to attention deficit hyperactivity disorder has been reviewed. It indicates small yet reliable aggregate effects (Nigg & Holton, 2014).

Vitamin D plays an important role in the development of Central Nervous System. A study assessed the relation between the deficiency of vitamin D during pregnancy and the ADHD symptoms in the child. It demonstrated an association between low maternal 25 (OH)D during pregnancy and an elevated risk for the offspring ADHD (Sucksdorff, et al., 2019).

Management

No treatments have been found to cure this disorder, but many treatments exist which can assist effectively with the management.

Pharmacological and non-pharmacological treatments are the two major categories of the treatment for ADHD.

Pharmacological treatment of ADHD

Pharmacological treatment is generally considered as the first line treatment for ADHD in children and adolescents. There is ample evidence suggesting the efficacy and safety of both stimulant and non-stimulants in treatment. Stimulants are approved by the Food and Drug Administration (FDA) to treat ADHD in children and adolescents, and are considered first line pharmacological agents in the treatment of ADHD (Pliszka, 2007).

Stimulants (Methylphenidate and amphetamines) increase the level of norepinephrine and dopamine, by facilitating their release in prefrontal cortex. Methylphenidate help increase level of dopamine by blocking its reuptake from synaptic cleft, and it also is a dopamine transporter. Amphetamines on the other hand increase the availability of norepinephrine and dopamine (Sheir, Reichenbacher, Ghuman, & Ghuman, 2012).

Ritalin is mostly prescribed medication for high school children with emotional and behavioural problems. This drug is found to be helpful in working more on aggressive behaviour in hyperactive children.

Non-stimulant drugs is generally not the first-line of pharmacological management. It is due to their robust response than the stimulant drugs. They are generally prescribed if the child fails to achieve the desired effects with the stimulants (Pliszka,2007).

Pemoline is another drug prescribed by the doctors. This drug particularly helps in improving the classroom behaviour by improving cognitive processing.

Due to well established efficacy and safety, psychostimulants have been prominent medications for ADHD. Yet there are chances of unacceptable side-effects and also the frequent dosing might be the issue. Most researched medication which is non-stimulant, has shown to reduce the symptoms of ADHD. These non-stimulant drugs are tricyclic antidepressants. Newer antidepressants like bupropion and venlafaxine might show promising results (Findling & Dogin, 1998).

However, taking any drug over longer period of time is a topic of concern. A thorough assessment and a prescription from an authorized professional should be taken. Also, timely observations from the parents and teachers can lead to a better understanding of how the medication is helping the child and it is also helpful to notice side effects, if any.

Non-pharmacological Treatment

Although, the effects of pharmacological stimulants have been observed, some investigators do have concerns regarding the long-term effects and side-effects of these medicines. For example pharmacological similarity of Ritalin and cocaine, has caused some investigators to be concerned about its use for the treatment of ADHD (Volkow, et al., 1995). Hence depending solely upon medication is not preferred in most of the cases. We can simply call these as psychosocial interventions. The psychosocial interventions can be delivered at different levels. Starting from family or parental education, management at school or classroom level and also one to one counselling.

Behavioural Interventions

Most recommended behavioural interventions are based on goals like increasing the time span of the child to sit at one place, appropriate behaviour in class while the teacher is teaching, cooperative behaviour with peers while playing. When we talk about behavioural interventions, behaviour modification has proven to be one of the evidence based treatment. In this the desired behaviour of the child which is in the form of the goals mentioned above, is reinforced and sometimes the behaviour that is supposed to reduce, is punished.

In a study, children were given a combination treatment that included Behaviour therapy and methylphenidate. After eight weeks the methylphenidate was replaced by placebo. The ratings from parents and teachers were taken. The results indicated that behaviour therapy given in school and home is not as effective as methylphenidate, but may be helpful as an adjunct to the methylphenidate in children with ADHD (Klein & Abikoff, 1997).

Neurofeedback

Neurofeedback is another emerging treatment which has shown positive results in managing the symptoms of ADHD in children.

In a meta-analysis, 14 controlled treatment studies conducted post year 1994 were identified. These included behaviour modification, neurofeedback therapy, multimodal psychosocial treatment, school based programs, working memory training, parent training and self- monitoring. It was observed that, amongst these, Behaviour modification and neurofeedback was most supported by the evidence (Hodgson, Hutchingson, & Denson, 2014).

Another strategy used in management of children with ADHD is that, counsellors or teachers or parents may help these children by giving them cues in mnemonic forms for how to behave in certain situations. An example of such cue could be "SLANT", where S means "Sit up Straight", L means "Lean Forward", A means " Activate thinking and Ask questions", N means "Name the key information and Nod your head to validate the teacher/speaker" and T means "Track the teacher/ speaker" (Mercer, Mercer, & Pullen, 2011).

Social Skills Training

Social skill training has also helped children with ADHD in managing their social interactions. In a study, social skill training was given to the children diagnosed with ADHD. It was found that, children suffering more with inattention improved in assertion skills. The social skills training led to greater improvements on parent's reports of their child's cooperation and assertion abilities. The children also reported empathy skills (Antshel & Remer, 2003).

A study revealed the role of social stories as an intervention for disruptive behaviours demonstrated by three children with ADHD. Social stories offered the children, alternative social responses, which in turn helped them in reducing the target behaviours like calling out of turn, rising out of the seat and aggressiveness. It was observed that the disruptive behaviours decreased in two out of the three children (Greenway, 2018).

Exercise

Physical exercise helps in boosting the Dopamine activity, which in turn helps in focusing attention. Activities like dance, gymnastics help these children; outdoor games involving other children might also help in developing better social skills. A meta-analysis of the literature suggested moderate to large effect of physical activity on children with ADHD, with significant effect for emotion/mood (Cornelius, Fedewa, & Ahn, 2017).

A regular schedule that takes care of the right timings for meals and bedtimes, providing enough quality sleep is also very important. Stimulant drugs might interfere with the child's sleep schedule. The parents need to look after that.

Family Therapy

Not much literature is available regarding the role of this particular therapy for the management of ADHD . Although in a study, parenting style and its relationship to functioning in children with and without ADHD was examined. Parenting style was assessed measures of consistency, warmth and anger, whereas, socio-emotional functioning for children was measured through parent, teacher reports and direct academic assessments. It was observed that generic parenting intervention, which promoted warmth, consistency and calm parenting may help the children with ADHD to alleviate the socio-emotional impairments (Bhide, Sciberras, Anderson, Hazell, & Nicholson, 2016).

A study was conducted in order to evaluate the efficacy of the Parent Child Interaction Therapy (PCIT) for Puerto Rican preschool children in age group 4-6, having the diagnosis of ADHD. The families that underwent the PCIT along with those who did not, completed pre and post treatment assessments. These assessments included the child's ADHD symptoms, behavioural problems, family functioning and the parent's satisfaction with the treatment. The mothers reported a significant decrease in hyperactivity and inattention, also the aggression was reduced and oppositional defiant variables were less than the pre-treatment. The parental stress associated with the child's behaviour was also reported to be reduced (Matos, Bauermeister, & Bernal, 2009).

Parent Training

The parents and the schools play a vital role in helping these children deal with their problems.

According to Dr. Russell Barkley, educating the family and the school staff about the disorder and its management plays an important role. Handling such children on a daily basis can lead to feelings of frustration from a parent's point of view. The first thing they need to do is understanding that this is not their fault, parents also need to tell themselves that they are not bad parents. As the symptoms of ADHD are quite observable, parents need to seek right help from the professionals in understanding why their child is behaving in a certain way. This will help in right diagnosis and early intervention.

Multimodal intervention was found to be a promising treatment for ADHD. It includes the pharmacological management of the disorder, parental counselling, attention enhancement training and parental training. It was seen that, with the help of these techniques, the symptoms of ADHD, behavioural issues at school and home were reduced and also the academic performance was improved (Rejani, Oommen, Srinath, & Kapur, 2012).

Parents attribute their high stress to their children's behaviour, unmet needs of support, and social stigma. Future interventions directly targeting their stress may provide wide range of benefits for themselves as well as their children and families (Leitch, et al., 2019).

Stress management techniques can also help parents by increasing their ability to deal with frustration, which in turn can help them deal with the child calmly (NIMH, 2016).

Training parents and providing them with number of tools to cope with and effectively manage their child's difficult behaviour. It helps the parents understand and use immediate, consistent and effective responses in terms of rewards or punishments for the given behaviour of their child. Training the parents about different behavioural strategies is important part of parental training.

A meta-analysis examined the effect of behavioural parent training on child and parental outcome for children with ADHD. It was observed that it is an effective intervention for children with ADHD. In spite of its effectiveness, its sustainability over time could be an issue and the effect of this intervention decreases in children with ADHD comorbid with other behavioural issues (Lee, Niew, Yang, Chen, & Lin, 2012).

Most of the parent training programmes focus on 'behavioural management', this involves learning how to plan and structure the activities, and to praise and encourage children for even a very small progress (Borrill, 2000).

Behavioural Parent Training has been documented to improve both child ADHD behaviour and maladaptive parent's behaviour (Chronis, Chacko, Fabiano, Wymbs, & Pelham, 2004). Parents can help their children by providing them with specific routines, by spending time with them by engaging in playful activities, asking questions which have specific answers, either one word, or yes or no answers. Help them giving short and precise instructions.

Handling temper tantrums of these children is not an easy job. Parents can use distractors to deal with anger outbursts of their children. Losing their cool makes it more difficult. Looking at a parents' anger the child learns to mirror the anger back. So staying calm during tantrums is very important. Here the Time-outs work. Time out is a technique under behavioural therapy.

As already mentioned above, children with ADHD are seen to face difficulties handling their emotions. Emotion dysregulation has been described as a central feature for ADHD. In a study, participants having ADHD and Borderline Personality Disorder along with healthy controls were assessed and compared on Emotion Regulation, based on components like 'being aware of emotions', 'making sense of emotions', ' modifying and accepting emotions', and 'confronting emotions with self-encouragement'. It was observed that, participants with ADHD faced difficulties in encouraging themselves to attend inner aversive experiences, without engaging in impulsive behaviour (Cavelti, et al., 2019).

Emotionally being supportive to the child regarding her/his academic performance is also one of the most important aspects of parenting. Children with ADHD are often seen to show poor academic performance. Not comparing your child with other children in her/his class is the key to achieve this in most of the situations.

Supporting and encouraging these children to engage in exercise as well as in recreational activities also helps them in terms of investing their energy in right things and also in relieving the stress.

Parent Support Groups can also help parents by giving them a platform to share their experiences and connect them to other parents facing similar problems (NIMH, 2016).

While the child is assessed properly and is taking treatment from professionals, it's also important for the parents to know the governmental rules, regulations, and about the certifications if required.

Role of Schools and Teachers

Schools can indeed be of a great help supporting children with ADHD and their parents. Teachers usually face no problem in identifying children who are facing difficulties fitting in the school structure . Observable symptoms of ADHD, like inability to sit at one place while the teacher is teaching, disturbing the class, over activity can be easily spotted by the teacher. The schools can refer these children to professionals who can assess these children on reliable psychological tools for reaching to a proper diagnosis. Once the diagnosis is made, the teacher can be a great support to the parents and the child.

After reaching to a right diagnosis, teachers can help such children by providing the modifications in the environment as well as in overall routine activities of the child.

Generally it is advised to the teachers to minimize the distractions in the child's surrounding (Borrill, 2000). The teacher may begin with re-arranging the child's sitting arrangement, by moving the child's desk to keep it nearer to the them and the blackboard. They can also help the child with different tailor-made sheets and worksheets put into simpler words and broken down in simple steps, to be better able to understand the concepts taught in the class.

Teachers also have to pay attention so that the other children in the class do not bully the child with ADHD for his behaviour or poor academic performance. Psychoeducation sessions for the class can be arranged by the teachers and counsellors in the school which will help the other kids to understand the nature of the disorder. This can also help to develop empathy in other children towards their friends facing different issues.

The schools can further arrange awareness programs for students, teachers as well as parents, where in professionals like psychiatrists, clinical psychologists, educational psychologists, special education teachers and remedial teachers can help them understand the problem with a holistic approach.

Dr. Russell Barkley has suggested different strategies regarding the accommodations that can be done for the children with ADHD in their classrooms. He suggests the use of brief, clear and visual mode of delivering the rules and instructions to the children helps them understand them better. To help them understand the association between the desired behaviour and the reward, he suggests that the rewards should be given to these children almost immediately and more frequently. Not only that, but these incentives should be more powerful than needed to manage the behaviour of other children. Dr. Barkley also places importance on the anticipation by the teachers, in terms of managing the behaviour of children with ADHD during the time like transition from one activity to other (Barkley, 2008).

To conclude, no single way of treatment has been proven to work alone for managing symptoms of ADHD, hence a combination of interventions can be used. Similarly, no single entity is enough to deal with disorders like ADHD. Parents, Teachers, Doctors, Psychiatrists, Clinical and educational psychologists, remedial teachers/ special educators have to work together in order to help these children deal with their issues.

REFERENCES

American Psychiatric Association. (2000). Diagnostic and Statistical Manual of Mental Disorders (4th ed.). Washington DC: Author.

American Psychiatric Association. (2013). *Diagnostic and Statistical Manual of Mental Disorders* (5th ed.). Author.

Antshel, K. M., & Remer, R. (2003). Social Skills Training in Children With Attention Deficit Hyperactivity Disorder: A Randomized Controlled Clinical Trial. *Journal of Clinical Child and Adolescent Psychology*, *32*(1), 153–165. doi:10.1207/S15374424JCCP3201_14 PMID:12611031

Arnold, L. E., & DiSilvestro, R. A. (2005). Zinc in Attention-Deficit/ Hyperactivity Disorder. *Journal of Child and Adolescent Psychopharmacology*, *15*(4), 619–627. doi:10.1089/cap.2005.15.619 PMID:16190793

Arnold, L. E., Hodgkins, P., Kahle, J., Madhoo, M., & Kewley, G. (2020). Long -Term Outcomes of ADHD: Academic Achievement and Performance. *Journal of Attention Disorders*, *24*(1), 73–85. doi:10.1177/1087054714566076 PMID:25583985

Arnold, L. E., Roy, A., Taylor, E., Hetchman, L., Margaret, S., Swanson, J. M., ... Rohde, L. A. (2019). Predictive Utility of Childhood Diagnosis of ICD-10 HKD: Adult outcomes in MTA and Effect of Comorbidity. *European Child & Adolescent Psychiatry*, *28*, 557–570. doi:10.100700787-018-1222-0 PMID:30232561

Ayuso, R., Maestu, F., & Gonzalez, M. J., RomoBarrientos, C., & Andrade, J. M. (2006). Executive Function in Attention Deficit Hyperactivity Disorder in Childhood. *Revista de Neurología*, •••, 265–271.

Azeredo, A., Moreira, D., & Barbosa, F. (2018, October). ADHD, CD, and ODD: Systematic review of genetic and environmental risk factors. *Research in Developmental Disabilities*, *82*, 10–19. doi:10.1016/j.ridd.2017.12.010 PMID:29361339

Banerjee, T. D., Middleton, F., & Faraone, S. V. (2007, September). Environmental risk factors for attention-deficit hyperactivity disorder. *Acta Paediatrica Nurturing the Child*, *96*(9), 1269–1274. doi:10.1111/j.1651-2227.2007.00430.x PMID:17718779

Barkley, R. A. (2002). Major Life Activity and Health Outcomes Associated with Attention Deficit/ Hyperactivity Disorder. *The Journal of Clinical Psychiatry*, *63*, 10–15. PMID:12562056

Barkley, R. A. (2008). Classroom Accommodations for Children with ADHD. *The ADHD Report*, *16*(4), 7–10. doi:10.1521/adhd.2008.16.4.7

Barry, T., Lyman, R. D., & Klinger, L. G. (2002). Academic Underachievement and Attention Deficit Hyperactivity Disorder: The Negative Impact of Symptom Severity on School Performance. *Journal of School Psychology*, *40*(3), 259–283. doi:10.1016/S0022-4405(02)00100-0

Bhide, S., Sciberras, E., Anderson, V., Hazell, P., & Nicholson, J. M. (2016). Association between parenting style and socio-emotional and academic functioning in children with and without ADHD: A community based study. *Journal of Attention Disorders*, *23*(5), 463–474. doi:10.1177/1087054716661420 PMID:27474160

Borrill, J. (2000). *All About ADHD*. Mental Health Foundation.

Brown, T. (2009, March). ADD/ADHD and impaired executive function in clinical practice. *Current Attention Disorders Reports*, *1*(1), 37–41. doi:10.100712618-009-0006-3

Bunford, N., Evans, S. W., & Langberg, J. M. (2014). Emotion Dysregulation Is Associated with Social Impairment Among Young Adolescents With ADHD. *Journal of Attention Disorders*, *22*(1), 66–82. doi:10.1177/1087054714527793 PMID:24681899

Cavelti, M., Corbisiero, S., Bitto, H., Moerstedt, B., Newwark, P., Faschina, S., ... Stieglitz, R. D. (2019). A Comparison of Self Reported Emotion Regulation Skills in Adults with Attention Deficit Hyperactivity Disorder and Borderline Personality Disorder. *Journal of Attention Disorders*, *23*(12), 1396–1406. doi:10.1177/1087054717698814 PMID:28367706

Chronis, A. M., Chacko, A., Fabiano, G. A., Wymbs, B. T., & Pelham, W. E. Jr. (2004). Enhancements to the Behavioural Parent Training Paradigm for Families of Children with ADHD: Review and Future Directions. *Clinical Child and Family Psychology Review*, *7*(1), 1–27. doi:10.1023/B:CCFP.0000020190.60808.a4 PMID:15119686

Coghill, D. R., Seth, S., & Matthews, K. (2014). A comprehensive assessment of memory, delay aversion, timing, inhibition, decision making, and variability in attention deficit hyperactivity disorder: Advancing beyond the three-pathway models. *Psychological Medicine*, *44*(9), 1989–2001. doi:10.1017/S0033291713002547 PMID:24176104

Comings, D. E., Gade-Andavolu, R., Gonzalez, N., Wu, S., Muhleman, D., Blake, H., ... MacMurray, J. P. (2000). Comparison of the role of dopamine, serotonin, and noradrenaline genes in ADHD, ODD and conduct disorder: Multivariate regression analysis of 20 genes. *Clinical Genetics*, *57*(3), 178–196. doi:10.1034/j.1399-0004.2000.570304.x PMID:10782925

Cornelius, C., Fedewa, A. L., & Ahn, S. (2017, January). The Effect Of Physical Activity on Children with ADHD: A Quantitative Review of the Literature. *Journal of Applied School Psychology*, *33*(2), 136–170. doi:10.1080/15377903.2016.1265622

Doernberg, E., & Hollander, E. (2016). Neurodevelopmental Disorders (ASD and ADHD): DSM-5, ICD-10, and ICD-11. *CNS Spectrums*, *21*(4), 295–299. doi:10.1017/S1092852916000262 PMID:27364515

Elbaz, F., Zahra, S., & Hanafy, H. (2017). Magnesium, Zinc and Copper estimation in children with attention deficit hyperactivity disorder (ADHD). *The Egyptian Journal of Medical Human Genetics*, *18*(2), 153–163. doi:10.1016/j.ejmhg.2016.04.009

Elia, J., & Devoto, M. (2007). ADHD genetics: 2007 update. *Current Psychiatry Reports*, *9*(5), 434–439. doi:10.100711920-007-0057-z PMID:17915085

Epstein, J. N., & Loren, R. E. (2013, October). Changes in the Definition of ADHD in DSM-5: Subtle but Important. *HHS Public Access: Neuropsychiatry (London)*, *3*(5), 455–458. doi:10.2217/npy.13.59 PMID:24644516

Faraone, S. V., Rostain, L., Blader, J., Busch, B., Childress, A. C., Connor, D. F., & Newcorn, J. H. (2019). Practitioner Review: Emotional Dysregulation in Attention Deficit/ Hyperactive Disorder- Implications For Clinical Recognition and Intervention. *Journal of Child Psychology and Psychiatry, and Allied Disciplines*, *60*(2), 133–150. doi:10.1111/jcpp.12899 PMID:29624671

Feldman, R. (2010). Middle Childhood. In Discovering The Life Span (p. 209). Pearson.

Findling, R. L., & Dogin, J. W. (1998). Psychopharmacology of ADHD: Children and adolescents. *The Journal of Clinical Psychiatry*, *59*(7), 42–49. PMID:9680052

Frankel, F., & Feinberg, D. (2002). Social Problems Associated with ADHD Vs. ODD in Children Referred For Friendship Problems. *Child Psychiatry and Human Development*, *33*(2), 125–146. doi:10.1023/A:1020730224907 PMID:12462351

Freeman, R. (2007). Tic disorder and ADHD: Answeres from a world-wide clinical dataset on Tourette syndrome. *European Child & Adolescent Psychiatry*, *16*(S1), 15–23. doi:10.100700787-007-1003-7 PMID:17665279

Gaub, M., & Carlson, C. L. (1997). Gender Differences in ADHD: A Meta-Analysis and a Critical Review. *Journal of the American Academy of Child and Adolescent Psychiatry*, *36*(8), 1136–1139. doi:10.1097/00004583-199708000-00023 PMID:9256583

Gomez, R., Vance, A., Watson, S., & Stavropoulos, V. (2019). *ROC Analysis of Relevant Conners' 3 - Short Forms, CBCL and TRF Scales for Screening ADHD and ODD*. Sage Journals., doi:10.1177/1073191119876023

Gonzalez, J., Dodds, A., Whitney, J., MacMillan, C., Waber, D., Faraone, S. V., ... Biederman, J. (2007). Psychiatric disorders and behavioral characteristics of pediatric patients with both epilepsy and attention deficit hyperactivity disoredr. *Epilepsy & Behavior, 10*(3), 384–388. doi:10.1016/j.yebeh.2007.01.010 PMID:17368109

Goodman, R. (1997). The Strengths and Difficulties Questionnaire: A Research Note. *Journal of Child Psychology and Psychiatry, and Allied Disciplines, 38*(5), 581–586. doi:10.1111/j.1469-7610.1997.tb01545.x PMID:9255702

Greenway, C. (2018). The Efficacy of Social Stories in the Classroom to Reduce Disruptive Behaviors in Children with ADHD. *Acta Psychopathologica, 4*.

Hodgson, K., Hutchingson, A. D., & Denson, L. (2014, May). Nonpharmacological Treatments for ADHD: A Meta-Analytic Review. *Journal of Attention Disorders, 18*(4), 275–282. doi:10.1177/1087054712444732 PMID:22647288

Hoogman, M., Bralten, J., Hibar, D., Mennes, M., Zweirs, M. P., Shweren, L. S., ... Franke, B. (2017, April). Subcortical brain volume differences in participants with attention deficit hyperactivity disorder in children and adults: A cross-sectional mega-analysis. *The Lancet. Psychiatry, 4*(4), 310–319. doi:10.1016/S2215-0366(17)30049-4 PMID:28219628

Jepsen, J., Fagerlund, B., & Mortensen, E. L. (2009). Do Attention Deficits Influence IQ Assessment in Children and Adolescents with ADHD? *Journal of Attention Disorders, 12*(6), 551–562. doi:10.1177/1087054708322996 PMID:18815437

Klein, R. G., & Abikoff, H. (1997, July). Behaviour therapy and methyphanidate in treatment of children with ADHD. *Journal of Attention Disorders, 2*(2), 89–114. doi:10.1177/108705479700200203

Lange, K. W., Reichl, S., Lange, K. M., Tucha, L., & Tucha, O. (2010). The History of Attention Deficit Hyperactive Disorder. *ADHD Attention Deficit Hyperactivity Disorders, 2*(4), 241–255. doi:10.100712402-010-0045-8 PMID:21258430

Langer, N., Benjamin, C., Becker, B., & Gaab, N. (2015, June). Comorbidity of reading disabilities and ADHD: Structural and functional brain characteristics. *Human Brain Mapping, 40*(9), 2677–2698. doi:10.1002/hbm.24552 PMID:30784139

Lawrence, V., Houghton, S., Douglas, G., Durkin, K., Whiting, K., & Tannock, R. (2004). Executive Function and ADHD: A comparison of children's performance during neuropsychological testing and real-world activities. *Journal of Attention Disorders, 7*(3), 137–149. doi:10.1177/108705470400700302 PMID:15260171

Lee, P. C., Niew, W., Yang, H., Chen, V. C., & Lin, K. (2012). A Meta-analysis: Behavioural Parent Training for Children with Attention Deficit Hyperactive Disorder. *Research in Developmental Disabilities, 33*(6), 2040–2049. doi:10.1016/j.ridd.2012.05.011 PMID:22750360

Lee, S. I., Schachar, R. J., Chen, S. X., Orstein, T. J., Charach, A., Barr, C., & Ickwoicz, A. (2008). Predictive Validity of DSM-IV and ICD-10 Criteria for ADHD and Hyperkinetic Disorder. *Journal of Child Psychology and Psychiatry, and Allied Disciplines*, *49*(1), 70–78. doi:10.1111/j.1469-7610.2007.01784.x PMID:17979965

Leitch, S., Scriberras, E., Post, B., Gerner, B., Rinehart, N., Nicholson, J. M., & Evans, S. (2019). Experience of stress in parents of children with ADHD: A qualitative study. *International Journal of Qualitative Studies on Health and Well-being*, *14*(1), 1690091. Advance online publication. doi:10.1080/17482631.2019.1690091 PMID:31713473

Linnet, K. M., Dalsgaard, S., Obel, C., Wisborg, K., Henriksen, T. B., Rodriguez, A., Kotimaa, A., Moilanen, I., Thomsen, P. H., Olsen, J., & Jarvelin, M. R. (2003). Maternal Lifestyle Factors in Pregnancy Risk of Attention Deficit Hyperactivity Disorder and Associated Behaviors: Review of the Current Evidence. *The American Journal of Psychiatry*, *160*(6), 1028–1040. doi:10.1176/appi.ajp.160.6.1028 PMID:12777257

Macey, K. D. (2003). Conners' Adult ADHD Rating Scales (CAARS). *Archives of Clinical Neuropsychology*, *18*(4), 431–437. doi:10.1016/S0887-6177(03)00021-0

Matos, M., Bauermeister, J. J., & Bernal, G. (2009). Parent-Child Interaction Therapy for Puerto Rican Preschool Children with ADHD and Behaviour Problems: A Pilot Efficacy Study. *Family Process*, *48*(2), 232–252. doi:10.1111/j.1545-5300.2009.01279.x PMID:19579907

Mayes, S. D., Waschbusch, D. A., Calhoun, S. L., & Mattison, R. E. (2019). How Common are Academic Overachievement and Underachievement in Children with Autism or ADHD? *Journal of Developmental and Physical Disabilities*. Advance online publication. doi:10.100710882-019-09719-8

McCoach, D. B., Siegle, D., & Rubenstein, L. D. (2020). Pay Attention to Innatention: Exploring ADHD Symptoms In A Sample Of Underachieving Gifted Students. *Gifted Child Quarterly*, *64*(2), 100–116. doi:10.1177/0016986219901320

Mercer, C. D., Mercer, A. R., & Pullen, P. C. (2011). *Teaching Students With Learning Problems* (8th ed.). Pearson.

Milberger, S., Biederman, J., Faraone, S. V., Chen, L., & Jones, J. (1997). ADHD Is Associated With Early Initiation of Cigarette Smoking in Children and Adolescents. *Journal of the American Academy of Child and Adolescent Psychiatry*, *36*(1), 37–44. doi:10.1097/00004583-199701000-00015 PMID:9000779

Mitchison, G. M., & Njardvik, U. (2019). Prevalence and Gender Difference of ODD, Anxiety and Depression in a Sample of Children with ADHD. *Journal of Attention Disorders*, *23*(11), 1339–1345. doi:10.1177/1087054715608442 PMID:26443719

Murray-Close, D., Hoza, B., Hinshaw, S. P., Arnold, L. E., Swanson, J., Jensen, P. S., ... Wells, K. (2010, November). Developmental Process in Peer Problems of Children with Attention-Deficit/ Hyperactivity Disorder in The Multimodal Treatment Study of Children with ADHD. *Development and Psychopathology*, *22*(4), 785–802. doi:10.1017/S0954579410000465 PMID:20883582

Naddar, T. S., Silberg, J. L., Eaves, L. J., Maes, H. H., & Meyer, J. M. (1998). Genetic Effects on ADHD Symptomatology in 7- to-13 Year-Old Twins: Results From Telephone Survey. *Behavior Genetics*, *28*(2), 83–99. doi:10.1023/A:1021686906396 PMID:9583234

Nigg, J. T. (2001). Is ADHD a disinhibitory disorder? *Psychological Bulletin*, *127*(5), 571–598. doi:10.1037/0033-2909.127.5.571 PMID:11548968

Nigg, J. T., & Holton, K. (2014, October). Restiction and Elimination Diets in ADHD treatment. *Child & Adolescent Psychiatric Clinics*, *23*(4), 937–953. doi:10.1016/j.chc.2014.05.010 PMID:25220094

NIMH. (2016). *Attention Deficit/ Hyperactivity Disorder (ADHD): The Basics*. NIH Publication.

Pheula, G. F., Rohde, L. A., & Schmitz, M. (2011). Are family variables associated with ADHD, inattentive type? A case-control study in schools. *European Child & Adolescent Psychiatry*, *20*(3), 137–145. doi:10.100700787-011-0158-4 PMID:21290154

Pliszka, S. (2007). Practice parameter for the assessment and treatment of the children and adolescents with attention deficit/ hyperactivity disorder. *Journal of the American Academy of Child and Adolescent Psychiatry*, *46*(7), 894–921. doi:10.1097/chi.0b013e318054e724 PMID:17581453

Polanczyk, G., Lima, M., Horta, B. L., Biederman, J., & Rohde, L. A. (2007). The Worldwide Prevalence of ADHD: A Systematic Review and Metaregression Analysis. *The American Journal of Psychiatry*, *164*(6), 942–948. doi:10.1176/ajp.2007.164.6.942 PMID:17541055

Reale, L., Bartoli, B., Cartabia, M., Zanetti, M., Costantino, M. P., Canevini, M. P., Termine, C., & Bonati, M.Lombardy ADHHD Group. (2017). Comobidity, Prevalence & Treatment Outcome in Children and Adolescents with ADHD. *European Child & Adolescent Psychiatry*, *26*(12), 1443–1457. doi:10.100700787-017-1005-z PMID:28527021

Rejani, T. G., Oommen, A., Srinath, S., & Kapur, M. (2012). Efficacy of Multimodal Intervention for Children with Attention Deficit Hyperactivity Disorder (ADHD)- An Indian Study. *Journal of Behavioral and Brain Science*, *2*(01), 117–127. doi:10.4236/jbbs.2012.21014

Shaw, P., Stringaris, A., Nigg, J., & Leinbenluft, E. (2014, March). Emotion Dysregulation in Attention-Deficit/Hyperactivity Disorder. *The American Journal of Psychiatry*, *171*(3), 276–293. doi:10.1176/appi.ajp.2013.13070966 PMID:24480998

Sheir, A. C., Reichenbacher, T., Ghuman, H. S., & Ghuman, J. K. (2012). Pharmacological Treatment of Attention Deficit Hyperactivity Disorder in Children and Adolescents: Clinical Strategies. *Journal of Central Nervous System Disease*, *5*, 1–17. doi:10.4137/JCNSD.S6691 PMID:23650474

Sibley, M. H., & Yeguez, C. E. (2018). The Impact of DSM-5 A-Criteria on Parent Ratings of ADHD in Adolescents. *Journal of Attention Disorders*, *22*(1), 83–91. doi:10.1177/1087054714526040 PMID:24626330

Silverstein, M. J., Faraone, S. V., Leon, T. L., Biederman, J., Spencer, T. J., & Adler, L. A. (2018). The Relationship Between Executive Function Deficits and DSM-5 Defined ADHD Symptoms. *Journal of Attention Disorders*, *24*(1), 41–51. doi:10.1177/1087054718804347 PMID:30296883

Siregar, J., & Wimbarti, S. (2018). Screening for the hyperkinetic disorder by using strength and difficulties questionnaire teacher report (SDQ-TR) in Indonesia school-aged children. *Global Journal of Psychology Research: New Trends and Current Issues, 8*(2), 76–87. doi:10.18844/gjpr.v8i2.3490

Sucksdorff, M., Brown, A. S., Chudal, R., Surcel, H. M., Salomaki, S. H., Postava, K. C., ... Sourander, A. (2019). Maternal Vitamin D Levels and the Risk of Offspring Attention-Deficit/ Hyperactivity Disorder. *Journal of the American Academy of Child and Adolescent Psychiatry*. Advance online publication. doi:10.1016/j.jaac.2019.11.021 PMID:31863882

Swanson, J. M., Kinsbourne, M., Nigg, J., Lanphear, B., Stephanatos, G. A., Volkow, N., ... Wadhwa, P. D. (2007). Etiological Subtypes of Attention Deficit/Hyperactivity Disorder: Brain Imaging, Molecular Genetic & Environmental Factors and the Dopamine Hypothesis. *Neuropsychology Review, 17*(1), 39–59. doi:10.100711065-007-9019-9 PMID:17318414

Timothy, W. e. (1997). Attention Deficit Hyperactivity Disorder (ADHD) is Associated with Early Onset Substance Use Disorders. *The Journal of Nervous and Mental Disease, 185*(8), 475–482. doi:10.1097/00005053-199708000-00001 PMID:9284860

Tripp, G., Luk, S. L., Schaughency, E. A., & Singh, R. (1999). DSM-IV and ICD-10: A Comparison of The Correlates of ADHD and Hyperkinetic Disorder. *Journal of the American Academy of Child and Adolescent Psychiatry, 38*(2), 156–164. doi:10.1097/00004583-199902000-00014 PMID:9951214

Tripp, G., & Wickens, J. R. (2009). Neurobiology of ADHD. *Neuropharmacology, 57*(7-8), 579–589. doi:10.1016/j.neuropharm.2009.07.026 PMID:19627998

Volkow, N. D., Ding, Y. S., Fowler, J. S., Wang, G. J., Logan, J., Gatley, J. S., ... Wolf, A. P. (1995). Is Methylphenidate Like Cocaine? *Archives of General Psychiatry, 52*(6), 456–463. doi:10.1001/archpsyc.1995.03950180042006 PMID:7771915

World Health Organization. (1992). *The ICD10 Classification of Mental and Behavioural Disorders: Clinical descriptions and diagnostic guidelines*. Author.

Zhang, W., Fan, L., & Jiang, Y. P. (2016). Memory Updating Deficit in Attention Deficit Hyperactivity Disorder (ADHD) Children. *Medicine and Biopharmaceutical*, 3-11. doi:10.1142/9789814719810_0001

Chapter 2
Attention Deficit Hyperactivity Disorder (ADHD):
Introduction, Mental Health Concerns, and Treatment

Shreyasi Vashishtha
Indian Institute of Technology, Kanpur, India

ABSTRACT

Attention deficit hyperactivity disorder (ADHD) is the most common psychiatric condition in children. It comprises three core characteristics, namely inattention, hyperactivity, and impulsivity. The current chapter highlighted the comorbidity of ADHD with other psychiatric conditions like autism spectrum, learning disorders, bipolar disorder, externalizing problems, and sleep difficulties along with familial and academic difficulties. It also focused on the behavioral manifestation of ADHD including mental health issues like anxiety, depression, poor self-esteem, suicide, substance use, and sensory processing deficits. The common treatment for ADHD includes both pharmacological and non-pharmacological methods. Psychological treatment follows the use of behavioral principles used in operant conditioning. Parent and teacher training methods aim to empower them in regulating antecedents and consequences to bring desired changes in behavior. Other interventions discussed in the chapter are cognitive behavioral therapy and physical activity training.

INTRODUCTION

ADHD is a neurobehavioral condition characterized by clinically high levels of inattention, hyperactivity, and impulsivity. Symptoms appear in early childhood and in two-third of the cases, symptoms continue in modified forms to adulthood (Faraone et al., 2006). Symptoms can also vary in different settings like home and School. Persistence of symptoms into adulthood brings disruption in developmentally appropriate social, academic, and occupational spheres of life (Mannuzza and Klein, 2000).

DOI: 10.4018/978-1-7998-5495-1.ch002

Hyperactivity in ADHD can be understood as restlessness or continuous fidgeting behavior, unable to sit quietly and excess movements like running, climbing, or talking. Impulsivity refers to impairment in the ability to delay response in the presence of the stimuli. Its behavioral manifestation would include difficulty waiting for their turn or standing in queues, interrupting other's speech, taking actions without giving proper thought. Inattention suggests the inability to maintain focus on a task, inability to provide close attention to details, and struggling with any other task requiring sustained attention span (Barkley, 1998).

Epidemiology

ADHD is one of the most common neurodevelopmental disorders of children. Epidemiological studies report ADHD to be present in 7-8 percent of the primary school-going children. It has a worldwide prevalence of 5-9 percent in children aged between 5-17 years. Prevalence in adults ranges from 2.5-4.4 percent. Studies indicate more prevalence in boys than girls with a ratio ranging from 3:1 to 9:1 (Polanczyk et al, 2014). First degree relatives of a child diagnosed with ADHD are more prone to be diagnosed than the general population.

Etiology

Historical theories of etiology focused on the 'minimal brain damage' hypothesis. Environmental and dietary factors were also focus of many etiological studies. Currently, studies focus on familial factors, genetic basis, and neuroimaging, neurochemical factors to determine a more specific cause of the condition (Gozal and Molfese, 2005).

Genetic studies indicate inheritability to be as high as 75 percent. Twin studies indicate a high concordance rate in monozygotic twins (51%) than dizygotic twins (33%). First degree relatives of ADHD child has increased risk of 2-8 times than the general population. Gene studies indicate the role of dopamine-related genes such as dopamine transporter gene or dopamine 4 receptor seven-repeat allele gene in the manifestation of ADHD. Another study support polygenic multiple threshold models, which states that ADHD is surfaced when an individual crosses the threshold level of liability (Rhee et al, 1999).

Neurochemical studies focus primarily on the role of dopamine in the prefrontal cortex indicated by its role in higher cognitive function and self-regulatory behavior. Higher accumulation of nor-adrenaline in the peripheral system provides dysfunctional feedback to the lower level of non-adrenaline in locus ceruleus (central noradrenergic system) is seen in the animal studies for inattention (Sadock and Sadock, 2015). This highlights the role played by the stimulant medication in the treatment of ADHD. The stimulant medication increases both dopamine and norepinephrine levels by increasing their release and blocking uptake (Engert and Pruessner, 2008). Studies using EEG data indicate increases beta and theta activity in the prefrontal cortex in youth with ADHD. These people also showed difficulty in emotional regulation (Clarke et al., 2011).

Many other studies question the methodological problems and interpretation in familial, twin adoption, and brain studies. Such studies postulate the potential role of non-genetic factors in the manifestation of ADHD (Furman, 2008). Developmental factors include premature birth, low birth weight, prenatal brain trauma, or inflammation due to infection prominently in the first trimester. Environmental factors involve exposure to toxins, lead, and maternal drinking and smoking during pregnancy.

MENTAL HEALTH CONCERNS IN ADHD

ADHD is a categorical yet continuous disorder this means that although it is outside the range of normal childhood behavioral patterns, it lies in continuum with normal childhood development. ADHD causes difficulties across different domains, these are:

A. Cognitive implications: Fleeting attention span and organizational skills make them vulnerable to poor performance on the time-dependent test. Based on data from these tests, historically, children with ADHD were misinterpreted as intellectually deficient due to poor academic performances (Gozal and Molfese, 2005).
B. Emotional Implications: Children with ADHD may learn to exhibit their anger in the form of temper outbursts and mood liability may be present. Anxiety and Depression can also be present (Taurines et al., 2010).
C. Social Implication: Some children have a problem reading social cues and are perceived as intrusive and insensitive for the needs of others (Mannuzza and Klein, 2000).
D. Academic Implications: Children with ADHD have considerable difficulties in the academic domain due to either direct interference of attentional or hyperactive problems or because of the higher rate of comorbidity between ADHD and specific learning difficulties (SLD) (Germano et al., 2010).

One major feature of ADHD is its higher comorbidity with other clinical conditions. Approximately 40-80 percent of children and adolescents diagnosed with ADHD are at risk for other psychiatric conditions. A study points out that 40 percent of children with ADHD are at risk for one psychiatric disorder, 32 percent are at risk for two psychiatric conditions, and 11 percent for three disorders (Szatmari. et., al 1992).

Figure 1. Comorbidities with ADHD (Reale et al., 2017)

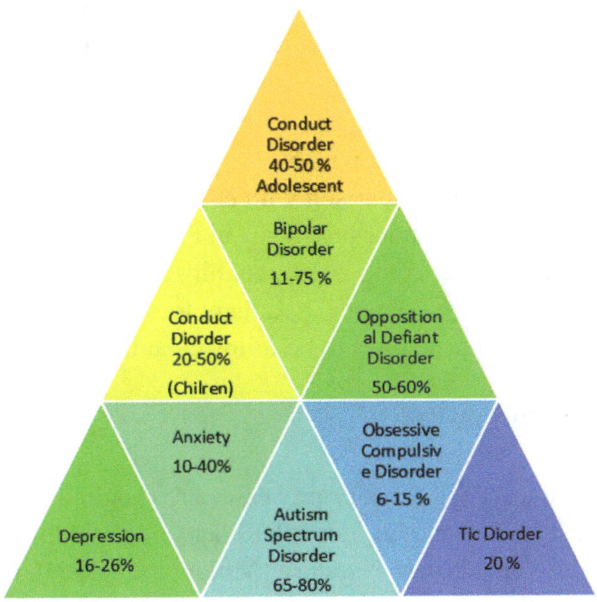

Externalizing Disorders: Oppositional Defiant Disorder and Conduct Disorder

A high prevalence rate is found in children with ADHD who meet the criteria for ODD and CD. This highlights the similarities in these disorders and questions their distinctions. Although ADHD can exist independently without disruptive behavior problems, the reverse is usually not true for ODD and CD. Studies indicate most of the time ADHD to be a precursor for these externalizing behavior. ADHD with comorbid ODD has a higher risk for the development of anxiety, depression, conduct, and antisocial personality disorder, thus it has a poor prognosis than ADHD alone (Noordermeer et al., 2017). Risk factors for such conditions include parental criticism, association with deviant peers, and socio-economic status. The development of CD from ADHD can be attributed to the inappropriate emotional expression such as frequent use of bad language, anger, and hostility (Barkley, 2014). Children with ADHD and CD have a higher risk for the development of antisocial personality disorder and criminal behavior (Storebo and Simonsen, 2016).

Autism Spectrum Disorder (ASD)

ASD is a lifelong developmental condition with difficulty in communication along with repetitive and restricted behavioral patterns. Diagnostic and Statistical Manual of Mental Disorders, 5th Edition (DSM-5) categorizes autistic disorder, Asperger's syndrome, and pervasive developmental disorder under ASD (APA, 2013). ADHD and ASD co-occur in 30-70 percent of cases (Rau et al., 2020). These two disorders overlap in terms of a). executive functioning, including working memory deficits, vigilance-impairment, response inhibition (Goldin et al., 2013), b).deficits in sensory processing in modalities including tactile, oral, auditory, vestibular, and visual deficits (Miller et al., 2009), c). emotional recognition and theory of mind (Kern et al.,2015; Leitner, 2014, Buitelaar et al., 1999; Johnson, 2012), d). sleep disturbance and anxiety (Kern et al,2015) e). pragmatic use of language (Leitner, 2014), and f). similar genetically functional pathways are also found in these conditions (Rivero et al., 2015; Lionel et al., 2014). The clinical presentation of ASD and ADHD also has common behavioral and cognitive features and therefore previously, ADHD was not diagnosed when Autism was present. It was considered as a part of autism. With the fifth version of DSM, they are regarded as co-occurring conditions that follow a distinct treatment approach (Mansour et al., 2017). ASD symptoms in ADHD can also be understood as the difficulty in social- communication reciprocity, while this is a core symptom of ASD diagnosis, it is present in a moderate to high range in children with ADHD with 50-60 percent of children with ADHD experiencing peer rejection (Barkley et al., 1990). In comparison with children who only have ASD, children with a co-diagnosis of ADHD with ASD have a poor prognosis in terms of mental health care (Frazier et al., 2001), executive functioning (Berenguer et al., 2018), cognitive delay (Sinzing et al., 2008) and social adaptivity (Ames and White, 2011). Psychological treatment for both these conditions include modules derived from behavioral theories and principles to be followed at home and school.

Sensory Processing Problems

To engage in day to day life functioning sensory processes are required for a successful and adaptive response to the incoming sensory information. It involves detecting, modulating, or organizing, and interpreting the stimuli to produce an adaptive response (Miller et al., 2009). Children with ADHD have problems of over or under sensitivity, sensation craving/seeking, sensory discrimination, and sensory-based motor disorder (Miller et al., 2006; Ghanizadeh, 2011). This occurs due to the problem in the ability to regulate the sensory stimuli. Children with the problem of over/hypersensitivity respond to the stimuli in a faster, more intense, or for a longer duration. This can lead to the perception of a slight unpleasant stimulus as highly irritating and a person may respond aggressively than a person with normal sensitivity. Children with the problem of under sensitivity fail to recognize the sensory stimuli available in the environment (Engel-Yeger & Ziv-On, 2011).

The sensory integrative approach is a treatment module used in occupational therapy to overcome sensory processing deficits. The sensory integration approach is based on the principle of neuroplasticity and targets to repetitively provide sensory stimulation in the brain to improve its ability for sensory processing (Lang et al., 2012). The fact that sensory integration therapy work as a functional intervention for both ADHD and ASD indicates the common neurological deficits in sensory processing (Little et al., 2017).

Bipolar Disorder

Approximately 10-40 percent of children and adolescent with ADHD shows comorbidity with mood disorders (Taurines et al., 2010). There exist a lot of ongoing debate in the scientific community about the diagnostic differentiation between ADHD and mania due to overlap in symptom presentation such as elevated mood, irritability, distractibility, talkativeness, and mood lability. It is the time-based difference that separates them as distinct conditions, wherein the onset of ADHD is in childhood, and mania occurs as a distinct episode for a discrete period followed by either a normal or depressive phase (Skirrow et al., 2012).

Depression and Anxiety

The inattentive type of ADHD is more likely to develop internalizing problems such as depression and anxiety than a combined type of ADHD (Weiss et al., 2003). A diagnosis of ADHD with comorbid ODD/CD is more prone to depression than ADHD alone (Ostrander and Herman, 2006). The presence of comorbid anxiety in children with ADHD leads to increased behavioral dysregulation (Sorensen et al., 2011), greater deficits in working memory and physical anxiety symptoms than the group with a diagnosis of only ADHD (Jarrett et al., 2016). In adults with ADHD, comorbidity of mood and anxiety disorder is greater, 57.3 percent, and 27.2 percent respectively (Taurines et al., 2010).

Suicide Risk

A review by Balazs and Kereszteny (2017) find a positive relation between ADHD and suicidality (attempt, ideation, and complete suicide) across gender and age groups. The prevalence rate for adolescents was found to be 5.7 percent and 16 percent for adults. Studies indicate that the presence of comorbid disorders poses an increased risk for suicide (Fitzgerald et al., 2019, Balaz and Kereszteny 2017, Yoshimasu, 2019). The psychiatric comorbidity of generalized anxiety disorder, hypomanic episode, and substance use disorder was found to have a significantly greater risk for suicide (Yoshimasu et al., 2019). In a study by Nigg (2013) girls with ADHD were at higher risk for suicide attempt and boys with ADHD have a greater risk for complete suicide. In terms of the type of ADHD, the combined type was found to have twice the risk for attempt and ideation than the inattentive type. Also, children and adolescents who have sadness and ODD are eight times more prone to suicide ideation and eleven times for suicide attempts than ADHD alone (Mayes et al., 2014).

Substance Use Disorder

ADHD and SUD are closely related conditions that affect the substantial clinical population both comorbidly and individually. Research suggests that these conditions have a lot in common which includes neurological factors such as the role of dopamine, common neural circuitry, and similar genetic factors. Children with ADHD have higher chances for the development of SUD (Lee et al., 2011; Charach et al., 2011). The prevalence of ADHD in SUD vary considerably, one meta-analysis review found that one in every four SUD patient has ADHD (Oortmerssen *et al, 2014)*. ADHD increases the risk for nicotine initiation by 2.4 fold and one out of two adolescents with ADHD and nicotine addiction develops SUD (Carrellas et al., 2016). However, the link between ADHD and SUD is not entirely predictable. The presence of comorbid conditions can also serve as a mediating factor in the progression of SUD (Estevez et al., 2016).

Academic Difficulties

Academic issues are often a persistent complaint in children and adolescents with ADHD since inattention, impulsivity, and hyperactivity may itself become too critical factors in academic achievement. Their presence can disrupt normal academic behavior. Many studies also claim genetic and neurodevelopmental similarities in ADHD and SLD (Pettersson et al., 2013). The relation between ADHD and SLD can be described using multiple deficit model, which explains that comorbidity develops due to the co-existence of multiple, probable, predicting variables and risk factors that are common across the development of these disorders (Pennington, 2006). Studies indicate that ADHD and SLD have similar genetic influences and neurological functioning such as processing speed, executive functioning, working memory, inhibition, and sustained attention (McGrath and Stoodley, 2019). Educational institutes across the globe now recognize the educational need of children with ADHD and SLD, many global universities assist mild impairment students in providing extra time, separate exam rooms, etc (Vickers, 2010). Also, students with ADHD are increasingly enrolling in higher education institutions, although fewer of them are finishing their graduation (Jansen et al., 2017).

Sleep Problems

Sleep problems are associated with ADHD children in about 70 percent of the cases. Major sleep problem includes insomnia, restless leg syndrome, periodic limb movement during sleep, and presence of sleep apnea is also being postulated (Schredl, 2007). It may look like that an ADHD child does not require large sleep, research indicates that they are more disruptive in the day time if their sleep disturbs (Harpin, 2005).

Family Difficulties

Researches indicate the presence of increased stress, conflict, poor parental monitoring, less authoritative parenting styles in a family of ADHD children compare to controlled population. Given the characteristic behavior of an ADHD child, attentional demands are very high at the caregiver's ends. An increased complication in the parent-child interactions is perceived in such families in comparison to controlled families (Barkley, Karlsson, & Pollard, 1985). Intrusive and hyperactive behavior of the children with ADHD can lead to the development of negative reactions from the other family members and can cause disturbances between parental relations as well. The presence of an ADHD child likely fluctuates the dynamics within the family members irrespective of the genetic predisposition among the other family members. If the family is at risk for genetic disposition factors, it can contribute to either amplification or maintenance of the disruptive behavior as the child grows. On the contrary scenario, the more responsive and sensitive family environment can serve as a protective factor by the development of self-controlling patterns in the child (Johnston and Mash, 2001). Family environment if not directly contributing to ADHD symptoms can also play a role in the development of other externalizing behavior such as defiant behavior or conduct issues.

Parental management factors such as control, consistency leads to functionally adaptive control-related beliefs in children. Children with ADHD who lack control-beliefs are more prone to develop depression later in their life, a faulty parent management system can mediate this process (Ostrander and Herman, 2006).

Social Difficulties

Children with ADHD experience vast difficulties in social interactions. The majority of them experience rejection by their peer in their early interaction with them. Their play behavior is considered to be intrusive, controlling/inattentive, or violating the rules of the organized game (Carpenter., et., al 2009). Social rejection adds to academic difficulties and it may cause poor self-esteem in children. Boys react more aggressively than girls.

Treatment

Treatment for ADHD includes both pharmacological and non-pharmacological management. The presence of comorbid disorders also complicates the clinical presentation and management approach in the overall treatment process of ADHD.

In terms of pharmacological management, the most successful treatment is seen with the stimulant medication of class amphetamines, common brand name- Adderall and methylphenidate, common brand name - Ritalin These preparations come under classified drugs and can be prescribed to children 6 years or older (Atkinson and Hollis, 2010). Stimulant drugs common side effects include headache, nausea, insomnia, daytime sleepiness, gastrointestinal symptoms, mood swings, increased blood pressure, increased pulse rates, and increased motor tics (in children with a history of motor tics). American Academy of child and adolescent psychiatry guidelines recommends parents of the children who are on stimulant medications to get their child's physical examination, pulse, weight, and height checked-up quarterly. Although medication does not directly affect academic learning in the child, an increased attention span, allows a child to focus more on the academic domain and a decrease in disruptive behavior creates more acceptance in the peer group which can lead to an improvement in the self-image of the child (Sadock and Sadock, 2015).

PSYCHOLOGICAL INTERVENTIONS FOR ADHD

Psychoeducation

It involves a detailed session with parents during which the diagnosis of ADHD is discussed. Parents are provided with support and their understanding of the problem is taken into consideration. Using the examples from the child's description given by the parents, the clinical picture of ADHD explained to them, the scientific meaning behind the symptoms is explained. Other factors such as a course of the disorder, etiological factors, family history, and treatment strategies along with foreseeable complications are deliberated. A psychoeducation program conducted for parents of children with ADHD demonstrated a positive impact on medication adherence and symptomatology of ADHD (Bai et al., 2015).

Behavioral Modification

Behavior modification in terms of Parent training programs is one of the key treatment strategies for ADHD. It involves the use of operant conditioning principals to manage the problematic behavior of the child and to provide a more organized and well-defined system of behavior that leads to the desired behavioral change. It is also called contingency management. This treatment module is both suitable in individual/couple format or group format. In his training program, Kazdin (1997) firstly taught parents with the learning principles behind the process of behavioral change, followed by specific techniques based on the principles and practice/skill-building sessions. They were asked to implement skills learned in the session at home with the child, and discuss its outcomes with the therapist in weekly sessions.

Positive Reinforcement

The skill of positive reinforcement is practically used by each parent, they all know when to praise a child when the child is behaving in a good manner. At the same time, this skill can be strategically used when a new behavior is required to be established. It refers to a system of providing rewards and incentives to the child when positive behavior is displayed., it is more about setting defined boundaries for the child. In the parent management training, the technique of positive reinforcement involves pre-designing a ***contract*** with the child, where expected behavior is discussed and clearly defined to the child. The child receives a (pre-decided) reward, either extrinsic or intrinsic when desired behavior goals are met or his privileges are removed (pre-decided) when he fails to complete the task. Examples of extrinsic rewards can include money, tokens, toys, or any object so desired by the child. Intrinsic rewards can include praise, pride, enjoyment gained through activities.

Using the principles of positive reinforcement, children can be asked to indulge in an activity which is disliked by them (Harwell and Jackson, 2008). A reward must be strong enough to work as an intrinsic motivational factor, for a child to indulge in the usually disliked activity and to finish it. This helps both in task completion and development of self-regulation in the child. The reward needs to be presented consistently, each time the desired behavior is performed (Kazdin, 1997). At the same time, it is made sure that the value the reward holds somewhat equal weightage to the amount of the effort paid by the child. If the reward has undervalued, it is not strong enough or if it is overly valued the effort loses its value.

Figure 2. Benefits of Positive reinforcements

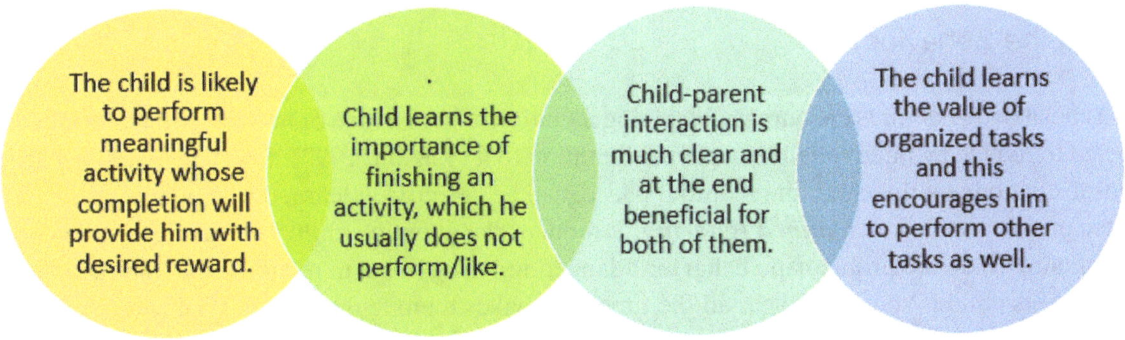

It can be designed in a game-format and degrees of reward can be defined wherein, each rewards value co-depends on the amount of effort paid or difficulty level of the child. Other forms of reward such as tokens, lotteries, special privileges, free time, etc. can also be used (Harwell and Jackson,2008).

Figure 3.

Tips for giving instructs to the child

- Ensure that child is paying attention. If not, the child is called by name and asked to pay attention
- Make sure that child maintains the eye contact during conversation.
- The message is stated in a steady tone, in brief and clear manner.
- State the message directly specifying the task behavior and not commenting or exaggerating the child's behavior. (For example: "Don't disturb your brother" is unclear whereas "Let your brother study and you sit here until he finishes" is more precise.)
- In case the child is not performing as mentioned. Clearly state the consequence (pre-decided) and it is important to practice the consequence rather than merely threatening the child with it. Also, any such consequences are clearly defined to the child, it can include a 2-3 minute time-out or loss of any privilege.

Managing Negative Behavior

Ignoring the Behavior

Such as positive behavior is encouraged by giving attention to it, negative or non-desired behavior can be expected to reduce by intentionally not paying attention to it (Kazdin, 1997). Few behaviors that are not purposefully done by the child, in the initial phase, can be selectively learned to ignore by the parents. This technique is called as ***Planned Ignoring.*** It reduces the attention child is getting as reinforcement by continuing to do the problematic behavior. Planned ignoring helps in reducing the comrade of critical comments child is so used to hear all the time and makes them feel accepted (Gable et al., 2009).

Timeout

Time out is initiated as a consequence of inappropriate behavior displayed by the child. It requires removing the child for a brief period from the activity he/she was involved in and placing him in a non-reinforcing place. It is important to give clear instructions to the child, what he is supposed to do in the timeout place, and when he/she can come out of the place. For instance "Go to timeout" is a vague phrase. Instruction can be like *"(Name of the child)! You need to stop disturbing your sibling when he is studying. Take a 2-minute timeout in the kitchen and come back and start making your school bag for tomorrow"*

Social Skills Training

An ADHD child has a problem in social skills, they often end up expressing themselves more aggressively and show tantrum, thus their social behavior is often problematic. Aim of the social skills training includes increasing the pro-social behavior that includes increasing cooperation, communication, participation, and validation (Forness and Kavale, 2001). Social skills training involves correctly identifying and responding to verbal and non-verbal behavior in social settings. It also involves establishing and picking up micro-skills in any social communication like noting, reflecting, attending behavior, etc. Social skills training aims to cognitively reframe the signals/triggers child assess in social communication. They learn to "read" social cues in a communication, such as recognizing emotion from tone and verbal expression, control impulse to speak, and learning others to complete their conversation (Mrug et al., 2001). Social skills training is most successful when used as a conjunctive treatment along with other behavioral or parent management intervention plan.

Academic Based Interventions

Teachers who work with ADHD children made an individualized suitable academic plan for the child more commonly known as the individualized education plan (IEP). Formulating an IEP involves assessment of individualized behavioral determinants of ADHD, their needs and strengths, identifying the academic instruction strategies to be applied along with behavioral intervention plans. It also consists of the classroom accommodation required for a child (Harwell and Jackson, 2008).

For conducting the class, the teacher needs to state behavioral expectations from the students during the class. It is also advisable to use audio-visual material and student-based activities while demonstrating the academic material. While assigning task both oral and written directions needs to be given. For example classroom activities, lesson numbers, the key highlight of the lesson, page number can be both orally directed and written on a whiteboard for a child to look in case his attention fleets in between the class. A lesson must always be divided into small manageable parts and revised each time when going to the next level (Pfiffner et al., 2006).

Forming pairs or buddy for the assignment can also be facilitated. It is advised to keep the group small only preferably 2-4 participants. To make learning more interesting, more engagement using colourful diagrams, or charts are often used. Worksheets and checklist also help keep students on track.

More significantly providing support and assistant to the child in a continuous manner is essential. Understanding that topic that may come handy to other children, although falling in the intellectual capacity of an ADHD child, can still be challenging for them. It is vital that teachers stay supportive and encouraging them during this process. Sometimes allowing the child to ventilate frustration healthily can also be helpful. The teacher can give them a small break or allowing some movement within the class to release their fidgety during the class. They can also be permitted to do some errands such as bringing a book from the teacher's desk or library, this will help them in ventilating their energy and coming back to class in a more focused manner (Harwell and Jackson, 2008).

Cognitive Behavioral Therapy (CBT)

CBT works successfully in the treatment of attention, both selective and sustained attention, impulsivity, and hyperactivity. The goal of CBT is to improve self-regulation in children by learning to self-monitor the behavior and to bring changes in the maladaptive behavior using the process of self-instruction. It is based upon Meichenbaum and Goodman's (1971) model of self-instruction training by learning to verbalize actions firstly aloud followed by an inner talk. CBT postulates that inability to self-control the behavior such as impulsivity is more due to cognitive than behavioral deficits. According to this ADHD child is unable to imply thinking process correctly before they act on, leading to a decreased inhibition, thus it focuses more on response-delay using cognitive strategies (Daly et al.,2007). Using self-instruction or self-praise while doing an activity reduces the frustration arising from delayed gratification, thus helping the child to organize their thought and helping in a response delay. Other strategies involve using self-reinforcing statements such as "*I know the line is lengthy in the ice-cream parlor, I will wait for my turn to get that full cone.*"

A CBT therapist is required to be well versed with the child's behavioural assessment and tailor-made the training program as per the individualized need of the child. Assessment involves behavioral analysis, level of impairment, reinforcing factors and other cognitive skills to form a complete cognitive-behavioral profile of the child. A therapist practices the self-instruction training using modeling it first and then eliciting the same from the child. A child learns problem-solving strategies such as first verbalizing the problem aloud, reviewing the possible options, choosing one option, finding out if the option is correct or not, if yes, then praising the self. If the option is incorrect, the child verbalizes what went wrong by reviewing all the steps and using self-motivation statements like "*I see and understand why the option I choose was wrong, I will try to do better next time*" (Flores, 2015).

The therapist provides praise as an immediate reward to the child in the successful completion of self-instruction. Possible social setting to further practice self-instruction is discussed with both child and parent, it can include child behavior during playtime, classroom behavior, or with a sibling. Parents are also given training in contingency management, wherein they learn to regulate antecedents and consequences of an event to bring the desired behavior in the child (Meichenbaum and Goodman, 1971).

Physical Activity Training

In children with ADHD, physical exercises are positively related in the reduction of core problematic symptoms and associated difficulties such as academic performances, self-esteem, cognitive functions, behavioral changes, social functioning, reduction in anxiety (Grassman et al., 2017; Hoza et al., 2016; Smith et al., 2013; Verret et al., 2012; Hillman et al., 2008). Even though children with ADHD are perceived as active due to the presence of restlessness and hyperactivity, it is a contrary fact that they are also at risk for deficits in both gross and fine motor skills functioning (Pan et al., 2019; Fliers et al., 2008; Harvey and Reid, 2003). Physical training of children with ADHD with consistently structured physical activities helps to overcome these motor skills deficits. The neurological benefit of physical and cognitive training is the increased blood flow in the brain, which can lead to increased brain tissue volume and when applied from a younger age can help to potentially change the long term complication of this disorder (Halperin and Healey, 2011). According to the review done by Grassman et al., (2017), the ideal amount of physical exercise for improvement in cognitive function is moderate to high intensity. In their study Pan et al., (2019) found that physical exercise benefited in the motor skills and executive skill deficits of the ADHD children. They concluded that physical exercise as a treatment module only bring positive changes in individual and possess more benefit and no harm in any possible manner.

Other Treatment

Some other treatments that work in conjugation with CBT or Behavioural treatment plan for ADHD include meditation practices, yoga, and attention building exercises such as deep breathing exercises, humming sounds. Many parents also find play therapy that uses art and another medium such as clay or puppet as an expressive medium to be useful.

ADHD is a complex condition that requires effort from all stakeholders including parents, teachers, medical health practitioners. The presence of comorbid conditions and the likelihood of difficulties at the familial level makes the treatment process further difficult. New treatment approaches can focus upon parental assessment and psychotherapy (Tuscano et al., 2017), more RCTs to compare singular and combined interventions strategies (Evans et al., 2018) and early intervention strategies at preschool level need to be focused (Murray et al., 2018).

REFERENCES

Alderson, R. M., Rapport, M. D., & Kofler, M. J. (2007). Attention-Deficit/Hyperactivity disorder and behavioral inhibition: A meta-analytic review of the stop-signal paradigm. *Journal of Abnormal Child Psychology, 35*(5), 745–758. doi:10.100710802-007-9131-6 PMID:17668315

American Psychiatric Association. (2013). *Diagnostic and statistical manual of mental disorders* (5th ed.). American Psychiatric Publishing.

Ames, C. S., & White, S. J. (2011). Brief report: Are ADHD traits dissociable from the autistic profile? Links between cognition and behavior. *Journal of Autism and Developmental Disorders, 31*(3), 357–363. doi:10.100710803-010-1049-0 PMID:20585847

Atkinson, M., & Hollis, C. (2010). NICE guideline: Attention deficit hyperactivity disorder. *Archives of Disease in Childhood - Education and Practice, 95*(1), 24–27. doi:10.1136/adc.2009.175943 PMID:20145015

Bai, G. N., Wang, Y. F., Yang, L., & Niu, W. Y. (2015). Effectiveness of a focused, brief psychoeducation program for parents of ADHD children: Improvement of medication adherence and symptoms. *Neuropsychiatric Disease and Treatment, 11*, 2721–2735. PMID:26604761

Balazs, J., & Kereszteny, A. (2017). Attention-deficit/hyperactivity disorder and suicide: A systematic review. *World Journal of Psychiatry, 7*(1), 44–59. doi:10.5498/wjp.v7.i1.44 PMID:28401048

Barkley, R. A. (1998). Attention-deficit/hyperactivity disorder. In E. Mash & R. Barkley (Eds.), *Treatment of childhood disorders* (2nd ed., pp. 55–110). Guilford Press.

Barkley, R. A. (Ed.). (2014). *Attention-deficit hyperactivity disorder: A handbook for diagnosis and treatment*. Guilford Publications.

Barkley, R. A., Karlsson, J., & Pollard, S. (1985). Effects of age on the mother-child interactions of ADD-H and normal boys. *Journal of Abnormal Child Psychology, 13*(4), 631–637. doi:10.1007/BF00923146 PMID:4078191

Berenguer, C., Roselló, B., Colomer, C., Baixauli, I., & Miranda, A. (2018). Children with autism and attention deficit hyperactivity disorder. Relationships between symptoms and executive function, the theory of mind, and behavioral problems. *Research in Developmental Disabilities, 83*, 260–269. doi:10.1016/j.ridd.2018.10.001 PMID:30368089

Brown, T. E. (2013). *A new understanding of ADHD in children and adults: Executive function impairments*. Routledge. doi:10.4324/9780203067536

Buitelaar, J. K., Van der Wees, M., Swaab-Barneveld, H., & Van der Gaag, R. J. (1999). Verbal memory and performance IQ predict theory of mind and emotion recognition ability in children with autistic spectrum disorders and in psychiatric control children. *Journal of Child Psychology and Psychiatry, and Allied Disciplines, 40*(6), 869–881. doi:10.1111/1469-7610.00505 PMID:10509882

Carpenter, R. E., Loo, S. K., Yang, M., Dang, J., & Smalley, S. L. (2009). Social Functioning Difficulties in ADHD: Association with PDD Risk. *Clinical Child Psychology and Psychiatry, 14*(3), 329–344. doi:10.1177/1359104508100890 PMID:19515751

Carrellas, N., Wilens, T. E., & Anselmo, R. (2016). Treatment of comorbid substance use disorders and ADHD in youth. *Current Treatment Options in Psychiatry, 3*(1), 15–27. doi:10.100740501-016-0072-y

Charach, A., Yeung, E., Climans, T., & Lillie, E. (2011). Childhood attention-deficit/hyperactivity disorder and future substance use disorders: Comparative meta-analyses. *Journal of the American Academy of Child and Adolescent Psychiatry, 50*(1), 9–21. doi:10.1016/j.jaac.2010.09.019 PMID:21156266

Chronis-Tuscano, A., Wang, C. H., Woods, K. E., Strickland, J., & Stein, M. A. (2017). Parent ADHD and evidence-based treatment for their children: Review and directions for future research. *Journal of Abnormal Child Psychology, 45*(3), 501–517. doi:10.100710802-016-0238-5 PMID:28025755

Clarke, A. R., Barry, R. J., Dupuy, F. E., Heckel, L. D., McCarthy, R., Selikowitz, M., & Johnstone, S. J. (2011). Behavioural differences between EEG-defined subgroups of children with attention-deficit/hyperactivity disorder. *Clinical Neurophysiology*, *122*(7), 1333–1341. doi:10.1016/j.clinph.2010.12.038 PMID:21247797

Engel-Yeger, B., & Ziv-On, D. (2011). The relationship between sensory processing difficulties and leisure activity preference of children with different types of ADHD. *Research in Developmental Disabilities*, *32*(3), 1154–1162. doi:10.1016/j.ridd.2011.01.008 PMID:21324640

Engert, V., & Pruessner, J. C. (2008). Dopaminergic and noradrenergic contributions to functionality in ADHD: The role of methylphenidate. *Current Neuropharmacology*, *6*(4), 322–328. doi:10.2174/157015908787386069 PMID:19587853

Estévez, N., Dey, M., Eich-Höchli, D., Foster, S., Gmel, G., & Mohler-Kuo, M. (2016). Adult attention-deficit/hyperactivity disorder and its association with substance use and substance use disorders in young men. *Epidemiology and Psychiatric Sciences*, *25*(3), 255–266. doi:10.1017/S2045796015000360 PMID:25989844

Evans, S., Ling, M., Hill, B., Rinehart, N., Austin, D., & Sciberras, E. (2018). Systematic review of meditation-based interventions for children with ADHD. *European Child & Adolescent Psychiatry*, *27*(1), 9–27. doi:10.100700787-017-1008-9 PMID:28547119

Faraone, S. V., Biederman, J., & Mick, E. (2006). The age-dependent decline of attention deficit hyperactivity disorder: A meta-analysis of follow-up studies. *Psychological Medicine*, *36*(2), 159–165. doi:10.1017/S003329170500471X PMID:16420712

Fitzgerald, C., Dalsgaard, S., Nordentoft, M., & Erlangsen, A. (2019). Suicidal behaviour among persons with attention-deficit hyperactivity disorder. *The British Journal of Psychiatry*, *215*(4), 615–620. doi:10.1192/bjp.2019.128 PMID:31172893

Fliers, E., Rommelse, N., Vermeulen, S. H. H. M., Altink, M., Buschgens, C. J. M., Faraone, S. V., Sergeant, J. A., Franke, B., & Buitelaar, J. K. (2008). Motor coordination problems in children and adolescents with ADHD rated by parents and teachers: Effects of age and gender. *Journal of Neural Transmission (Vienna, Austria)*, *115*(2), 211–220. doi:10.100700702-007-0827-0 PMID:17994185

Forness, S. R., & Kavale, K. A. (2001). ADHD and a return to the medical model of special education. *Education & Treatment of Children*, 224–247.

Frazier, J. A., Biederman, J., Bellordre, C. A., Garfield, S. B., Geller, D. A., Coffey, B. J., & Faraone, S. V. (2001). Should the diagnosis of attention-deficit/hyperactivity disorder be considered in children with a pervasive developmental disorder? *Journal of Attention Disorders*, *4*(4), 203–211. doi:10.1177/108705470100400402

Furman, L. M. (2008). Attention-deficit hyperactivity disorder (ADHD): Does new research support old concepts? *Journal of Child Neurology*, *23*(7), 775–784. doi:10.1177/0883073808318059 PMID:18658077

Gable, R. A., Hester, P. H., Rock, M. L., & Hughes, K. G. (2009). Back to basics: Rules, praise, ignoring, and reprimands revisited. *Intervention in School and Clinic*, *44*(4), 195–205. doi:10.1177/1053451208328831

Germanò, E., Gagliano, A., & Curatolo, P. (2010). Comorbidity of ADHD and dyslexia. *Developmental Neuropsychology, 35*(5), 475–493. doi:10.1080/87565641.2010.494748 PMID:20721770

Ghanizadeh, A. (2011). Sensory processing problems in children with ADHD, a systematic review. *Psychiatry Investigation, 8*(2), 89. doi:10.4306/pi.2011.8.2.89 PMID:21852983

Goldin, R. L., Matson, J. L., Tureck, K., Cervantes, P. E., & Jang, J. (2013). A comparison of tantrum behavior profiles in children with ASD, ADHD and comorbid ASD and ADHD. *Research in Developmental Disabilities, 34*(9), 2669–2675. doi:10.1016/j.ridd.2013.04.022 PMID:23764824

Gozal, D., & Molfese, D. L. (2005). *Attention Deficit Hyperactivity Disorder*. Humana Press. doi:10.1385/1592598919

Grassmann, V., Alves, M. V., Santos-Galduróz, R. F., & Galduróz, J. C. F. (2017). Possible cognitive benefits of acute physical exercise in children with ADHD: A systematic review. *Journal of Attention Disorders, 21*(5), 367–371. doi:10.1177/1087054714526041 PMID:24621460

Halperin, J. M., & Healey, D. M. (2011). The influences of environmental enrichment, cognitive enhancement, and physical exercise on brain development: Can we alter the developmental trajectory of ADHD? *Neuroscience and Biobehavioral Reviews, 35*(3), 621–634. doi:10.1016/j.neubiorev.2010.07.006 PMID:20691725

Harpin, V. A. (2005). The effect of ADHD on the life of an individual, their family, and community from preschool to adult life. *Archives of Disease in Childhood, 90*(suppl 1), i2–i7. doi:10.1136/adc.2004.059006 PMID:15665153

Harvey, W. J., & Reid, G. (2003). Attention-deficit/hyperactivity disorder: A review of research on movement skill performance and physical fitness. *Adapted Physical Activity Quarterly; APAQ, 20*(1), 1–25. doi:10.1123/apaq.20.1.1

Harwell, J. M., & Jackson, R. W. (2008). *The complete learning disabilities handbook: Ready-to-use strategies and activities for teaching students with learning disabilities*. John Wiley & Sons.

Hillman, C. H., Erickson, K. I., & Kramer, A. F. (2008). Be smart, exercise your heart: Exercise effects on brain and cognition. *Nature Reviews. Neuroscience, 9*(1), 58–65. doi:10.1038/nrn2298 PMID:18094706

Hoza, B., Martin, C. P., Pirog, A., & Shoulberg, E. K. (2016). Using physical activity to manage ADHD symptoms: The state of the evidence. *Current Psychiatry Reports, 18*(12), 113. doi:10.100711920-016-0749-3 PMID:27807701

Jansen, D., Petry, K., Ceulemans, E., van der Oord, S., Noens, I., & Baeyens, D. (2017). Functioning and participation problems of students with ADHD in higher education: Which reasonable accommodations are effective? *European Journal of Special Needs Education, 32*(1), 35–53. doi:10.1080/08856257.2016.1254965

Jarrett, M. A., Wolff, J. C., Davis, T. E. III, Cowart, M. J., & Ollendick, T. H. (2016). Characteristics of children with ADHD and comorbid anxiety. *Journal of Attention Disorders, 20*(7), 636–644. doi:10.1177/1087054712452914 PMID:22863769

Johnson, M. H. (2012). Executive function and developmental disorders: The flip side of the coin. *Trends in Cognitive Sciences*, *16*(9), 454–457. doi:10.1016/j.tics.2012.07.001 PMID:22835639

Johnston, C., & Mash, E. J. (2001). Families of children with attention-deficit/hyperactivity disorder: Review and recommendations for future research. *Clinical Child and Family Psychology Review*, *4*(3), 183–207. doi:10.1023/A:1017592030434 PMID:11783738

Kaiser, N. M., & Pfiffner, L. J. (2011). Evidence-based psychosocial treatments for childhood ADHD. *Psychiatric Annals*, *41*(1), 9–15. doi:10.3928/00485713-20101221-03

Kazdin, A. (1997). Parent management training: Evidence, outcomes, and issues. *Journal of the American Academy of Child and Adolescent Psychiatry*, *36*(10), 1349–1356. doi:10.1097/00004583-199710000-00016 PMID:9334547

Kern, J. K., Geier, D. A., Sykes, L. K., Geier, M. R., & Deth, R. C. (2015). Are ASD and ADHD a continuum? A comparison of pathophysiological similarities between the disorders. *Journal of Attention Disorders*, *19*(9), 805–827. doi:10.1177/1087054712459886 PMID:23074304

Knouse, L. E., & Safren, S. A. (2013). Psychosocial treatment for adult ADHD. In *ADHD in adults* (pp. 119–136). Humana Press. doi:10.1007/978-1-62703-248-3_7

Lang, R., O'Reilly, M., Healy, O., Rispoli, M., Lydon, H., Streusand, W., ... Didden, R. (2012). Sensory integration therapy for autism spectrum disorders: A systematic review. *Research in Autism Spectrum Disorders*, *6*(3), 1004–1018. doi:10.1016/j.rasd.2012.01.006

Lee, S. S., Humphreys, K. L., Flory, K., Liu, R., & Glass, K. (2011). Prospective association of childhood attention-deficit/hyperactivity disorder (adhd) and substance use and abuse/dependence: A meta analytic review. *Clinical Psychology Review*, *31*(3), 328–341. doi:10.1016/j.cpr.2011.01.006 PMID:21382538

Leitner, Y. (2014). The co-occurrence of autism and attention deficit hyperactivity disorder in children–what do we know? *Frontiers in Human Neuroscience*, *8*, 268. doi:10.3389/fnhum.2014.00268 PMID:24808851

Lionel, A. C., Tammimies, K., Vaags, A. K., Rosenfeld, J. A., Ahn, J. W., Merico, D., & Gazzellone, M. J. (2014). Disruption of the ASTN2/TRIM32 locus at 9q33. 1 is a risk factor in males for autism spectrum disorders, ADHD and other neurodevelopmental phenotypes. *Human Molecular Genetics*, *23*(10), 2752–2768. doi:10.1093/hmg/ddt669 PMID:24381304

Little, L. M., Dean, E., Tomchek, S., & Dunn, W. (2018). Sensory processing patterns in autism, attention deficit hyperactivity disorder, and typical development. *Physical & Occupational Therapy in Pediatrics*, *38*(3), 243–254. doi:10.1080/01942638.2017.1390809 PMID:29240517

Luoni, C., Balottin, U., Zaccagnino, M., Brembilla, L., Livetti, G., & Termine, C. (2013). Reading difficulties and attention deficit hyperactivity behaviours: Evidence of an early association in a non-clinical sample. *Journal of Research in Reading*, *38*(1), 73–90. doi:10.1111/j.1467-9817.2013.01555.x

Mannuzza, S., & Klein, R. G. (2000). Long-term prognosis in attention-deficit/hyperactivity disorder. *Child and Adolescent Psychiatric Clinics of North America*, *9*(3), 711–726. doi:10.1016/S1056-4993(18)30114-7 PMID:10944664

Mansour, R., Dovi, A. T., Lane, D. M., Loveland, K. A., & Pearson, D. A. (2017). ADHD severity as it relates to comorbid psychiatric symptomatology in children with autism spectrum disorders (ASD). *Research in Developmental Disabilities*, *60*, 52–64. doi:10.1016/j.ridd.2016.11.009 PMID:27889487

Mayes, S. D., Calhoun, S. L., Baweja, R., Feldman, L., Syed, E., Gorman, A. A., & Siddiqui, F. (2015). Suicide ideation and attempts are associated with co-occurring oppositional defiant disorder and sadness in children and adolescents with ADHD. *Journal of Psychopathology and Behavioral Assessment*, *37*(2), 274–282. doi:10.100710862-014-9451-0

McGrath, L. M., & Stoodley, C. J. (2019). Are there shared neural correlates between dyslexia and ADHD? A meta-analysis of voxel-based morphometry studies. *Journal of Neurodevelopmental Disorders*, *11*(1), 31. doi:10.118611689-019-9287-8 PMID:31752659

Meichenbaum, D. H., & Goodman, J. (1971). Training impulsive children to talk to themselves: A means of developing self-control. *Journal of Abnormal Psychology*, *77*(2), 115–126. doi:10.1037/h0030773 PMID:5550424

Miller, L. J. (2006). *Sensational Kids: Help and Hope for Children with Sensory Processing Disorder*. Putnam.

Miller, L. J., Nielsen, D. M., Schoen, S. A., & Brett-Green, B. A. (2009). Perspectives on sensory processing disorder: A call for translational research. *Frontiers in Integrative Neuroscience*, *3*, 22. doi:10.3389/neuro.07.022.2009 PMID:19826493

Montoya, A., Colom, F., & Ferrin, M. (2011). Is psychoeducation for parents and teachers of children and adolescents with ADHD efficacious? A systematic literature review. *European Psychiatry*, *26*(3), 166–175. doi:10.1016/j.eurpsy.2010.10.005 PMID:21292454

Mrug, S., Hoza, B., & Gerdes, A. C. (2001). Children with attention-deficit/hyperactivity disorder: Peer relationships and peer-oriented interventions. *New Directions for Child and Adolescent Development*, *2001*(91), 51–78. doi:10.1002/cd.5 PMID:11280014

Murray, D. W., Lawrence, J. R., & LaForett, D. R. (2018). The Incredible Years® Programs for ADHD in young children: A critical review of the evidence. *Journal of Emotional and Behavioral Disorders*, *26*(4), 195–208. doi:10.1177/1063426617717740

Nigg, J. T. (2013). Attention-deficit/hyperactivity disorder and adverse health outcomes. *Clinical Psychology Review*, *33*(2), 215–228. doi:10.1016/j.cpr.2012.11.005 PMID:23298633

Noordermeer, S. D., Luman, M., Weeda, W. D., Buitelaar, J. K., Richards, J. S., Hartman, C. A., Hoekstra, P. J., Franke, B., Heslenfeld, D. J., & Oosterlaan, J. (2017). Risk factors for comorbid oppositional defiant disorder in attention-deficit/hyperactivity disorder. *European Child & Adolescent Psychiatry*, *26*(10), 1155–1164. doi:10.100700787-017-0972-4 PMID:28283834

Ostrander, R., & Herman, K. C. (2006). Potential cognitive, parenting, and developmental mediators of the relationship between ADHD and depression. *Journal of Consulting and Clinical Psychology*, *74*(1), 89–98. doi:10.1037/0022-006X.74.1.89 PMID:16551146

Pan, C. Y., Tsai, C. L., Chu, C. H., Sung, M. C., Huang, C. Y., & Ma, W. Y. (2019). Effects of physical exercise intervention on motor skills and executive functions in children with ADHD: A pilot study. *Journal of Attention Disorders, 23*(4), 384–397. doi:10.1177/1087054715569282 PMID:25646023

Pennington, B. F. (2006). From single to multiple deficit models of developmental disorders. *Cognition, 101*(2), 385–413. doi:10.1016/j.cognition.2006.04.008 PMID:16844106

Pettersson, E., Anckarsäter, H., Gillberg, C., & Lichtenstein, P. (2013). Different neurodevelopmental symptoms have a common genetic etiology. *Journal of Child Psychology and Psychiatry, and Allied Disciplines, 54*(12), 1356–1365. doi:10.1111/jcpp.12113 PMID:24127638

Pfiffner, L. J., Barkley, R. A., & DuPaul, G. J. (2006). Treatment of ADHD in school settings. *Attention deficit hyperactivity disorder: A handbook for diagnosis and treatment, 3*, 547-589.

Polanczyk, G. V., Willcutt, E. G., Salum, G. A., Kieling, C., & Rohde, L. A. (2014). ADHD prevalence estimates across three decades: An updated systematic review and meta-regression analysis. *International Journal of Epidemiology, 43*(2), 434–442. doi:10.1093/ije/dyt261 PMID:24464188

Purdie, N., Hattie, J., & Carroll, A. (2002). A review of the research on interventions for attention deficit hyperactivity disorder: What works best? *Review of Educational Research, 72*(1), 61–99. doi:10.3102/00346543072001061

Rau, S., Skapek, M. F., Tiplady, K., Seese, S., Burns, A., Armour, A. C., & Kenworthy, L. (2020). Identifying comorbid ADHD in autism: Attending to the inattentive presentation. *Research in Autism Spectrum Disorders, 69*, 101468. doi:10.1016/j.rasd.2019.101468

Reale, L., Bartoli, B., Cartabia, M., Zanetti, M., Costantino, M. A., Canevini, M. P., Termine, C., & Bonati, M.Lombardy ADHD Group. (2017). Comorbidity prevalence and treatment outcome in children and adolescents with ADHD. *European Child & Adolescent Psychiatry, 26*(12), 1443–1457. doi:10.100700787-017-1005-z PMID:28527021

Rhee, S. H., Waldman, I. D., Hay, D. A., & Levy, F. (1999). Sex differences in genetic and environmental influences on DSM–III–R attention-deficit/hyperactivity disorder. *Journal of Abnormal Psychology, 108*(1), 24–41. doi:10.1037/0021-843X.108.1.24 PMID:10066990

Rivera-Flores, G. W. (2015). Self-instructional cognitive training to reduce impulsive cognitive style in children with Attention Deficit with Hyperactivity Disorder. *Electronic Journal of Research in Educational Psychology, 13*(1), 27–46.

Rivero, O., Selten, M. M., Sich, S., Popp, S., Bacmeister, L., Amendola, E., ... Schmitt, A. G. (2015). Cadherin-13, a risk gene for ADHD and comorbid disorders, impacts GABAergic function in hippocampus and cognition. *Translational Psychiatry, 5*(10), e655. doi:10.1038/tp.2015.152 PMID:26460479

Sadock, B. J., Kaplan, H. I., & Sadock, V. A. (2007). *Kaplan &Sadock's synopsis of psychiatry: Behavioral sciences/clinical psychiatry* (10th ed.). Wolter Kluwer.

Sadock, B. J., Sadock, V. A., & Ruiz, P. (2015). *Kaplan & Sadock's synopsis of psychiatry: Behavioral sciences/clinical psychiatry* (11th ed.). Wolters Kluwer.

Schredl, M., Alm, B., & Sobanski, E. (2007). Sleep quality in adult patients with attention deficit hyperactivity disorder (ADHD). *European Archives of Psychiatry and Clinical Neuroscience*, *257*(3), 164–168. doi:10.100700406-006-0703-1 PMID:17131215

Sinzig, J., Morsch, D., & Lehmkuhl, G. (2008). Do hyperactivity, impulsivity inattention have an impact on the ability of facial affect recognition in children with autism and ADHD? *European Child & Adolescent Psychiatry*, *17*(2), 63–72. doi:10.100700787-007-0637-9 PMID:17896119

Skirrow, C., Hosang, G. M., Farmer, A. E., & Asherson, P. (2012). An update on the debated association between ADHD and bipolar disorder across the lifespan. *Journal of Affective Disorders*, *141*(2-3), 143–149. doi:10.1016/j.jad.2012.04.003 PMID:22633181

Smith, A. L., Hoza, B., Linnea, K., McQuade, J. D., Tomb, M., Vaughn, A. J., Shoulberg, E. K., & Hook, H. (2013). Pilot physical activity intervention reduces severity of ADHD symptoms in young children. *Journal of Attention Disorders*, *17*(1), 70–82. doi:10.1177/1087054711417395 PMID:21868587

Sorensen, L., Plessen, K. J., Nicholas, J., & Lundervold, A. J. (2011). Is behavioral regulation in children with ADHD aggravated by comorbid anxiety disorders? *Journal of Attention Disorders*, *15*(1), 56–66. doi:10.1177/1087054709356931 PMID:20071639

Storebö, O. J., & Simonsen, E. (2016). The Association between ADHD and Antisocial Personality Disorder (ASPD): A Review. *Journal of Attention Disorders*, *20*(10), 815–824. doi:10.1177/1087054713512150 PMID:24284138

Szatmari, P. (1992). The epidemiology of attention-deficit hyperactivity disorders. In G. Weiss (Ed.), *Child and adolescent psychiatry clinics of North America: Attention deficit disorder* (pp. 361–372). W. B. Saunders.

Taurines, R., Schmitt, J., Renner, T., Conner, A. C., Warnke, A., & Romanos, M. (2010). Developmental comorbidity in attention-deficit/hyperactivity disorder. *Attention Deficit and Hyperactivity Disorders*, *2*(4), 267–289. doi:10.100712402-010-0040-0 PMID:21432612

Vaidya, C. J. (2012). Neurodevelopmental abnormalities in ADHD. *Current Topics in Behavioral Neurosciences*, *9*, 49–66. doi:10.1007/7854_2011_138 PMID:21541845

Van Emmerik-van Oortmerssen, K., van de Glind, G., van den Brink, W., Smit, F., Crunelle, C. L., Swets, M., & Schoevers, R. A. (2012). Prevalence of attention-deficit hyperactivity disorder in substance use disorder patients: A meta-analysis and meta-regression analysis. *Drug and Alcohol Dependence*, *122*(1-2), 11–19. doi:10.1016/j.drugalcdep.2011.12.007 PMID:22209385

Verret, C., Guay, M. C., Berthiaume, C., Gardiner, P., & Béliveau, L. (2012). A physical activity program improves behavior and cognitive functions in children with ADHD: An exploratory study. *Journal of Attention Disorders*, *16*(1), 71–80. doi:10.1177/1087054710379735 PMID:20837978

Vickers, M. Z. (2010). *Accommodating College Students with Learning Disabilities: ADD, ADHD, and Dyslexia*. John William Pope Center for Higher Education Policy (NJ1).

Weiss, M., & Murray, C. (2003). Assessment and management of attention-deficit hyperactivity disorder in adults. *Canadian Medical Association Journal*, *168*(6), 715–722. PMID:12642429

World Health Organization. (2004). *The ICD-10 Classification of mental and behavioral disorders*. WHO.

Yoshimasu, K., Barbaresi, W. J., Colligan, R. C., Voigt, R. G., Killian, J. M., Weaver, A. L., & Katusic, S. K. (2019). Psychiatric comorbidities modify the association between childhood ADHD and risk for suicidality: A population-based longitudinal study. *Journal of Attention Disorders*, *23*(8), 777–786. doi:10.1177/1087054717718264 PMID:28689473

Chapter 3
Pre-, Peri-, and Post-Natal Risk Factors in ADHD

Pangajam Ponnuswamy
SRM Medical College Hospital and Research Centre, India

Ann Sarah Paul
SRM Medical College Hospital and Research Centre, India

Aneesha Brigitte Jose
SRM Medical College Hospital and Research Centre, India

ABSTRACT

Attention deficit/hyperactivity disorder (ADHD) is a neurodevelopmental disorder most commonly found in childhood with its core symptoms manifesting as inattention, impulsiveness, and hyperactivity. As ADHD generates a substantial rate of burden to the society in terms of economic and medical resources used, priority is given to explore the risk factors that contributes towards the multifactorial origin of this disorder to offer possible preventive and therapeutic interventions. With heritability accounting for 75% to 80% of the variability seen in ADHD, the remaining are explained through environmental risk factors that are exposed during critical period of pre-, peri-, and postnatal development. Though literature on the risk factors have been mostly controversial, certain associations have been made with regards to ADHD pathophysiology.

INTRODUCTION

Attention Deficit/ Hyperactivity Disorder (ADHD) is the most common neurodevelopmental disorder which manifests in early childhood and persists mostly into adolescence and adulthood (Sagiv et al, 2013). It is characterized by its core symptoms of inattention, impulsiveness and hyperactivity and accessory symptoms such as disorganization, affect control, hot temper and affective liability (Tole et al, 2019; Zappitelli, Pinto and Grizenko, 2001). Children with ADHD show considerable variation in their symptom severity, degree of impairment and presence of other co-morbid conditions (Linnet et al, 2003).

DOI: 10.4018/978-1-7998-5495-1.ch003

Prevalence varies from 5% to 10% in children (Sagiv et al, 2013) and approximately 3% in adulthood (Tole et al, 2019) with more inattentiveness exhibited and less of hyperactivity and impulsivity. ADHD generates a substantial burden on the quality of life and psychosocial functioning of affected children and their family members along with a considerable strain on medical, educational and social resources and therefore, high priority is given to study and investigate the risk factors associated with it(Tole et al, 2019; Sagiv et al, 2013).

The etiology of ADHD is multifaceted with an interplay of gene, development and environmental factors (Sagiv et al, 2013). Heritability has been considered as the strongest factor in the development of ADHD with genetic factors responsible for approximately three-quarters of the variability found in ADHD; that is, up to 75%-80% of symptoms seen in ADHD individuals are due to genetic component (Mill and Petronis, 2008; Grizenko et al, 2008). First-degree relatives of the affected person have a 2 to 8-fold risk for developing this disorder (Grizenko et al, 2008). The remaining were due to environmental factors which includes several pre-, peri- and postnatal risk factors. Previous literature has shown that insults that transpires during critical pre- and perinatal period of development tend to have a direct effect on the fetal brain leading to neurochemical alterations that are commonly associated with ADHD and other psychiatric conditions (Zappitelli, Pinto and Grizenko, 2001). As per the programming hypothesis, unfavorable intrauterine environment increases the susceptibility to disorders in later life (Linnet et al, 2003). However, research on various influences that may predispose to neonatal brain trauma in the etiology of ADHD has come out to be controversial (Zappitelli, Pinto and Grizenko, 2001).

Prenatal Stressors

The focus on the impact of in utero toxins on the developing fetus has been on three exposures; mainly, cigarette smoking, alcohol intake and use of illicit drugs. The neurochemical hypothesis on the pathogenesis of ADHD describes a dysfunction of dopaminergic systems in the prefrontal cortex areas of the brain (Zappitelli, Pinto and Grizenko, 2001). According to animal studies, rats and pups that have been exposed to nicotine during their prenatal period exhibited a decrease in their striatal dopaminergic receptor binding sites. Existing evidence on prenatal risk factors and etiology of ADHD is considered to have a genetic origin. Approximately 10-40% of the variance is associated to environmental causes. There is insufficient literature to support a causal relationship between prenatal risk factors and the development of the disorder. It is difficult to separate the effect of prenatal risk from postnatal risk factors such as social adversity, mental health of the parent and inherited factors transmitted from the mother (Emma Sciberras et al, 2017).Mothers who experienced emotional problems and stress during pregnancy lead to Attention Deficit hyperactivity Disorder of their children(Simon2016).

A study (Knopik et al., 2005) conducted through diagnostic telephone interview, focused on the contributions of parental alcoholism, prenatal substance abuse and genetic transmission as risk factors for ADHD. They conducted a twin study on female adolescents so /as to see the separate effects of both genetic and environmental factors. The results found the following as risk factors among the sample:

- Parental alcoholism: There was an increased risk of the child developing ADHD if alcoholism was prevalent among the parents.
- Parental substance use and perinatal risk factors: It was seen that smoking during pregnancy was associated with an increased chance of low birth weight in the child. These associations remained even when smoking was controlled during the period of pregnancy. Results showed that there

was a greater likelihood of ADHD to be developed among those whose mothers reported heavy alcohol drinking during pregnancy, in fathers who engaged in substance abuse and those with low birth weight.

- Genetic influence on the risk of ADHD: Results show that having a twin with ADHD increases the risk factor to develop the disorder in the case of both monozygotic and dizygotic twins. Non-shared environmental factors seem to account for about 14% of the variability after prenatal and parental factors were controlled.

Substance Use

Maternal substance usage during pregnancy is associated with the symptoms of ADHD (Langley et al 2012) A history of alcohol usage disorders in the parents also found a linage with elevated symptoms of the disorder among the children. Even drinking prior to the birth of the child seems to be related to the risk. This is suggestive of a germ cell mutation within the child (Infante et., al 2015). Children who were exposed to alcohol prenatally revealed attention deficit between the ages of 7 to 14 years. They were less accurate in response which resulted in more omission errors, slow and inconsistent respond lead to variability in response time during Continuous performance test (CPT) when compared to children who were not exposed to alcohol prenatally. Children who were exposed to alcohol were more active than children who were not exposed to alcohol.

Consumption of alcohol and maternal smoking at the time of pregnancy has increased the prevalence of ADHD by 1.55 times, 2.64 times respectively. Moreover, Passive smoking and alcohol intake during pregnancy have increased the occurrence of ADHD by 1.58 times. This shows that simultaneous alcohol usage and passive smoking during pregnancy increases the risk of ADHD (Han et al., 2015; Golmirzaei et., al2013). Nicotine is linked to both DNA and RNA synthesis within the brain of the fetus. This could disrupt the normal brain development and may result in the development of symptoms of the disorder (Silva et al 2014,). Wang et., al (2019) found that the vulnerability of ADHD genotypes carriers might increase when the children having the history of in- utero to cigarette smoking.

Smoking

Studies have proposed two mechanisms through which prenatal smoking impacts fetal neurodevelopment:

- Nicotine causing disturbance to dopaminergic system as mentioned above
- Fetal hypoxia; it has been hypothesized that prenatal smoking causes elevation in carboxyhemoglobin levels in both pregnant mothers and their fetuses leading to decreased oxygen delivery to fetal tissues (Zappitelli, Pinto and Grizenko, 2001).

A review study conducted by Zappitelli, Pinto and Grizenko (2001) showed that maternal smoking was independently associated childhood behavior problem, especially ADHD. Few prospective studies have shown that smoking during, and not after, pregnancy was linked with higher ADHD ratings even when confounding variables (such as maternal age, sex, socioeconomic status and maternal stress) were controlled for. Tole et., al. (2019) in their study with 42 ADHD individuals confirmed previous literature about the link between with prenatal smoking and later diagnosis of ADHD; however, the authors demonstrated that parents affected with psychiatric disorders tends to carry greater risk for hyperactivity and inattention in the child than smoking, Other studies too have confirmed the impact of prenatal smoking is raising the risk for developing ADHD with significantly higher reports of ADHD in children who were exposed to heavy smoking (greater than 10 cigarettes per day) during prenatal period (Pohlabeln et al., 2017: Motlagh et al., 2010; Huang et al., 2017).

Literature has shown few evidences of genetic factors confounding the association between maternal smoking during pregnancy and ADHD diagnosis in children, while other studies have been able to bring about the relationship between smoking during pregnancy and low birth weight in both unrelated and related mother-child pairs (Ketzer et al., 2012). Likewise, in a meta-analytical study by Linnet et al, 2003, the authors found that there was four times the higher risk of ADHD in the children who were exposed to tobacco in utero independently of maternal ADHD; in addition, they were able to demonstrate that the majority of studies they reviewed showed an association between prenatal smoking and inattention and hyperactivity (Linnet et al., 2003; Pohlabeln et al., 2017).

A study (Motlagh et al., 2010) conducted at Yale Child Study Centre on the effect of severe psychosocial stress and cigarette smoking during the period of pregnancy on ADHD as well as Tourette syndrome. They examined both pre and perinatal risk factors that are often associated with the disorders as they often tend to co-occur. The study focused on the effect of increased level of maternal smoking, maternal stress, reduced birth weight and other perinatal events. The results depicted that those with ADHD alone had the greatest rate of heavy smoking among the mothers during pregnancy. Maternal psychosocial stress was seen in around 27% of the children with ADHD and this was much higher as compared to the control group. The ADHD group was strongly associated with exposure to maternal smoking and psychosocial stress during pregnancy. The group seemed to have a limited ability to cope with the stress. This is in line with previous research, though several studies have shown that this association is often due to genetic factors.

Alcohol Consumption and Illicit Drug Use

Research on the relationship between child's exposure to prenatal alcohol and ADHD has been an important area of interest since children with fetal alcohol syndrome (FAS) show signs of attention and memory deficits; however, the findings have been inconclusive (Sagiv et al., 2013; Zappitelli, Pinto and Grizenko, 2001).Animal studies on monkeys exposed to moderate levels of ethanol in utero revealed that ethanol tends to boosts the migration of nerve cells hypothesized to be involved in behavioral difficulties along with production of certain neurochemical hormones that disturbs brain development (Linnet et al., 2003). Maternal alcohol usage leads to the development of ADHD symptoms, but not to the extent of clinical diagnosis of ADHD as it has a minor role among the other risk factors (Eilertsen et al., 2017).

Prenatal alcohol exposure has an association with increased number of symptoms of inattention and hyperactivity of children with ADHD. The children who were exposed to alcohol prenatally showed differences in neurophysiological processes as in comparison with the children who were not exposed to alcohol prenatally (Burden et al., 2010). Prenatal exposure to alcohol has created calculation difficulties specifically number processing among the adolescents with ADHD. This number processing deficit is due to poorer function of the executive brain system. However, it can be mediated by IQ and executive function but not magnitude comparison (Jacobson et al, 2011).

Zappitelli, Pinto and Grizenko (2001) in their review found that relation existed between ADHD and familial risk for alcoholism more so than prenatal exposure to alcohol and a significant association was only seen in a dose-dependent fashion. The authors suggested that controversy exist on this subject because there is no clear pathophysiologic event that relates ethanol consumption during prenatal period and specific abnormalities exhibited by ADHD children. Moreover, there are several confounding variables such as dietary, genetic factors, presence of maternal psychiatric illness with maternal smoking and alcohol consumption acting in a collinear manner which makes it a difficult risk factor to study (Linnet et al., 2003; Zappitelli, Pinto and Grizenko, 2001). Linnet et al. (2003) review study confirmed previous literature which had hypothesized the contribution of alcohol on central nervous system impairment but not per se ADHD for which the findings were inconsistent.

Difficulties on interpreting studies on the impact of drug use during pregnancy on ADHD have been noted because it is often seen with other risk factors such as cigarette smoking and alcohol consumption. Though the negative effect of drugs on fetal development is known, its exact relation to ADHD is still unclear; most studies have shown that the serious consequence of drug abuse to be secondary to the effect of smoking (Linnet et al., 2003). Maternal use of illicit drug prior to birth has been associated with traits of inattention but without leading to ADHD diagnosis (Sagiv et al., 2013). Children with ADHD had deficits in daily living skills and socialization due to Prenatal exposure to alcohol . It was expressed in difficulty attaining age appropriate self-care, handling money, going to places independently, observing rules, picking up social cues and avoiding risky social situations (Ware et al.2014).

Croker et al. (2009) studied adaptive function impairments among children with prenatal exposure to alcohol, ADHD without alcohol exposure and children without ADHD. They found that children who were exposed to alcohol had shown impairments in adaptive function which is portrayed by an arrest in development, and supported by a lack of improvement in socialization and communication assessment scores. Children with ADHD without prenatal exposure to alcohol also shown delay in development, but their assessment scores improved with age but not at the level of children without ADHD.

Pagnin et al. (2018) conducted a longitudinal study on prenatal alcohol use as a risk for developing attention deficit hyperactivity disorder (ADHD). Logical regression was used to check the effect of alcohol on different trimesters as well as the effect of binge drinking. The prevalence of alcohol use among women have increased through the years and statistics show that one in ten pregnant women consume alcohol. It is also seen that among those studies, there are cases where alcohol is consumed at a level that may have serious consequences. Most common mental disorders that are seen among children who have been exposed to prenatal alcohol use are externalizing disorders. With regard to the results, it can be seen that the prevalence rates of ADHD in children who were exposed to alcohol were much higher when compared to the general population. Alcohol consumption was seen as a risk when consumed at any trimester even if the consumption was to a low to moderate level. Clinical interviews as well as prospective designs were used that show that alcohol use was a risk factor in the development of externalizing behaviors as well as inattention and hyperactivity within a child. It was also found that the risk of ADHD increased close to five times when the mother engaged in binge drinking where four to five drinks were consumed at one single occasion. Other factors that increased the risk of developing the disorder included genetic factors and the mental health of the mother. Boys were more likely to develop ADHD and suffer from foetal alcohol syndrome disorders.

Environmental Toxins

Polychlorinated Biphenyl (PCB) are toxins that can pass directly into the placenta of the fetus and tends to exert neurotoxic effects on the developing brain by causing alterations in thyroid functioning, neurotransmitter levels especially metabolism of dopamine (Mill and Petronis, 2008). A study that focused on the relationship between prenatal exposure to polycyclic aromatic hydrocarbons (PAH), a carcinogenic and neurotoxic combustion by-product and ADHD, revealed that high levels of PAH with any material hardship (any unmet basic needs) significantly increased the odds of exhibiting ADHD symptoms in children (Perera et al.,2017). Thus, being from a socioeconomically disadvantage family elevates the risk of developing ADHD both directly and indirectly.Skogheima et al. (2020) in their longitudinal studyassessed the of organic pollutant perfluoroalkyl substances' associationwith ADHD among preschool children belonging to Norwegian mothers. He found that prenatal exposure to perfluoroalkyl substances did not have any association with symptoms of ADHD or cognitive symptoms.In a large Cohort study done by Bashash (2018) in Mexican countryamong 6-12 years of children found a strong association between higher prenatal fluoride exposure and more behavioral symptoms of inattention but then not hyperactivity or impulse control. This strengthens the evidence of neurotoxicity of early life exposure to fluoride and related ADHD.ADHD is a brain-based disorder that can be mediated through environmental factors but not directly caused by such factors (Pearson and Crowley 2012.

Maternal Stress

Exposure to severe stress during pregnancy time increases the incidence of ADHD and other comorbid disorders especially bipolar disorder; psychological stress impacts the hypothalamic-pituitary-adrenal (HPA) axis, secretion of glucocorticoid hormones and the protective capacity of the placenta. Moreover, stress experienced tends to alter the gene expression by influencing fetal microRNA regulation (Tole et al., 2019; Linnet et al., 2003; Motlagh et al., 2010). Reduced amount of catecholamine in the cortical and subcortical regions of brain have been offered as link to ADHD symptoms (Grizenko et al., 2008). Motlagh et al. (2010) in their sample found that approximately 27% of children with ADHD had mothers who had experienced severe psychosocial stress.

Stress during the late first and second trimester has been implicated in the development of psychiatric disorder, including ADHD since prenatal time is a crucial period for brain development (Tole et al., 2019). Linnet et al. (2003), in their review of studies found stress to be exerting a small but significant association with regards to attentional difficulties and hyperactivities; the authors had reviewed a prospective study with a large cohort sample which revealed the time of experiencing maternal stress has a direct impact on behavioral dysfunction thereby confirming with other researches (Linnet et al., 2003). An explanation given by Grizenko et al (2008) for the above findings is that vulnerable fetuses that undergoes stress during the first trimester is likely to get aborted with only resilient ones surviving past it.

Furthermore, Grizenko et al. (2008) revealed that prenatal stress has a direct impact on the severity of the ADHD symptomatology with children scoring higher on Child Behavioral Checklist (CBCL) when mothers experienced moderate to severe stress as compared to mothers with low stress or no stressors. However, fascinatingly, literature has shown that the impact of prenatal stress can be cushioned if they handled with care postnatally by mothers or even primary caregivers; thus if help is lend to mother during pregnancy or early postnatal period on how to deal effectively with stress, it can have positive impact on further development (Grizenko et al., 2008).

Maternal Characteristics During Pregnancy

Literature has suggested various maternal factors seen during pregnancy that correlates with ADHD symptomatology. Young maternal age was one of the aspects that had been studied with regards to

ADHD characteristics; studies have shown that mothers who are younger than 25 at the time of child's birth and mothers not in their first marriage tend to have children referred for ADHD diagnosis (Zappitelli, Pinto and Grizenko, 2001). In addition, Sagiv et al. (2013) found a protective association for older maternal age at birth and ADHD; an explanation given for this finding is that young mothers tend to be impulsive and more stressed that can possible transfer to the child (Sagiv et al., 2013; Pohlabeln et al., 2017). Furthermore, young mothers are more at social and economic disadvantage (due to pregnancy interrupting education) which are also independently associated with poor outcomes for the children including ADHD and comorbid antisocial behavior (Pohlabeln et al., 2017: Russell et al., 2015)

Other factors that have been linked with subsequent ADHD diagnosis are poor maternal pregnancy health, eclampsia, lower parental education and maternal mental health (Zappitelli, Pinto and Grizenko, 2001; Sagiv et al., 2013). With regards to parental education, Sagiv et al.(2013) found that paternal education was associated with behavioral rating scale measures while maternal education and household income were associated with ADHD diagnosis. Gestational hypertension is another aspect that has been studied with respect to ADHD, with studies showing that mothers who were diagnosed with gestational hypertension increasing the risk for hyperkinetic disorder two-folds; moreover, medication used in the treatment may influence the functional development in children (Pohlabeln et al., 2017).

Perinatal Stressors

The role of complications arising during perinatal period in the development of ADHD has been quite controversial since it has not been established whether it is associated with a specific diagnoses or it is considered as a general risk for psychiatric disorders; nevertheless, together with other genetic, pre and postnatal factors, certain perinatal factors has been correlated with the etiology of ADHD (Tole et al., 2019).ADHD was associated with the first born status (Bhatia, Choudry and Sidhana 1998).

Hypoxia

As mentioned before, since dysfunction in dopamine transmission in prefrontal cortex and striatum has been associated with ADHD, it has been suggested that perinatal trauma which results in hypoxia can cause brain ischemia and abnormalities in dopaminergic system. Confirming to the hypothesis, ADHD has been correlated with infants who had received CardiffBag Resuscitation with low Apgar score 5 and below; children who experienced hypoxia at neonatal period had shown cerebral hypoperfusion of the frontal lobe thereby suggesting a link between ADHD and early hypoxic-ischemic damage (Zappitelli, Pinto and Grizenko, 2001; Tole et al., 2019). This hypothesis came in place from animal studies which demonstrated that when rats were exposed to intra uterine anoxia resulting from caesarean section, they exhibited hyperactivity and mesolimbic mesocoritical dopamine activation impairments in left prefrontal cortex (Zappitelli, Pinto and Grizenko, 2001; Ketzer et al., 2012). In humans, perinatal asphyxia can cause neurological and intellectual dysfunction along with psychiatric conditions. Furthermore, having cranial ultrasound abnormalities near birth tends to independently increases the risk of being diagnosed with ADHD in the future even when neonatal complications, prenatal factors and socioeconomic status were controlled (Zappitelli, Pinto and Grizenko, 2001). Ketzer et al., (2012) in their study of 248 children and adolescents with ADHD inattentive type, confirmed that disruptive behaviors were significantly associated with complications to maternal physical problems that arises during pregnancy and delivery specifically anoxia and hypoxia.

Fetal distress during birth due to obstetrical abnormalities such as prolapsed umbilical cord, multiple pregnancies or abnormal fetal position, prolonged labor and neonatal factors such as prematurity, respiratory distress and cardiopulmonary abnormalities have been reported more in mothers of children who have been diagnosed with hyperactivity when compared to healthy normal. Freitag et al., (2011) was able to demonstrate the association of bleeding during pregnancy has towards the risk of inattentive symptoms in their sample.

Low Birth Weight (LBW) and Pre-term Baby

Similar to the effect of maternal consumption of alcohol during pregnancy, the role of low birth weight in its contribution towards ADHD symptoms has been contradictory. Though a majority of studies have reported that low birth weight (as more of an indicator of prematurity and intrauterine issues) being associated with intellectual and learning disabilities and not ADHD, few studies have demonstrated that higher rates of ADHD being reported in children with LBW and extreme LBW (ELBW) than normal birth weight children, especially in urban population (Zappitelli, Pinto and Grizenko, 2001).

Similarly, Groen-Blakhuis et al. (2011) were able to show an inverse relationship between birth weight and attentional problems. In their study, they found that when children weighed between 1.5 to 2 kg, they score higher on scales that measured attentional problem and interestingly, this trend was seen in both term-born and preterm babies. The authors indicated that this finding suggested birth weight as an independent risk factor. Animal studies have shown that growth restriction in utero (IUGC) which shows as LBW has an impact on brain volume; in humans, IUGC was connected with reduction in volume in inferior dorsal prefrontal cortex and less activation of bilateral temporal lobe during neuropsychological test (Groen-Blakhuis et al., 2011). On the other hand, Motlagh et al., (2010) could not replicate the influence of low birth weight in ADHD children. van Mil et al., (2015) studied the connection of birth weight on ADHD, but like other studies, they studied birth weight as a continuum; their findings showed that relationship between these two variables were in a curvilinear manner where higher birth weight was associated with less attentional problems but as the weight approached 3.6 kg or more, it did not reduce the risk of attentional problems.

Tole et al., (2019) in their study mentioned that there was an increased rate of reporting of pre-term birth in patients of ADHD. Other studies too have found the susceptibility that preemies have in increasing the risk for ADHD; an interesting finding that literature has shown is that gestational hypertension is a risk factor for preterm infants which can mean that the link between preterm birth and ADHD risk is partly mediated by gestational hypertension

Postnatal Stressors

Venkatesh et al., (2012) studied the cognitive and behavioral markers of ADHD symptoms in Indian children. They found that cognitive and behavioral markers of ADHD symptoms are present in children prior to entry into formal schooling, but current behavioral screeners are not developmentally sensitive to these differences in infancy and toddlerhood. Speech delay was reported in around 55% of children with ADHD. Risk factors for Attention Deficit Hyperactivity Disorder among Indian children are identified as poor maternal health, maternal stress and speech delay (Simon 2016). ADHD is commonly prevalent in preschool children and toddlers. ADHD was most widely present in children who are from nuclear families, parents' anxiety and tension lead to behavioral problems in children. Behavioral problems exhibited due to emotional issues due to frustration and failures. Speech and language delay may be the pointer to ADHD. Single parenting, substance use of parents, mental illness are not the major causative factors in children with ADHD compared to western studies. Socioeconomic status, prematurity and perinatal adversity does not have significant association with ADHD.

Quality of Parent-child Relationship

Early relationship between ADHD individuals and their parents have been stated as being more complicated when compared to controls, in terms less warmth and affection, and more quarrelling; in addition, postnatal bonding were reported as less in ADHD children as they were found to be more crybabies (Tole et al., 2019). Likewise, Freitag et al., (2011), confirmed the impact of familial risk factors on ADHD; apart from the above-mentioned factors, variables such as child maltreatment, scapegoating, parental separation or divorce, neglect and difficult communication patterns have been observed in families with ADHD individuals. Stress experienced in the last trimester as well in the early postnatal period has shown to hamper mother-child relationship and literature has supported the predisposition a child has for developmental and behavioral problems in such cases (Grizenko et al., 2008).

Socioeconomic Factors and Adverse Childhood Experiences

Russell et al. (2015) revealed financial difficulty, an indicator of socioeconomic status, associated with increased risk of ADHD diagnosis; however, this association was mediated by family factors such as parental involvement. The odds of receiving ADHD diagnosis was higher in children who had parents who were less involved along with at least one family adversity. Findings from their study suggests that a number of socioeconomic risk factors act in a cumulative manner in mediating the pathway towards ADHD development (18). Brown et al. (2014) revealed that presence of one or more adverse and traumatic childhood experiences in individuals diagnosed with ADHD. Parental psychopathology and socioeconomic hardship had been connected with parent reported ADHD symptoms and their findings confirm with Russell et al. (2015) conclusions about the cumulative effect of risk factors in the pathogenesis of ADHD.

Respiratory Disorders and Infections

Researches have shown there is an elevation in risk of developing ADHD in children with neonatal respiratory disorders and infections acquired during the first 4 weeks after birth; abnormalities in white matter development was given as a possible explanation given to this observation (Pohlabeln et al., 2017). Interestingly, it exposes that though postnatal infections as a risk factor for altered brain development, it can be prevented (Pohlabeln et al., 2017).

Thus, research has shown that pre-, peri- and postnatal stressors interacts with genetic factors in the pathogenesis of ADHD regardless of comorbid disorders; but it still remains unclear which of those stressors plays a major role in the abnormal development of dopaminergic systems. There are certain limitations to these above-mentioned studies which explains the difficulty in determining the causal relationship such as most being retrospective studies where biases are highly likely in recalling critical information. When it comes to matters such as prenatal smoking and alcohol consumption, mothers tend to purposely withhold information due to the stigma that are associated with it. Moreover, confounding variables, especially family risk for ADHD, are difficult to be controlled for in these studies making it difficult to find the causal relationship between environmental risk factors and ADHD pathophysiology. Regardless, research on epigenetic factors, which are heritable but reversible changes to genomic functions independent of DNA sequence, have demonstrated that phenotypic expression of ADHD tends to be mediated by environmental toxins (tobacco, alcohol, PCBS) thereby offering possibilities for preventive and therapeutic interventions in the future (Mills and Petronis, 2008).

REFERENCES

Bhatia, M. S., Choudry, S., & Sidhana, A. (1998). Attention Deficit hyperactive disorder among Psychiatric patients. *Indian Pediatrics*, *36*, 583–587. PMID:10736588

Brown, N. M., Brown, S. N., Briggs, R. D., Germán, M., Belamarich, P. F., & Oyeku, S. O. (2017). Associations between adverse childhood experiences and ADHD diagnosis and severity. *Academic Pediatrics*, *17*(4), 349–355. doi:10.1016/j.acap.2016.08.013 PMID:28477799

Burden, M. J., Jacobson, J. L., Westerlund, A., Lundahl, L. H., Morrison, A., Dodge, N. C., & Jacobson, S. W. (2010). An Event-Related Potential Study of Response Inhibition in ADHD With and Without Prenatal Alcohol Exposure. *Alcoholism, Clinical and Experimental Research*, *34*(4), 617–627. doi:10.1111/j.1530-0277.2009.01130.x PMID:20102568

Crocker, N., Vaurio, L., Riley, E. P., & Mattson, S. N. (2009). Comparison of Adaptive Behavior in Children With Heavy Prenatal Alcohol Exposure or Attention-Deficit/Hyperactivity Disorder. *Alcoholism, Clinical and Experimental Research*, *33*(11), 2015–2023. doi:10.1111/j.1530-0277.2009.01040.x PMID:19719794

Eilertsen, E. M., Gjerde, L. C., Reichborn-Kjennerud, T., Ørstavik, R. E., Knudsen, G. P., Knudsen, C., ... Ystrom, E. (2017). Maternal alcohol use during pregnancy and offspring attention-deficit hyperactivity disorder (ADHD): A prospective sibling control study. *International Journal of Epidemiology*, *46*(5), 1633–1640. doi:10.1093/ije/dyx067 PMID:28449133

Freitag, C. M., Hänig, S., Schneider, A., Seitz, C., Palmason, H., Retz, W., & Meyer, J. (2011). Biological and psychosocial environmental risk factors influence symptom severity and psychiatric comorbidity in children with ADHD. *Journal ofNeural Transmission (Vienna, Austria)*, *119*(1), 81–94. doi:10.100700702-011-0659-9 PMID:21626412

Grizenko, N., Shayan, Y. R., & Polotskaia, A. (2008). Relation of maternal stress during pregnancy to symptom severity and response to treatment in children with ADHD. *Journal of Psychiatry & Neuroscience*, *33*, 10–16. PMID:18197267

Groen-Blokhuis, M. M., Middeldorp, C. M., Van Beijsterveldt, C. E., & Boomsma, D. I. (2011). Evidence for a causal association of low birth weight and attention problems. *Journal oftheAmericanAcademy of Child &. Adolescent Psychiatry*, *50*(12), 1247–1254. doi:10.1016/j.jaac.2011.09.007

Huang, L., Wang, Y., Zhang, L., Zheng, Z., Zhu, T., Qu, Y., & Mu, D. (2017). Maternal Smoking and Attention-Deficit/Hyperactivity Disorder in Offspring: A Meta-analysis. *Pediatrics*, *141*(1). doi:10.1542/peds

Infante, M. A., Moore, E. M., Nguyen, T. T., Fourligas, N., Mattson, S. N., & Riley, E. P. (2015). Objective assessment of ADHD core symptoms in children with heavy prenatal alcohol exposure. *Physiology & Behavior, 148*, 45–50. doi:10.1016/j.physbeh.2014.10.014 PMID:25447751

Ketzer, C. R., Gallois, C., Martinez, A. L., Rohde, L. A., & Schmitz, M. (2012). Is there an association between perinatal complications and attention-deficit/hyperactivity disorder-inattentive type in children and adolescents? *Revista Brasileira de Psiquiatria (Sao Paulo, Brazil), 34*(3), 321–328. doi:10.1016/j.rbp.2012.01.001 PMID:23429778

Knopik, V. S., Sparrow, E. P., Madden, P. A., Bucholz, K. K., Hudziak, J. J., Reich, W., Slutske, W. S., Grant, J. D., McLAUGHLIN, T. L., Todorov, A., Todd, R. D., & Heath, A. C. (2005). Contributions of parental alcoholism, prenatal substance exposure, and genetic transmission to child ADHD risk: A female twin study. *Psychological Medicine, 35*(5), 625–635. doi:10.1017/S0033291704004155 PMID:15918339

Linnet, K. M., Dalsgaard, S., Obel, C., Wisborg, K., Henriksen, T. B., Rodriguez, A., Kotimaa, A., Moilanen, I., Thomsen, P. H., Olsen, J., & Jarvelin, M. (2003). Maternal lifestyle factors in pregnancy risk of attention deficit hyperactivity disorder and associated behaviors: Review of the current evidence. *The American Journal of Psychiatry, 160*(6), 1028–1040. doi:10.1176/appi.ajp.160.6.1028 PMID:12777257

Mill, J., & Petronis, A. (2008). Pre- and Peri-natal environmental risks for attention-deficit hyperactivity disorder (ADHD): The potential role of epigenetic processes in mediating susceptibility. *Journal of Child Psychology and Psychiatry, and Allied Disciplines, 49*(10), 1020–1030. doi:10.1111/j.1469-7610.2008.01909.x PMID:18492038

Motlagh, M. G., Katsovich, L., Thompson, N., Lin, H., Kim, Y., Scahill, L., Lombroso, P. J., King, R. A., Peterson, B. S., & Leckman, J. F. (2010). Severe psychosocial stress and heavy cigarette smoking during pregnancy: An examination of the pre- and perinatal risk factors associated with ADHD and Tourette syndrome. *European Child & Adolescent Psychiatry, 19*(10), 755–764. doi:10.100700787-010-0115-7 PMID:20532931

Pagnin, D., Grecco, M. L., & Furtado, E. F. (2018). Prenatal alcohol use as a risk for attention-deficit/hyperactivity disorder. *European Archives of Psychiatry and Clinical Neuroscience*. Advance online publication. doi:10.100700406-018-0946-7 PMID:30353263

Pearson, G. S., & Crowley, A. A. (2013). Attention deficit hyperactivity disorder (ADHD). *Child and Adolescent Behavioral Health*, 139-152. doi:10.1002/9781118704660.ch7

Perera, F. P., Wheelock, K., Wang, Y., Tang, D., Margolis, A. E., Badia, G., Cowell, W., Miller, R. L., Rauh, V., Wang, S., & Herbstman, J. B. (2018). Combined effects of prenatal exposure to polycyclic aromatic hydrocarbons and material hardship on child ADHD behavior problems. *Environmental Research, 160*, 506–513. doi:10.1016/j.envres.2017.09.002 PMID:28987706

Pohlabeln, H., Rach, S., De Henauw, S., Eiben, G., Gwozdz, W., & Pigeot, I. (2017). Further evidence for the role of pregnancy-induced hypertension and other early life influences in the development of ADHD: Results from the IDEFICS study. *European Child & Adolescent Psychiatry, 26*(8), 957–967. doi:10.100700787-017-0966-2 PMID:28258320

Russell, A. E., Ford, T., & Russell, G. (2015). Socioeconomic associations with ADHD: Findings from a mediation analysis. *PLoS One*, *10*(6), e0128248. doi:10.1371/journal.pone.0128248 PMID:26030626

Sagiv, S. K., Epstein, J. N., Bellinger, D. C., & Korrick, S. A. (2012). Pre- and postnatal risk factors for ADHD in a nonclinical pediatric population. *Journal of Attention Disorders*, *17*(1), 47–57. doi:10.1177/1087054711427563 PMID:22298092

Sciberras, E., Mulraney, M., Silva, D., & Coghill, D. (2017). Prenatal risk factors and the etiology of ADHD—Review of existing evidence. *Current Psychiatry Reports*, *19*(1), 1. Advance online publication. doi:10.100711920-017-0753-2 PMID:28091799

Simon, A. (2016). Prenatal, Perinatal and Postnatal Risk Facotrs for Attention Deficit Hyperactivity Disorder in India- A Retrospective Analysis. *Indian Journal of Applied Research*, *6*(4).

Skogheima, T. S., Villangera, G. D., Vegard, K., Weydea, S. M., Engelb, P. S., Øiec, M. G., ... Aasea, H. (2020). Prenatal exposure to perfluoroalkyl substances and associations with symptoms of attention-deficit/hyperactivity disorder and cognitive functions in preschool children. *International Journal of Hygiene and Environmental Health*, 223. PMID:31653559

Tole, F., Kopf, J., Schröter, K., Palladino, V. S., Jacob, C. P., Reif, A., & Kittel-Schneider, S. (2019). The role of pre-, peri-, and postnatal risk factors in bipolar disorder and adult ADHD. *Journal of Neural Transmission (Vienna, Austria)*, *126*(9), 1117–1126. doi:10.100700702-019-01983-4 PMID:30758784

Van Mil, N. H., Steegers-Theunissen, R. P., Motazedi, E., Jansen, P. W., Jaddoe, V. W., Steegers, E. A., Verhulst, F. C., & Tiemeier, H. (2015). Low and high birth weight and the risk of child attention problems. *The Journal of Pediatrics*, *166*(4), 862–869.e3. doi:10.1016/j.jpeds.2014.12.075 PMID:25681197

Venkatesh, C., Andal, A., Ravikumar, T., & Virudhagirinathan, B. (2012). Attention-deficit/Hyperactivity disorder in children: Clinical profile and Co-morbidity. *Indian Journal of Psychological Medicine*, *34*(1), 34. doi:10.4103/0253-7176.96155 PMID:22661805

Wang, M., Zhao, Q., Kang, H., & Zhu, S. (2019). Attention deficit hyperactivity disorder (ADHD) in children with epilepsy. *Irish Journal of Medical Science*. Advance online publication. doi:10.100711845-019-02042-3 PMID:31187336

Ware, A. L., Glass, L., Crocker, N., Deweese, B. N., Coles, C. D., Kable, J. A., May, P. A., Kalberg, W. O., Sowell, E. R., Jones, K. L., Riley, E. P., & Mattson, S. N. (2014). Effects of Prenatal Alcohol Exposure and Attention-Deficit/Hyperactivity Disorder on Adaptive Functioning. *Alcoholism, Clinical and Experimental Research*, *38*(5), 1439–1447. doi:10.1111/acer.12376 PMID:24655090

Zappitelli, M., Pinto, T., & Grizenko, N. (2001). Pre-, peri-, and postnatal trauma in subjects with attention-deficit hyperactivity disorder. *Canadian Journal of Psychiatry*, *46*(6), 542–548. doi:10.1177/070674370104600609 PMID:11526811

Chapter 4
ADHD in Children:
Assessment and Management

Sandamita Choudhury
151 Base Hospital, Guwahati, India

ABSTRACT

Attention deficit/hyperactivity disorder (ADHD) is among the most common neurobehavioral disorders presenting for treatment in children and adolescents. ADHD is often chronic with prominent symptoms and impairment spanning into adulthood. During the past decade, epidemiological studies have documented high rates of comorbid conditions among individuals with ADHD. In the absence of adequate identification of its comorbidities and secondary symptoms, it has an impact on the behavioural and academic outcomes in the long run. Research highlights the psycho educational effectiveness that focused on the relative/caregivers of ADHD as better understanding and knowledge of the disorder improves treatment adherence, quality of life, and decreased symptoms of ADHD. Therefore, the chapter intends to throw light on the classification of ADHD, its assessment, and psychological management for better outcomes in children.

DEFINING ADHD

Attention-deficit/hyperactivity disorder (ADHD) is a childhood- onset neuropsychiatric disorder characterized by a combination of age-inappropriate levels of inattention, impulsive behaviour and hyperactivity (Thapar & Cooper, 2016). The symptoms of ADHD must cause significant impairments in more than one setting, e.g., at school or work, or with family and peers (APA, 2013).

According to The Diagnostic and Statistical Manual of mental disorders (DSM V), Attention deficit/ hyperactivity disorder (ADHD) is characterized by three subtypes namely: the predominantly inattentive type (IA), the predominantly hyperactive/impulsive type (HI) and the combined type (C).

DOI: 10.4018/978-1-7998-5495-1.ch004

Children of the IA/HI type should show six (or more) out of the nine relevant symptoms specified persistently for at least 6 months to a degree that is inconsistent with developmental level and that negatively impacts directly on social and academic/occupational activities:

The Predominantly Inattentive Type (ADHD-IA)

- Makes careless mistakes/lacks attention to detail
- Difficulty sustaining attention
- Does not seem to listen when spoken to directly
- Fails to follow through on tasks and instructions
- Exhibits poor organization
- Avoids/dislikes tasks requiring sustained mental effort
- Loses things necessary for tasks/activities
- Easily distracted (including unrelated thoughts)
- Is forgetful in daily activities

The Predominantly Hyperactive/Impulsive Type (ADHD-HI)

- Fidgets with or taps hands or feet, squirms in seat
- Leaves seat in situations when remaining seated is expected
- Experiences feelings of restlessness
- Has difficulty engaging in quiet, leisurely activities
- Is "on-the-go" or acts as if "driven by a motor"
- Talks excessively
- Blurts out answers
- Has difficulty waiting their turn
- Interrupts or intrudes on others

The Combined Type (AHD-C)

If combined presentation of symptoms of both Inattention and hyperactivity are present persistently for at least 6 months.

It also specifies the severity level by classifying into the following subtypes:

- **Mild:** Few, if any, symptoms in excess of those required to make the diagnosis are present, and symptoms result in only minor functional impairments.
- **Moderate:** Symptoms or functional impairment between "mild" and "severe" are present.
- **Severe:** Many symptoms in excess of those required to make the diagnosis, or several symptoms that are particularly severe, are present, or the symptoms result in marked impairment in social or occupational functioning. (APA, 2013)

COMORBID CONDITIONS ASSOCIATED WITH ADHD

Early comorbidities concurrent with ADHD may include tic disorder, anxiety disorder, autism spectrum disorder, communication and specific learning or motor disorders and intellectual disability. Long-term follow-up studies from childhood to adulthood found that children with ADHD, were more impaired in psychosocial, educational, motor incoordination, dysgraphia and had higher risks for substance abuse, delinquent behaviour, antisocial disorders, major depression and anxiety disorders as adults (Biederman, Petty &Monuteaux, 2010) (Hodgkins, 2012; Molina, 2007). Study conducted by Kadesjo&Gillberg (2001)

Figure 1. Functional problems associated with attention-deficit/hyperactivity disorder using the International Classification of Functioning, Disability, and Health conceptual model
(Reprinted from Leo, I. M., & Feldman, H. M.(2007). Academic and educational outcomes of children with ADHD (Special issue). Journal of Paediatric Psychology, 32, 643-654)

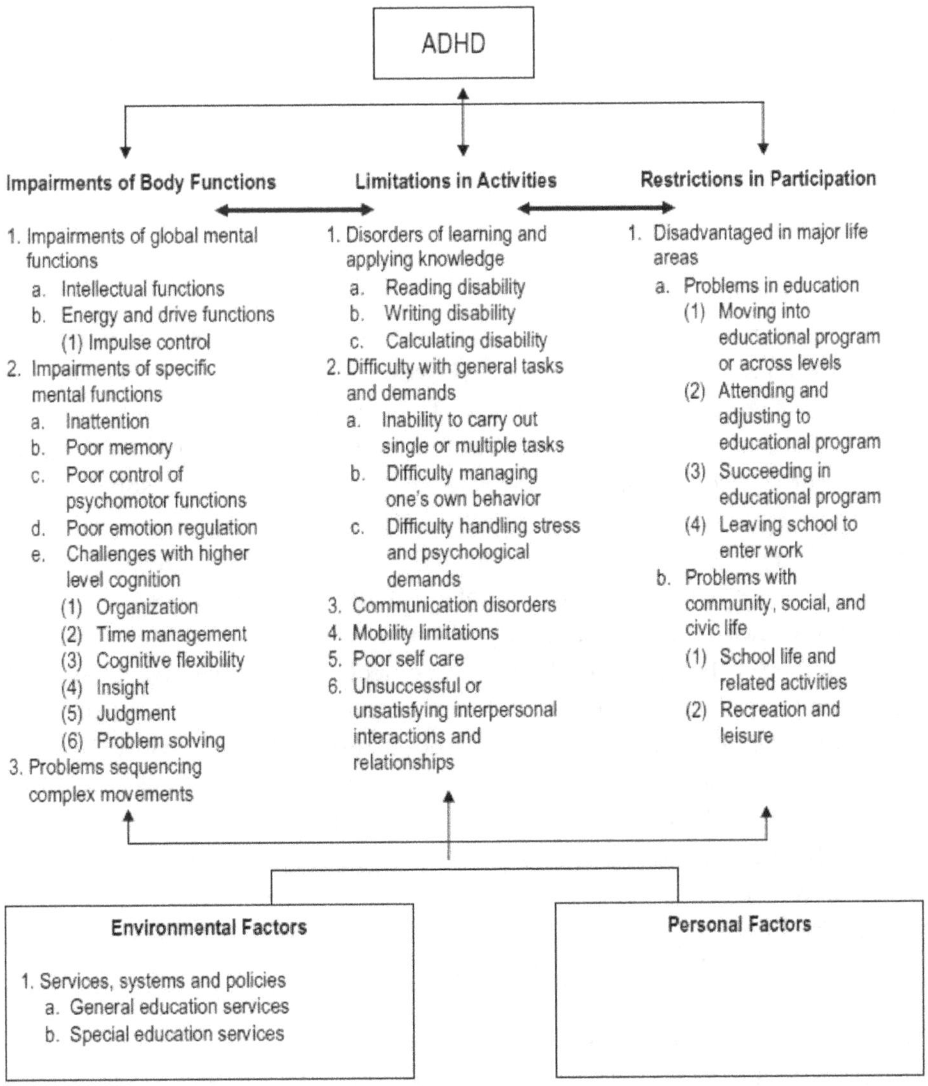

suggested that around 60% of children with ADHD, compared to up to 35% normal children may have poor motor coordination or developmental coordination disorder. There is also indication of manifesting deficits in handwriting and in the perceptual- motor components related to the skills (Hickey &Fricker, 1999).Therefore,it is essential to screen for the secondary symptoms and co-occurring or comorbid problems during the initial assessment as young people could often benefit from psychosocial interventions and referral to allied health professionals, including psychologists and speech and occupational therapists. Parental management skills and mental health should also be assessed to ensure parents are able to implement any management recommendations for their children (Wither, 2015).

Leo & Feldman (2007) categorised the functional impairment faced by ADHD children in terms of their academics by employing International Classification of Functioning, Disability, and Health

Under ICF framework, health conditions can impact functions at 3 mutually interacting levels of analysis i.e. Body Functions & Structures, Activities of Daily Living and Social Participation.

Leo and Feldman (2007) also reported that children with ADHD-IA are more likely to be rated as below average or failing in school compared with the children with ADHD-C and ADHD-HI subtype (Baumgaertel et al., 1995). ADHD-IA children are described as having a sluggish cognitive tempo, leading to the assumption that there is a higher prevalence of learning disorders in the ADHD-IA than the ADHD-C populations. Barkleyet. al (1990) found more children with ADHD-IA than children with ADHD-C in classrooms.

CLINICAL ASSESSMENT OF ADHD

Most diagnostic guidelines require that ADHD be assessed and diagnosed by relying on information provided via a variety of methods (e.g., clinical interviews, observations and ratings) and collected from multiple sources (e.g., parents and teachers). However, Edwards et.al., (2007) pointed that using of subjective measures always incorporates the risk of informant biases, which was supported by Van &Verhulst (2005) notion that clinicians are often confronted with great inconsistencies between ratings obtained from different sources. In order to investigate the effectiveness of subjective (rating scale/ screening tool) and objective measures (assessment battery/tool), Toplak and colleagues in 2013 argue that one important difference between ratings/subjective measure and objective test is that the former measure typical performance (i.e., how an individual normally performs), whereas tests usually capture optimal performance (i.e., how well an individual performs under relatively optimal conditions) which is free of situational influences. Thus, the combination of objective and subjective measures may provide additional information than objective measures alone as it has been argued that tests and ratings may capture at least partly different constructs and should not be used interchangeably.

The case history and assessment should focus on comprehensive evaluation and identification of the chief complaint, symptoms of ADHD, academic-behavioural issues, and the level of functional impairment (French, 2015). Because ADHD has a strong genetic propensity, it is important to obtain a complete family medical and psychiatric history.Importance should be given on identification of the presence of risk factors or comorbid conditions.

Few Risk factors that could be noted are as follows:

- Family medical history of ADHD or another mental health disorder
- Prenatal and perinatal factors, including premature birth and low birth weight

- Genetic disorders such as fragile X syndrome, tuberous sclerosis
- Sleep disorders including obstructive sleep apnea and inadequate sleep
- Seizure disorders or other neurologic disorders
- Socioeconomic and environmental risk factors include parenting practices, teacher-child interactions, exposure to adverse childhood experiences/stressors, child maltreatment, malnourishment, poverty, parental pathology, exposure to severe, early social deprivation.
- Maternal exposure to harmful toxins, drug use, alcohol use, or smoking during pregnancy (Substance Abuse and Mental Health Services Administration, 2016)

A comprehensive social history, including an understanding of the child's environment and how ADHD is affecting family members, should be obtained. How the child is functioning in the home, school, and community will provide the mental health professional with insight into the severity of ADHD symptoms. A complete physical exam, including a neurologic exam, should be obtained for all children being evaluated for an ADHD diagnosis (Wolraich et al. 2011) (French, 2015).The next step in the assessment is to obtain symptom documentation over time and in more than one major setting (for example, home and preschool/ school) which may be obtained through rating scales handed out to teachers/caregivers.

In addition, viewing the child's report cards and samples of the child's schoolwork; any formal testing performed by school personnel; a description of the child's behavior in the classroom; the child's learning patterns; how the symptoms affect the child's progress at school; ways the teacher has adapted the classroom program to help the child; and whether other conditions contribute to or affect the symptoms are found to be helpful in diagnosis (Wesemann, 2018).

It is essential to screen for the secondary symptoms of attention deficit hyperactivity disorder (ADHD), such as social, learning and behavioural difficulties, which holds to be crucial for the long-term prognosis of young people and can persist even with pharmacological treatment. Further, areas of effectiveness of psychosocial intervention may be sought with exploration into it.

Following are few standardised assessment tools which may be used in combination or as an individual tool/battery collaborating with a comprehensive case history to formulate an appropriate diagnosis:

- **Conners-3 parent/teacher ratings:** The Conners-3 parent/teacher ratings are two questionnaires assessing ADHD symptoms and associated problems like oppositional behavior or learning problems in children and adolescents aged 6–18 years. The long version contains 105/111 items (parent/teacher) rated on a 4-point Likert-scale from 0 (not at all/never) to 3 (very much/very frequently). The Conners 3 incorporates the following ten scales: inattention, hyperactivity/impulsivity, learning problems, executive functions, aggression, peer relations (content scales); DSM IV-inattention, DSM IV-hyperactivity/impulsivity, DSM IV-conduct disorder, DSM IV-oppositional defiant disorder (symptom scales); ADHD index, Global index (Conners CK., 2008). The German version has revealed good to very good internal consistency (Cronbach's α = .74–.96) (Christiansen, Hirsch, Drechsler, Wanderer S, Knospe, Gunther, et al. 2016)
- **Swanson, Nolan and Pelham Questionnaire (SNAP-IV, Swanson et al., 1983):** SNAP-IV is a 26 item rating scale used to obtain ratings from two sources, parents and teachers. It includes 18 ADHD symptoms (9 for inattentive, 9 for hyperactive/impulsive) and 8 opposition/defiance disorder(ODD) symptoms specified in the DSM-IV. Items are rated on a 4-point scale from (0) not at all to (3) very much. Average rating-per-item (ARI) subscale scores for both parent and teacher scales are calculated for the inattention, hyperactivity/impulsivity, and opposition/defi-

Figure 2. Areas to be assessed in Young People with ADHD to identify the comorbidity
(Adapted from Winther, Jo. (2015) Attention deficit hyperactivity disorder psychosocial interventions for young people, Medicine Today, Volume 16)

AREAS FOR ASSESSMENT IN YOUNG PEOPLE WITH ADHD

A .Social skills difficulties

• Is your child able to make friends? • Is your child able to keep friends?

• How many friends does your child have? • Does your child have a best friend?

B. Learning and study skill difficulties

• How is your child going academically (oral and reading comprehension, spelling and maths)?

• What are their communication skills like (expressing their thoughts and knowledge; understanding what others are saying, particularly for school tasks)?

•What are their study habits like (note taking, time management, test taking)? • What support strategies are used and do they work?

C. School behavioural issues

• How many schools have they attended? • What is their attendance rate like? • What is their relationship like with the teachers? • Have they had any involvement with school support services? • Do they understand behavioural instructions and processes?

D. Working memory difficulties

• Is your child able to remember things? • How many instructions at a time are they able to remember?

• Are they able to hold information in their mind and use it immediately (e.g. 5+5=10) or remember key facts over time? • Is 'poor memory' due to poor comprehension?

E. Coexisting conditions

• Does your child worry a lot? • Are there more days than not when they are down or irritable?

• Do you have any behavioural concerns with your child?

• Do they have language and speech difficulties? (e.g. poor story structure, not understanding abstract ideas, difficulties creating a sentence such as mixing up words, forgetting words, unclear words)

• What are their gross and fine motor skills like?

F. Parenting styles

• Are you able to remain calm when dealing with misbehaviour or do you argue with your child?

• Do you have the energy you need to parent your child? • Do you enjoy spending time with your child? • Do you talk to your child about their problems?

G. Parental psychopathology

• Do you ever feel down or irritable for long periods of time? • Do you ever feel low in energy or have lost interest in things? • Do you ever feel nervous or shaky inside or worry about things too much?

• Do you have any physiological symptoms such as headaches; hot or cold spells; poor appetite; constipation or loose bowel motions and/or sleep difficulties?

ance domains, resulting in six SNAP-IV subscale scores that can range from 0 to 3, abbreviated subsequently as P-Inatt, P-Hyp/Imp, P-Odd, T-Inatt, T-Hyp/Imp and T-Odd.

- **Vanderbilt Assessment Scale (Wolraich, 2003):** The Vanderbilt ADHD Diagnostic Rating Scale (VADRS) is a psychological assessment tool for parents of children aged 6 to 12 designed to measure the severity of attention deficit hyperactivity disorder (ADHD) symptoms. Developed by Mark Wolraich at the Oklahoma Health Sciences Center, this rating scale also includes items related to other disorders which are frequently comorbid with ADHD such as Oppositional Defiant Disorder, Conduct Disorder, Anxiety, and Depression, disorders. There are two versions available: a parent form that contains 55 questions, and a teacher form that contains 43 questions.
- **AD/HD Rating Scale-IV:** The AD/HD Rating Scale-IV (DuPaul, Power et al., 1998) is an 18-item parent and teacher rating scale that focuses exclusively on AD/HD. It presents the 9 inattention and 9 hyperactive-impulsive symptoms from DSM-IV in an alternating fashion: inattention in odd-numbered positions and hyperactive-impulsive in even-numbered positions.The AD/HD Rating Scale-IV is a psychometrically sound instrument showing substantial reliability and validity across many peer reviewed studies (e.g., DuPaul, Power, McGoey, Ikeda, &Anastopoulos, 1998). Parent and teacher ratings are internally consistent, stable over a 4-week period, and significantly correlated with observations of classroom behaviour, as well as with corresponding subscales on the Conners' Parent and Teacher Rating Scales (DuPaul et al., 1997).
- **Academic Performance Rating Scale:** The APRS is a 19-item scale that was developed to reflect teachers' perceptions of children's academic performance and abilities in classroom settings. Teachers answered each item using a 1 (never or poor) to 5 (very often or excellent) Likert scale format. Seven APRS items (i.e., nos. 12, 13, 15- 19) were reverse- keyed in scoring so that a higher total score corresponded with a positive academic status. (DuPaul, 1991)
- **The Color Cancelation Test (Kapur, 1974)**: It is a measure of visual scanning and sustained attention. This test has been used with normal children and those with attention deficit hyperactivity disorder. It is sensitive to behavioural deficits in sustained attention (Kapur, 1974). This test consists of 150 circles in red, blue, yellow, black, and gray. The participants were required to cancel only the yellow and red circles as fast as possible. The time taken to complete the test comprised the score. Variations of this test include picture cancellation, letter cancellation, number cancellation and symbol cancellation
- **The Color Trails Test (D'Elia et al., 1996): It** is a measure of focused attention. Children aged 5–16 years show a steady age-dependant progression on this test. It is sensitive to the effects of frontal damage (Williams et al., 1995). In the Color Trails Test 1, the participant was asked to serially connect the numbers 1–25 printed in two colors without regard to the color. In the Color Trails Test 2, the participants were required to connect the numbers serially from 1 to 25, alternating between pink and yellow circles and disregarding the numbers in circles of the alternate color. The time taken to complete each part comprised the score.
- **Bender Visuo motor gestalt test (BGT) (Koppitz, 1975):** It is a test of visuo motor integration, developed by Bender (1938) consisting of 9 cards with abstract designs, subject is required to copy the design one at a time, on a blank paper. Designs are scored for distortion of shape, rotation, perseveration, overlapping. A high score indicates imperfections while a low BGT score reflects good performance. Hyperkinetic boys made more errors of distortion, rotation, integration and perseveration, scoring a lower age equivalent than the normal boys of the same age.

- **Seguin Form board (Cattell, 1953):** This consists of a large wooden board from which ten geometrical shapes are cut. The subject is instructed to replace the blocks in their right places as fast as they can. Three trails are given and the time taken is noted. The visuomotor coordination of the subject is assessed on this test. Timings on the three trials also show us whether the child is able to learn from experience and improve his performance through trial and error. Hyperkinetic children took longer time than the normal boys, giving the former group a lower mental age. (Oommen, 1993)
- **Porteus Maze test (Porteus, 1965):** It consists of 11 mazes arranged in order of increasing difficulty for children aged 3-14 years. The child is asked to draw a line between the lines carefully without touching the sides. The score reveals haphazard, impulsive or over confident habits/actions often seen in hyperkinetic children
- **Quantified Behavior Test for children aged 6–12 (QbTest)** The QbTest is a computerized neuropsychological tests consisting that assess the three core symptoms of ADHD using a continuous performance test (CPT) and a parallel registration of the participants' movements with an infrared camera following a reflective marker attached to a headband. Stimuli are in the form of either a target (a gray circle) ornon-target (graycircle with a cross) presented in random order of appearance. The target/non-target ratio is 50/50. The task is to press a button as quickly as possible when the target appears.

Since during performance, the participant's head movements are recorded with an infrared camera, total of nine parameters are obtained which corresponds to the three core ADHD symptoms. Parameters includes: time active, Distance, area, micro events and motion simplicity. Inattention is measured by the following parameters: reaction time (RT), RT variability and omission errors (Ulberstad, 2012). Reh et al explained 76% of the total variance and reliability estimates ranging from $\alpha = .60$ (impulsivity) to $\alpha = .95$ (hyperactivity) for these factors.

Along with assessment of ADHD, it is essential to evaluate the others areas of functioning such as intelligence, academic achievement levels, speech and language problems, learning disorders, working memory, and other types of executive and neuropsychological functioning since comorbid conditions may affect the overall functioning of the individual. Thus, it has been supported by studies of Emser et al, 2018 that prediction using the objective measures did not produce as accurate a classifier as the combined objective and subjective measures in children. However, predicting an ADHD diagnosis using only the objective measures was still significant with 78% accuracy.

Management of ADHD

Regardless of the developmental stage, treatment for people with this disorder involves a combination of medication (to minimize the symptoms of inattention, hyperactivity and impulsivity) and the adoption of psychological/psychosocial interventions including behaviour modification, environmental accommodations, parental counselling and educational intervention aimed to develop strategies to deal with residual symptoms (Mongolia &Hechtman, 2016; Sprich, Safren, Finkelstein, Remmert, &Hammerness, 2016). Basic focus should be on planning of individualised programmes specific to each child strengths and needs. However, due to the incredible fluctuating performance children with ADD show, therefore behaviour and work expectations should be within the child's capabilities with parents, teacher and therapist working together (Hirisave, OOmmen, Kapur, 2002). While non-adherence to treatment may range from 13.2% to 64.0% (McCarthy, 2014), factors related to non-adherence may range from lack of knowledge of ADHD, medication characteristics, and treatment goals (Charach& Fernandez, 2013). Therefore, providing information about these aspects to patients and their families is important for the mental health professional to seek and maintain adequate treatment.

- **Psychoeducation:** Psychoeducation is the process which aims to broaden the knowledge of the patient/ family member about the diagnosis, etiology, functioning, treatment and prognosis, as well as to clarify the doubts and corrections of distorted information (Menezes& Souza, 2012; Swadi, Bobier, Price, & Craig, 2010). Interaction should focus on the use of appropriate language in a Didactic manner with the target population ranging from caregivers, parents, teachers, family members, relatives to empower them in dealing with the issues related to the client. Psychoeducational intervention assesses perceptions of the disorder and treatment (Bussing et al., 2012; Young, 1999), and then provides information about ADHD and coping strategies in a systematic and didactic way. The transmission of such knowledge can be done in different forms, individually or in groups, and include lectures, conversation wheels, manuals, videos or bibliotherapy (self-help manuals) (Bai, Wang, Yang, &Niu, 2015). Psychoeducation presents various beneðts, such as increased knowledge about the disorder, motivation for change, participation in treatment, satisfaction with psychological treatment, greater adherence to it, and relapse reduction (Burlingame, Ridge, Matasuno, Hwang, &Ernshaw, 2006; Knapp, 2004; Nussey, Pistrang, & Murphy, 2013; Ferrin, et al., 2014; Hogue et al., 2014; Montoya et al., 2011). The parents have observed to acknowledge and value the efforts of the service providers to psychoeducate them. However, there have been depicted a varied preference of the parents concerning the amount of information received and the way information was made available with some parents preferring detailed information in the form of a pamphlet and/or the internet, while others preferred brief information transmitted orally by health professionals (Coletti et al., 2012).
- **Psychosocial Intervention:** For preschool-aged children (ages 4 to 5 years), parent- or teacher-administered behavioural intervention should be the ðrst line of treatment; medication may be considered if ðrst-line treatments are not available or insufðcient. For children ages 6 to 11 years, the combination of medication and behavioural interventions have proved to be the best outcome considering the level of ADHD. For adolescents (ages 12 to 18 years), an FDA-approved medication should be prescribed, preferably along with behaviour therapy. (Wolraich M, Brown L, Brown RT, et al., 2011).

Successful programs for children with ADHD should incorporate the following components such as Accommodations, Instruction and Intervention.

Accommodation involves what can be done to make learning easier for students with ADD/ADHD. *Instruction* involves the strategies/methods incorporated for better teaching. *Intervention* involves management of maladaptive behaviours that disrupt concentration or distract other students.

Students whose ADHD impairs their learning may qualify for special education under the Individuals with Disabilities Education Act or for a Section 504 plan (for children who do not require special education) under the Rehabilitation Act of 1973. Children with ADHD can benefit from study skills instruction, changes to the classroom setup, alternative teaching techniques and a modified curriculum (APA, 2017)

TEACHING AND ACCOMMODATIONS: (SEGAL, J.,2019)

Seating

Seat the child with ADD/ADHD in a distraction free and structured environment away from door/ windows, preferably making him seated in the front desk near a "study buddy" wherein a classmate may assist innote taking, organization of material.Seating in rows facing the teacher helps in individual attention.

Information Delivery

Give single, precise instruction at a time and repeat as necessary for feedback. Pair written instruction with oral instructions. Carefully observe the child in order to determine when the child is particularly focused and attentive (e.g., early in the day, after recess, before lunch)accordingly schedule his most difficult and challenging assignments and activities at these times by using of visual charts, pictures, colour coding, creating of outlines for note-taking that helps in organization. Materials/Instructions may be organized and classified for better understanding by asking for feedback of the information to review its understanding. Teach at a tolerance level which is easier for the child to work as opposed to teaching at a frustration level. Use transitional strategies such as(e.g. buzzers, visual timers, verbal warnings, 'first/then' instructions, physical contact which may be hand on the shoulder or directing of arm and hand movements) to ensure the person does not become distracted between tasks and to help him remind of time.

Organization

The child should be encouraged to maintain a master notebook with separate sections for separate subjects. Consider homework areas are to be arranged in an orderly manner and belongings are easily accessible as required. Make organization of books, desk, locker, and book bag a regular routinized part of his day by use of checklist as independently as possible with assistance initially. Merely telling her to "straighten out your book bag" will not be effective. He should be assigned to spend a few minutes organizing at the beginning, middle, and end of the school day (Brock, 2010).

Make sure the child writes down assignments and important dates and follows it. Create worksheets and tests with fewer items or multiple choice format or orally asking at frequent intervals rather than long tests. Reduce the number of timed tests. Divide long-term projects into segments and assign smaller achievable goal for each segment. Avoid multiple tasks/assignment at a time. For example, if the child is assigned twenty math problems, give them to him five at a time. As he completes one set, give him the next five. This will be less intimidating and overwhelming. Gradually, increase the length of the segments. Help the person to prioritise assignments and activities by use of flow charts, visual cues.

During exams, explain the questions in simple words, overlooking the spelling mistakes and focus on the content instead while marking. Try alternative methods of assessment, such as oral testing or demonstration testing. Written tests and assessments will present particular difficulty for children with attentional problems because of the children's language and organizational weaknesses. Encourage him to work accurately rather than hastily completing his work and making sure that he gets into the habit of always checking finished work. Teach skills on what to do before beginning a task or leaving (e.g. asking: Do I have all I need? Did I put everything away?); the important part is get the young person to stop and think. Error monitoring exercises such as COPS works wherein it stands for C: capital, O: overall appearance, P: punctuation, S: spelling) (Hirisave, Oommen, & Kapur, 2002).

Teaching techniques that help students with ADD/ADHD focus and maintain their concentration on your lesson and their work can be beneficial to the entire class.

Attention Enhancement Strategies

Growing evidence have suggested that attention training programme could be highly beneficial for children with attention issues so the first critical step lies in enhancing more complex cognitive skills, especially memory. With impaired attention skills, the child may not pay attention to new information; leading to difficulty in retrieving it later. Intervention may improve their attention span over time, which could help them to be more productive across different conditions. (Morris, 1998)

Certain strategies include stringing beads-big to small, matching/ sorting, join dots,letter number sequencing, finger dexterity games, colouring within lines, mazes, painting within lines, cutting pictures and sticking them, jigsaw puzzles, letter/number cancellation,letter number and letter- symbol substitution, hocus-focus (find the difference), identifying repeated designs/ letter/ number, watching video, listening to stories and narrating them in own words (Hirisave, Oommen, & Kapur, 2002).

Another emerging technique to enhance attention is practising mindfulness. Applications of mindfulness training to child and adolescent samples with ADHD have been delivered in different formats (i.e., the child or adolescent receives training only, or caregivers receive concurrent mindfulness instruction as well). Practicing mindfulness exercises is all about paying attention and focusing. At the intervention level, mindfulness meditation practices involve focusing attention on a particular object (e.g., one's own breath) and returning to this object after becoming distracted. This is proposed to improve attentional control abilities. That is, this practice requires top-down regulation of attention and conflict detection, which can be thought of as a regulatory approach to attention that improves executive processes (Chiesa, Calati, & Serretti, 2011). Studies have shown that mindfulness can help kids improve their behaviour and their ability to focus in school. One way to practice is to sit quietly and focus on breathing in and out. Taking even a few deep breaths before class or a test could make a difference. (Keng, Smoski, & Robins, 2011).

Starting a Lesson

Signal the start of a lesson with an aural cue, such as an egg timer, or a horn. Also, subsequent cues to show the remaining time for the lesson to completing. Clearly outline the main heading of the lessons (what they are going to learn), rules, limits, and expectations on the board. Mention the materials they'll need during the lesson. Establish eye contact with any child who has ADD/ADHD. (Raggi & Chronis, 2006)

Conducting the Lesson

Keep instructions simple and structured. Vary the pace and include different kinds of activities. Many students with ADD do well with competitive games or other activities that are rapid and intense. Use props, charts, and other visual aids. Have an unobtrusive cue set up with the student who has ADD/ADHD, such as a touch on the shoulder or placing a sticky note on the student's desk, to remind the student to stay on task. Allow the child frequent productive breaks by assigning responsible chores in classroom, group activities such as helping the teacher with books, cleaning the black board and praising for the effort to boost his self-esteem and channelizing his energy . Let the child doddle or squeeze a rubber ball or tap something that doesn't make noise as a physical outlet, take informed breaks in between tasks but also given the responsibility to come back to the task assigned. Try not to ask a student with ADD/ ADHD perform a task or answer a question publicly that might be too difficult.

Ending the Lesson

Summarize key points. If you give an assignment, have three different students repeat it, then have the class say it in unison, and put it on the board. Use chunking, rehearsal, generating mental images and rote learning to remember key information. Look for signs or stress/ memory overload and provide encouragement for practice of segment learnt. Practice dictation exercises to help the young person develop auditory memory skills.

Parental Behavioural Training

The children get bored easily so keep up their interest and motivation with adequate and immediate reinforcements. Never take good behaviour for granted. Identify the child's desired behaviour and consistently reinforce the behaviour by behavioural reward systems, acceptance, affection, avoiding criticism, positive play and building empathy. Praise and reinforce the child for not interrupting, for working patiently, remaining in his seat, staying on task, cooperating. Be firm and consistent by not giving in to the child's tendency to escape a task he has lost interest in but you know he is capable of performing. Visible signs of hyperactive behaviours during seat work (e.g., drumming fingers, pencil tapping, squirming in seat, fidgeting) are actually a release for the child's hyperactivity and distractibility. Unless the movements are distracting or disruptive for others, ignore them. Use time out for misbehaviour.

Incorporation of Daily Report Cards (DRC) or school-home based notes acts as a means of communication between teachers and parents which allow for parents to know what occurred in the classroom on a daily basis and in most cases to be involved in the reward or consequence that occurs due to the report. Sample of DRC have been shown below:

Evidences show that enhancing problem-solving skills among children with ADHD leads to better outcomes and relapse prevention. The components of effective problem solving module include generating alternative solutions, evaluating options, considering consequences of each option and providing self-rewards. Parental emotional regulation and self-care should focus on anger management by recognising triggers of anger and anxiety related to the child's behaviour, practising of relaxation skills, engaging in pleasant events/tasks, maintaining effective partner support and adequate division of roles/responsibilities.

Maintaining Motivation

A difficult task caregivers and teachers struggle with ADHD children is to motivate the young ones to maintain an appropriate behaviour. A child's performance and motivation are influenced by three major factors: his degree of interest in the activity, the difficulty of the activity, and the duration of the task. Studies show that curriculum that is stimulating and relevant to the child's life experiences, which allows him to use creativity/novelty, allows him choice/options are more likely to keep the interests and motivation of the child. The presentation should be creative, colourful, multimodal, and enjoyable.

Figure 3. Daily report card

Daily Behavior Report Card

Name:______________________ Date:______________

Paid Attention In Class	**YES**	**SO-SO**	**NO**
Followed Directions	**YES**	**SO-SO**	**NO**
Sat Still In Seat	**YES**	**SO-SO**	**NO**
Got Along With Classmates	**YES**	**SO-SO**	**NO**

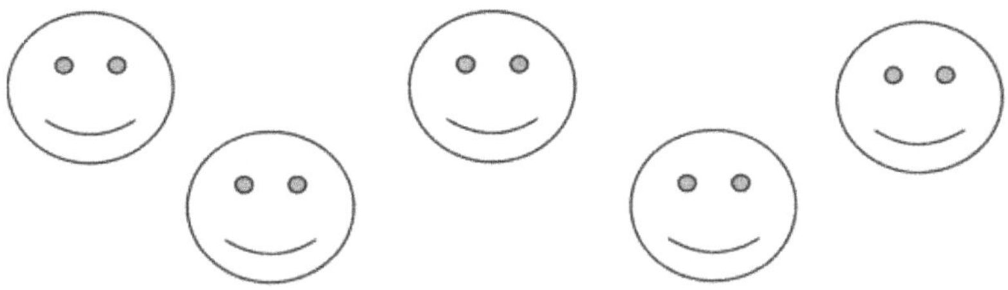

Teacher Comments: ____

Total Points for Note: ________________ (YES = 2, SO-SO = 1, NO = 0, ☺ = 1)

Good Report Card? (Yes or No)__________ Reward Earned: ________________

Parent Signature ____________________

As much as possible, the curriculum should be stimulating. Research has shown that a curriculum that is irrelevant to the student's social and economic interests generally results in disruptive behaviour, poor academic performance, limited progress, and dropping out. It is extraordinarily difficult for a child with ADD to remain engaged in a curriculum that is not interesting or challenging. These children live very much in the present. Therefore, long-term goals and rewards (e.g., grades and report cards) are often ineffective motivator.

The child with ADD will respond more positively to a curriculum that allows him choices and options. He will also be more likely to participate actively in tasks when there is a degree of creativity and novelty (e.g., presenting a history review using a Jeopardy! game). In order to maintain the motivation of this child, the teacher must simultaneously consider what is being taught and how it is being taught. The content alone is unlikely to hold the child's attention or motivation for an extended period. The content should be stimulating and relevant. The content alone is unlikely to hold the child's attention or motivation for an extended period of time. The presentation should be creative, colourful, multimodal, and enjoyable.

One of the effective tool in helping a child with ADD/ADHD is to maintain a positive attitude by making the child your partner by saying, "Let's figure out ways together to help you get your work done." Assure the child that you'll be looking for good behaviour and quality work, and when you see it, reinforce it with immediate and sincere praise. Finally, look for ways to motivate a student with ADD/ADHD by offering rewards on a point or token system.

CONCLUSION

Thus, treatment of young children with ADHD is most effective when a combination of behavioural management strategies, school support and medication is used with allied health referral. These relatively well established treatments are being supplemented by a number of new, innovative treatment approaches that offer considerable potential to broaden the range of treatment options available and to enhance both the breadth of coverage and intensity of effects obtained.

REFERENCES

APA. (2013). Diagnostic and statistical manual of mental disorders-fifth edition (DSM-5). Arlington: American Psychiatric Publishing, Inc.

Biederman, J., Petty, C. R., Monuteaux, M. C., Fried, R., Byrne, D., Mirto, T., Spencer, T., Wilens, T. E., & Faraone, S. V. (2010). Adult psychiatric outcomes of girls with attention deficit hyperactivitydisorder: 11-year follow-up in a longitudinal case-control study. *The American Journal of Psychiatry*, *167*(4), 409–417. doi:10.1176/appi.ajp.2009.09050736 PMID:20080984

Bussing, R., Fernandez, M., Harwood, M., & Hou, W. (2008). Parent and teacher SNAP-IV ratings of attention deficit hyperactivity disorder symptoms: Psychometric properties and normative ratings from a school district sample. *Assessment*, *15*(3), 317–328. doi:10.1177/1073191107313888 PMID:18310593

Conners, C. K. (2008). *Conners* (3rd edition: manual). Multi-Health Systems.

Edwards, M., Gardner, E., Chelonis, J., Schulz, E., Flake, R., & Diaz, P. (2007). Estimates of the validity and utility of the Conners' continuous performance test in the assessment of inattentive and/or hyperactive-impulsive behaviors in children. *Journal of Abnormal Child Psychology*, *35*(3), 393–404. doi:10.100710802-007-9098-3 PMID:17295064

Emser, T. S., Johnston, B. A., Steele, J. D., Kooij, S., Thorell, L., & Christiansen, H. (2018). Assessing ADHD symptoms in children and adults: Evaluating the role of objective measures. *Behavioral and Brain Functions*, *14*(1), 11. doi:10.118612993-018-0143-x PMID:29776429

French, W. P. (2015). Assessment and treatment of attention-deðcit/hyperactivity disorder part 1. *Pediatric Annals*, *44*(3), 114–120. doi:10.3928/00904481-20150313-13 PMID:25806728

Hickey, G., & Fricker, P. (1999). Attention deficit hyperactivity disorder, CNS stimulants and sport. *Sports Medicine (Auckland, N.Z.)*, *27*(1), 11–21. doi:10.2165/00007256-199927010-00002 PMID:10028130

Hirisave, U., Oommen, A., & Kapur, M. (2002). *Psychological Assessment of Children in the clinical setting*. Published at NIMHANS.

Hodgkins, P., Arnold, L. E., Shaw, M., Caci, H., Kahle, J., Woods, A. G., & Young, S. (2012). A systematic review of global publication trends regarding long-term outcomes of ADHD. *Frontiers in Psychiatry, 2*, 84. doi:10.3389/fpsyt.2011.00084 PMID:22279437

Keng, S. L., Smoski, M. J., & Robins, C. J. (2011). Effects of mindfulness on psychological health: A review of empirical studies. *Clinical Psychology Review, 31*(6), 1041–1056. doi:10.1016/j.cpr.2011.04.006 PMID:21802619

Lavoie, R. (2010). *Motivating the Child with Attention Deficit Disorder*. Retrieved from http://www.ldonline.org/article/19975

Leo, I. M., & Feldman, H. M. (2007). Academic and educational outcomes of children with ADHD [Special issue]. *Journal of Pediatric Psychology, 32*(6), 643–654. doi:10.1093/jpepsy/jsl054 PMID:17569716

Morris, J. (1998). *Facing AD/HD: A Survival Guide for Parents of Children with Attention Deficit/Hyperactivity Disorder*. Research Press.

Oliveira, C. T., & Dias, A. C. G. (2018). Psychoeducation for Attention Deðcit/Hyperactivity Disorder: What, How and Who Shall We Inform? *Trends in Psychology/TemasemPsicologia, 26*(1), 263-281.

Substance Abuse and Mental Health Services Administration. (2016). *Co-occurring disorders*. Received from www.samhsa.gov/disorders/co-occurring

Thapar, A., & Cooper, M. (2016). Attention deficit hyperactivity disorder. *Lancet, 387*(10024), 1240–1250. doi:10.1016/S0140-6736(15)00238-X PMID:26386541

Toplak, M. E., West, R. F., & Stanovich, K. E. (2013). Practitioner review: Do performance based measures and ratings of executive function assess the same construct? *Journal of Child Psychology and Psychiatry, and Allied Disciplines, 54*(2), 131–143. doi:10.1111/jcpp.12001 PMID:23057693

Van der Ende, J., & Verhulst, F.C. (2005). Informant, gender and age differences in ratings of adolescent problem behaviour. *European Child* and *Adolescent Psychiatry, 14*, 117–126.

Wolraich, M., Brown, L., Brown, R. T., DuPaul, G., Earls, M., Feldman, H. M., Ganiats, T. G., Kaplanek, B., Meyer, B., Perrin, J., Pierce, K., Reiff, M., Stein, M. T., & Visser, S. (2011). Subcommittee on attention-deðcit/ hyperactivity disorder; Steering Committee on quality improvement and management. ADHD: Clinical practice guideline for the diagnosis, evaluation, and treatment of attention-deðcit/hyperactivity disorder in children and adolescents. *Pediatrics, 128*(5), 1007–1022. doi:10.1542/peds.2011-2654 PMID:22003063

Wolraich, M., Lambert, W., Doffing, M., Bickman, L., Simmons, L., & Worley, K. (2003). Psychometric Properties of the Vanderbilt ADHD Diagnostic Parent Rating Scale in a Referred Population. *Journal of Pediatric Psychology, 28*(8), 559–568. doi:10.1093/jpepsy/jsg046 PMID:14602846

Chapter 5
Adolescents and Attention Deficit Hyperactivity Disorder (ADHD):
Symptoms, Causes, Assessment, and Treatment

Kalpana Raman
Auckland University of Technology, New Zealand

ABSTRACT

This chapter attempts to individually understand the concept of adolescence and ADHD before it combines to the understanding of the progression of ADHD as a neurodevelopmental and behavioural disorder moving through the lifespan in different formats/symptoms. This understanding would provide the clinicians and academicians clarity to follow the golden rule of 'early diagnosis early intervention' by identifying the progressive nature in terms of genetic, biochemistry, psycho-social, and personality aspects maintaining the disorder. Finally, this chapter would also provide an overview about the possible interventions and treatment plans available and briefly discusses the recent issues and trends throughout the chapter.

INTRODUCTION

The two main components namely attention deficit/inattention and hyperactivity/impulsivity marks the disorder of ADHD. The age of adolescents ascertained by the standards of World Health Organization (WHO) is between the ages of 10-19 years(Encyclopedia Britannica). It is a phase when an individual tends to undergo overall growth and development in terms of biological (puberty, primary and secondary sexual characteristics, voice box modulation etc.); cognitive (understanding and possess developed meanings, preparing to gradually become independent etc.); behavioural (levels of energy, coping mechanisms etc); social (group formations, affiliation, social norms, traditions and folklores etc.). It is considered

DOI: 10.4018/978-1-7998-5495-1.ch005

to be a mid-phase wherein an individual is learning and experiencing the transitional roles from childhood to adulthood through various means. In general, the age of adolescence from epidemiological and psychological perspectives is indicative of engaging into increased behaviours involving risk-taking, high impulsivity, substance abuse, self-harming tendencies (Hafner&An Der, 1997), gradually moving towards marked mental health issues such as affective disorders, anxiety disorders, and personality disorders etc. (Goodwin, 2009; Park et al, 2006) resulting in lack of resources to deal effectively, poor self-efficacy, lack of life skills etc. (Young et al, 2005).

Attention Deficit Hyperactivity Disorder is commonly abbreviated and denoted as ADHD in the world. ADHD is a neurodevelopmental disorder (Sparrow &Erhardt, 2014) as well as classified under behavioral disorder (International Classification of Diseases- ICD 10). The defining subtypes according to DSM-IV (Diagnostic Statistical Manual- IV edition) in ADHD classification are: Hyperactive/impulsive, inattention and combined; dimensionally they have been classified under 'inattention and hyperactive'. In ICD-10 they have been coded at F90 as 'Hyperkinetic disorders'. Global prevalence has been estimated to be around 2-7% (Sayal et al, 2018). As per the DSM-IV manual the prevalence in males is higher than the females with the ratio of one male in every three males compared to one female in every nine females, symptoms usually presenting by the age of 3-6 years. The review paper by the same authors Sayal et al (2018) have summarized that the recent trends are indicative of increasing prevalence in female sample. Various causal factors have been attributed to the manifestation of symptoms in patients with ADHD diagnosis but no single causal factor can be isolated and held responsible. Thus understanding of bio-psycho-social perspective to any disorder is vital in planning of careful and appropriate assessment and intervention. The initial and basic medical model to any disorder/illness has been criticized and the need for understanding the psychosocial perspectives has been underlined. In the forthcoming headings, understanding of ADHD specifically in the context of adolescents' age range has been addressed.

Lifespan Perspective-ADHD in Adolescence

Till recent years, ADHD was considered to be a childhood behavioral disorder and not much scientific interest was laid to the age related transactional changes in ADHD symptoms (Becker & Barley, 2019). But, recently the rising incidents of road accidents, reckless driving(Barkley, 2015), impulsivity, self-harming tendencies and other core personality traits have drawn everyone's attention towards the developmental psychopathology perspective of ADHD (Hinshaw, 2017).

The developmental psychopathology model/framework has focused on the interaction between the predisposing, precipitating and perpetuating factors of the disorder which provides clarity in the development of symptoms and explains the causation of the disorder in multi-modal format. The guiding principles of the framework includes delineating between normalcy and difficulty and disordered state, continuities and discrepancies or gaps, risk factors, various process models "reciprocal, transactional, ontogenic" and various vulnerabilities levels (Pg. 8-12; See Becker & Barkley, 2019 for further details).

As obsessive-compulsive disorder has been defined as a heterogeneous group of disorders, similarly due to marked transitions in symptoms and their manifestations as the growth and development occurs in individuals, ADHD has also been classified as heterogeneous group of disorders wherein there is a possible change in manifestation of hyperactivity in childhood to increased impulsivity, fidgety, inattention during adolescence and adulthood (Marsh & Williams, 2004).

A study done by Caye et al (2016) suggested that approximately 70% of children diagnosed with ADHD in childhood tends to manifest these moderate-severe symptoms later in the stages even till adulthood- a concept descriptive about the nature of lifespan maintenance of ADHD symptoms. The comorbid conditions identified with ADHD also are indicative of lifespan development(Asherson, Buitelaar, Faraone& Rohde, 2016) of the disorder such as the transition from conduct or oppositional disorder to antisocial traits of personality, delinquency to substance dependence or abuse etc. (Elia, Ambrosini&Berrettini, 2008). Thus, various researches suggest that in order to appropriately devise a treatment plan, awareness of symptoms and utilization of accurate assessment tools is vital (Becker & Barkley, 2019).

Symptoms, Comorbidity and Effects of ADHD in adolescence

The American Psychiatric Association (APA, 2000) explained that the individuals with ADHD tend to exhibit the defining three symptoms mentioned above: hyperactive, impulsive and inattentive throughout the lifespan as per the developmental psychopathology perspective in varied formats (Barkley, Fischer, Smallish & Fletcher, 2002)which as any psychiatric disorder has its lasting effects on their routine functioning such as occupational, educational, social, emotional, physical health etc.

The symptoms checklist to be able to diagnose in children is clearly laid out in ICD-10 and DSM-IV and V (latest) but the evolvement of symptoms is less understood. The challenges posited in this understanding relate to the reliable and authentic informant, tool used to ascertain the diagnosis and the parent-teacher rater agreement during adolescence (Sibley et al, 2012). It is believed that ADHD present in adolescence may or may not have been diagnosed in childhood due to the financial burden it carries for assessment and intervention and also that the symptoms such as hyperactivity (running, jumping, squirming etc.) in childhood might be manifested differently during adolescence and adulthood such as restlessness, jumping to conclusions, impulsivity, self-harm etc. (Wender, 1990).

Generally, the symptoms mentioned in the previous chapters of this book and the DSM-IV or V and ICD-10 (F90.0) are followed throughout the world for diagnosing. Commonly agreed upon criteria are extracted from DSM as checklist which highlights presence of at least six symptoms to be accurately matched in either inattention or hyperactivity. DSM V has brought about certain changes with respect to the presence of symptoms at a certain age (17 years and older) and number of symptoms to be present (variable between 5 or 6) for diagnostic purposes which have assisted the clinicians in diagnosing ADHD during adolescence. A liberal approach has been adopted by DSM V wherein the manual acknowledges the potential of no harm or significant threat caused during childhood due to the symptoms but adopted developmental approach that the symptoms exhibited currently could be treated as symptoms present during the adolescent period and may be unavailable/undetected during childhood (Brahmbhatt, 2016).

The important criteria to note is that ADHD is not curtailed to individual setting but is dispersed throughout various settings causing impairment in social, occupational, academic and daily functioning (Teichner, 2016).Due to its impact on various settings of individual life, it can be diagnosed as disorder. ADHD during adolescence and adulthood has been described to be overloaded with the difficulties in interpersonal relationships (commonly known as interpersonal stressors), marital conflict, difficulties in sustaining or maintaining meaningful relationships, occupation/education related difficulties (as the comorbid conditions in childhood is suggestive of specific learning disorders, autism spectrum, oppositional defiant, conduct disorder), antisocial tendencies, behavioral difficulties, drop out and attrition, increased criminal/risk taking behavior, reckless sexual behavior etc(Thompson, Molina, Pelham, &Gnagy, 2007; Kent et al, 2011; Flory, Molina, Pelham, Gnagy, & Smith, 2006; Sibley et al, 2011).Also, the issues highlighted by various authors are inattention, inability to sustain attention in daily activities (DSM-V, 2013) due to which there is decrease/lack or poor performance in any given setting such as education/academic/ occupation (Breslau et al, 2009; Scholtens, Rydell& Yang, 2013), inability to initiate and maintain effective peer relations, depression and suicidal ideations/thoughts(Patros et al, 2013), physical and medical illness (smoking, body image related difficulties like obesity, non-compliance) and burden(Nigg, 2013), core symptoms of depression manifest like decreased/low self-esteem (Harpin et al, 2013), lack of cohesiveness(Klein, Mannuzza, &Olazagasti, 2012; Leo & Feldman, 2007), diminished social functioning etc.

Commonly, the comorbid conditions and the presentation of symptoms during adolescence age makes the diagnosis challengingas the appropriate and accurate diagnosis of ADHD requires adequate assessment of the past history related to symptomatology, traces of difficulty areas which are invariably dependent on the parents and adolescent's responses on the rating scales. Few researchers have focused on this challenge of accurate diagnosis as based on the developmental framework of the disorder, the symptoms of hyperactivity (jumping from one place to another: example) gradually weans during adolescence and more prominent symptoms could be fidgeting, impulsivity or inattentiveness (Brahmbhatt, 2016).The comorbid conditions identified with ADHD during adolescence are anxiety disorders, affective disorders, substance dependence/abuse, tic disorders etc. (Young &Bramham, 2012).Although the symptoms decrease and change their manifestations as per age, the impulsive traits (signifying personality disorders if developed for longer period of time) and inattention (a symptom associated with majority of psychiatric disorders) persists and may lead to severe to chronic undesirable to debilitating conditions (Wolraich et al., 2005).Thus, the various researchers and authors have considered the adolescence ADHD as the most demanding and puzzling disorder to understand, assess and treat in order to alleviate the symptoms and improve the quality of life and wellbeing of the individuals with ADHD and their immediate family (Sibley et al, 2012). Various causal factors have been attributed to the study and development of ADHD such as biological studies inclusive of genetic, biochemistry, adoption studies, and psycho-social correlates etc. which have been briefly outlined in the following section.

Etiological/Causal Factors of ADHD

Every psychiatric, behavioral, neuro-developmental disorder tends to have overlay of various causal factors resulting in the disorder. Usually they have been characterized under three sections broadly as outlined in the Figure 1 Multi Factorial Etiological representation of disorders.The figure reflects the various factors (multifactor) in each section which may contribute in the development of any disorder.

While an attempt is made to ascertain the causation of the disorder, at times it is difficult to clearly determine the cause responsible for the disorder. ADHD is one of those disorders wherein vast number of researches (Nigg, 2006, 2013; Thapar et al, 2013) has focused on determining the accurate causation throwing some light but future research areas are open to explore which would assist in defining ADHD and provide a definitive factor which precipitates and maintain the disorder. Thus, ADHD is considered to be a multi-causal disorder.

As the previous chapters has discussed the various causal factors of ADHD, the same follows in the developmental perspective of ADHD during adolescence period. Thus, brief key etiology is presented here. Steinhausen (2009) in his approach to explore genetic basis in ADHD had revealed that ADHD is highly inheritable and the risk of inheriting ADHD is higher in the probands of first degree relatives (Willcutt, 2012).Willcutt had determined the risk to be six to eight multifold times for inheriting.

Figure 1. Multi-factorial etiological representation of disorders

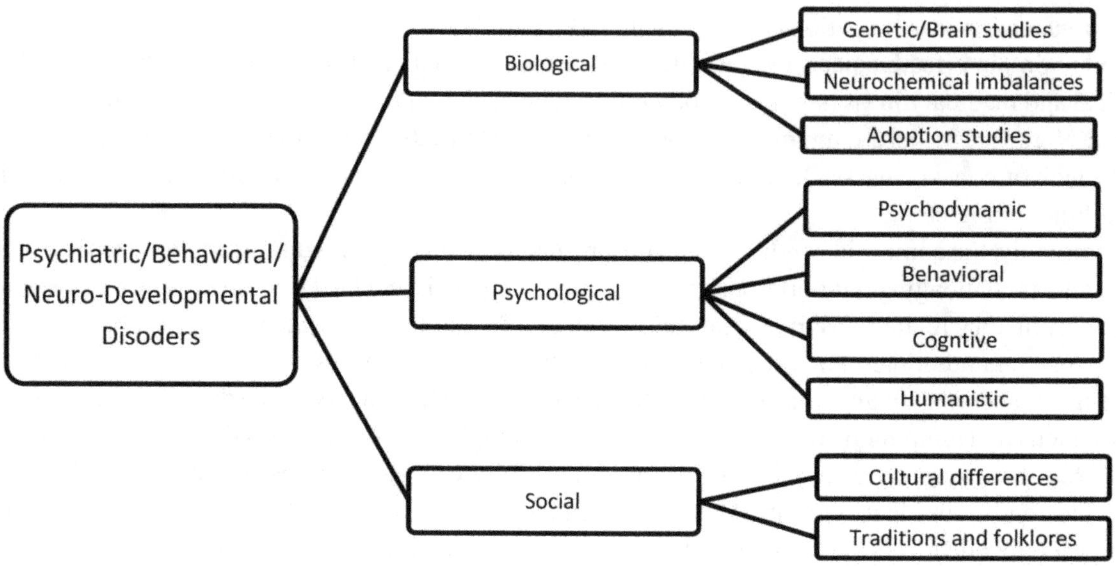

Willcutt et al (2013 & 2014) conducted a study at the Colorado Learning Disabilities Research Centre to estimate whether there is any difference in the inheritance rates in probands in childhood and adolescence and found that the values were same for both in childhood and adolescence. The twin studies have also furthered the role of genes in the development of ADHD by determining high concordance rates "58-82%" in monozygotic twins compared to dizygotic in both children and adolescence (Willcutt et al, 2010). Neurochemical roles have been seen in the dopamine(Spencer et al, 2005) and serotonin transmitters (Stergiakouli&Thapar, 2010).

It has been long debated to conclude the role of genes and environment. The environmental factors responsible for ADHD in childhood are "preterm birth, low birth weight, trauma during birth, maternal depression, smoking, drinking and substance use during pregnancy" (Young &Bramham, 2012). The brain studies suggest changes in both the structure and functions of the brain in children and adolescents with ADHD. The role of prefrontal region has been ascertained in ADHD disorder as two theories defining ADHD symptoms are motivation deficit and executive functions dys-regulation especially difficulty in tasks involving set shifting, working memory and response inhibition (Pennington &Ozonoff, 1996; Nigg, 2001; Willcutt, 2005).The social factors are similar across all nations in both developing and developed nations (Polanczyk et al, 2007). The other factors responsible are "early attachment issues, adversities, deprivation" (Rutter, 2005). Thus, the study and understanding of the bio-psycho-social markers of ADHD is considered important. Knowledge of the causal factors is important but assessing and treatment is more vital of ADHD for the enhancement of performance, quality of life and wellbeing.

Assessing ADHD

The main goal of assessment of ADHD is to determine the extent of impairment, level of pervasiveness and stability of the disorder in an individual, progressive course of disorder, maintaining factors, prognostic rate, and negative history to be able to exclude other comorbid disorders and be assured of the diagnosis if required through various sources. Especially in ADHD assessment the sources identified for the purpose of authenticity and honest information gathering although not always definite are self, parents and tutors/teacher. The ratings on symptoms by self are considered to be important during adolescence due to the knowledge possessed (Smith et al, 2000). Recently, the potential challenges reported by various researchers which have been stated by various clinicians is the questionable credibility of the information provided by adolescents as they have tendency of under rating their symptoms and reporting falsely (Epstein et al, 2008); the retrospective memory of parents cannot be assessed with detail (Miller, Newcorn & Halperin, 2010) as the majority of symptoms especially hyperactivity (a key symptom of ADHD diagnosis) tends to modify into impulsivity during adolescence. A review paper by Wolraich, Wibblesman& Brown (2005) also highlighted a pertinent issue with the amount of time spent during childhood with parents is significantly more than during adolescence which makes it more difficult to rely on their memory to report current symptoms without being overwhelmed by the childhood symptoms. A study conducted by Keeley et al (2018) addressed the relevance of combined approach towards the assessment of ADHD specifically in adolescence. They assessed the psychometric validity of six item ADHD self-report scale (ASRS-6) which is a shorter version of the original ASRS-18 item version on 89 (N=89) adolescents and parents and found that the adolescents rating was suggestive of social anxiety symptoms more than the depressive symptoms reporting wherein a conflict was seen between the parent-adolescent leading to disagreement between them which made the researchers to conclude and mark the relevance of self-parent-teacher assessment to be able to comprehensively diagnose and plan the further course.

The assessment approach of ADHD during adolescence has been described as “multi-informant, multi-setting and multi-modal” by Sparrow & Erhardt in their book published in 2014 addressing the major concerns associated with assessment and treatment of ADHD in adolescence. The issue and relevance of multi-informant have been addressed above. Similarly, multi-setting refers to situations not only confined to home setting but to provide a generalized perspective of the symptoms and effects of the disorder in an individual to suggest the pervasive spread across the various phases of life. Any disorder whether physical or psychiatric, behavioral or neuro-developmental employs various approaches/modes to finalize the course of further treatment such as history taking, interviews, examination of past history and records, further assessments (if physical then analysis of blood samples, brain scans etc. and if psychiatric then cognitive functioning, personality assessment and psychopathology assessment, field visits, use of rating scales etc) are conducted. The assessment tools should be carefully chosen keeping in view the goals of assessment, culture sensitivity, intellectual functioning, level of education, socio-economic conditions etc. in order to extract maximum information for the planning of intervention (Miller et al, 2009; Nigg, 2013).

The valid and reliable structured and semi-structured interview schedules based on the latest diagnostic manual DSM-V available for furthering our understanding of ADHD in adolescence are Barkley & Murphy’s ADHD interview (2006) for teenagers; Diagnostic Interview for Children and Adolescence-version IV abbreviated as DICA-IV by Reich (2000); Diagnostic Interview Schedule for Children –IV abbreviated as DISC-IV (Columbia DISC Development Group, 1997); K-SADS for comorbidity issues which is a Schedule for Affective Disorders and Schizophrenia for School-Age Children developed by Kaufman et al (1996). The age range for all the schedules are 6-17 years of age and are available as either pencil-paper or computerized versions for the ease of utilization. Following the interview, careful selection of rating scales and further assessments should be done. Although the rating scales are not considered to be diagnostic tools but information provided in the rating scales consisting of problematic behaviors checklist assists in planning and employing behavioral therapy techniques in the alleviation of symptoms. The most commonly and widely used ADHD rating scales are Conners ADHD rating scale Version 3 & Conners CBRS which is Comprehensive Behavior Rating scales (Conners, 2008) for the age range of 6-18 years; Behavior Assessment System for Children edition 2 abbreviated as BASC-2 (Reynolds &Kamphaus, 1992); Brown ADD scales for Children specifically for attention deficit symptoms in childhood and adolescence (Brown, 2001). Each domain can be individually assessed based on the goal and need for assessment such as utilizing neuro-cognitive tasks like Stroop test for response inhibition, Wisconsin Card Sorting Test for set shifting, Tower of London test, n-back tasks for attention and concentration, Rey Osterrieth Complex Figure test (Meyers & Meyers, 1995) & Continuous Performance Tests (CPT) etc. as these assessment tools can assist in determining the role of prefrontal region and planning of cognitive rehabilitation of the individual accordingly. Intellectual functioning assessment tools can be selected to rule out comorbidities of intellectual disability and specific learning disability based on the level of education and age of the individual such as NIMHANS Index of SLD; Wechsler Intelligence scales based on the age range of the individual and Raven's Standard Progressive matrices etc.

Another new scale developed by Swanson et al. (2001) named Swanson, Nolan, and Pelham Rating scale-IV (SNAP-IV). It has 26 items out of which 18 items are worded as symptoms of ADHD equally divided into 9 each for inattention and hyperactivity and 8 items of oppositional-defiant disorder (ODD). The rating has to be completed on a 4-point Likert scale ranging from not at all to very much. The assessment is similar to Conners ADHD rating scale and has to be completed by the individual with ADHD (adolescent), parents and teacher to be able to quantify with average weights and understand qualitatively for further progress. A study conducted by Nichols et al (2017) attempted to ascertain the factor structure (work on psychometrics) and find the best model fit for the assessments in adolescence with ADHD. They recruited 588 participants from who were carefully extracted and recruited from the "NIMH Multimodal treatment Study of Children (MTA)" (Pg.629) who was followed up for 8 years and were assessed on various measures: SNAP-IV (Swanson et al, 2001) specifically designed for the MTA for this purpose; Children's Depression inventory (CDI; Kovacs, 1995), Multidimensional Anxiety Scale for Children (MASC; March et al, 1997); Columbia Impairment Scale (CIS; Bird et al, 1993); Social Skills rating scale (SSRS; Gresham & Elliot, 1990); Wechsler Individual Achievement Test (WIAT; Wechsler, 1992) as scales to determine the participants to be excluded from the sample. The researchers found the best model fit with second order three-factor model for ADHD in adolescence using teacher rating whereas second order two-factor model for self and parents rating. The paper discusses the key issues related to utilisation of assessment tools for the purpose of diagnostics in adolescence ADHD and concluded that clarity of understanding of identifying and diagnosing ADHD is vital for clinicians and can be achieved only by giving special attention and reforming/restructuring of the disorder specific to adolescence.

Smith & Martel (2019) conducted a novice study by conducting personality tests to understand and plot the trait profiles of adolescents and young adults' pattern of ADHD which can further assist in the awareness of comorbidity and prognostic clarity which forms a basis for psycho-education as the foremost step during psychological interventions. They assessed 182 adolescents and 287 young adults on the measures of ADHD rating scale: adolescents were given and asked to complete the ADHD rating scale by DuPaul, Power, Anastopoulos, & Reid (1998); Youth Self-Report (Achenbach, 1991) to evaluate the issues pertaining to "internalizing-externalising" (Pg.443); and a Q-sort measurement was used with parents known as the California Child Q-sort (CCQ) developed by Caspi et al (1992). The researchers found similarities between childhood profiles and adolescent and young adulthood profiles on traits of personality. They found patterns pertaining to low and high extraversion and high neuroticism linked to ADHD in adolescence and adulthood. Based on each test's interpretive abilities and normative data representative of the individual being assessed, a report is finalized which assists in goal setting of the intervention.

The abovementioned studies provide information about the possible utility, relevance and psychometric validity of few scales specific to the context of adolescents. Many studies have focused on childhood patterns and understanding of symptoms as ADHD was considered to be childhood disorder for long but recently the growing interest and recognition of symptoms during adolescence and adulthood has channeled attention of clinicians and researchers to understand better and assist the clients, parents, relatives and the education providers with possible intervention plans which has been detailed in the next section.

Treatment & Intervention of ADHD

Based on the diagnosis, comorbidity, assessment reports, clinical observation, pervasiveness, level of impairment, readiness towards therapy, commitment and parental/informants involvement, therapeutic approach is devised for the adolescent with ADHD.

Usually, depending on the pervasiveness of the disorder and the generalized impairment, pharmacological treatment is determined which includes stimulant medications: methylphenidate such as Ritalin etc. and amphetamine medications such as Adderall etc. (Heal, Smith &Findling, 2012); non-stimulant medications: alpha-adrenergic agonist, Wellbutrin etc. as adjunct (Banaschewski et al, 2004). Well documented evidence is available signifying the increase in the prescribed stimulants medications for the treatment of ADHD especially in the recent decades.

A study done by Visser et al (2014) in the pool of understanding the increase in trend of prescribing stimulant medications found an increase of five-times more prescriptions of stimulant medications between the years of 2007-2010 than 1988-1994. Many general public and researchers have raised their humane concerns suggesting over-prescription of stimulant medications in recent years which might be problematic to the growing children at a later run (LeFever, Arcona & Antonuccio, 2003). In contrast to the increased prescription of these ADHD medications, few studies specific to the geographical regions of the United States of America (USA) found that it is not always true about the over-prescription (Connor, 2011) but few states and regions such as North Carolina there is a trend reflecting the increased prescriptions of such medications (Angold, Erkanli, Egger, & Costello, 2000). Studies have also ascertained the efficacy of medications in the treatment of ADHD especially in the symptoms of academic achievement and efficiency, decreased disturbance in occupational and educational settings and also improved markings on rating scales by family and teachers (Nigg & Barkley, 2014). Stimulant medications have been found to improve performance in few neuropsychological measures especially attention and vigilance tasks (Quinlan, 2000).

Non-pharmacological treatment options are psychosocial therapeutic approaches depending on the case formulation of the individual. Various approaches specifically behavioral therapy, cognitive behavioral therapy (CBT by Beck, 2011) and mindfulness meditation and techniques (Review by Leeth, Villarreal & Styck, 2019) has been extensively researched and proved their efficacy in the treatment of adolescence with ADHD.

Evans et al (2014) categorized psychological therapeutic approaches into "behavioral treatments" and "training interventions" (Pg.354) wherein token economy based on behavioral therapy principles of rewards and punishments to unlearn a maladaptive behavior and inculcate a desirable behavior has been detailed under the category of behavioral treatments and life skills training utilizing deeper theoretically rooted principles of social skills training, problem solving skills (Barkley, Edwards, Lanery et al, 2001), CBT (Sprich et al, 2016), mindfulness approaches (as outlined in the book by Becker & Barkley, 2019) have been detailed. Behavioral interventions have laid their focus on the functionality aspect of ADHD and alleviate the symptoms associated with it. Thus, many studies have documented the efficacy of behavioral interventions in childhood as that is the major treatment plan followed by clinicians apart from medications during childhood disorders. One such study by Evans, Owens, and Bunford (2014) have found that the behavioral interventions involving multi-person and multi-level intervention module namely parental management training (PMT), peer related (skills training), and other important skills (Evans et al, 2014) to have deeper effects when followed aptly at the home and school/occupational settings in amelioration of functional symptoms of ADHD.

PMT specifically utilizes strategies of psycho-educating the immediate famiy and relatives of the individual with ADHD to be informed and educate about ADHD, its progressive nature, etiology, prognostic criteria's and rates, homework difficulty, academics, occupational difficulties, instructions, medications and treatment complains and adherence, token economy (contingency management), techniques involved in contingency management such as time out, negative or positive reinforcement and punishment etc. (Chronis, Chacko, Fabiano, Wymbs, & Pelham, 2004). The techniques in social skills training are tailored depending on the level of skills already present and have to be modified or adapted or inculcated gradually involving communication skills, verbal and non-verbal language, problem solving skills, decreasing anger outbursts/irritability/suggestibility, concept and formation of groups, cooperation/competition/negotiation/bargaining etc. to name a few (Daly, Hildenbrand, & Brown, 2015). Grogan & Weitzman (2015) devised a 12 step intervention plan for parents of ADHD adolescents wherein the parents play a role as coach. The major steps are "..acceptance, surrender to higher power, inventory: daily review, crisis de-briefing, daily prayer of staying focused on goals, admit to others the exact nature of our wrongs, making restrictions for infarctions.: (Pg 370-374).

The role of cognitive retraining or neuropsychological rehabilitation in ADHD has also been researched because of the two underlying theories underpinning the explanation of development of ADHD namely the executive dysfunction and motivation deficit/emotion dys-regulation. In order to enhance executive functioning (pre-frontal region of the brain), two basic principles guide the enhancement of executive functioning in brain which are neuroplasticity and neurogenesis. Based on these principles, cognitive tasks coupled with behavioral therapy have been found to be beneficial to improve attention, sustain it and also improve the brain functions (Van der Oord et al, 2014). Initially paper-pencil cognitive tasks were more popularized but in the recent decades computerized cognitive retraining also known as brain games has been reviewed with its widespread usage such as Brain function therapy, Cogmed, Lumosity, Happy Neuron, Nintendo, Cognifit etc (Sibley, Kurian, Evans, Waxmonsky, & Smith, 2014).

A cognitive behavioral model of ADHD in adults has been popularized by Young & Bramham (2012) in their book which acts as catalyst in case formulation and treatment planning of individuals with ADHD by the psychologists. The stages of therapy have been outlined in their work known as "The Young-Bramham Schedule" (Pg.14; See Young & Bramham book on CBT guide, 2012) and each module of therapy have been explained in their book. It provides basic to advanced levels of treatment modules pertaining to psychological therapy. Emilsson (2011) found that CBT was highly efficacious in amelioration of ADHD symptoms and also the symptoms suggestive of comorbid conditions. With the growing literature about effectiveness of CBT approaches in the treatment of ADHD symptoms, iCBT

(Internet CBT) which is a self-help program was launched and disseminated by Petterson, Soderstrom, Edlund-Soderstrom&Nilson (2017). Reviewing the efficacy of video therapy/video-conference therapy, Sibley, Comer, & Gonzalez (2017) delivered tailor made modules of therapy via video-conferencing format to the parents and adolescents (teenagers) and they found improvement in ADHD symptoms in teenagers especially in symptoms related to organization, planning etc.

CBT treatment protocol for adults has been modified for utilization with adolescents by Safren, Sprich, Perlman & Otto (2005 & 2017) and they have published "therapist guide and client workbook" (Pg.356) for easy reference usually consisting of twelve sessions lasting for 45-50 minutes with the modules focusing on effective psycho-education, cognitive restructuring, organization and planning, distraction as coping strategies, parental and teacher involvement etc.

Parental management training during childhood ADHD, psycho-education and behavioral techniques have proven to be beneficial and well documented during childhood but there is dearth of literature focusing on adolescence ADHD development, treatment and prognosis. Combining pharmacological and non-pharmacological approaches have been seen consistently in other psychiatric conditions to improve the prognosis rates by lowering the relapse rates in individuals and recent advancements have been made in this area and still progressing especially in the area of ADHD in adolescence years.

ACKNOWLEDGMENT

This chapter received no specific grant from any funding agency in the public, commercial, or not-for-profit sectors. The access to books, journal articles, and research articles was supported by the online library facilities of the Auckland University of Technology.

REFERENCES

Achenbach, T. M. (1991). *Integrative guide for the 1991 CBCL/4-18, YSR, and TRF profiles*. University of Vermont, Department of Psychiatry.

American Psychiatric Association. (2000). Diagnostic and Statistical Manual of Mental Disorders. APA.

American Psychiatric Association. (2013). *Diagnostic and Statistical Manual of Mental Disorders* (5th ed.). American Psychiatric Association.

Angold, A., Erkanli, A., Egger, H. L., & Costello, E. J. (2000). Stimulant treatment for children: A community perspective. *Journal of the American Academy of Child and Adolescent Psychiatry*, *39*(8), 975–984. doi:10.1097/00004583-200008000-00009

Asherson, P., Buitelaar, J., Faraone, S. V., & Rohde, L. A. (2016). Adult attentiondeficit hyperactivity disorder: Key conceptual issues. *The Lancet. Psychiatry*, *3*(6), 568–578. doi:10.1016/S2215-0366(16)30032-3

Banaschewski, T., Roessner, V., Dittmann, R. W., Santosh, P. J., & Rothenberger, A. (2004). Non-stimulant medications in the treatment of ADHD. *European Child & Adolescent Psychiatry*, *13*(1), 102–116.

Barkley, R., Fischer, M., Smallish, L., & Fletcher, K. (2002). The persistence of attention deficit hyperactivity disorder into young adulthood as a function of reporting source and definition of disorder. *Journal of Abnormal Psychology, 111*(2), 279–289. doi:10.1037/0021-843X.111.2.279

Barkley, R., Fischer, M., Smallish, L., & Fletcher, K. (2006). Young adult outcome of hyperactive children: Adaptivefunctioning in major life activities. *Journal of the American Academy of Child and Adolescent Psychiatry, 45*(2), 192–202. doi:10.1097/01.chi.0000189134.97436.e2

Barkley, R. A. (2015b). Etiologies of ADHD. In R. A. Barkley (Ed.), *Attention-deficit hyperactivity disorder: A handbook for diagnosis and treatment* (4th ed., pp. 356–390). Guilford Press.

Barkley, R. A., Edwards, G., Laneri, M., Fletcher, K., & Metevia, L. (2001). The efficacy of problem-solving communication training alone, behavior management training alone, and their combination for parent– adolescent conflict in teenagers with ADHD and ODD. *Journal of Consulting and Clinical Psychology, 69*(6), 926–941. doi:10.1037/0022-006X.69.6.926

Barkley, R. A., & Murphy, K. R. (2006). *Attention Deficit Hyperactivity Disorder: A Clinical Workbook* (3rd ed.). Guilford Publications.

Beck, J. S. (2011). *Cognitive behavior therapy: Basics and beyond* (2nd ed.). Guilford Press.

Becker, S. P., & Barley, R. A. (2019). *ADHD in Adolescents: Development, Assessment, and Treatment*. Guilford Publications.

Bird, H. R., Shaffer, D., Fisher, P., & Gould, M. S. (1993). The Columbia impairment scale (CIS): Pilot findings on a measure of global impairment for children and adolescents. *International Journal of Methods in Psychiatric Research, 3*, 167–176.

Brahmbhatt, K., Hilty, D. M., Hah, M., Han, J., Angkustsiri, M. D., & Schweitzer, J. (2016). Diagnosis and Treatment of ADHD during Adolescence in the Primary care setting: Review and Future Directions. *The Journal of Adolescent Health, 59*(2), 135–143. doi:10.1016/j.jadohealth.2016.03.025

Breslau, J., Miller, E., Breslau, N., Bohnert, K., Lucia, V., & Schweitzer, J. (2009). The impact of early behavior disturbances on academic achievement in high school. *Pediatrics, 123*(6), 1472–1476. doi:10.1542/peds.2008-1406

Brown, T. E. (2013). *A new understanding of ADHD in children and adults: Executive function impairments*. Routledge. doi:10.4324/9780203067536

Caspi, A., Block, J., Block, J. H., Klopp, B., Lynam, D., Moffitt, T. E., & Stouthamer-Loeber, M. (1992). A" common-language" version of the California Child Q-Set for personality assessment. *Psychological Assessment, 4*(4), 512–523. doi:10.1037/1040-3590.4.4.512

Caye, A., Spadini, A. V., Karam, R. G., Grevet, E. H., Rovaris, D. L., Bau, C. H., Rohde, L. A., & Kieling, C. (2016). Predictors of persistence of ADHD into adulthood: A systematic review of the literature and meta-analysis. *European Child & Adolescent Psychiatry, 25*(11), 1151–1159. doi:10.100700787-016-0831-8

Chronis, A. M., Chacko, A., Fabiano, G. A., Wymbs, B. T., & Pelham, W. E. Jr. (2004). Enhancements to the behavioral parent training paradigm for families of children with ADHD: Review and future directions. *Clinical Child and Family Psychology Review*, *7*(1), 1–27. doi:10.1023/B:CCFP.0000020190.60808.a4

Conners, C. K. (2008). *Conners* (3rd ed.). Multi-Health Systems.

Connor, D. F. (2011, August 11). Problems of overdiagnosis and overprescribing in ADHD. *The Psychiatric Times*.

Daly, B. P., Creed, T., Xanthopoulos, M., & Brown, R. T. (2007). Psychosocial treatments for children with attention deficit/hyperactivity disorder. *Neuropsychology Review*, *17*(1), 73–89. doi:10.100711065-006-9018-2

Daly, B. P., Hildenbrand, A. K., & Brown, R. T. (2015). *ADHD in Children and Adolescents*. Hogrefe Publishing.

DeFries, J. C., & Fulker, D. W. (1985). Multiple regression analysis of twin data. *Behavior Genetics*, *15*(5), 467–473. doi:10.1007/BF01066239

DeFries, J. C., & Fulker, D. W. (1988). Multiple regression analysis of twin data: Etiology of deviant scores versus individual differences. *ActaGeneticaeMedicaeetGemellologiae*, *37*, 205–216.

DuPaul, G. J., Power, T. J., Anastopoulos, A. D., & Reid, R. (1998). *ADHD rating scale–IV (for children and adolescents): Checklists, norms, and clinical interpretation*. Guilford.

Elia, J., Ambrosini, P., & Berrettini, W. (2008). ADHD characteristics: I. Concurrent co-morbidity patterns in children and adolescents. *Child and Adolescent Psychiatry and Mental Health*, *2*(1), 15. doi:10.1186/1753-2000-2-15

Emilsson, B., Gudjonsson, G., Sigurdsson, J. F., Baldursson, G., Einarsson, E., Ofafsdottir, H., & Young, S. (2011). Cognitive behaviour therapy in medication-treated adults with ADHD and persistent symptoms: A randomized controlled trial. *BMC Psychiatry*, *11*(1), 116. doi:10.1186/1471-244X-11-116

Epstein, J. N., Langberg, J. M., Lichtenstein, P. K., Mainwaring, B. A., Luzader, C. P., & Stark, L. J. (2008). Community-wide intervention to improve the attention-deficit/hyperactivity disorder assessment and treatment practices of community physicians. *Pediatrics*, *122*(1), 19–27. doi:10.1542/peds.2007-2704

Evans, S. W., Owens, J. S., & Bunford, N. (2014). Evidence-based psychosocial treatments for children and adolescents with attention-deficit/hyperactivity disorder. *Journal of Clinical Child and Adolescent Psychology*, *43*(4), 527–551. doi:10.1080/15374416.2013.850700

Evans, S. W., Pelham, W. E., Smith, B. H., Bukstein, O., Gnagy, E. M., Greiner, A. R., Altenderfer, L., & Baron-Myak, C. (2001). Dose-response effects of methylphenidate on ecologically valid measures of academic performance and classroom behavior in adolescents with ADHD. *Experimental and Clinical Psychopharmacology*, *9*(2), 163–175. doi:10.1037/1064-1297.9.2.163

Fischer, M., Barkley, R. A., Smallish, L., & Fletcher, K. (2002). Young adult follow-up of hyperactive children: Self-reported psychiatric disorders, comorbidity, and the role of childhood conduct problems and teen CD. *Journal of Abnormal Child Psychology*, *30*(5), 463–475. doi:10.1023/A:1019864813776

Flory, K., Molina, B., Pelham, W. Jr, Gnagy, E., & Smith, B. (2006). Childhood ADHD Predicts Risky Sexual Behaviorin Young Adulthood. *Journal of Clinical Child and Adolescent Psychology*, *35*(4), 571–577. doi:10.120715374424jccp3504_8

Goodwin, G. M. (2009). Evidence-based guidelines for treating bipolar disorder: Revised second edition recommendations from the British Association of Psychopharmacology. Journal of Psychopharmacology, 4, 346– 388.

Gresham, F. M., & Elliot, S. N. (1990). *Social skills rating system manual*. American Guidance Service.

Grogan, M., & Weitzman, J. (2015). Using the 12-steps as a Parenting intervention with ADHD Adolescents. *The American Journal of Family Therapy*, *43*(4), 364–377. doi:10.1080/01926187.2015.1051904

Hafner, H., & An Der, H. W. (1997). Epidemiology of Schizophrenia. *Canadian Journal of Psychiatry*, *42*(2), 139–151. doi:10.1177/070674379704200204

Harpin, V., Mazzone, L., Raynaud, J. P., Kahle, J., & Hodgkins, P. (2013). Long-Term Outcomes of ADHD: A Systematic Review of Self-Esteem and Social Function. *Journal of Attention Disorders*.

Heal, D. J., Smith, S. L., & Findling, R. L. (2012). ADHD: Current and future therapeutics. *Current Topics in Behavioral Neurosciences*, *9*, 361–390. doi:10.1007/7854_2011_125

Hinshaw, S. P. (2017). Developmental psychopathology as a scientific discipline: A 21st-century perspective. In T. P. Beauchaine & S. P. Hinshaw (Eds.), *Child and adolescent psychopathology* (3rd ed., pp. 3–32). Wiley.

Kaufman, J., Birmaher, B., Brent, D., Rao, U., & Ryan, N. (1996). *Kiddie-Sads-present and Lifetime version (K-SADS-PL)*. University of Pittsburgh, School of Medicine.

Keeley, L. M., Makol, B. G., Qasmieh, N., Deros, D. E., Karp, J. N., Lipton, M. F., Augenstein, T. M., Truong, M. L., Racz, S. J., & Reyes, A. D. L. (2018). Validity of Adolescent and Parent Reports on the Six-Item ADHD Self Report Scale (ASRS-6) in Clinical Assessments of Adolescent Social Anxiety. *Journal of Child and Family Studies*, *27*(4), 1041–1053. doi:10.100710826-017-0950-y

Kent, K. M., Pelham, W. E., Molina, B. S. G., Waschbusch, D. A., Yu, J., Sibley, M. H., & … . (in press). The academicexperience of male high school students with ADHD. Paper submitted for publication. *Journal of Abnormal Child Psychology*.

Klein, R. G., Mannuzza, S., Olazagasti, M. A., Roizen, E., Hutchison, J. A., Lashua, E. C., & Castellanos, F. X. (2012). Clinical and functional outcome of childhood attention-deficit/hyperactivity disorder 33 years later. *Archives of General Psychiatry*, *69*(12), 1295–1303. doi:10.1001/archgenpsychiatry.2012.271

Kovacs, M. (1995). *Manual: The Children's Depression Inventory*. Multi-Health Systems.

Leeth, C. D., Villarreal, V., & Styck, K. M. (2019). Mindfulness Interventions for Children and Adolescents with ADHD: A Review of Objectives and Skills. *Journal of Creativity in Mental Health*, *14*(4), 436–446. doi:10.1080/15401383.2019.1625840

LeFever, G. B., Arcona, A. P., & Antonuccio, D. O. (2003). ADHD among American schoolchildren: Evidence of overdiagnosis and overuse of medication. *The Scientific Review of Mental Health Practice, 2*, 49–60.

Loe, I.M., & Feldman, H.M. (2007).Academic and educational outcomes of children with ADHD. *Ambulatory Pediatrics: The Official Journal of the Ambulatory Pediatric Association, 7*(1), 82–90.

March, J. S., Parker, J. D. A., Sullivan, K., Stallings, P., & Conners, K. (1997). The multidimensional anxiety scale for children (MASC): Factor structure, reliability, and validity. *Journal of the American Academy of Child and Adolescent Psychiatry, 36*(4), 554–565. doi:10.1097/00004583-199704000-00019

Marsh, P. J., & Williams, L. M. (2004). An investigation of individual typologies of AttentionDeficit Hyperactivity Disorder using cluster analysis of DSM-IV criteria. *Personality and Individual Differences, 36*(5), 1187–1195. doi:10.1016/S0191-8869(03)00210-1

Meyers, J. E., & Meyers, K. R. (1995). *Rey complex figure test and recognition trial.* Psychological Assessment Resources.

Miller, C. J., Newcorn, J. H., & Halperin, J. M. (2010). Fading memories: Retrospective recall inaccuracies in ADHD. *Journal of Attention Disorders, 14*(1), 7–14. doi:10.1177/1087054709347189

Molina, B. S. G., Pelham, W. E., Gnagy, E. M., Thompson, A. L., & Marshal, M. P. (2007). Attention-deficit/hyperactivitydisorder risk for heavy drinking and alcohol use disorder is age specific. *Alcoholism, Clinical and Experimental Research, 31*, 643–654.

Nichols, J. Q. V. A., Shoulberg, E. K., Garner, A. A., Hoza, B., Burt, K. B., Close, D. M., & Arnold, L. E. (2017). Exploration of the Factor Structure of ADHD in Adolescence through Self, Parent, and Teacher Reports of Symptomatology. *Journal of Abnormal Child Psychology, 45*(3), 625–641. doi:10.100710802-016-0183-3

Nigg, J. T. (2013). Attention-deficit/hyperactivity disorder and adverse health outcomes. *Clinical Psychology Review, 33*(2), 215–228. doi:10.1016/j.cpr.2012.11.005

Nigg, J. T., & Huang-Pollock, C. L. (2003). An early-onset model of the role of executive functions and intelligence in conduct disorder/delinquency. In B. B. Lahey, T. E. Moffitt, & A. Caspi (Eds.), *Cause of conduct disorder and juvenile delinquency* (pp. 227–253). Guilford Press.

Otto, M. W. (2000). Stories and metaphors in cognitive-behavioral therapy. *Cognitive and Behavioral Practice, 7*(2), 172–177. doi:10.1016/S1077-7229(00)80027-9

Park, M. J., Paul Mulye, T., Adams, S. H., Brindis, C. D., & Irwin, C. E. Jr. (2006). The health status of young adults in the United States. *The Journal of Adolescent Health, 39*(3), 305–317. doi:10.1016/j.jadohealth.2006.04.017

Patros, C. H., Hudec, K. L., Alderson, R. M., Kasper, L. J., Davidson, C., & Wingate, L. R. (2013). Symptoms of attention-deficit/hyperactivity disorder (ADHD) moderate suicidal behaviors in college students with depressed mood. *Journal of Clinical Psychology, 69*(9), 980–993. doi:10.1002/jclp.21994

Pennington, B. F., & Ozonoff, S. (1996). Executive functions and developmental psychopathology. *Journal of Child Psychology and Psychiatry, and Allied Disciplines*, *37*(1), 51–87. doi:10.1111/j.1469-7610.1996.tb01380.x

Pettersson, R., Soderstrom, S., Edlund-Soderstrom, K., & Nilsson, K. W. (2017). Internet-based cognitive behavioral therapy for adults with ADHD in outpatient psychiatric care: A randomized trial. *Journal of Attention Disorders*, *21*(6), 508–521. doi:10.1177/1087054714539998

Polanczyk, G., de Lima, M. S., Horta, B. L., Biederman, J., & Rohde, L. A. (2007). The worldwide prevalence of ADHD: A systematic review and metaregression analysis. *The American Journal of Psychiatry*, *164*(6), 942–948. doi:10.1176/ajp.2007.164.6.942

Quinlan, D. M. (2000). Assessment of attention-deficit/hyperactivity disorder and comorbidities. In T. E. Brown (Ed.), *Attention-deficit disorders and comorbidities in children, adolescents, and adults* (pp. 455–508). American Psychiatric Press.

Reich, W. (2000). Diagnostic Interview for Children and Adolescents (DICA). *Journal of the American Academy of Child and Adolescent Psychiatry*, *39*(1), 59–66. doi:10.1097/00004583-200001000-00017

Reynolds, C. R., & Kamphaus, R. W. (2015). *Behavior Assessment System for Children. 3*. Pearson.

Rutter, M. (2005). Environmentally mediated risks for psychopathology: Research strategies and findings. *Journal of Child Psychology and Psychiatry, and Allied Disciplines*, *44*(1), 3–18.

Safren, S. A., Perlman, C. A., Sprich, S. E., & Otto, M. W. (2005). *Mastering your adult ADHD: A cognitive behavioral treatment program, therapist guide*. Oxford University Press.

Sibley, M. H., Comer, J. S., & Gonazalez, J. (2017). Delivering Parent-Teen Therapy for ADHD through Videoconferencing: A preliminary investigation. *Journal of Psychopathology and Behavioral Assessment*, *39*(3), 467–485. doi:10.100710862-017-9598-6

Sibley, M. H., Kuriyan, A. B., Evans, S. W., Waxmonsky, J. G., & Smith, B. H. (2014). Pharmacological and psychosocial treatments for adolescents with ADHD: An updated systematic review of the literature. *Clinical Psychology Review*, *34*(3), 218–232. doi:10.1016/j.cpr.2014.02.001

Sibley, M. H., Pelham, E. M., Molina, B. S. G., Gnaggy, E. M., Waschbusch, D. A., Garefino, A. C., & … . (2012). Diagnosing ADHD in Adolescence. *Journal of Consulting and Clinical Psychology*, *80*(1), 139–150. doi:10.1037/a0026577

Sibley, M. H., Pelham, W. E., Molina, B. S. G., Gnagy, E. M., Waschbusch, D. A., Biswas, A., MacLean, M. G., Babinski, D. E., & Karch, K. M. (2011). TheDelinquency Outcomes of Boys with ADHD with and without comorbidity. *Journal of Abnormal Child Psychology*, *39*(1), 21–32. doi:10.100710802-010-9443-9

Smith, B. H., Pelham, W. E. Jr, Gnagy, E., Molina, B., & Evans, S. (2000). The reliability, validity, and unique contributions of self-report by adolescents receiving treatment for attention-deficit/hyperactivity disorder. *Journal of Consulting and Clinical Psychology*, *68*(3), 489–499. doi:10.1037/0022-006X.68.3.489

Smith, T. E., & Martel, M. M. (2019). Trait-Based Profiles of ADHD in Adolescents and Young Adults. *Journal of Clinical Child and Adolescent Psychology*, *48*(3), 440–454. doi:10.1080/15374416.2018.1491004

Sparrow, E. P., & Erhardt, D. (2014). *Essentials of ADHD Assessment for Children and Adolescents.* John Wiley & Sons.

Spencer, T. J. (2004). ADHD treatment across the life cycle. *The Journal of Clinical Psychiatry, 65*(3), 22–26.

Sprich, S. E., Safren, S. A., Finkelstein, D., Remmert, J. E., & Hammerness, P. (2016). A randomized controlled trial of cognitive behavioral therapy for ADHD in medication treated adolescents. *Journal of Child Psychology and Psychiatry, and Allied Disciplines, 57*(11), 1218–1226. doi:10.1111/jcpp.12549

Steinhausen, H.-C. (2009). The heterogeneity of causes and courses of attention-deficit hyperactivity disorder. *Acta Psychiatrica Scandinavica, 120*(5), 392–399. doi:10.1111/j.1600-0447.2009.01446.x

Stergiakouli, E., & Thapar, A. (2010). Fitting the pieces together: Current research on the genetic basis of attention-deficit/hyperactivity disorder (ADHD). *Journal of Neuropsychiatric Disease and Treatment, 6*, 551–560. doi:10.2147/NDT.S11322

Stroop, J. R. (1935). Studies of interference in serial verbal reactions. *Journal of Experimental Psychology, 18*(6), 643–662. doi:10.1037/h0054651

Swanson, J. M., Schuck, S., Mann, M., Carlson, C., Hartman, K., Sergeant, J. A., & Wigal, T. (2001). *Categorical and dimensional definitions and evaluations of symptoms of ADHD: the SNAP and SWAN ratings scales.* Academic Press.

Teichner, G. (2016). *Attention-Deficit/Hyperactivity Disorder in Children and Adolescents: A DSM-5 Handbook for Medical and Mental Health Professionals.* Momentum Press.

Thapar, A., Harrington, R., & McGuffin, P. (2001). Examining the comorbidity of ADHD-related behaviours and conduct problems using a twin study design. *The British Journal of Psychiatry, 179*(3), 224–229. doi:10.1192/bjp.179.3.224

Thompson, A., Molina, B., Pelham, W., & Gnagy, E. (2007). Risky driving in adolescents and young adults withchildhood ADHD. *Journal of Pediatric Psychology, 32*(7), 745–759. doi:10.1093/jpepsy/jsm002

Van der Oord, S., Ponsioen, A. J. G. B., Geurts, H. M., Brink, E. L. T., & Prins, P. J. M. (2014). A pilot study of the efficacy of a computerized executive functioning remediation training with game elements for children with ADHD in an outpatient setting: Outcome on parentand teacher-rated executive functioning and ADHD behavior. *Journal of Attention Disorders, 18*(8), 699–712. doi:10.1177/1087054712453167

Visser, S. N., Danielson, M. L., Bitsko, R. H., Holbrook, J. R., Kogan, M. D., Ghandour, R. M., & Blumberg, S. J. (2014). Trends in the parent-report of health care provider-diagnosed and medicated attention-deficit/hyperactivity disorder: United states, 2003– 2011. *Journal of the American Academy of Child and Adolescent Psychiatry, 53*(1), 34–46. doi:10.1016/j.jaac.2013.09.001

Wechsler, D. (1992). *Wechsler individual achievement test: Manual.* Psychological Corp.

Wechsler, D. (2004). *WISC-IV: Wechsler Intelligence Scale for Children, Integrated: Technical and interpretive manual.* Harcourt Brace.

Willcutt, E. G. (2012). The prevalence of DSM-IV attention-deficit/hyperactivity disorder: A meta-analytic review. *Neurotherapeutics; the Journal of the American Society for Experimental NeuroTherapeutics, 9*(3), 490–499. doi:10.100713311-012-0135-8

Willcutt, E. G., Betjemann, R. S., McGrath, L. M., Chhabildas, N. A., Olson, R. K., DeFries, J. C., & Pennington, B. F. (2010). Etiology and neuropsychology of comorbidity between RD and ADHD: The case for multiple-deficit models. *Cortex, 46*(10), 1345–1361. doi:10.1016/j.cortex.2010.06.009

Willcutt, E. G., Betjemann, R. S., Pennington, B. F., Olson, R. K., DeFries, J. C., & Wadsworth, S. J. (2007). Longitudinal study of reading disability and attentiondeficit/hyperactivity disorder: Implications for education. *Mind, Brain and Education: the Official Journal of the International Mind, Brain, and Education Society, 4*(4), 181–192. doi:10.1111/j.1751-228X.2007.00019.x

Willcutt, E. G., Pennington, B. F., Duncan, L., Smith, S. D., Keenan, J. M., Wadsworth, S. J., DeFries, J. C., & Olson, R. K. (2010). Understanding the complex etiology of developmental disorders: Behavioral and molecular genetic approaches. *Journal of Developmental and Behavioral Pediatrics, 31*(7), 533–544. doi:10.1097/DBP.0b013e3181ef42a1

Wolraich, M. L., Wibbelsman, C. J., & Brown, T. E. (2005). Attention-deficit/hyperactivity disorder among adolescents: A review of the diagnosis, treatment, and clinical implications. *Pediatrics, 115*(6), 1734–1746. doi:10.1542/peds.2004-1959

Young, S. (2005). Coping strategies used by adults with ADHD. *Personality and Individual Differences, 38*(4), 809–816. doi:10.1016/j.paid.2004.06.005

Young, S., & Bramhan, J. (2012). *Cognitive-Behavioural Therapy for ADHD in Adolescents and Adults: A Psychological Guide to Practice* (2nd ed.). John Wiley & Sons. doi:10.1002/9781119943440

ADDITIONAL READING

Buitelaar, J. K. (2017). Optimising treatment strategies for ADHD in Adolescence to minimize 'lost in transition' to adulthood. *Epidemiology and Psychiatric Sciences, 26*(5), 448–452. doi:10.1017/S2045796017000154

Chimiklis, A. L., Dahl, V., Spears, A. P., Goss, K., Fogarty, K., & Chacko, A. (2018). Yoga, Mindfulness, and Meditation Interventions for Youth with ADHD: Systematic Review and Meta-Analysis. *Journal of Child and Family Studies, 27*(10), 3155–3168. doi:10.100710826-018-1148-7

Derefinko, K. J., Hayden, A., Sibley, M. H., Duvall, J., Milich, R., & Lorch, E. P. (2014). A Story Mapping intervention to improve narrative comprehension deficits in adolescents with ADHD. *School Mental Health, 6*(4), 251–263. doi:10.100712310-014-9127-7

Kiani, B., Hadianfard, H., & Mitchell, J. T. (2017). The impact of Mindfulness meditation training on executive functions and emotion dysregulation in an Iranian sample of female adolescents with elevated attention-deficit/hyperactivity disorder symptoms. *Australian Journal of Psychology, 69*(4), 273–282. doi:10.1111/ajpy.12148

Schultz, B. K., & Evans, S. W. (2015). *A Practical Guide to Implementing School-Based Interventions for Adolescents with ADHD*. Springer. doi:10.1007/978-1-4939-2677-0

Sciberras, E., Mulraney, M., Mensah, F., Oberklaid, F., Efron, D., & Hiscock, H. (2019). Sustained impact of sleep intervention and moderators of treatment outcome for children with ADHD: A randomised controlled trial. *Psychological Medicine*, *50*(2), 210–219. doi:10.1017/S0033291718004063

Sibley, M. H., Pelham, W. E. Jr, Derefinko, K. J., Kuriyan, A. B., Sanchez, F., & Graziano, P. A. (2013). A Pilot Trial of Supporting Teens' Academic Needs Daily (STAND): A Parent-Adolescent Collaborative Intervention for ADHD. *Journal of Psychopathology and Behavioral Assessment*, *35*(4), 436–449. doi:10.100710862-013-9353-6

Weyandt, L. L., & DuPaul, G. J. (2013). *College Students with ADHD: Current Issues and Future Directions*. Springer. doi:10.1007/978-1-4614-5345-1

Chapter 6
Inattention and Hyperactivity in Adults:
Incorporating New Developments in Existing Scenario of Adult ADHD

Chirag D. Parmar
Gujarat Institute of Mental Health, India

Krunal H. Patel
Gujarat Institute of Mental Health, India

ABSTRACT

This chapter focuses on ADHD in the adult population. The authors of this chapter incorporate new developments in existing understanding of the disorder. This chapter includes journey of 'ADHD diagnosis in adults' to current practice. Understanding of newer aspect of etiological research and its application in identification of adult ADHD is given utmost importance in this chapter. Core parts of the disorder like clinical features, diagnosis, comorbidity, and management are discussed in detail, keeping in mind disease progression from childhood to adulthood. Finally, the authors discussed a lacunae in current scenario and possible future interventions that can improve overall outcome of functional impairments in adults.

INTRODUCTION

Attention-deficit hyperactivity disorder (ADHD) was originally conceptualized as a developmental delay in behavioural control during childhood that was usually outgrown by adolescence. Several lines of evidence support the recognition that ADHD is a disorder across the life span. Seminal work in the 1970s by Paul Wender and colleagues at the University of Utah identified a group of adults with persistent childhood ADHD symptoms who exhibited a response to stimulant treatment similar to that seen in ADHD children. During this same period, longitudinal follow-up studies of adults who had been diagnosed with childhood hyperactivity described the persistence of ADHD symptoms in 40 to 60 percentages of

DOI: 10.4018/978-1-7998-5495-1.ch006

subjects. In the early 1990s, several publications in the lay press spurred widespread public awareness of adult ADHD. These early investigations and the increased public demand for clinical care led to growing interest in the phenomenology, causes, and treatment of adult ADHD. Adult attention-deficit hyperactivity disorder (ADHD) is a mental health disorder that includes a combination of persistent problems, such as difficulty paying attention, hyperactivity and impulsive behaviour. Adult ADHD can lead to unstable relationships, poor work or school performance, low self-esteem, and other problems.

Although ADHD in adulthood is widely acknowledged, some clinicians and investigators continue to question the existence of the disorder. Principal objections include perceptions that ADHD symptoms decline with time; assessment is difficult; the disorder is often confused or coexisting with other psychopathology; and patients' bias clinical reporting to receive a diagnosis that is deemed popular. Nonetheless, several reviews demonstrate that adult ADHD is a valid disorder, can be reliably diagnosed, and predicts treatment response. American Psychiatric Association has included ADHD as a Diagnosable disorder in DSM-5 .Pharmacological, neurocognitive, brain imaging, and genetics studies in adults have replicated findings seen in ADHD children.

Definition and History

Originally, attention-deficit hyperactivity disorder (ADHD; formerly called minimal brain damage) was considered to be a childhood disorder and was therefore not diagnosed in adults. In the second edition of DSM (DSM-II American Psychiatric Association, 1968) the condition now known as ADHD was referred to as hyperkinetic reaction of childhood, with no consideration of an adult disorder. This concept that ADHD was a child-only disorder began to change in the 1970s. For the first time, preliminary reports in 1976 on the nature of ADHD symptoms and psychosocial impairments in adults with a past history of childhood ADHD argued that ADHD might not always be outgrown in adulthood. Authors wood et al.(1976) and Hechtman et al.(1976) emphasized many similarities between ADHD in children and in adults in patterns of core symptoms and comorbidity, association with impairments and cognitive performance measures, and response to medication . Subsequently, in 1980, the category of attention deficit disorder (ADD), residual type, was defined in DSM-III (American Psychiatric Association, 1980); this category provided the first opportunity to make a formal diagnosis of ADHD in adults with a past history of ADD and persisting attention and concentration problems, without a requirement of persisting hyperactivity symptoms. This DSM-III category inherently implied that adults could not meet full diagnostic criteria. This diagnostic possibility must have served a purpose in practice, because its removal in the DSM-III-R (American Psychiatric Association, 1987) led to a request from a number of researchers and clinicians to restore it, efforts followed to define appropriate diagnostic criteria for ADHD in adults (Wender,1987). Although the category of ADD, residual type, was not restored in the DSM-IV, the DSM-IV ADHD criteria were modified in such a way that they could be applied more easily to adults (American Psychiatric Association, 1994). Since then, the acceptance of adult ADHD by the professional community and the general public has been growing (Jaffe, 1995). The Current version of DSM-5 (American Psychiatric Association, 2013) continues to have adult ADHD as diagnostic entity. Several longitudinal follow-up studies convincingly showed that ADHD symptoms persisting significant proportion of adults with a history of childhood ADHD (Mannuzza, Klein, Bessler, Malloy, & LaPadula, 1993 ; Mannuzza, Klein, Bessler, Malloy, & LaPadula, 1998; Weiss & Hechtman, 1993). These studies were important in establishing that ADHD often persisting to adulthood, with age-related changes in the way that the characteristic symptoms of the disorder present in adults.

EPIDEMIOLOGY

Epidemiological studies suggest that ADHD is a prevalent disorder, affecting between 4 and 5 percent of school-aged children. Accurate epidemiological sampling for ADHD in adults is difficult due to the frequency with which it is confused with other conditions and the potential loss of affected individuals among the incarcerated and homeless. Based on the expected persistence of ADHD in 50 to 70 percent of childhood cases, investigators have estimated the prevalence of adult ADHD in the range of 2 to 4 percent. Recent evidence supports a prevalence rate of 4 percent, suggesting that adult ADHD is a major public health concern.

Prevalence of ADHD in Women

As ADHD in adults became more widely recognized and treated in the mid-1990s; a number of adult ADHD clinics were established. Informal reports emerging from these clinics initially suggested that the percentage of women self-referred to these clinics was much higher than the percentage of males with ADHD previously reported in the literature. More recent studies investigating gender ratios of adults with ADHD have found that the difference in prevalence rates for males and females may diminish in adulthood (Faraone et al., 2000). Although the rearing reliable data on the number of women with ADHD or the true male-to-female ratio of adults with ADHD, all of these reports strongly suggest that women with ADHD represent a more significant proportion of adults with ADHD than has been previously recognized.

ETIOLOGY

ADHD is principally a genetic disorder. Twin and family genetics studies demonstrate that the mean heritability of ADHD exceeds 80 percent. Approximately one-third of adults with ADHD have at least one child with the disorder, and similarly, one-third of children with ADHD have at least one affected parent. Evidence suggests that ADHD is a complex behavioural phenotype resulting from multiple genes, each contributing additive risk for the condition. Molecular genetic studies have identified numerous candidate genes, many of which appear to play a role in brain catecholamine activity, that are possibly associated with ADHD. Several teams of investigators have independently demonstrated an increased association of the 7-repeat allele polymorphism at the dopamine type 4 receptor (DRD4) gene located on chromosome 11 with ADHD. This increased association of DRD4 has been identified in both juveniles and adults with ADHD. Early reports of major gene effects from other potential risk factor alleles require further replication.

Twin Studies in Adults

Despite the high heritability reported from child and adolescent twin samples this has not been the case for comparable studies in adults which show heritability in the region of 0.30 to 0.40 (Boomsma et al. 2010). The reasons for this discrepancy are not yet fully understood but may be due, at least in part, to the use of self-rated data in the adult studies rather than informant-rated data used in most child and adolescent studies. This has been shown in the child and adolescent literature where studies that have included self-ratings of ADHD symptoms find far lower heritability that those based on parent and teacher reports. One study that investigated this question used parent, teacher, and self-ratings in a sample of 11 to 16 year olds and found no evidence of a heritable phenotype using self-report of ADHD symptoms (Scourfield, M. & McGuffin, P. 2002). In this study, correlations for MZ and DZ pairs were 0.73 and 0.25 for parent ratings and 0.81 and 0.38 for teacher ratings, respectively–giving high estimates of heritability in the region of 0.7–0.8. However, the correlation for self-rated ADHD symptoms among the same 11 to 16 year olds were 0.29 for both MZ and DZ twin pairs, indicating no genetic effects at all and only a moderate familial effect due entirely to environmental factors. Although the self-ratings of ADHD symptoms in this study used a comparatively short scale consisting of only a few broad symptom items, the difference in heritability estimates for self-ratings compared to informant ratings was very striking.

The general conclusion of low heritability for self-rated current ADHD symptoms in adults is further supported by a large sample of Swedish adult twins that estimated heritability to be around 0.35 (Larsson, Chang, D'Onofrio, & Lichtenstein, 2014).This finding is again consistent with that of the adolescent study of self-reported symptoms from Ehringer and colleagues (2006) and the recent adult twin study from Boomsma (2010).

In conclusion several published and unpublished studies confirm that heritability for self-rated ADHD in adult population samples is around 30%, with the majority of the phenotypic variance accounted for by unique environmental factors and measurement error. One explanation for the relatively low heritability could be low test–test reliability of self-reported ratings of ADHD symptoms in adults.

However, there can be potential sources of error that might give rise to low heritability estimates in self-ratings of ADHD symptoms in adults and require further exploration. First, as discussed earlier, self-ratings of current ADHD symptoms in adolescence confirm the importance of ratter effects because we know there is a major discrepancy in heritability estimates derived from self-and informant ratings during adolescence. Second, another potentially important factor is age of onset of the reported symptoms. Self-rating scales should therefore be used with caution in genetic epidemiological studies of ADHD in adults. Studies of ADHD in adults should focus on reporter ratings (spouse, close relative, employer) in addition to self-ratings and on the continuity of symptoms from childhood through to adulthood.

Adoption Studies of Adult ADHD

Another important source of information on the genetic influences on adult ADHD is derived from adoption data. Several reports have suggested that the familial risk for ADHD in adults is mediated predominantly by genetic and not environmental influences, based on different rates of ADHD among biological and non-biological (adoptive) parents of children with ADHD. Initial reports from early family studies found that adoptive parents of hyperactive children were less likely than biological parents to have hyperactivity or associated disorders (Cantwell, 1972; Morrison & Stewart, 1971).

Adult ADHD symptoms reported by both self and informant reports were found to be higher among the parents of children with ADHD, with increased levels of inattentiveness and cognitive problems, hyperactivity and restlessness, impulsivity, and emotional lability. The sample contained both biological and nonbiological parents, and the informant data showed that among the parents of ADHD children levels of inattention, cognitive problems, impulsivity, and emotional lability were higher for biological parents compared to non-biological parents. The informant data but not the self-ratings of ADHD symptoms therefore supported the hypothesis that the familial association of parent ADHD with offspring ADHD is the result of biological factors and therefore likely to be explained by genetic factors shared between parent and offspring.

Persistence of Symptoms and the Genetics of ADHD

One family studies of ADHD in adults (Biederman et al., 1995) found that the risk of ADHD among the offspring of adults with ADHD was much higher than the risk of ADHD among relatives of children with ADHD. For example, the 57% prevalence of ADHD among children of parents with adult ADHD was much higher than the 15% prevalence of ADHD among siblings of children with ADHD (Biederman et al., 1995). This high familial loading of adult ADHD suggests that genes, or other familial risk factors, may play a greater role in the aetiology of persistent ADHD than they do for remitting ADHD. This "persistence" hypothesis was tested in two ways.

In a prospective study, 140 ADHD boys and 120 non-ADHD boys were examined at a baseline assessment and completed a 4-year follow-up study. By mid–adolescence, 85% of the ADHD boys continued to have the disorder, whereas 15% showed remission of symptoms. The prevalence of ADHD was significantly higher among the relatives of persistent ADHD probands compared to the relatives of remitted ADHD probands (Biederman et al., 1996). Parents of persistent ADHD probands had a recurrence rate of ADHD of 16.3% compared to 10.8% for parents of non-persistent ADHD probands, whereas siblings of persistent ADHD probands had a recurrence rate of ADHD of 24.4% compared to 4.6% among siblings of non-persistent ADHD probands (Biederman et al., 1995; Faraone, Biederman, & Friedman, 2000).

In a retrospective study, ADHD adolescents having retrospectively reported childhood-onset ADHD were compared with ADHD children. The relatives of adolescent probands had higher rates of ADHD compared with the relatives of child probands (Biederman et al., 1995).

Thus, a prospective study of children and a retrospective study of adolescents suggest that, when ADHD persists in to adolescence and adulthood, it shows greater familial loading for ADHD than do non-persistent forms of ADHD. Taken together, these data suggest that, from a familial perspective, not only is the adult ADHD diagnosis valid, but it might actually be more valid than the childhood diagnosis – because the familial transmission of ADHD seems to be greater for adults than children with ADHD. This leads to the straightforward prediction that familial transmission is greater when examining ADHD symptoms in adult relatives than it is when examining symptoms in non-adult relatives.

Molecular Genetic Findings:

We have already described how international research has established that there is a strong genetically inherited contribution to ADHD. It is established that certain alleles (sequence variants) of the gene coding for the dopamine D4 receptor (DRD4) occur more frequently in children with ADHD than in healthy controls, and other DNA changes associated with ADHD have been found as well.

Several linkage studies that scan the entire human genome have been completed that indicate suggestive target regions containing one or more risk genes for ADHD. More recently, enormous expectations have been generated by the development of very high-density genetic marker maps that enable scans of the human genome for association with common genetic variations, using single-nucleotide polymorphism (SNP) arrays that assay hundreds of thousands of markers in one experiment.

Several Genome Wide Association Studies (GWAS) have been initiated for ADHD, and initial data have identified several potential genes associated with ADHD that were not the target of previous candidate gene studies (Franke, Neale, & Faraone, 2009). The strongest of these initial findings is perhaps the association with the Cadherin 13 gene (CDH13). This gene lies within the region of linkage on chromosome 16 identified in the meta-analysis of linkage studies (Zhou,et al., 2008). SNPs within the CDH13 gene region were reported to be associated with ADHD in are analysis of the genome wide association scan study from the IMAGE sample using a two-stage approach (Lasky-Su, et al. 2008) .

Functional MRI studies in ADHD

Task-dependent functional deficits in adults with ADHD: Studies have shown both regional and network-wide deficits during the performance of working memory tasks by adults with ADHD. Decreased activation, compared to healthy controls, has been found in the left inferior frontal gyrus, the occipital gyrus, and the cerebellum (Valera, Faraone, Biederman, Poldrack, & Seidman, (2005); Wolf et al.,2009) as well as the right insula and the medial frontal gyrus (Wolf et al.,2009), whereas increased activation at the right cerebellum was associated with lower ADHD symptoms.

Adults with ADHD have also shown abnormal functional connectivity patterns in nodes of working memory/executive function and attention networks, such as the inferior and superior frontal gyri, the anterior cingulate cortex, and the superior parietal lobule (Wolf et al., 2009). Enhanced functional connectivity of the right inferior frontal gyrus was associated with improved task performance in the high load condition in the ADHD group (Wolf et al., 2009). An interesting study has suggested that the commonly observed executive function deficits in ADHD may be partly caused by deficits in more fundamental processes (Hale, Bookheimer, McGough, Phillips, & McCracken, 2007).

Adults with ADHD showed atypical brain activation in task-related networks while performing both variations so fat ask that differed in their load on executive functions. Digit span backward is considered to be an executive function/ working memory task, whereas digit span forward involves a single component process requiring the simple repetition of a series of numbers. The authors suggested that deficits in higher mental processes, such as executive functions, may stem from dysfunction in more fundamental neural systems engaged in "access to, or generation of, phonologically represented in formation" (Hale et al., 2007). Thus ADHD may be associated with a dysfunction in fundamental neural systems that may lead to a deficit in higher order executive functions such as inhibitory control.

ADHD adults studied with positron emission tomography (PET) exhibited decreased prefrontal cortex glucose metabolism. Several studies using single photon emission tomography (SPECT) demonstrated increased dopamine transporter (DAT) binding densities in the striatal regions. This is a particularly interesting finding, given that methylphenidate blocks DAT activity, possibly leading to normalized DAT functioning, and is consistent with reports implicating the DAT gene with ADHD.

Electrophysiological Studies of Adult ADHD

Investigations of adult ADHD, which use electrophysiological techniques (electroencephalography [EEG] and event-related potential [ERPs]), have indicated persistence of neurophysiological abnormalities in ADHD. Electrophysiology measures neural activation with millisecond resolution, which allows precise tracking of differential steps in information processing. This constitutes a significant advantage of these methods over behavioural and brain imaging techniques (e.g. PET, fMRI), which have a temporal resolution in the order of seconds. However, electrophysiological methods are more limited than neuroimaging techniques for localizing brain processes.

The most consistent finding from EEG studies in ADHD is that children, adolescents, and adults with the disorder exhibit increased theta activity when compared with controls, particularly relative to other frequencies during the eyes-closed resting condition (Bresnahan, Anderson & Barry, 1999; Chabot & Serfontein, 1996; Koehler et al., 2009) This slow-wave activity occurs in the frequency band of 3.5–7.5 cycles per second (Hz) range and is associated with drowsiness and cortical under arousal.

A number of studies suggest increased alpha activity in adults with ADHD (Bresnahan, Anderson, & Barry,1999; Koehler et al., 2009), both during eyes-closed resting and task conditions. There is inconsistency in the findings related to delta activity in adult ADHD, with one study reporting increased activity (Bresnahan, Barry, Clarke, & Johnstone, 2006.; Hermens et al., 2004), one reporting a reduction in activity(Clarke et al. 2008), and another reporting no differences in delta activity between cases and controls (Koehler et al.,2009).

Environmental Factors in ADHD

Several environmental variables contribute increased risk for development of childhood ADHD, notably maternal use of nicotine during pregnancy, birth before completion of 32 weeks' gestation, and increased serum lead levels. Although it appears that between 30 and 50 percent of children demonstrate remission from the full ADHD syndrome, it is unclear which factors contribute to the persistence of ADHD into adulthood. Adverse factors such as paternal incarceration, parental mental illness, financial stress, foster care, and child abuse increase risk for more severe adult outcomes, whereas higher intelligence and consistent structure at home and school appear to decrease risk. Further elucidation of specific risk factors for adult persistence may facilitate development of preventative strategies and improved long-term outcomes.

CLINICAL FEATURES AND DIAGNOSIS

Clinical Significance of ADHD in Adults:

If adult ADHD is a clinically significant disorder, then adults with ADHD should show functional impairments in multiple domains. The ADHD adults had fewer years of education and lower rates of professional employment. Compared with the non-ADHD adults, more ADHD adults had had their driver's license suspended, had performed poorly at work, and had quit or been fired from their job. Barkley et al. (1996) evaluated the motor vehicle driving knowledge and skills and negative driving outcomes of older teens and young adults with ADHD. Although the young adults with ADHD showed no deficits in driving knowledge, they had elevated rates of speeding citations, suspended licenses, crashes, and accidents causing bodily injury compared to those without ADHD. They were more likely to be rated by themselves and others as having poorer driving habits. In addition, on a computer-simulated driving test, young adults with ADHD had more crashes, scrapes, and erratic steering.

Given that academic underachievement is a well-known correlate of ADHD in childhood (Hinshaw, 1992), ADHD adults ought to have histories reflecting school problems. Several studies have shown this to be so. Compared with control adults, ADHD adults had significantly higher rates of repeated grades, tutoring, placement in special classes, and reading disability. In one survey of 1001 ADHD and non-ADHD adults in the United States (Biederman et al., 2006), which had the largest sample of community-diagnosed adults with ADHD ever studied, showed that adults with self-reported ADHD in the community suffer from significant impairments across multiple domains of functioning. Adult ADHD to be associated with histories of school failure, occupational impairment, substance use, traffic violations, arrests, decreased quality of life, and sexual problems. Taken together, these findings support the idea that, even in those adults diagnosed in the community, ADHD is a clinically significant and highly disabling disorder (Biederman et al., 2006).

Recognition of ADHD in Adults

Recently in Diagnostic and Statistical Manual of Mental Disorder edition 5, the diagnosis of adult ADHD has been acknowledged. Diagnosis of ADHD in child requires six or more inattentive or hyperactive/impulsive symptoms from any of those domains; this requirement was decreased to five symptoms in either domain for diagnosis of patients aged 17 years and older. Apparently those symptoms should have been started before the age of 12 year.

Inattention Symptom Examples:

- Does not pay close attention to details or makes careless mistakes
- Has trouble keeping attention on activities
- Does not seem to listen when spoken to directly
- Does not follow through no instructions and fails to finish tasks
- Has difficulty organizing tasks and activities
- Avoids, dislikes, or is reluctant to do tasks requiring sustained mental effort
- Loses things necessary to do tasks or activities
- Is easily distracted
- Is forgetful in daily activities

Hyperactivity or Impulsiveness Symptom Examples:

- Fidgets with hands or feet or squirms in seat
- Leaves seat at times when remaining seated is expected
- Feels restless
- Has difficulty taking part in leisure activities
- Is "on the go" or acts as if "driven by a motor"
- Talks excessively
- Blurts out answers before questions have been completed
- Has difficulty awaiting turn
- Interrupts conversations or intrudes on other's activities

Clinicians use DSM symptoms to determine retrospectively if criteria for ADHD were met in childhood. If there is evidence of a childhood diagnosis, patients are questioned as to the on-going persistence of DSM symptoms. A diagnosis of adult ADHD is made if patients meet retrospective childhood and current ADHD criteria. Information derived from third-party sources, such as interviews with parents or older siblings, school records, and employment evaluations, can provide collaborative support for the diagnosis.

Interpretation of DSM criteria, while assessment of an adult can be used liberally if concerned physician find it suitable. History of ADHD in childhood, current symptoms of ADHD and significant functional impairment can be the influencing point while considering liberal use of criteria. Clinicians are encouraged to incorporate well-standardized ADHD rating scales into adult assessments to quantify patient deviance from population norms. Clinicians are also find it appropriate to offer the treatment to patients with clear childhood histories and on-going ADHD-related difficulties, even if current symptoms fall below the threshold required for a formal diagnosis. A diagnosis of ADHD in partial remission is allowed for patients who met criteria in childhood and currently experience on-going symptoms and impairment but fall short of full diagnostic criteria. Assessment of adult ADHD requires careful consideration of the potential for other comorbid psychopathology.

Utah Criteria

Wender(1995, pp 122-43) had developed criteria for adult ADHD, which is also known as the Utah criteria. This criterion focuses on the distinct nature of the disorder in adults. For diagnosis of adult ADHD, as a primary requirement ADHD symptoms must been consistently present during childhood in absence of any therapy. In adulthood primary symptoms like hyperactivity and poor concentration must be present. Additionally there should be presence two symptoms out of the five symptoms: affective lability; hot temper; inability to complete tasks and disorganization; stress intolerance; and impulsivity.

Utah criteria are used widely in clinical practice. Nonetheless, the criteria have several limitations. First, with subsequent editions of the DSM, Utah criteria have increasingly diverged from current conceptualizations of the childhood ADHD. Second, Utah criteria make a diagnosis only in patients who experience both inattention and hyperactivity. By definition, this excludes those patients with the primarily inattentive ADHD subtype and those patients whose hyperactive symptoms, but not inattentive symptoms, remit. Third, Utah criteria do not allow a diagnosis in the presence of significant coexisting psychopathology. Utah criteria are highly useful in identification of relatively homogeneous patient groups that respond well to ADHD medications. However, the criteria are over restrictive and insensitive to many adult patients who would benefit from ADHD treatment.

Table 1. Rating Scales and Diagnostic Instruments for Adult ADHD

Sr. no.	Instruments	Type of Instrument
1	ADHD-IV Rating Scale Childhood Self-Report	Retrospective childhood assessment-Rating scale
2	WHO Adult ADHD Self Report Scale	Rating scale
3	Barkley Adult ADHD Rating scale-IV	
4	ADHD-IV Rating Scale Current Self-Report	
5	Conners' Adult ADHD Rating Scales (CAARS): self and observer reports	
6	Brown Adult Attention Disorders Scale	
7	Diagnostic Interview for ADHD Adults (DIVA)	Diagnostic interview
8	Conner's Adult ADHD Diagnostic Interview	
9	Brown Adult ADHD Diagnostic Interview	
10	Adult ADHD Clinical Diagnostic Scale	

Rating Scales and Diagnostic Instruments:

Several commonly used rating scales and structured diagnostic interviews used in adult assessment are summarized in Table 1.

Laboratory Studies

There are insufficient data to support the use of neuropsychological tests, computerized tests of attention, or brain imaging modalities in the diagnosis of adult ADHD. Neuropsychiatric testing can be useful in differentiating ADHD from specific learning disabilities and other cognitive impairments, particularly in the presence of predominately inattentive symptoms and history of school failure. However, neuropsychiatric testing has no demonstrated value in assessment of ADHD itself. Although current research using electroencephalography (EEG), SPECT, and PET imaging suggests the presence of unique features in adults with ADHD, these studies do not have sufficient evidence to support claims of clinical diagnostic utility. Adult ADHD remains a clinical diagnosis derived through careful history taking, adherence to clinical criteria, and differential diagnosis of other psychopathology

DIFFERENTIAL DIAGNOSIS & COMORBIDITIES

Several ADHD symptoms, like problems with attention, motor restlessness or pacing, increased rate of speech, and "on the go attitude" are common in other psychiatric disorders. Core symptoms of ADHD seen in adult population put considerable challenge for diagnosis purpose when they are presented in attenuated form and in the absence of full diagnostic criteria. The prominent differentiation point is the pervasive nature of the symptoms in ADHD. Another important point to remember is the likelihood of dual diagnosis in the presented patients. It is projected that, with reference to dual diagnosis, 70% of adults with ADHD have at least one co morbid disorder, and many have several (Wilens, Biederman, & Spencer, 2002). These disorders often complicate the functional impairment in adult ADHD and may hinder with their treatment; for example, the use of stimulants in patients having co morbid anxiety disorders or histories of stimulant dependence.

Mood Disorders

Depressive syndromes presenting with prominent poor concentration or psychomotor agitation are separated from ADHD on the basis of presence of dysphoric or sad mood and disinterest in surrounding. Presence of Vegetative and cognitive symptoms during a distinct episode can substantiate the diagnosis of depressive syndrome. While considering dual diagnosis of depressive disorders with ADHD one must document the presence of disturbing core symptoms of ADHD outside of the defined mood episode.

Similarly bipolar mood disorder presented in mania may have pressured speech or impulsivity is seen with elevated or irritable mood. Person presented with hypomania may not have prominent grandiosity or flights, will need a great deal of evaluation. There may be a significant overlap of symptoms in these conditions. A clear past history suggesting of mood episode along with significant family history may hint towards bipolar disorder. Also, difficulties with impulsivity and hyperactivity in ADHD will last beyond defined episode of mood disorder. A currently established diagnostic criterion for ADHD does not show any problem with mood or emotional regulation. Many investigator had sawn that person with Adhd have issues regarding emotion prominently regulation. Wender's (1995) Utah Criteria for ADHD include "affective liability," "hot temper, and "overreacts" among symptoms of ADHD in adults. Barkley (2010) described emotional regulation as the core problem of persons with ADHD. Considering this Utah criteria as well as data from Barkley differentiation of ADHD from mood disorder will need careful assessment in adults who had history of ADHD symptoms in childhood. Significant number of patients with ADHD has been showing current major depressive disorder. As reported by Mcgough (2017), Evidence suggest that the prevalence of MDD in adults having childhood ADHD is up to 16 percent, but prevalence estimates of major depressive disorder (MDD) in samples of adults with ADHD range from 16 to 31% (Wilens, Nierenberg, Rostain, & Spencer, 2008).

Anxiety Disorders

Pacing or psychomotor agitation Shawn in anxiety disorder should be differentiated from symptoms of ADHD by presence of subjective sense of worry or apprehension. Feeling of restlessness and 'on the go' nature of ADHD can also be felt in anxiety disorder. Person with any of these disorders also reports difficulties in controlling thoughts. While In generalized anxiety disorders the uneasiness with worry is generalized while it can be situation specific in certain other anxiety diagnosis, person with ADHD may not recognize subjective sense of worry or apprehensions as the core nature of their illness. Presence of Prominent autonomic symptoms may help to settle down diagnosis of anxiety disorders in many cases. One important point to note here is should ADHD be seen as a risk factor for anxiety disorder. This can be particularly the case when person with ADHD identifies his or her symptoms of ADHD as a reason for failure in particular settings. Like students with ADHD worry about getting less marks in examination secondary to ADHD. Empirical research into the epidemiology of ADHD and anxiety in children has found that up to one-third of patients with ADHD have a comorbid anxiety disorder (Biederman, Faraone, & Lapey, 1992) and the same has been found for adults (Kessler et al., 2006; McGough et al., 2005).

Neurodevelopmental Disorder

Adults showing difficulties in attention in the absence of hyperactivity must arise suspicion of specific learning disabilities. Careful history could find academic difficulties in those adults having SLD. Adults having inattention can be due to lack of interest out of frustration due to limited ability. Learning disability in adults does not impair life outside of academic and working environment.

An adult with developmental disabilities or intellectual disabilities may present with some of the symptoms seen in ADHD patients. But these are the conditions which are presented for evaluation in childhood period and psychological testing will reveal significant neurocognitive deficits in those individuals (Gillig et al.2005).

While putting diagnosis of Autistic spectrum disorder, the social, communication is seen as the core feature, but it has been seen that having few or no friends is also very common in ADHD(Barkley, 1998; Bauermeister et al., 2005). Keeping this in mind eccentric behavior in ASD can be differentiating symptoms in adult. The social dysfunction as well as peer rejection in ADHD can be separated from ASD by focused assessment on social isolation and disengagement. An indifference to verbal and nonverbal cues often seen in communications is very evident in ASD. A high rate of ADHD in Asperger syndrome was reported by Ghaziuddin et al.(1998). Rasmussen & Gillberg (2000) has also provided some insights in to ASD and ADHD, the authors reported that 75% of those children who had shown ADHD with ASD at age 7 years continued to meet criteria for Asperger syndrome or atypical autism at age 22 years. In one large study of 273 adult patients, roughly 41% had ADHD as the "major" clinical diagnosis, 47% had ASDs as the major diagnosis, and 12% had other diagnoses. Almost 40% of those with ASDs also met criteria for ADHD. The vast majority of all the patients with ASDs or ADHD also met criteria for one or more (often several) personality disorders (Anckarsater et al., 2006).

Substance Use Disorders

Substance use disorder usually starts in adolescence and till that time ADHD manifestation have already been present in child. Adults with ADHD and Substance use disorders have been reported to have an earlier onset of Substance use disorders relative to adults without ADHD (Wilens, Biederman, Mick, Faraone, & Spencer, 1997) as well as higher risk of Substance use disorders (Schubiner et al.,2000). This is significant in the sense as ADHD can be seen as a risk factor for Substance use disorder. The presence of ADHD also appears to influence the transition into Substance use disorders (Wilens et al., 1997). As same study (Wilens et al., 1997) also indicates that ADHD accelerate the transition from less severe drug or alcohol abuse to more severe dependence (1.2 years in ADHD versus 3 years in non-ADHD controls. An interesting correlation was found in non alcohol substance use disorders, which were increased in early adulthood (mean age, 25 years) of affected in individuals with ADHD but only in those who had developed conduct disorder during adolescence (Mannuzza et al.1993 & Mannuzza et al, 1998).

Personality Disorders

Borderline personality disorder and ADHD in adults share many symptoms, which include impulsivity, affective lability, and angry outbursts, the impulsivity and anger in ADHD is usually brief and inconsiderate, while symptoms in the borderline patient are more interpersonal and ongoing. Patients with ADHD do not show prominent conflicted relationships, suicidal preoccupation, self-mutilation, identity disturbances, or feelings of abandonment which are whole mark of borderline personality disorder (Gillig, Gentile, & Atiq, 2005). Storebø & Simonsen (2016) has found increased risk of antisocial personality disorder in children with ADHD with or without co occurring conduct disorder. Biederman et al. (2011) also found increased antisocial aliments in girls having ADHD in 11 year controlled follow up study.

Organic Pathology

Some medical conditions, such as thyroid problems and seizure disorders, can cause symptoms that resemble ADHD symptoms. A medical examination does not confirm ADHD but is extremely important in helping to rule out other conditions or problems. Similarly medication induced hyperactivity and in attention is also common with the use of isoniazid, bronchodialtors, neuroleptics or thyroid supplements. Psychoactive substance use can also produce symptoms that can mimic clinical picture of ADHD, so one need to carefully evaluate for use of substance in attenuated or altered form of ADHD symptoms. A detail history and careful medical examinations along with use of laboratory tests can differentiate these conditions from adult ADHD.

Other Important Conditions

It is very difficult to differentiate between early developments of conduct disorder with ADHD in childhood. Many researchers see ADHD and Conduct disorder a related condition. During adulthood conduct disorder may convert in to antisocial personality disorder both of which also have kind of similar presentation with adult ADHD. Hyperactivity, risk taking behavior, impulsivity can also be seen as part of conduct disorder but severe aggression, violation of rights of others and patterns of deceit points towards conduct disorder. ADHD with comorbid conduct disorder has poor outcome than outcome of either condition alone as reported by Connor (2017). Co morbidity with conduct disorder increases the risk of substance use disorder as well as antisocial personality disorder in adults. There is an increased risk for children with ADHD with or without comorbid cunduct disorder to develop later onset of antisocial personality disorder as shown by Storebø & Simonsen (2016).

COURSE AND PROGNOSIS

Transition of childhood ADHD to adult ADHD has been always seen as a reduction of symptoms severity. Previously ADHD was not studied adequately to understand consequence illness on adult's life. But now ADHD has been recognized as a serious medical condition with long-term consequences (Curatolo, D'Agati, & Moavero, 2010; Davis, Cheung, Takahashi, Shinoda, & Lindstrom, 2011; Lecendreux, Konofal, & Faraone, 2011 ; Wilcox, Washburn, & Patel,2007). It is important to note that diagnostic criteria for ADHD is specifically developed keeping children and adolescents in mind. They have never been prepared for adults, making it difficult to understand what it means by "criteria for adult ADHD". In DSM 5, diagnosis of adult ADHD requires five instead of six symptoms in both inattention and hyperactivity domain. ADHD in partial remission is also a possible diagnosis for adults who had previously met the full criteria for diagnosis but not able to meet those full criteria since last 6 months. These changes in DSM 5 are an attempt to understand and identify adult ADHD as a disorder of a concern, as new research in this field suggests ADHD to be a lifelong illness. In many individuals with ADHD, disorder can remain present over lifespan and produce devastating effect on social and occupational domain of an individual. On the other hand reduction in number of symptoms for full diagnosis of adult ADHD in DSM 5 also signifies the reduction of ADHD symptoms along with age. But residual symptoms can produce functional impairments in many of the adults. So this syndrome remission from childhood to adulthood can also be viewed as a more of a function of syndrome definition only.

Long Term Follow-Up Studies

A follow up study by Barbaresi et al. 2013, has shown that one third of 232 children with ADHD had fulfilled criteria for adult ADHD at around age of 27.There were no difference in persistence across gender in this study. In another long term follow-up study specifically on boys by Biedermanet al. (2010), showed 78% of the boys have some ADHD symptoms as a young adult, 35 percent have full DSM IV criteria while 22 percent have subsyndromal ADHD. Out of rest 15% have some functional impairment and 6% were in remission but still under treatment. Biederman et al.(2010), had also studied 140 girls in 11 year follow up study, in which researcher found 62% of girls had impairing ADHD symptoms in their young adulthoods. Researcher also found higher risk for antisocial disorder, major depression and anxiety disorder compare to girls without ADHD Owens et al. (2015) has reported 50% to 80% persistence of ADHD from childhood to adolescence and 35% to 65% in to adulthood in their work.

Three core symptoms – inattention, hyperactivity, and impulsivity –which are present in children are shifted to inattention primarily in adulthood. Along with inattention, affective labiality, irritability, and dysphoria, emerge as more prominent symptoms than in childhood (Riccio et al., 2005; Wender, Reimherr, Wood, & Ward, 1985). Although new research are emerging for long term consequences of ADHD in adult life but still outcome studies of ADHD-affected children are limited, and there are Insufficient data to draw conclusions regarding the developmental course of ADHD from early to middle adulthood.

Prognosis With Co-Morbid Psychopathology

Adults with ADHD demonstrate significant rates of co-occurring psychopathology. Around 70% of adults with ADHD have at least one co-morbid disorder, and many have several (Wilens et al., 2002). Presence of co morbid psychopathology can limit the ability of affected individual to use alternative measures to cope up with the core deficits. This can lead to further decline in functional ability of an individual. As reported by Mcgough(2017), available research of substance use with ADHD shows that those who are drug dependant have a more difficult time achieving sobriety than individuals without ADHD. Similarly, adults with ADHD initiate nicotine use at earlier ages, demonstrate higher rates of lifetime nicotine addiction, and have more difficulty in maintaining smoking cessation. Prospective research study of Rasmussen & Gillberg (2000) which followed up children with ADHD into early adulthood (ages 21-27 years), have found higher rates of ADHD symptoms and antisocial personality disorders (ASPDs) in those with childhood ADHD compared with those without ADHD. The differential impact of co morbid psychopathology on long-term ADHD outcome is still in need for further research.

Functional Impairments As Long Term Outcome

ADHD confers significant risk for lifetime functional impairments in terms of social functioning, relationship difficulties. Adult with ADHD show that they have significantly higher rates of marital dissatisfaction and discord, higher divorce rate, and parenting difficulties. (Barkley & Fischer, 2010; Eakin et al. 2004). Work related problems also affect the long term outcome, as adult with ADHD are found to quiet or lose the job more often, have history of poor educational performance and less formal training (barkley & Murphey 2010). Adult with ADHD may show the risk of involvement in high-risk activities, unprotected sex, and unsafe driving which can be evident by their poor choices regarding own safety and health (Mcgough, 2017). Conversely, some of these affected individuals succeed in making lifestyle adjustments that minimize evidence of impairment. Individuals find occupations for which they are well suited, can live alone or find suitable close relationships, or can utilize other talents that compensate for ADHD related difficulties. Education above high school level (>12 years) and work participation were associated with lower rates of comorbid disorders (Anker, Bendiksen, & Heir, 2018) Additional research is required to identify predictive Factors that mitigate these impairments.

MANAGEMENT

Adult attention-deficit hyperactivity disorder (ADHD) has been increasingly recognized in the clinical and scientific literature as a valid clinical entity (Spencer, Biederman, Wilens, & Faraone, 1994). Once diagnosis of adult ADHD is made patient should also be evaluated for co morbidities as there is very high percentage of patients are suffering from concurrent psychopathology. Patients should be provided all the option for treatment and therapy should be designed in a way that fulfill the need of the patients. Management of adult ADHD can include psycho education, pharmacotherapy, management of co morbidity, psychotherapy and other alternative methods. Evidence for pharmacotherapy is quit robust and it has been the primary treatment method for nearly all patients.

Psychoeducation

Psycho education about the illness remains the mainstay of management in adult ADHD. Understanding the biological nature of the disease is well accepted by adults and leads to more significant understanding of own illness. But psycho education also relies upon more skill based approaches such as empowering patients and teaching them how to cope. Major psycho education points are acknowledgment of the symptoms, acknowledgment of the constructive aspects of ADHD, becoming aware of the functional disabilities due to ADHD, cost of having ADHD on different areas of life (work, social life, relationship, parenting), learning how to find reliable information on ADHD, learning to think in a constructive way how to deal with the problems related to ADHD.

Pharmacological Management

Pharmacological Management of Adult ADHD involves pharmacotherapy for ADHD as well as management for co morbidities. Those medications which are very effective in children and adolocescence are also effective in adult ADHD. Medicines used for treatment are methylphenidate, lisdexamfetamine, dexmethylphenidate, desipreamine, dextroamphetamine, mixed amphetamine, pemoline, bupropion, nicotine agonists, modafinil, monoamine oxidase inhibitors, guanfacine and atomoxetine. Not all of the above medicines are approved by US FDA for adult ADHD. Conventionally stimulant medication is more commonly used for its potent effect.

Table 2. Commonly Used Medication with Adult Doses

Type	Name	Dose	Regimen
Stimulant	Methylphenidate	5-30mg	OD to QID
	Dexmethylphenidate	2.5 to 20 mg	OD to QID
	Dextroamphitamine	5 to 30 mg	OD to TID
Nonstimulant	Atomoxetine	25 to 80 mg	OD to BD
	Bupropion	75 to 100mg	TDS
	Guanfacine	1 to 3mg	OD

There has been a shift use of pharmacotherapy as use of non stimulant medication has been increasing. Particularly Atomoxetine, an effective noradrenergic reuptake inhibitor having very less side effects shown to be potent medication for adult ADHD. The reason behind this shift is mainly due to its potency along with less chance of recreational diversion of prescription. Modafinil may also be a viable alternative to conventional stimulants for the treatment of adults with ADHD (Taylor & Russo, 2000). Commonly used medication with their adult doses and regimen are shown in Table 2.

Concerns With Stimulant Medication

For adequate coverage for whole day might require multiple dosing regimens. Stimulants are also available with extended release form which is useful for effective control of symptoms throughout the day. Another important concern is about misuse of stimulant medication. Prominently stimulants are used by college students for better academic performance. One review characterized this pattern of use by college students in an effort to stay up later, to sharpen mental skills and study harder (Weiner, 2000). But recreational use is also possible as both methylphenidate and amphetamine both has reinforcing property. Extended release preparation are helpful in curb this recreational use as slow and steady release of these preparation are less likely to produce the high in users as against the older immediate release preparation.

Management of Co-Morbidity

Adult ADHD is seen along with much co-morbidity. Major depressive disorder, anxiety disorder, substance use disorder and personality disorders are frequently accompany adult ADHD. An important management issue is the sequence of therapy for the condition. Research suggest that those condition should be treated first which is producing more disturbance in person's life. Looking at this principal depressive disorder or anxiety should be treated first with appropriate medicines. This approach may also be true for substance use disorder. While considering treatment of personality disorder it is advisable to treat ADHD first as reduction in impulsivity and in attention can also help in therapy part of personality disorder management. Use of stimulant medication for adult ADHD in presence of substance use disorder is producing quite a thought in treating consultants. In general it is advisable not to use stimulant in substance use disorder involving use of psychostimulant like cocaine or methamphetamine. Active substance use disorder should also be considered as contraindicated for stimulant use. Non-stimulant medication is always a safe alternative for ADHD in co morbid substance use disorder. Non-stimulant are also preferred in persons with tics or anxiety disorder.

General Principals of Management in Adult ADHD with Medication

Treatment planning should be customized for need of the patient. Individuals should be encouraged for having life modification like, balanced diet, exercise, daily planner, considering support from friends/family (if not involved already) and quitting any substance use. They should be provided all the option for therapy including non pharmacological therapy. Risk versus benefit ratio of the chosen medication/plan should be explained and documented.

Baseline Assessment of an Individual's Before Starting Medicines

- Review the diagnostic criteria whether they are still fulfilled by an individual or note, and document it along with severity.
- Use standardized tool for assessment of severity and impairment
- A review of current mental health for co occurring conditions including neuro-developemental condition should be done.
- Social/functional circumstances should be evaluated which can include current educational, and employment circumstances, risk assessment for substance misuse, drug diversion and care needs.
- Evaluate physical health which includes a detailed medical history, contraindicated medications, current medication, weight, baseline pulse and blood pressure, a cardiovascular assessment.

Medication

- Offer the stimulants medication as first line of medication with ADHD, Give at least 6 week trial on adequate dose before switching in case of not deriving enough benefit.
- Offer non stimulant to adults if they cannot tolerate stimulant or symptoms have not responded to separate trials of stimulants for sufficient time, preferably 6 weeks, having considered alternative preparations and adequate doses.
- Stimulant should be prescribed very carefully especially if risk of drug misuse is evident in the form of recreational use, as a cognition enhancer or appetite suppressants.
- When prescribing stimulants for ADHD, think about slow-release once-daily preparations for the reasons like convenience, improving adherence, reducing stigma (as it decreases the need to take medicines at workplace), the risk of stimulant misuse and diversion with immediate-release preparations.

Co-occurring Condition

- If adults with ADHD have an acute psychotic or manic episode then stop any medication for ADHD, consider restarting or starting new ADHD medication only after the episode has resolved, review risk versus benefit ration in this situation before starting medication.
- Offer the medication to patients with anxiety disorder, tic disorder or autism spectrum disorder to individual with ADHD same as individual without ADHD.
- If a person taking stimulants develops tics which are possibly due to stimulants related, reduce the stimulant dose, or consider changing to atomoxetine, clonidine or stop the medication.
- If a person with ADHD develops new seizures or a worsening of existing seizures, review their ADHD medication and stop any medication that might be contributing to the seizures. Reintroduce the antiepileptic only if they are not found to be the causative agent.

Dose Titration and Monitoring

- if any of the condition is present along with ADHD then dose titration should be slow and monitoring should be more frequent ; neuro-developemental disorders (for example, autism spectrum disorder, tic disorders, learning disability, intellectual disability), mental health conditions (for example, anxiety disorders, schizophrenia or bipolar disorder, depression, personality disorder, eating disorder, post-traumatic stress disorder, substance misuse), physical health conditions (for example, cardiac disease, epilepsy or brain injury)
- Evaluate changes in weight at regular period in adults and consider monitoring of BMI of adults with ADHD if there has been weight change as a result of their treatment.

- ◦ Monitor heart rate and blood pressure and at every dose change and at regular interval. Consider referring to physician if sustained tachycardia, arrhythmia or increase in systolic blood pressure is noticed. Reduction of their doses of stimulant might be the requirement.
- ◦ Monitor adults with ADHD for any side effects like sexual dysfunction- erectile/ejaculatory dysfunction on atomoxetine or changes in sleep pattern on stimulants.

Treatment Adherence

- ◦ Symptoms of ADHD itself may be responsible for non adherence to medication. Make sure that individuals with ADHD understand the risk versus benefit ratio for the treatment and educate them about all possible apprehension that can reduce the adherence.
- ◦ Educate patients for being responsible regarding their own health, including taking their medication as needed.
- ◦ Give clear instructions about how to take the, which may include information on dose, duration, adverse effects, dosage schedule. Find new ways to give instructions like use of audio-visual methods.
- ◦ Using visual reminders to take medication regularly for example, apps, alarms, clocks, pill dispensers, or notes on calendars or fridges are very effective in reminders.
- ◦ Explain individuals for taking medication as part of their daily routine like, before meals or after brushing teeth which can also increases the adherence.

Review of the Current Plan of Treatment.

ADHD medication should be reviewed periodically and discuss with the person with adhd(and their families /caregivers if appropriate) whether medication should be continued. The review should include evaluation following points:

- Choices made by an adult with ADHD (and their family or caregivers if needed)
- Benefits towards symptoms reduction, improvements in day to day activities, work efficiency and improvements in social situations buy current medication.
- adverse effects
- Clinical need of the individuals and whether optimized dose will be beneficial or not.
- Effects of missed doses, planned dose reductions and periods of no treatment
- Effect of medication on existing physical and mental conditions.
- Need for support and type of support (for example, psychological, educational, and social).

Non-Pharmacological measures

Non-pharmacological treatment should be advised first for adults with ADHD who have made informed decision to use non pharmacological measure over medication. Persons who are not able to tolerate the medication or medication is not effective in them should also advised to have non pharmacological measure. Certain people are not able to adhere to the pharmacology oriented therapy due to variety of reason; they can also get benefit from these measures. One should consider non-pharmacological treatments in combination with medication for adults with ADHD who have benefited from medication but whose symptoms are still causing functional impairment. Support adherence to non-pharmacological treatments by discussing the balance of risks and benefits (for example, how the treatment can have a positive effect on ADHD symptoms).

Newer research is encouraging for cognitive behavior therapy for treatment of adult ADHD. Other then CBT, mindfulness based therapy, coaching, neurofeedback, meditation are gaining attention for alternative approach in therapy. Although there is lack of substantial evidence to show their effectiveness in general but individual approach for certain patients may be helpful. In cognitive behavioral model emphasis is given to identify how core neuropsychiatric deficit are leading functional impairment. Underachievement secondary to this core deficit leads to dysfunctional cognition and secondary anxiety/depression. Core deficit can also hinder person's ability to use alternative measure to overcome deficits in many cases. Ultimately this lead to functional impairment which is main target for intervention through CBT. In adult ADHD, targeted, skills-based interventions have a role in effectively treating this disorder (Knouse & Safren, 2010). CBT has demonstrated efficacy for major depression (Bockting, Spinhoven, Koeter, Wouters, & Schene, 2006; DeRubeis, Gelfand, Tang, & Simons, 1999) and anxiety (Siev & Chambless, 2007; van Apeldoorn et al., 2008) and shows promise in substance abuse (Kadden, Cooney, Getter, & Litt, 1989, Kadden, Litt, Kabela-Cormier, & Petry, 2007; Najavits & Weiss, 1994), all disorders that are highly comorbid with ADHD in adults.

The concept of ADHD coaching was developed by E. M.Hallowell and John J. Ratey. Focus of ADHD Coaching is to build corporation among the coach and patient with the aim of to reduce functional impairment by putting effective plan. Coaching deals with daily problems and tries to sort out those with the help of time management, priority setting or organizing skills. Self regulation and emotional support also important aspect of coaching. A coach helps people with ADHD carry out the practical activities of daily life in an organized, goal-oriented and timely fashion. Coaching itself is different from CBT as CBT is focused on modification of cognitive and behavioral process. Coaching is viewed as a wellness model and not designed to help a client heal or deal with psychological barriers to growth.

Neurofeedback uses EEG as a medium for feedback. Normal brainwave patterns have been found to correspond to various mental states. Slow-wave activities are categorized in to delta, 0–3 Hz; theta, 4–7 Hz; and alpha, 8–12 Hz. Delta is characterized by sleep; theta and alpha are characterized by drowsiness, relaxation, and internal orientation. States of focus and alertness have a frequency range from 12–20 Hz, high beta ranging from 20–34 Hz usually correspond to ruminating and anxiety. Alpha rhythm is the dominant activity in healthy controls in rest;. Theta and delta are believed to originate from sub cortical layers. ADHD is seen as producing deregulated brainwave functioning, The theory of neurofeedback is based on data showing that many patients with ADHD have more slow wave (especially theta, 3.5–8 Hertz) power in their EEG spectral analysis than normal controls and conversely less beta (12–20 Hz) power (V. Monastra, D. Monastra, & George,2002). Neurofeedback training is intended to reduce low-wave activity and augment faster activity (beta)(12 to 20Hz) but at the same time restricting the high beta activity(20-34) .

FUTURE DIRECTIONS

As of now we are still unsure of causative factor for ADHD, similarly longitudinal outcome in adult ADHD is still needed to be evaluated. Neuroscientists and genetic researchers will make use of newer advances in the field of research to explore the underlying causes of ADHD, which in turn will aid in the development and study of new and improved management practices. One particular interesting focus is endophenotype which is a holding key between gene and phenotype. The ROCFT and WISC endophenotypes (Mastronardiet et al. 2016), visuo-spatial and verbal working (Rommelse et al.,*2008),* time reproduction (Toplak, Dockstader, & Tannock, 2006 ; Rommelse, Oosterlaan, Buitelaar, Faraone, & Sergeant,2007) might be a significant endophenotype in ADHD which can shape the future assessment and management aspect of ADHD. Growing research also point out the role of micronutrients in as possible cause of ADHD or as a role in management. Important micronutrients which are subject to research are zinc, copper, magnesium, iron, vitamin c, vitamin D, vitamin B6 (Darling, Eggleston, Retallick-Brown, & Rucklidge, 2019; Greenblatt & Delane, 2017)

Incresing awareness of impairments occurring in all domains of adult life associated with ADHD will force the development of better instruments for assessment to identify and quantify neuropsychological and functional impairments and to measure treatment response. This will lead us to more concrete instrument from just symptom checklists. There is also need for change in current clinical practice focusing on change in the viewing adult ADHD as a special condition with its co morbidity. It is increasingly clear that although individuals may share a diagnosis of ADHD, there is tremendous variability in developmental trajectories, domains of impairment, and comorbidity patterns. Adult ADHD research should continue to focus on various life transitions and challenges faced during the course of adult development. Certain questions are very important to answer as these domains of the illness have not been studied adequately.

- Is the incidence rate increasing for ADHD?
- What are numbers of affected individual have co morbidity and whether these conditions being correctly diagnosed and managed? What can be the best management for these situations?
- What social and economic impacts does ADHD have on families, education, workplace, judicial matter and health systems?
- Are people with ADHD able to access appropriate and timely treatment?
- How effective are the treatments and what are their long-term effects?

There should be considerable change in current medication regimen as these regimens are having limitation in the form of duration of action, abuse potential and side effects. In future potent medicines with longer duration of action and less abusive potential are needed to effectively manage the core symptoms of the illness. Apart from medicine newer aspect of therapy should also be sought for managing overall outcome of quality of life of an individual with ADHD.

Promising adjunctive psychosocial and other non-pharmacological therapeutic approaches will undergo more sophisticated and rigorous study to establish their effectiveness and unique contribution to treatment regimens designed for adult ADHD. Similar to CBT, ADHD coaching has shown good outcome in management of daily activity of an affected adult individual. Good randomized comparative studies are needed to put more evidence forward, so that coaching can become a standard therapy in management of an affected adult individual.

Technology is the future and it has also its say in management of ADHD in adults. People with ADHD usually have issues with failure to pay attention to details, time management, completing tasks, and organization. Mobile applications and computer programs can improve organization skills, help to reach goals, and even fight the urge to succumb to distraction in people with ADHD. Digital tools can help people with ADHD improve focus, increase productivity, and remember to turn their work in on time, if used effectively. Similarly applications are also useful for medicines reminder leading to proper dosing regimen in working adult. It is also important to prevent overuse of digital media, so the concept of media-free times (meals and celebrations) and media-free zones (bedrooms, outdoor spaces, etc.) are important to set limits on this kind of overuse. EEG neuro-fedback is also gaining popularity in management of ADHD as it has shown the effectiveness in core deficit. Mobile neuro-feedback system which can be home-based training tool is a way forward for neurofeedback. With a low-cost home-based neurofeedback technology may have potency to reduce symptoms (e.g., enhancing attention, reducing impulsive behavior) in adults with ADHD. Neurofeedback can be provided via a conventional theta beta protocol in which individuals train using tasks, videos, or audio clips in a tablet-based app, and receive positive visual/auditory feedback when their brainwaves are in the desired range.

CONCLUSION

ADHD in adults was first noted in the research literature as far back as 50 years ago, but it did not gain widespread acceptance until the 1990s. It's prevalence range from 2 to 4 percent in Adults. Research found that genetic factors are primarily responsible for it. Several inattention and hyperactive-impulsive symptoms help in diagnosis. Adults with ADHD face many academic, occupational, relational and social problems. Early identification is necessary for timely intervention. Adult ADHD can be confused with variety of psychiatric conditions but one need to keep in mind that these conditions can also be a co morbid diagnosis. Mood disorder, anxiety disorder, substance use disorder and personality disorder are prominent one to mention here. Keeping those conditions in mind not only helps in relieving difficulties in affected individuals but addressing these conditions can promise the better long term outcome of an individual. Long term studies have shown that substantial number of adults who had ADHD during childhood does have some functional impairment. Long term outcome of an affected individual is still a research question and considerable research to establish definite prognostic factors. Pharmacological as well as non pharmacological measures does have role in shaping long-term outcome. While stimulant remain the main pharmacotherapy non stimulant medication are also found to be effective. CBT particularly helps to address co morbid conditions and has a definitive role in management of adult ADHD. An important agenda for adult ADHD research in the next decade, as we see it, will be to identify clinically useful ADHD "profiles," to determine if these different profiles are empirically valid, and to study whether they respond differentially to particular treatments for adult ADHD.

ACKNOWLEDGMENT

This research received no specific grant from any funding agency in the public, commercial, or not-for-profit sectors.

This research was supported by Gujarat Institute of Mental Health.

Authors also thanks Dr Ajay Chauhan & Mr Krunal Makwana for their support.

REFERENCES

American Psychiatric Association. (1968). *Diagnostic and statistical manual of mental disorders* (2nd ed.). American Psychiatric Association.

American Psychiatric Association. (1980). *Diagnostic and statistical manual of mental disorders* (3rd ed.). American Psychiatric Association.

American Psychiatric Association. (1987). *Diagnostic and statistical manual of mental disorders* (3rd ed. rev.). American Psychiatric Association.

American Psychiatric Association. (1994). *Diagnostic and statistical manual of mental disorders* (4th ed.). American Psychiatric Association.

American Psychiatric Association. (2013). *Diagnostic and statistical manual of mental disorders* (5th ed.). American Psychiatric Association.

Anckarsater, H., Stahlberg, O., Larsson, T., Hakansson, C., Jutblad, S. B., Niklasson, L., ... Rastam, M. (2006). The impact of ADHD and autism spectrum disorders on temperament character and personality development. *The American Journal of Psychiatry*, *163*(7), 1239–1244. doi:10.1176/ajp.2006.163.7.1239 PMID:16816230

Anker, E., Bendiksen, B., & Heir, T. (2018). Comorbid psychiatric disorders in a clinical sample of adults with ADHD, and associations with education, work and social characteristics: a cross-sectional study. *BMJ open, 8*(3). Attention-deficit/hyperactivity disorder in adults: an overview. *Biological Psychiatry*, *48*(1), 9–20.

Barbaresi, W. J., Colligan, R. C., Weaver, A. L., Voigt, R. G., Killian, J. M., & Katusic, S. K. (2013). Mortality, ADHD, and psychosocial adversity in adults with childhood ADHD: A prospective study. *Pediatrics*, *131*(4), 637–644. doi:10.1542/peds.2012-2354 PMID:23460687

Barkley, R., Murphy, K., & Kwasnik, D. (1996). Psychological adjustment and adaptive impairments in young adults with ADHD. *Journal of Attention Disorders*, *1*(1), 41–54. doi:10.1177/108705479600100104

Barkley, R. A. (1998). *Attention Deficit Hyperactivity Disorder: A Handbook for Diagnosis and Treatment*. Guilford Press.

Barkley, R. A. (2010). Deficient emotional self-regulation is a core component of attention-deficit/hyperactivity disorder. *Journal of ADHD & Related Disorders*, *1*(2), 5–37.

Barkley, R. A., & Fischer, M. (2010). The unique contribution of emotional impulsiveness to impairment in major life activities in hyperactive children as adults. *Journal of the American Academy of Child and Adolescent Psychiatry*, *49*, 503–513. PMID:20431470

Barkley, R. A., & Murphy, K. R. (2010). Impairment in occupational functioning and adult ADHD: The predictive utility of executive function (EF) ratings versus EF tests. *Archives of Clinical Neuropsychology*, *25*(3), 157–173. doi:10.1093/arclin/acq014 PMID:20197297

Barkley, R. A., Murphy, K. R., & Fischer, M. (2010). *ADHD in Adults: What the Science Says*. Guilford Press.

Bauermeister, J. J., Matos, M., Reina, G., Salas, C. C., Martinez, J. V., Cumba, E., & Barkley, R. A. (2005). Comparison of the DSM-IV combined and inattentive types of ADHD in a school-based sample of Latino/Hispanic children. *Journal of Child Psychology and Psychiatry, and Allied Disciplines*, *46*(2), 166–179. doi:10.1111/j.1469-7610.2004.00343.x PMID:15679525

Biederman, J., Faraone, S., Milberger, S., Curtis, S., Chen, L., Marrs, A., Ouellette, C., Moore, P., & Spencer, T. (1996). Predictors of persistence and remission of ADHD into adolescence: Results from a four-year prospective follow-up study. *Journal of the American Academy of Child and Adolescent Psychiatry, 35*(3), 343–351. doi:10.1097/00004583-199603000-00016 PMID:8714323

Biederman, J., Faraone, S. V., & Lapey, K. (1992). Comorbidity of diagnosis in attention deficit hyperactivity disorder. *Child and Adolescent Psychiatric Clinics of North America, 1*(2), 335–360. doi:10.1016/S1056-4993(18)30591-1

Biederman, J., Faraone, S. V., Mick, E., Spencer, T., Wilens, T., Kiely, K., ... Warburton, R. (1995). High risk for attention deficit hyperactivity disorder among children of parents with childhood onset of the disorder: A pilot study. *The American Journal of Psychiatry, 152*(3), 431–435. doi:10.1176/ajp.152.3.431 PMID:7864271

Biederman, J., Faraone, S. V., Spencer, T. J., Mick, E., Monuteaux, M. C., & Aleardi, M. (2006). Functional impairments in adults with self-reports of diagnosed ADHD: A controlled study of 1001 adults in the community. *The Journal of Clinical Psychiatry, 67*(4), 524–540. doi:10.4088/JCP.v67n0403 PMID:16669717

Biederman, J., Petty, C. R., Clarke, A., Lomedico, A., & Faraone, S. V. (2011). Predictors of persistent ADHD: An 11-year follow-up study. *Journal of Psychiatric Research, 45*(2), 150–155. doi:10.1016/j.jpsychires.2010.06.009 PMID:20656298

Biederman, J., Petty, C. R., Evans, M., Small, J., & Faraone, S. V. (2010). How persistent is ADHD? A controlled 10-year follow-up study of boys with ADHD. *Psychiatry Research, 177*(3), 299–304. doi:10.1016/j.psychres.2009.12.010 PMID:20452063

Biederman, J., Petty, C. R., Monuteaux, M.C., Fried, R., Byrne, D., & Mirto, T.,….Faraone, S. V. (2010). Adult Psychiatric Outcomes of Girls With Attention Deficit Hyperactivity Disorder: 11-Year Follow-Up in a Longitudinal Case-Control Study. *Journal of Psychiatry, 167*(4), 409–417. PMID:20080984

Bockting, C. L., Spinhoven, P., Koeter, M. W., Wouters, L. F., & Schene, A. H. (2006). Prediction of recurrence in recurrent depression and the influence of consecutive episodes on vulnerability for depression: A 2-year prospective study. *The Journal of Clinical Psychiatry, 67*(5), 747–755. doi:10.4088/JCP.v67n0508 PMID:16841624

Boomsma, D. I., Saviouk, V., Hottenga, J. J., Distel, M. A., de Moor, M. H., Vink, J. M., Geels, L. M., van Beek, J. H. D. A., Bartels, M., de Geus, E. J. C., & Willemsen, G. (2010). Genetic epidemiology of attention deficit hyperactivity disorder (ADHD index) in adults. *PLoS One, 5*(5), e10621. doi:10.1371/journal.pone.0010621 PMID:20485550

Bresnahan, S. M., Anderson, J. W., & Barry, R. J. (1999). Age-related changes in quantitative EEG in attention-deficit/hyperactivity disorder. *Biological Psychiatry, 46*(12), 1690–1697. doi:10.1016/S0006-3223(99)00042-6 PMID:10624551

Bresnahan, S. M., Barry, R. J., Clarke, A. R., & Johnstone, S. J. (2006). Quantitative EEG analysis in dexamphetamine-responsive adults with attention-deficit/hyperactivity disorder. *Psychiatry Research, 141*(2), 151–159. doi:10.1016/j.psychres.2005.09.002 PMID:16343642

Cantwell, D. P. (1972). Psychiatric illness in the families of hyperactive children. *Archives of General Psychiatry*, *27*(3), 414–417. doi:10.1001/archpsyc.1972.01750270114018 PMID:5051632

Chabot, R. J., & Serfontein, G. (1996). Quantitative electroencephalographic profiles of children with attention deficit disorder. *Biological Psychiatry*, *40*(10), 951–963. doi:10.1016/0006-3223(95)00576-5 PMID:8915554

Clarke, A. R., Barry, R. J., Heaven, P. C., McCarthy, R., Selikowitz, M., & Byrne, M. K. (2008). EEG in adults with attention-deficit/hyperactivity disorder. *International Journal of Psychophysiology: Official Journal of the International Organization of Psychophysiology, 70*(3), 176–183.

Connor, D. F. (2017). Disruptive Behavior Disorders in Children and Adolescents. In B. J. Sadock, V. A. Sadock, & P. Ruiz (Eds.), *Kaplan & Sadock's comprehensive textbook of psychiatry* (10th ed., Vol. 2, p. 3618). Wolters Kluwer.

Curatolo, P., D'Agati, E., & Moavero, R. (2010). The neurobiological basis of ADHD. *Italian Journal of Pediatrics*, *36*(1), 79. doi:10.1186/1824-7288-36-79 PMID:21176172

Darling, K. A., Eggleston, M., Retallick-Brown, H., & Rucklidge, J. J. (2019, November). Mineral-Vitamin Treatment Associated with Remission in Attention-Deficit/Hyperactivity Disorder Symptoms and Related Problems: 1-Year Naturalistic Outcomes of a 10-Week Randomized Placebo-Controlled Trial. *Journal of Child and Adolescent Psychopharmacology*, *29*(9), 688–704. doi:10.1089/cap.2019.0036 PMID:31343273

Davis, J. M., Cheung, S. F., Takahashi, T., Shinoda, H., & Lindstrom, W. A. (2011). Cross-national invariance of attention-deficit/hyperactivity disorder factors in Japanese and U.S. university students. *Research in Developmental Disabilities*, *32*(6), 2972–2980. doi:10.1016/j.ridd.2011.05.004 PMID:21624817

DeRubeis, R. J., Gelfand, L. A., Tang, T. Z., & Simons, A. D. (1999). Medications versus cognitive behavior therapy for severely depressed outpatients: Mega-analysis of four randomized comparisons. *The American Journal of Psychiatry*, *156*(7), 1007–1013. PMID:10401443

Eakin, L., Minde, K., Hechtman, L., Ochs, E., Krane, E., Bouffard, R., Greenfield, B., & Looper, K. (2004). The marital and family functioning of adults with ADHD and their spouses. *Journal of Attention Disorders*, *8*(1), 1–10. doi:10.1177/108705470400800101 PMID:15669597

Ehringer, M. A., Rhee, S. H., Young, S., Corley, R., & Hewitt, J. K. (2006). Genetic and environmental contributions to common psychopathologies of childhood and adolescence: A study of twins and their siblings. *Journal of Abnormal Child Psychology*, *34*(1), 1–17. doi:10.100710802-005-9000-0 PMID:16465480

Faraone, S. V., Biederman, J., & Friedman, D. (2000). Validity of DSM-IV subtypes of attention-deficit/hyperactivity disorder: A family study perspective. *Journal of the American Academy of Child and Adolescent Psychiatry*, *39*(3), 300–307. doi:10.1097/00004583-200003000-00011 PMID:10714049

Franke, B., Neale, B. M., & Faraone, S. V. (2009). Genome-wide association studies in ADHD. *Human Genetics*, *126*(1), 13–50. doi:10.100700439-009-0663-4 PMID:19384554

Ghaziuddin, M., Weidmer-Mikhail, E., & Ghaziuddin, N. (1998). Comorbidity of Asperger syndrome: A preliminary report. *Journal of Intellectual Disability Research, 42*(4), 279–283. doi:10.1111/j.1365-2788.1998.tb01647.x PMID:9786442

Gillig, P. M., Gentile, J. P., & Atiq, R. (2005). Attention-deficit hyperactivity disorder in adults. *Hospital Physician, 9*(2), 1–11. PMID:15737940

Grenblatt, J. M., & Delane, D. D. (2017). Micronutrient Deficiencies in ADHD: AGlobal Research Consensus. *Journal of Orthomolecular Medicine, 32*(6).

Hale, T. S., Bookheimer, S., McGough, J. J., Phillips, J. M., & McCracken, J. T. (2007). Atypical brain activation during simple & complex levels of processing in adult ADHD: An fMRI study. *Journal of Attention Disorders, 11*(2), 125–140. doi:10.1177/1087054706294101 PMID:17494829

Hechtman, L., Weiss, G., Finklestein, J., Werner, A., & Benn, R. (1976). Hyperactives as young adults: Preliminary report. *Canadian Medical Association Journal, 115*(7), 625–630. PMID:974949

Hechtman, L., Weiss, G., & Perlman, T. (1984). Hyperactives as young adults: Past and current substance abuse and antisocial behavior. *The American Journal of Orthopsychiatry, 54*(3), 415–442. doi:10.1111/j.1939-0025.1984.tb01507.x PMID:6331769

Hinshaw, S. P. (1992). Academic underachievement, attention deficits, and aggression: Comorbidity and implications for intervention. *Journal of Consulting and Clinical Psychology, 60*(6), 893–903. doi:10.1037/0022-006X.60.6.893 PMID:1460150

Jaffe, P. (1995). History and overview of adulthood ADD. In K. G. Nadeau (Ed.), *A Comprehensive Guide to Attention Deficit Disorder in Adults: Research, Diagnosis, and Treatment.* Brunner/Mazel.

Kadden, R. M., Cooney, N. L., Getter, H., & Litt, M. D. (1989). Matching alcoholics to coping skills or interactional therapies: Posttreatment results. *Journal of Consulting and Clinical Psychology, 57*(6), 698–704. doi:10.1037/0022-006X.57.6.698 PMID:2557364

Kadden, R. M., Litt, M. D., Kabela-Cormier, E., & Petry, N. M. (2007). Abstinence rates following behavioral treatments for marijuana dependence. *Addictive Behaviors, 32*(6), 1220–1236. doi:10.1016/j.addbeh.2006.08.009 PMID:16996224

Kessler, R.C., Adler, L., Barkley, R., Biederman, J., Conners, C. K., Demler, O., … Zaslavsky, A.M. (2006).The prevalence and correlates of adult ADHD in the United States: results from the National Comorbidity Survey Replication. *American Journal of Psychiatry, 163*(4), 716–23.

Knouse, L. E. & Safren, S. A. (2010). Current statusof cognitive behavioural therapy for adult attention deficit hyperactivity disorder. *Psychiatric Clinic of North America, 33*(3), 497-509.

Koehler, S., Lauer, P., Schreppel, T., Jacob, C., Heine, M., Boreatti-Hümmer, A., … Herrmann, M. J. (2009). Increased EEG power density in alpha and theta bands in adult ADHD patients. *Journal of Neural Transmission, 116*(1), 97–104.

Larsson, H., Chang, Z., D'Onofrio, B. M., & Lichtenstein, P. (2014). The heritability of clinically diagnosed attention deficit hyperactivity disorder across the lifespan. *Psychological Medicine, 44*(10), 2223–2229. doi:10.1017/S0033291713002493 PMID:24107258

Lasky-Su, J., Anney, R. J., Neale, B. M., Franke, B., Zhou, K., Maller, J. B., … Faraone, S. V. (2008). Genome-wide association scan of the time to onset of attention deficit hyperactivity disorder. *American Journal of Medical Genetics. Part B, Neuropsychiatric Genetics: The Official Publication of the International Society of Psychiatric Genetics, 147B*(8), 1355–1358.

Lecendreux, M., Konofal, E., & Faraone, S. V. (2011). Prevalence of attention deficit hyperactivity disorder and associated features among children in France. *Journal of Attention Disorders, 15*(6), 516–524. doi:10.1177/1087054710372491 PMID:20679156

Mannuzza, S., Klein, R. G., Bessler, A., Malloy, P., & LaPadula, M. (1993). Adult outcome of hyperactive boys: Educational achievement, occupational rank, and psychiatric status. *Archives of General Psychiatry, 50*(7), 565–576. doi:10.1001/archpsyc.1993.01820190067007 PMID:8317950

Mannuzza, S., Klein, R. G., Bessler, A., Malloy, P., & LaPadula, M. (1998). Adult psychiatric status of hyperactive boys grown up. *The American Journal of Psychiatry, 155*(4), 493–498. doi:10.1176/ajp.155.4.493 PMID:9545994

Martin, N., Scourfield, J., & McGuffin, P. (2002). Observer effects and heritability of childhood attention-deficit hyperactivity disorder symptoms. *The British Journal of Psychiatry, 180*(3), 260–265. doi:10.1192/bjp.180.3.260 PMID:11872519

Mastronardi, C. A., Pillai, E., Pineda, D. A., Martinez, A. F., Lopera, F., Velez, J. I., Palacio, J. D., Patel, H., Easteal, S., Acosta, M. T., Castellanos, F. X., Muenke, M., & Arcos-Burgos, M. (2016). Linkage and association analysis of ADHD endophenotypes in extended and multigenerational pedigrees from a genetic isolate. *Molecular Psychiatry, 21*(10), 1434–1440. doi:10.1038/mp.2015.172 PMID:26598068

McGough, J. J. (2017). Adult Manifestations of Attention-Deficit/Hyperactivity Disorder. In B. J. Sadock, V. A. Sadock, & P. Ruiz (Eds.), *Kaplan & Sadock's comprehensive textbook of psychiatry* (10th ed., Vol. 2, p. 3601). Wolters Kluwer.

McGough, J. J. (2017). Adult Manifestations of Attention-Deficit/Hyperactivity Disorder. In B. J. Sadock, V. A. Sadock, & P. Ruiz (Eds.), *Kaplan & Sadock's comprehensive textbook of psychiatry* (10th ed., Vol. 2, p. 3602). Wolters Kluwer.

McGough, J. J. (2017). Adult Manifestations of Attention-Deficit/Hyperactivity Disorder. In B. J. Sadock, V. A. Sadock, & P. Ruiz (Eds.), *Kaplan & Sadock's comprehensive textbook of psychiatry* (10th ed., Vol. 2, p. 3602). Wolters Kluwer.

McGough, J. J., Smalley, S. L., McCracken, J. T., Yang, M., Del'Homme, M., Lynn, D. E., & Loo, S. (2005). Psychiatric comorbidity in adult attention deficit hyperactivity disorder: Findings from multiplex families. *The American Journal of Psychiatry, 162*(9), 1621–1627. doi:10.1176/appi.ajp.162.9.1621 PMID:16135620

Monastra, V. J., Monastra, D. M., & George, S. (2002). The effects of stimulant therapy, EEG biofeedback, and parenting style on the primary symptoms of attention-deficit/ hyperactivity disorder. *Applied Psychophysiology and Biofeedback, 27*(4), 231–249. doi:10.1023/A:1021018700609 PMID:12557451

Morrison, J. R., & Stewart, M. A. (1971). A family study of the hyperactive child syndrome. *Biological Psychiatry, 3*(3), 189–195. PMID:5163807

Najavits, L. M., & Weiss, R. D. (1994). The role of psychotherapy in the treatment of substance-use disorders. *Harvard Review of Psychiatry*, *2*(2), 84–96. doi:10.3109/10673229409017121 PMID:9384886

Owens, E., Cardoos, S., & Hinshaw, S. (2014). Developemental Progression and Differences among Individuals with ADHD. In Attention deficit Hyperactive Disorder: A Handbook for Diagnosis and Treatment, (4th ed., pp. 223-255). New York, NY: Guilford Press.

Rasmussen, P., & Gillberg, C. (2000). Natural outcome of ADHD with developmental coordination disorder at age 22 years: A controlled, longitudinal, community-based study. *Journal of the American Academy of Child and Adolescent Psychiatry*, *39*(11), 1424–1431. doi:10.1097/00004583-200011000-00017 PMID:11068898

Riccio, C. A., Wolfe, M., Davis, B., Romine, C., George, C., & Lee, D. (2005). Attention deficit hyperactivity disorder: Manifestation in adulthood. *Archives of Clinical Neuropsychology*, *20*(2), 249–269. doi:10.1016/j.acn.2004.07.005 PMID:15708734

Rommelse, N. N., Oosterlaan, J., Buitelaar, J., Faraone, S. V., & Sergeant, J. A. (2007). Time reproduction in children with ADHD and their nonaffected siblings. *Journal of the American Academy of Child and Adolescent Psychiatry*, *46*(5), 582–590. doi:10.1097/CHI.0b013e3180335af7 PMID:17450049

Rommelse, N. N., Van der Stigchel, S., Witlox, J., Geldof, C., Deijen, J. B., Theeuwes, J., Oosterlaan, J., & Sergeant, J. A. (2008). Deficits in visuo-spatial working memory, inhibition and oculomotor control in boys with ADHD and their non-affected brothers. *Journal of Neural Transmission (Vienna, Austria)*, *115*(2), 249–260. doi:10.100700702-007-0865-7 PMID:18253811

Schubiner, H., Tzelepis, A., Milberger, S., Lockhart, N., Kruger, M., Kelley, B. J., & Schoener, E. P. (2000). Prevalence of attention-deficit/hyperactivity disorder and conduct disorder among substance abusers. *The Journal of Clinical Psychiatry*, *61*(4), 244–251. doi:10.4088/JCP.v61n0402 PMID:10830144

Siev, J., & Chambless, D. L. (2007). Specificity of treatment effects: Cognitive therapy and relaxation for generalized anxiety and panic disorders. *Journal of Consulting and Clinical Psychology*, *75*(4), 513–522. doi:10.1037/0022-006X.75.4.513 PMID:17663606

Spencer, T., Biederman, J., Wilens, T., & Faraone, S. (1994). Is attention deficit hyperactivity disorder in adults a valid disorder? *Harvard Review of Psychiatry*, *1*(6), 326–335. doi:10.3109/10673229409017099 PMID:9384867

Storebø, O. J., & Simonsen, E. (2016). The Association between ADHD and Antisocial Personality Disorder (ASPD): A Review. *Journal of Attention Disorders*, *20*(10), 815–824. doi:10.1177/1087054713512150 PMID:24284138

Taylor, F. B., & Russo, J. (2000). Efficacy of modafinil compared to dextroamphetamine for the treatment of attention deficit hyperactivity disorder in adults. *Journal of Child and Adolescent Psychopharmacology*, *10*(4), 311–320. doi:10.1089/cap.2000.10.311 PMID:11191692

Toplak, M. E., Dockstader, C., & Tannock, R. (2006). Temporal information processing in ADHD: Findings to date and new methods. *Journal of Neuroscience Methods*, *151*(1), 15–29. doi:10.1016/j.jneumeth.2005.09.018 PMID:16378641

Valera, E. M., Faraone, S. V., Biederman, J., Poldrack, R. A., & Seidman, L. J. (2005). Functional neuroanatomy of working memory in adults with attention-deficit/hyperactivity disorder. *Biological Psychiatry, 57*(5), 439–447. doi:10.1016/j.biopsych.2004.11.034 PMID:15737657

Van Apeldoorn, F. J., Van Hout, W. J., Mersch, P. P., Huisman, M., Slaap, B. R., Hale, W. W., Visser, S., van Dyck, R., & den Boer, J. A. (2008). Is a combined therapy more effective than either CBT or SSRI alone? Results of a multicenter trial on panic disorder with or without agoraphobia. *Acta Psychiatrica Scandinavica, 117*(4), 260–270. doi:10.1111/j.1600-0447.2008.01157.x PMID:18307586

Weiner, A. L. (2000). Emerging drugs of abuse in Connecticut. *Connecticut Medicine, 64*(1), 19–23. PMID:10697361

Weiss, G., & Hechtman, L. (1993). *Hyperactive Children Grow Up* (2nd ed.). Guilford.

Wender, P. H. (1995). *Attention-Deficit Hyperactivity Disorder in Adults*. Oxford University Press.

Wender, P. H., Reimherr, F. W., Wood, D., & Ward, M. (1985). A controlled study of methylphenidate in the treatment of attention deficit disorder, residual type, in adults. *The American Journal of Psychiatry, 142*(5), 547–552. doi:10.1176/ajp.142.5.547 PMID:3885760

Wilcox, C. E., Washburn, R., & Patel, V. (2007). Seeking help for attention deficit hyperactivity disorder in developing countries: A study of parental explanatory models in Goa, India. *Social Science & Medicine, 64*(8), 1600–1610. doi:10.1016/j.socscimed.2006.11.032 PMID:17267087

Wilens, T., Nierenberg, A. A., Rostain, A., & Spencer, T. J. (2008). Adult attention-deficit hyperactivity disorder and the role of depression. *CNS Spectrums, 13*(5), 2–17.

Wilens, T. E., Biederman, J., Mick, E., Faraone, S. V., & Spencer, T. (1997). Attention deficit hyperactivity disorder (ADHD) is associated with early onset substance use disorders. *The Journal of Nervous and Mental Disease, 185*(8), 475–482. doi:10.1097/00005053-199708000-00001 PMID:9284860

Wilens, T. E., Biederman, J., & Spencer, T. J. (2002). Attention deficit/hyperactivity disorder across the lifespan. *Annual Review of Medicine, 53*(1), 113–131. doi:10.1146/annurev.med.53.082901.103945 PMID:11818466

Wolf, R. C., Plichta, M. M., Sambataro, F., Fallgatter, A. J., Jacob, C., Lesch, K. P., Herrmann, M. J., Schönfeldt-Lecuona, C., Connemann, B. J., Grön, G., & Vasic, N. (2009). Regional brain activation changes and abnormal functional connectivity of the ventrolateral prefrontal cortex during working memory processing in adults with attention-deficit/hyperactivity disorder. *Human Brain Mapping, 30*(7), 2252–2266. doi:10.1002/hbm.20665 PMID:19107748

Wood, D. R., Reimherr, F. W., Wender, P. H., & Johnson, G. E. (1976). Diagnosis and treatment of minimal brain dysfunction in adults: A preliminary report. *Archives of General Psychiatry, 33*(12), 1453–1460. doi:10.1001/archpsyc.1976.01770120057005 PMID:793563

Zhou, K., Dempfle, A., Arcos-Burgos, M., Bakker, S. C., Banaschewski, T., Biederman, J., … Asherson, P. (2008). Meta-analysis of genome-wide linkage scans of attention deficit hyperactivity disorder. *American Journal of Medical Genetics. Part B, Neuropsychiatric Genetics: The Official Publication of the International Society of Psychiatric Genetics, 147B*(8), 1392–1398.

ADDITIONAL READING

American Psychiatric Association. (2013). *Diagnostic and statistical manual of mental disorders* (5th ed.). American Psychiatric Association.

Barkley, R. A. (2015). *Attention-Deficit Hyperactivity Disorder: A handbook for Diagnosis and Treatment* (4th ed.). Guilford Press.

Barkley, R. A., Murphy, K. R., & Fischer, M. (2010). *ADHD in Adults: What the Science Says*. Guilford Press.

Brown, T. E. (2013). *A New Understanding of ADHD in Children and Adults: Executive Function Impairments*. Routledge. doi:10.4324/9780203067536

Kooij, S. (2013). *Adult ADHD: Diagnostic Assessment and Treatment* (3rd ed.). Springer. doi:10.1007/978-1-4471-4138-9

Surman, C. (2014). *ADHD in Adults: A Practical Guide to Evaluation and Management (Current Clinical Psychiatry)*. Humana press.

Wender, P. H. (1995). *Attention-Deficit Hyperactivity Disorder in Adults*. Oxford University Press.

Wender, P. H. (2001). *ADHD: Attention Deficit Hyperactivity Disorder in Children, Adolescents and Adult*. Oxford University Press.

KEY TERMS AND DEFINITIONS

Adult ADHD: A disorder of inattention and hyperactivity symptoms in adults which is fulfilling the diagnostic criteria of ADHD as per DSM V.

Co-Morbidity: A presentation of two or more psychopathology together, fulfilling diagnostic criteria of each one independently.

Electrophysiological Studies: A study of neurophysiologic events with help of brain waves recordings by EEG and evoked potential.

Genetic Factors: Various etiological factors related to human genome.

Non-Pharmacological Measures: A treatment modalities which does not include bioactive substance induction in the human body.

Subsyndromal ADHD: A presented form of the ADHD disorder in which full ADHD diagnostic criteria is not met.

Chapter 7
Assessment of ADHD for Children, Adolescents, and Adults

Aarzoo Gupta
Government Medical College and Hospital, Chandigarh, India

Archana Kashyap
Government Medical College and Hospital, Chandigarh, India

ABSTRACT

The chapter highlights the role of comprehensive assessment and its meaningful elements to construe ADHD in terms of diagnosis and management. The cognitive, affective, and behavioral symptoms must not be attributed to emotional or mood disturbance or psycho-social adjustments. The chapter explains an assessment pyramid explaining of multi-level assessment and domains with an acronym of CTP depicting cognitive, temperament, and psychopathology. Assessment may be more precise when a professional has knowledge of developmental theories. Attention hyperactivity disorder (ADHD) entails a detailed assessment, involving varied social agents, to understand the dynamic manifestation of different ages as well as the dysfunction caused by it. The current chapter emphasizes psycho-social factors, comorbidities, and dual-diagnosis issues that may exacerbate or mask the presentation of ADHD in children, adolescents, and adults.

INTRODUCTION

A misdiagnosed condition usually gives rise to divergent management strategies. A comprehensive assessment is key to the treatment, outcome, and rehabilitation. Attention hyperactivity disorder (ADHD) is one such condition that entails a detailed assessment, involving varied social agents, to understand the dynamic manifestation of different ages as well as the dysfunction caused by it. The exhibited signs and ramifications of ADHD may go unnoticed and might gain attention due to its comorbidities as in the case of personality disorders (World Health Organization [WHO], 2004). This simile has greater application

DOI: 10.4018/978-1-7998-5495-1.ch007

especially in those cases of ADHD where families displayed tolerance for symptoms in childhood or the individual in his growing years carved out strategies to deal with ADHD and its sequel. This evolving environment during the development years is followed by poorer adjustment to social roles and norms in adulthood. This longitudinal and persistent maladjustment can significantly contribute to comorbid mood and anxiety disturbances (Kooij et al., 2010), being one of the causes for this population to access mental health services. Therefore, a disorder with an externalizing nature transforms into a covert presentation in adulthood. Further, the attention of the professional is concentrated on the management of the comorbidities than exploring underlying psychogenesis requiring a life-span developmental approach. The research and teaching related to ADHD also create the mind-set to explore ADHD in the paediatric population with minimum attention to its identification in adults or individuals having dual-diagnosis or comorbid conditions (Ginsberg, Quintero, Anand, Casillas, & Upadhyaya, 2014).

Many factors determine the course and prognosis of any psychiatric disorder. Intelligence, personality, family practices, choice of occupation, etcetera (etc.) are few such factors that interweave in revealing ADHD and its associated malfunction (Biederman et al., 1996). Therefore, the assessment of ADHD must include these factors that build one's strength or limitation to cope with the condition and subsequent impairments. The overall prognosis of ADHD is reported to be poor in the textbooks and knowing the factors encapsulated in Table 1 may be advisable to grasp the course of ADHD. It is shown in research that ADHD is an either underdiagnosed or over-diagnosed condition (Ginsberg et. al., 2014; Paris, Bhat, & Thombs, 2015), this finding also emphasizes the need to review its evaluation process considering theories of factors affecting the clinical indicators or how individuals try to resolve and cope with resulting difficulties.

Another unpinning issue is who all should be involved in the assessment. Does ADHD become a domain of mental health professionals alone? The proportion of inaccuracy in its diagnosis, due to its concealed nature, is the evidence that identification and diagnosis must be multi-disciplinary teamwork. The involvement of a multidisciplinary team approach will facilitate an expansive and in-depth comprehensive assessment. The inputs form class in-charge, extracurricular activity or sports in-charge, school psychologists, special educators, clinical psychologist, psychiatrist, paediatrician, neurologist, are crucial to recognizing ADHD symptoms. A multi-disciplinary team approach might help in early identification and intervention considering the current view of ADHD being a neurodevelopmental disorder. The changes in the structure and functioning of the brain corroborating with the psychological testing and clinical findings can strengthen the reliability of the assessment of ADHD. The intervention should not only be focusing on the management but long-term rehabilitation as ADHD is a chronic causing pervasive impairment. The long-term intervention emphasizing concentration, organizational, and impulse-modulation skills can help an adult with ADHD to function more adaptively (Katya, 2018). Therefore the prognosis and outcome can be determined by programs targeting brain deficits thru brain stimulation therapies based on the principle of brain plasticity (Merzenich, Vleet, & Nahum, 2014); along with individual (van Doren et al., 2019; Catalá-López et al., 2017), school-based as well as parent training intervention programs (Charach et al., 2013; DuPaul & Eckert, 1997; DuPaul, Eckert, & Vilardo, 2012).). A holistic assessment plan for persons having ADHD might help enhance the quality of day-to-day functioning and minimize the disease burden on the healthcare system (Fabiano, Schatz, Aloe, Chacko, & Chronis-Tuscano, 2015).

Historical Perspective

The history of ADHD can be traced back to the 18th century, its first mention appeared in a medical book (Barkley, 2012). Till the beginning of the 20th century, there had been some cases reporting use of labels such as 'fidgety Phil' (Lange, Reichl, Lange, Tucha, & Tucha, 2010) or 'problem of moral control; these described groups of traits or behaviours namely; aggression, defiance, passionate, inhibitory volition, low moral consciousness (Rafalovich, 2001). It was after the encephalitis epidemic of 1917-18 (Barkley, 2015), that behavioural disorders comprising of symptoms similar to what is now known as conduct or oppositional defiant disorders were recognized to be existing but Bender in 1940s identified that brain damage leads to ADHD (Lange et al., 2010). Strauss and Lehtinen in 1947 developed a program that was adopted in Public Schools of the United States and later they extended their work for children having ADHD with comorbid mental retardation and those with cerebral palsy (Barkley, 2015). It was the classic work of Denhoff Chess summarising that ADHD resolved by puberty (Mayes & Rafalovich, 2008) with a few shreds of evidence of persistence of ADHD symptoms in adolescence (Barkley, Fischer, Edelbrock, & Smallish, 1990). Later DSM-III/-R in 1980 and 1987 elaborated on diagnostic categories namely, ADD +H and ADD-H, with greater significance to ADD+H (Matthews, Nigg, & Fair, 2014). Before this, DSM-II mentioned hyperkinetic reaction but no further elaboration was given. It was DSM-IV that introduced evidence-based criteria to diagnose ADHD (Epstein & Loren, 2013) keeping in view the historical view on ADHD. The defined criteria were drawn from webbing and analysing the work of clinicians and researchers of the past two centuries. It is of importance to observe that the trends and developments in the assessment, as well as management, were greatly influenced by the social and medical advancements. The pioneering work was on children showing externalized signs and this trend continued for decades due to concealed manifestation of the subtypes of the disorder. There are few follow-ups or longitudinal studies providing evidence of ADHD symptoms being persistent through adolescence and adulthood (Biederman, Petty, Evans, Small, & Faraone, 2010) but identification of ADHD in adults is still ambiguous and demands more research and clarity in future studies.

Nosology of ADHD

The criteria presented in the diagnostic manuals such as Diagnostic and Statistical Manual of Mental Disorders (DSM) and The ICD 10 classification of mental and behavioural disorder: Clinical descriptions and diagnostic guidelines (ICD) has been through various revisions since it made its entry in the manuals. But training and research created a bias among the professionals to elicit and diagnose ADHD in school going or child population. Its presentation or prevalence has not been highlighted in those who have not been attending school or have finished school education. The most recent revisions of the manuals guide their user's to adopt a life-span approach to identify and diagnose ADHD. The definition of ADHD is common in both the revised manuals and there is no exact age of onset mentioned.

DSM, Fifth Edition (DSM-5) 5 elaborate on examples of the manifestation of ADHD in adolescence and adulthood. The *evidence of symptoms* is given more importance than *evidence of impairment*. The types of subtypes of the disorder are referred to as presentations with defined severity categorized as mild, moderate, or severe. There is a greater emphasis on symptoms affecting the quality of social, occupational, academic functioning than dysfunction. The ICD 11 would prioritize cultural and contextual factors; and avoid arbitrary cut-offs, precise criteria containing symptom count or duration. One major change in ICD11 would be that ADHD is not seen as a disorder of behaviour and will be classified as a neurodevelopmental disorder (Reed et al., 2019). This implies that the onset of ADHD is during the development period and certain functions are acquired and executed differently since the beginning. Consequently, difficulties in cognitive processes, emotional reactions, and behavioural regulation persist even in later years of life. Therefore inattention, hyperactivity or impulsivity, and other symptoms are to be traced back to childhood with an attempt to find evidence of its implications. The revised diagnostic guidelines shall excavate the advancement of research in the assessment of ADHD and breed more evidence-based interventions.

Assessment

Assessment is a detailed process to identify symptoms, factors contributing to the psychopathology, and its psychosocial consequences. The assessment findings corroborated from multiple sources and occasions are reliable and give direction to management. Diagnosis is an important component and aim of the assessment based on the conclusion of clinical interview aimed at elicitation of psychopathology and; psychological testing revealing the diagnostic clarification, symptom severity, associated and resulting difficulties in functioning; and behavioural observation of signs and symptoms. The challenges in the assessment are ruling out differentials and identify comorbidities with precedence. These challenges grow bigger when the manifestation of the primary diagnosis is camouflaged by the florid presentation of the comorbid conditions (Ghirwati et a., 2017).

The differential and comorbid diagnostic dilemmas must be contemplated and be resolved over time as the clinician develops a better view of the individual and his psycho-social environment. Therefore, multiple interviews and longitudinal observation is usually helpful in reviewing the diagnostic possibilities. The assessment must be corroborated by clinical interview, psychological use of tools, and observation; involving the index case as well as significant others to gather adequate information and clarification. The entire process of assessment is time-consuming and demands the patience of all stakeholders. But the increased need for mental health services in thickly populated societies has to lead a few Clinicians to bypass this process and initiate the treatment based on the presenting complaints. This approach delays the distinguishing ADHD from the displayed morbidity that becomes the focus of intervention. For example, the academic difficulties of childhood might cause poor social adjustment which creates low self-esteem or poor self-concept. The persistence of this negative self-concept contributes to distress, which when precipitated may lead to some psychiatric disorder that one seeks consultation for (Houck, Kendall, Miller, Morrell, & Wiebe, 2010).

The manifestation and dysfunction of any disorder vary with differences in sociodemographics, family factors, socio-economic status, and social roles that an individual plays. Many of those with ADHD go unnoticed as their compromised functioning does not get the attention of parents or teachers or other significant agents as impairment is not obvious. But as the individuals mature and enter new social roles, the pressure to meet the challenges of routine functioning can be either subtle or severe. This knowledge directs the Clinician to take account of developmental and psychosocial changes in the diagnosis and prognosis of ADHD (Freitag et al., 2012). The psychological assessment must be followed after ruling out issues related to sensory deficits or medical conditions which might be contributing to ADHD like symptoms (Adesman, 2001).

Planning Assessment

The authors are proposing an assessment pyramid in ADHD (APA, figure 1) which depicts the top-to-bottom approach to assessment. The top layer is similar to the tip of the iceberg but there is a lot more as you dig deeper. The individual problems can also be due to a dysfunctional family environment or social adjustment issues in phases of psychosocial development. The knowledge and understanding of developmental theories (Morgan, King, Weisz, & Schopler, 1993) can be adjacent and complementary to the assessment plan. It's conducive to barring age and psychosocial differences in manifestation as well as functioning in diverse domains of one's life (Ford-Jones, 2015). When an individual is presented with ADHD like symptoms, factors inducing emotional disturbance in the family or school environment must be ruled out (Vrijsen et al., 2018). Poor attention is a cognitive reflection of emotional disturbance. Lack of concentration and distractibility are common cognitive symptoms associated with emotional state reflected as negligence in behaviour. Similarly, over activity or hyperactivity may also be seen as a behavioural revelation of emotional disturbance. The children having emotional issues may express aggressive and disorganized behaviour depending upon their temperament or character which may be the result of both internal as well as external factors in one's environment (Hernandez, Smith, Day, Neal, & Dunsmore, 2018). The in-depth assessment of the family and school functioning is necessary as children have this tendency to imitate not only behaviours but also emotional reactions of a person in their environment (Jester et al., 2005). The individuals adopt reactions and cognitive patterns from various social agencies namely; family, neighbourhood, school, etc., that one comes across in the process of socialization (Arnon, Shamai, & Ilatov, 2008). Therefore it is beneficial to identify temperament, personality, habits, and reaction patterns as well as the psychopathology of significant others; as the individual might be internalizing and displaying many signs that may not be interpreted as symptom unless the quality of functioning is significantly compromised. The impulsivity or novelty-seeking in children can also be a temperamental trait inherited or learned as it is closely linked with parenting practices (Lynn et al., 2005). The research highlights that children with superior intelligence are more vigilant and productivity in the area of interest should be considered while interpreting distractibility (Carter & Swanson, 1995). There might be some similarities in the presentation of symptoms in children as well as adolescents and adults. The psychological assessment of individuals must follow the thumb-rule of CTP (Figure 2), that is, cognitive, temperament, or personality, and psychopathology. In the case of children, a test of multiple intelligence may suffice whereas in adults choice can be made from a test of intelligence or neurocognitive functioning or both. The process of assessment must hold an opinion on the source of referral and purpose of assessment. A comprehensive assessment is interpreted based on the following:

Clinical Interview

A detailed interview focusing on various aspects of one's life both cross-sectional and longitudinal is usually helped along with mental status examination (Manley, 2000). The elicitation of signs, symptoms, and treatment history and the most important diagnostic labels attached by other consultations is of great importance. Besides, information must be collected related to family and personal history, mental status examination, and lastly personality or temperament profile. The clinicians who usually rush to gather all of the mentioned information in the first contact without summating it with other sources are more vulnerable to misdiagnose ADHD or miss the diagnosis of ADHD. The three important things to remember is, the interview should be lengthy and vast; persistence and pervasiveness must be enquired with descriptive examples, the interpretation must be in light of socio-cultural norms.

Functional Assessment

The purpose of the assessment does not end with the diagnosis and initiation of treatment. It's a continuous process and a professional may need to revise the assessment of any component at any level. The functional assessment (FA) evolved out of applied behaviour analyses and is an effective method to monitor the progress of the treatment (Dixon, Vogel, & Tarbox, 2012). FA has its roots in operant conditioning and it surveys the contingencies acting upon the target behaviours (DuPaul & Ervin, 1996). The FA sights reinforcers that either cause or maintain any behaviour (Horner & Oregon, 1994). The FA significantly contributes to the treatment outcome and planning rehabilitation in social, educational, or occupational functioning.

Psychological Assessment

It includes diagnostic, severity, and assessment of associated or resulting difficulties. A vast assessment of cognitive, socio-emotional, and behavioural domains can be beneficial in a comprehensive plan for psychological intervention. Therefore, including tests of the neuropsychological profile, peer relations, emotional reactivity, temperament, conflicts, etc. help in identifying the change in functioning due to ADHD and comorbidities, if any. The psychological tools can also be used to monitor the progress of the outcome of the intervention. The selection of the tool is based on age and there is an option of self or clinician-administered measures (Table 2) (Emser et al., 2018; Ramsey, 2017; Pelham, Fabiano, & Massetti, 2005). To develop a holistic management plan it's suggested to use psychological tests for objective assessment of the family environment, peer or social adjustment, etc.

Observation

One should be vigilant to notice any discrepancies in reporting and observation (Adler & Cohen, 2004; McConaughy, Ivanova, & Antshel, 2009). The reasons must be skilfully explored for discrepant information. Most important, differences in intellectual capacities, interest, career choices or personality factors impacting one's information processing and resulting behaviours must be carefully recorded. Also to overcome subjectivity in observation, one can select applicable tools for observation (Table 3), (Emser et al., 2018) and take note of observation of other people in the social environments of the individual.

To summarise, a panoramic assessment with meaningful elements (Figure 3) can coach professionals and researchers to construe ADHD in terms of diagnosis and management.

Issues and Recent Trends in Assessment

Childhood

The childhood presentation is mostly around academic difficulties (Adesman, 2001). It is important to assess intelligence and specific learning disabilities (DuPaul, Gormley, & Laracy, 2012). The manifestation should not be understood only in terms of academics and symptoms, and its effects must be explored in all domains namely; peer relations, cooperative team participation, the perusal of interests and hobbies, etc. Symptoms attributed by emotional disturbance or abuse must not be labelled as ADHD as these might resemble those of ADHD. Whereas ADHD is a neurodevelopmental disorder and not a result of emotional disturbance or trauma. It has been noticed in current clinical settings that children with superior intelligence may be easily mistaken as ADHD by amateur professionals or by those who have limited exposure to manifestation of disorders among high-functioning individuals. Individuals with superior intelligence usually have a gush of physical and mental energy. This should not be confused with hyperkinetic and must be differentiated from high intelligence (Lovecky, 1999).

Adolescence

It's a phase of experimentation and shaping the notions or beliefs that one has learned or internalized in growing years. An individual's independent thinking starts crystallizing in adolescence and in the process many 'hit and trial' actions might be presented as impulsive acts. Another component is emotional regulation (ER) that one is learning ER through his social interactions and relationships (Sanchez, Lavigne, Romero, & Elosegui, 2019) The dilemmas and gullibility related to career choices is another important aspect which can sometimes mislead the professionals. A direct interview with the individual can help the clinician to understand the intention behind one's actions and these insights can be beneficial while diagnosing an adolescent with ADHD.

Adulthood

The most complex diagnosis of ADHD is in adulthood. In most of the cases, the person with ADHD seeks consultation for comorbidities (Wilens & Spencer, 2010). In such a scenario the clinician must be attentive to identify and rule out signs of ADHD in childhood history. The dissatisfactory treatment response to the comorbid condition could also be an indicator of covert ADHD. The manifestation of personality issues can be another misleading factor contributing to the misdiagnosis of ADHD (Storebo & Simonsen, 2013). The history must be reconnoitred for childhood diagnosis of ADHD which got resolved by adolescence. Further, there could be cases having a childhood diagnosis of ADHD requiring precedence over the current diagnosis. Finally, there could be those who were misdiagnosed in childhood with ADHD. All mentioned cases will need an investigation of risk and protective factors (Montoya et al., 2014).

CONCLUSION

There are three possibilities of target populations: one, children and adolescents seeking consultation for deteriorated functioning; two, adults seeking consultation due to socio-occupational difficulties and history revealing ADHD; three, children or adolescents or adults in consultation for the comorbid condition with underlying ADHD. The first two populations groups can be identified with the detailed clinical interview but the third group of the population might require the clinicians to have skills and knowledge of differentials and comorbid conditions to identify ADHD. Also, one should always be observant while eliciting family or marital history, if a family member of the index case shows the manifestation of 'never identified' ADHD and contributes to family psychopathology or disturbed family functioning. Assessment is a dynamic process influenced by ever-changing socio-eco-cultural systems and hence requiring revisions (Slobodin & Crunelle, 2019).

Table 1. Prognostic factors

Source	Good Prognostic Factors	Poor Prognostic Factors
Nigg & Nikolas, 2008	· Stronger reading ability · Absence of aggressive behaviour · Positive peer relations · Effective parenting	· Low socio-economic status · Parental axis I disorders · Marital conflict · Family stress
Schachar & Ickowicz, 2003		· Adverse psychosocial circumstances (e.g. Poverty, overcrowding, hostility in the parent–child relationship) · Parents with ADHD or other psychiatric disorders · Severe and persistent symptoms comorbid conduct, or a language or learning disorder in early development · Problematic social interactions
Gelder, Mayou, & Cowen, 2001		· Associated learning difficulties · Anti-social behaviour · Low intelligence
McCracken, 2000		· High rates of delinquent behaviours · Poorer self-esteem · Lower academic achievement · New diagnoses of conduct disorder, and greater substance abuse
Note: The factors are reported in various research studies and summarised in tabular form.		

Figure 1. Assessment Pyramid of ADHD (APA)
Note: The assessment of individual is only tip of the iceberg.

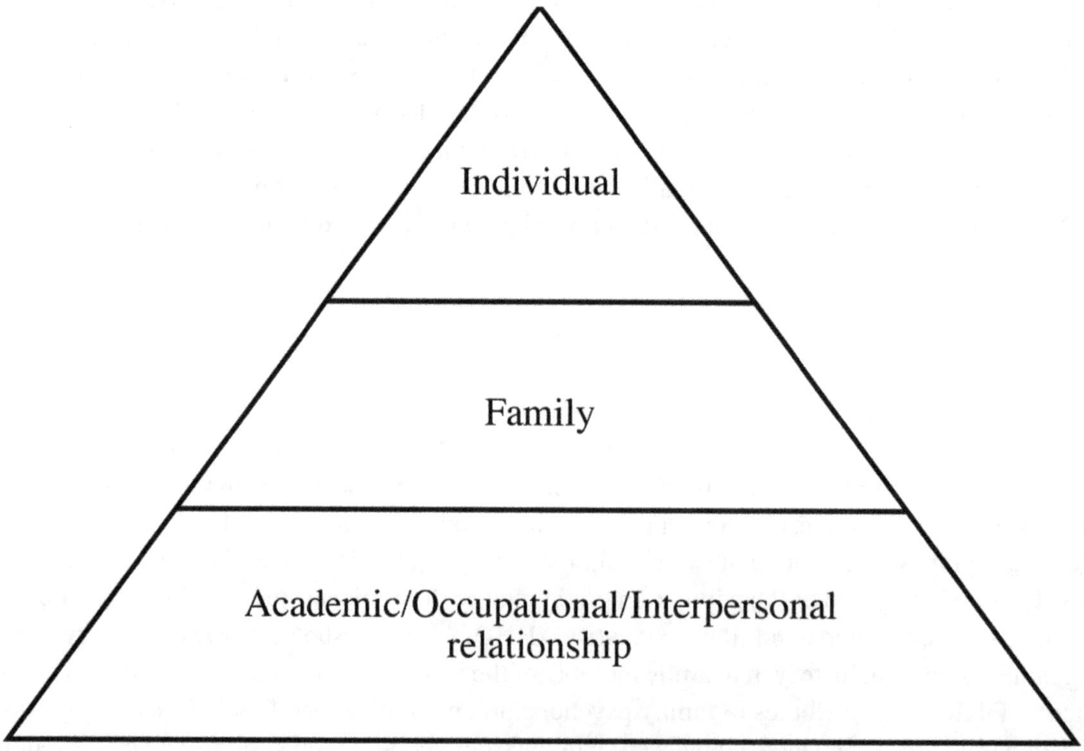

Figure 2. CTP domains of psychological assessment in ADHD
Note: The acronym CTP implies Cognitive, Temperament/Personality and Psychopathology.

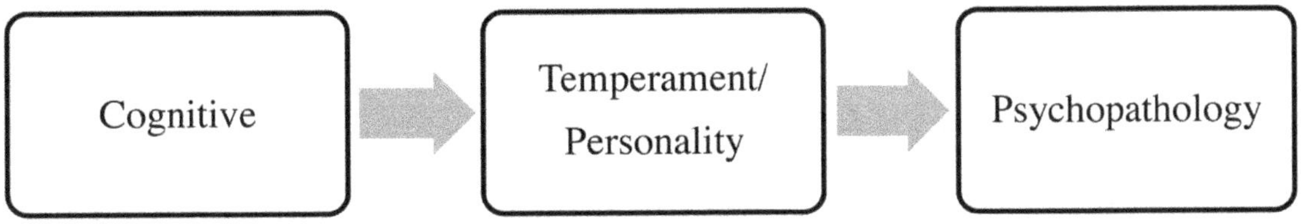

Table 2. List of tools used to diagnose or assess the severity of ADHD

Children and Adolescents	ADHD Child Evaluation (ACE) Vanderbilt ADHD Rating Scale (VADRS) ADHD Rating Scale (ADHD-RS) Swanson, Nolan, and Pelham Rating Scale (SNAP-IV) Child Behaviour Checklist (CBCL) Conners' Rating Scales
Adults	The Adult ADHD Clinical Diagnostic Scale (Adult ACDS) ADHD Lifespan Functioning Interview (ALFI) Conners' Adult ADHD Diagnostic Interview for DSM-IV (CAADID) Diagnostic Interview of ADHD in Adults (DIVA) Structured Clinical Interview for DSM-5 (SCID-5)- Adult ADHD Module Adult ADHD Self-Report Scale (ASRS) Symptom Checklist Barkley Adult ADHD Rating Scale-IV (BAARS-IV) Wender-Reimherr Adult Attention Deficit Disorder Scale (WRAADDS) Wender Utah Rating Scale (WURS) Barkley Adult ADHD Rating Scale-IV (BAARS-IV) Young ADHD Questionnaire (YAQ) Brown Attention Deficit Disorders Scales – Adult Version (BADDS) Conners' Adult ADHD Rating Scales (CAARS)
Note: Mentioned measures are to be chosen according to the sociodemographic of the case or population under study with copyright permission as applicable.	

Table 3. List of tools for Observation

Observation	Classroom Observations of Conduct and Attention Deficit Disorders (COCADD)
	Classroom Behaviour Code
	Response Class Matrix
	Playroom Observations
	STP Point System
	Individualized Target Behaviour Evaluation (ITBE)
Note: To be selected discretely as per the requirement and copyright permission as applicable.	

Figure 3. Components of Assessment
Note: Accurate assessment is central to sound diagnosis and feasible management.

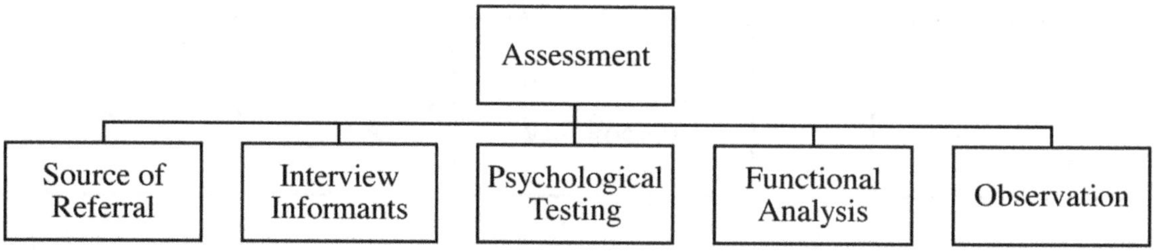

Highlights

- A compressive assessment entails clinical interview, psychological testing and pertinent observation.
- Clinical interview drawn upon developmental theories of Psychology endorses and streamlines the elicitation.
- Interview process guided by Assessment Pyramid of ADHD (APA) rectifies judgment.
- Psychological testing encompassing cognitive, temperament or personality, psychopathology (CTP) domains supports precision.
- Selection of measurement tools must be deliberated upon.
- Testing may be expanded to any of aspect of APA.
- Longitudinal observation in structured and unstructured setting is favourable.
- The assessment is to be interpreted in view of sociodemographics.
- A detailed assessment facilitates precedence of disorders in case of comorbidities
- The cognitive, affective and behavioural symptoms must not be attributed to emotional or mood disturbance or psycho-social adjustments
- Dual diagnosis in adults with ADHD may exacerbate or mask its symptoms.

REFERENCES

Adesman, A. R. (2001). The diagnosis and management of attention-deficit/hyperactivity disorder in pediatric patients. *The Journal of Clinical Psychiatry*, *3*(2), 66–77. doi:10.4088/pcc.v03n0204 PMID:15014618

Adler, L., & Cohen, J. (2004). Diagnosis and evaluation of adults with attention-deficit/hyperactivity disorder. *The Psychiatric Clinics of North America*, *27*(2), 187–201. doi:10.1016/j.psc.2003.12.003 PMID:15063992

American Psychiatric Association. (2013). *Diagnostic and Statistical Manual of Mental Disorders*. 5th. Author.

Arnon, S., Shamai, S., & Ilatov, Z. (2008). Socialization agents and activities of young adolescents. *Adolescence*, *43*, 373–397. PMID:18689107

Barkley, R. A. (2015). History of ADHD. In R. A. Barkley (Ed.), *Attention-Deficit Hyperactivity Disorder: A Handbook for Diagnosis and Treatment* (4th ed., p. 6). Guilford.

Barkley, R. A., Fischer, M., Edelbrock, C. S., & Smallish, L. (1990). The adolescent outcome of hyperactive children diagnosed by research criteria: I. An 8-year prospective follow-up study. *Journal of the American Academy of Child and Adolescent Psychiatry, 29*(4), 546-57. doi: 00007 doi:10.1097/00004583-199007000-

Barkley, R. A., & Peters, H. (2012). The earliest references to ADHD in the medical literature? Melchior Adam Weikard's description in 1775 of "attention deficit" (Mangel Der Aufmerksamkeit, Attnentio Volubilis). *Journal of Attention Disorders, 16*(8), 623–630. doi:10.1177/1087054711432309 PMID:22323122

Biederman, J., Faraone, S., Milberger, S., Curtis, S., Chen, L., Marrs, A., Ouellette, C., Moore, P., & Spencer, T. (1996). Predictors of persistence and remission of ADHD into adolescence: Results from a four-year prospective follow-up study. *Journal of the American Academy of Child and Adolescent Psychiatry, 35*(3), 343–351. doi:10.1097/00004583-199603000-00016 PMID:8714323

Biederman, J., Petty, C. R., Evans, M., Small, J., & Faraone, S. V. (2010). How persistent is ADHD? A controlled 10-year follow-up study of boys with ADHD. *Psychiatry Research, 177*(3), 299–304. doi:10.1016/j.psychres.2009.12.010 PMID:20452063

Carter, J. D., & Swanson, H. L. (1995). The relationship between intelligence and vigilance in children at risk. *Journal of Abnormal Child Psychology, 23*(2), 201–220. doi:10.1007/BF01447089 PMID:7642834

Catalá-López, F., Hutton, B., Núñez-Beltrán, A., Mayhew, A. D., Page, M. J., Ridao, M., Tobías, A., Catalá, M. A., Tabarés-Seisdedos, R., & Moher, D. (2017). The pharmacological and non-pharmacological treatment of attention deficit hyperactivity disorder in children and adolescents: Protocol for a systematic review and network meta-analysis of randomised controlled trials. *Systematic Reviews, 4*(1), 19. doi:10.118613643-015-0005-7 PMID:25875125

Charach, A., Carson, P., Fox, S., Ali, M. U., Beckett, J., & Lim, C. G. (2013). Interventions for preschool children at high risk for ADHD: A comparative effectiveness review. *Paediatrics, 131*(5), 1–21. doi:10.1542/peds.2012-0974 PMID:23545375

Dixon, D. R., Vogel, T., & Tarbox, J. (2012). A brief history of functional analysis and applied behavior analysis. In J. L. Matson (Ed.), *Autism and Child Psychopathology Series* (pp. 3–24). doi:10.1007/978-1-4614-3037-7_2

DuPaul, G. J., & Eckert, T. L. (1997). The effects of school-based interventions for attention deficit hyperactivity disorder: A meta-analysis. *School Psychology Review, 26*, 5–27.

DuPaul, G. J., Eckert, T. L., & Vilardo, B. (2012). The effects of school-based interventions for attention deficit hyperactivity disorder: A meta-analysis 1996-2010. *School Psychology Review, 41*, 387–412.

DuPaul, G. J., & Ervin, R. A. (1996). Functional assessment of behaviours related to attention-deficit/hyperactivity disorder: Linking assessment to intervention design. *Behavior Therapy, 27*(4), 601–622. doi:10.1016/S0005-7894(96)80046-3

Dupaul, G. J., Gormley, M. J., & Laracy, S. D. (2012). Comorbidity of LD and ADHD: Implications of DSM-5 for assessment and treatment. *Journal of Learning Disabilities*. Advance online publication. doi:10.1177/0022219412464351 PMID:23144063

Emser, T. S., Johnston, B. A., Steele, J. D., Kooij, S., Thorell, L., & Christiansen, H. (2018). Assessing ADHD symptoms in children and adults: Evaluating the role of objective measures. *Behavioral and Brain Functions*, *14*(11), 18. doi:10.118612993-018-0143-x PMID:29776429

Epstein, J. N., & Loren, R. E. A. (2013). Changes in the definition of ADHD in DSM-5: Subtle but important. *Neuropsychiatry*, *3*(5), 455–458. doi:10.2217/npy.13.59 PMID:24644516

Fabiano, G. A., Schatz, N. K., Aloe, A. M., Chacko, A., & Chronis-Tuscano, A. (2015). A systematic review of meta-analyses of psychosocial treatment for attention- deficit/hyperactivity disorder. *Clinical Child and Family Psychology Review*, *18*(1), 77–97. doi:10.100710567-015-0178-6 PMID:25691358

Ford-Jones, P. C. (2015). Misdiagnosis of attention deficit hyperactivity disorder: 'Normal behaviour' and relative maturity. *Paediatrics & Child Health*, *20*(4), 200–202. doi:10.1093/pch/20.4.200 PMID:26038639

Freitag, C. M., Hänig, S., Schneider, A., Seitz, C., Palason, H., Retz, W., & Meyer, J. (2012). Biological and psychosocial environmental risk factors influence symptom severity and psychiatric comorbidity in children with ADHD. *Journal of Neural Transmission (Vienna, Austria)*, *119*(1), 81–94. doi:10.100700702-011-0659-9 PMID:21626412

Gelder, M., Mayou, R., & Cowen, P. (2001). *Shorter Oxford Textbook of Psychiatry* (4th ed.). Oxford University Press.

Ghriwati, N. A., Langberg, J. M., Gardner, W., Peugh, J., Kelleher, K. J., Baum, R., ... Epstein, J. N. (2017). Impact of comorbid conditions on the community-based pediatric treatment and outcomes of children with ADHD. *Journal of Developmental and Behavioral Pediatrics*, *38*(1), 20–28. doi:10.1097/DBP.0000000000000359 PMID:27902542

Ginsberg, Y., Quintero, J., Anand, E., Casillas, M., & Upadhyaya, H. P. (2014). Underdiagnosis of attention-deficit/hyperactivity disorder in adult patients: A review of the literature. *The Primary Care Companion for CNS Disorders*, *16*(3), PCC.13r01600. doi:10.4088/PCC.13r01600

Hernandez, E., Smith, C. L., Day, K. L., Neal, A., & Dunsmore, J. C. (2018). Patterns of parental emotion-related discourse and links with children's problem behaviours: A person-centred approach. *Developmental Psychology*, *54*(11), 2077–2089. doi:10.1037/dev0000602 PMID:30284881

Horner, R. H. (1994). Functional assessment: Contributions and future directions. *Journal of Applied Behavior Analysis*, *27*(2), 401–404. doi:10.1901/jaba.1994.27-401 PMID:16795831

Houck, G., Kendall, J., Miller, A., Morrell, P., & Wiebe, G. (2010). Self concept in children and adolescents with ADHD. *Journal of Pediatric Nursing*, *26*(3), 239–247. doi:10.1016/j.pedn.2010.02.004 PMID:21601148

Jester, J. M., Nigg, J. T., Adams, K., Fitzgerald, H. E., Puttler, L. I., Wong, M. M., & Zucker, R. A. (2005). Inattention/hyperactivity and aggression from early childhood to adolescence: Heterogeneity of trajectories and differential influence of family environment characteristics. *Development and Psychopathology*, *17*(1), 99–125. doi:10.1017/S0954579405050066 PMID:15971762

Katya, R. (2018). Cognitive neuroscience of attention deficit hyperactivity disorder (ADHD) and its clinical translation. *Frontiers in Human Neuroscience*, *12*, 100-123. doi:10.3389/fnhum.2018.00100

Kooij, S. J. J., Bejerot, S., Blackwell, A., Caci, H., Casas-Brugué, M., Carpentier, P. J., … Fayyad, J. (2010). European consensus statement on diagnosis and treatment of adult ADHD: The european network adult ADHD. *BMC Psychiatry, 67.* Retrieved from https://www.biomedcentral.com/1471-244X/10/67

Lange, K. W., Reichl, S., Lange, K. M., Tucha, L., & Tucha, O. (2010). The history of attention deficit hyperactivity disorder. *Attention Deficit and Hyperactivity Disorders*, *2*(4), 241–255. doi:10.100712402-010-0045-8 PMID:21258430

Lovecky, D. (1999). *Gifted Children with ADHD*. Program of the 11th Annual CHADD International. Conference, Washington, DC. Retrieved from https://australiangiftedsupport.com/ccmword/wp-content/uploads/2014/12/1352289425.pdf

Lynn, D. E., Lubke, G., Yang, M., McCracken, J. T., McGough, J. J., Ishii, J., ... Nelson, S. F. (2005). Temperament and character profiles and the dopamine D4 receptor gene in ADHD. [Doi]. *The American Journal of Psychiatry*, *162*(5), 906–913. doi:10.1176/appi.ajp.162.5.906 PMID:15863792

Manley, M. R. S. (2000). Psychiatric interview, history, and mental status examination. In B. J. Sadock & V. A. Sadock (Eds.), *Kaplan & Sadock's Comprehensive Textbook of Psychiatry* (7th ed., pp. 1426–1455). Lippincott.

Matthews, M., Nigg, J. T., & Fair, D. A. (2014). Attention deficit hyperactivity disorder. *Current Topics in Behavioral Neurosciences*, *16*, 235–266. doi:10.1007/978-3-662-45758-0_249 PMID:24214656

Mayes, R., & Rafalovich, A. (2008). Suffer the restless children: The evolution of ADHD and paediatric stimulant use, 1900–80. *History of Psychiatry*, *18*(72), 435–457. doi:10.1177/0957154X06075782 PMID:18590022

McConaughy, S. H., Ivanova, M. Y., Antshel, K., Eiraldi, R. B., & Dumenci, L. Standardized observational assessment of attention deficit hyperactivity disorder combined and predominantly inattentive subtypes. II. Classroom observations. *School Psychology Review*, 38(3), 362–381. Retrieved from https://www.ncbi.nlm.nih.gov/pmc/articles/PMC2929014/

Mccracken, J. T. (2000). Attention-deficit disorders. In B. J. Sadock & V. A. Sadock (Eds.), *Kaplan & Sadock's Comprehensive Textbook of Psychiatry* (7th ed., pp. 5540–5541). Lippincott.

Merzenich, M., van Vleet, T. M., & Nahum, M. (2014). Brain plasticity-based therapeutics. *Frontiers in Human Neuroscience*, *8*, 385-401. Doi:10.3389/fnhum.2014.00385

Montoya, A., Quail, D., Anand, E., Cardo, E., Alda, J. A., & Escobar, R. (2014). Prognostic factors of improvement in health-related quality of life in atomoxetine-treated children and adolescents with attention-deficit/hyperactivity disorder, based on a pooled analysis. *Attention Deficit and Hyperactivity Disorders*, *6*(1), 25–34. doi:10.100712402-013-0119-5 PMID:24142305

Morgan, C. T., King, R. A., Weisz, J. R., & Scholper, J. (1993). *Introduction to psychology* (7th ed.). Tata McGraw-Hill.

Nigg, J., & Nikolas, M. (2008). Attention- deficit /hyperactivity disorder. In T. P. Beauchaine & S. P. Hinshaw (Eds.), *Child and Adolescent Psychopathology* (pp. 323–325). John Wiley.

Paris, J., Bhat, V., & Thombs, B. (2015). Is adult attention-deficit hyperactivity disorder being over diagnosed? *Canadian Journal of Psychiatry*, *60*(7), 324–328. doi:10.1177/070674371506000705 PMID:26175391

Pelham, W. E. Jr, Fabiano, G. A., & Massetti, G. M. (2005). Evidence-based assessment of attention deficit hyperactivity disorder in children and adolescents. *Journal of Clinical Child and Adolescent Psychology*, *34*(3), 449–476. doi:10.120715374424jccp3403_5 PMID:16026214

Rafalovich, A. (2001). The conceptual history of attention deficit hyperactivity disorder: Idiocy, imbecility, encephalitis and thc child deviant, 1877–1929. *Deviant Behavior*, *22*(2), 93–115. doi:10.1080/016396201750065009

Ramsay, J. R. (2017). Assessment and monitoring of treatment response in adult ADHD patients: Current perspectives. *Neuropsychiatric Disease and Treatment*, *13*, 221–232. doi:10.2147/NDT.S104706 PMID:28184164

Reed, G. M., First, M. B., Kogan, C. S., Hyman, S. E., Gureje, O., Gaebel, W., Maj, M., Stein, D. J., Maercker, A., Tyrer, P., Claudino, A., Garralda, E., Salvador-Carulla, L., Ray, R., Saunders, J. B., Dua, T., Poznyak, V., Medina-Mora, M. E., Pike, K. M., ... Saxena, S. (2019). Innovations and changes in the ICD-11 classification of mental, behavioural and neurodevelopmental disorders. *World Psychiatry; Official Journal of the World Psychiatric Association (WPA)*, *18*(1), 3–19. doi:10.1002/wps.20611 PMID:30600616

Sánchez, M., Lavigne, R., Romero, J. F., & Elósegui, E. (2019). Emotion regulation in participants diagnosed with attention deficit hyperactivity disorder, before and after an emotion regulation intervention. *Frontiers in Psychology*, *10*, 10. doi:10.3389/fpsyg.2019.01092 PMID:31178779

Schachar, R., & Ickowicz, A. (2003). Attention-deficit hyperkinetic disorders in childhood and adolescence. In M. G. Gelder, J. J. Lopez-Ibor, N. Andreasen, & J. J. Lopez-Idor (Eds.), *New Oxford Textbook of Psychiatry* (pp. 1365–1366). Oxford University Press.

Slobodin, O., & Crunelle, C. L. (2019). Mini review: Socio-cultural influences on the link between ADHD and SUD. *Frontiers in Public Health*, *7*, 173–186. doi:10.3389/fpubh.2019.00173 PMID:31294015

Storebø, O. J., & Simonsen, E. (2013). The association between ADHD and antisocial personality disorder (ASPD): A review. *Journal of Attention Disorders*. Advance online publication. doi:10.1177/1087054713512150 PMID:24284138

Van Doren, J., Arns, M., Heinrich, H., Vollebreat, M. A., Strehl, U., & Loo, S. K. (2019). Sustained effects of neurofeedback in ADHD: A systematic review and meta-analysis. *European Child & Adolescent Psychiatry*, *28*, 293–305. doi:10.100700787-018-1121-4 PMID:29445867

Vrijsen, J. N., Tendolkar, I., Onnik, M., Hoogman, M., Schene, A. H., & Fernández, G. (2018). ADHD symptoms in healthy adults are associated with stressful life events and negative memory bias. *Attention Deficit and Hyperactivity Disorders*, *10*(2), 151–160. doi:10.100712402-017-0241-x PMID:29081022

Wilens, T. E., & Spencer, T. J. (2010). Understanding attention-deficit/hyperactivity disorder from childhood to adulthood. *Postgraduate Medical Journal*, *122*(5), 97–109. doi:10.3810/pgm.2010.09.2206 PMID:20861593

World Health Organization. (2004). *The ICD 10 classification of mental and behavioural disorder: Clinical descriptions and diagnostic guidelines*. https://www.who.int/classifications/icd/en/bluebook.pdf

Chapter 8
Pharmacological Treatment of ADHD

Prateek Yadav
Government Hospital, India

ABSTRACT

The pharmacological treatment for ADHD has been researched well and we have efficacious drugs. Drugs are the mainstay of treatment particularly for over 6 years of age. There are two broad classes of drugs that are used in the treatment, psychostimulants and non-stimulants. Transcranial current stimulation and neurofeedback are other mechanisms that have been tried. There are various formulations and doses available for each and only certain drugs are available in India. The various guidelines broadly put stimulant Methylphenidate as the first choice and recommend early shift to a longer acting formulation. Treatment, various comorbidities, and side-effects of these drugs have to be kept in mind and dealt accordingly. Further psychosocial treatments should be used concurrently to improve the outcome.

INTRODUCTION

The pharmacological treatment for ADHD has been researched and rehearsed quite well, we have efficacious drugs and further search into new molecules is ongoing. Efficacy of both types of interventions i.e. psychosocial and medication is well established, however, drugs are the mainstay of treatment particularly for over 6yrs of age *(NICE, 2005)*. The Multimodal Treatment for ADHD study (MTA) established medication as a more effective modality compared to behavioural treatment *(MTA Cooperative Group, 1999)*

Studies have shown that children diagnosed with ADHD, being treated with medications, are academically closer to the normal children when compared to ADHD without medication and discontinuation of medication, has negative effects on academic performance. *(Keilow, Holm & Fallesen 2018)*. There are two broad classes of drugs that are used in the treatment, Psychostimulants and the Non-stimulants, which contain apart from Atomoxetine, drugs from other classes with mode of action different from the stimulants. Apart from this there are clinical procedures which help in alleviating the symptoms.

DOI: 10.4018/978-1-7998-5495-1.ch008

STIMULANTS

Psychostimulants are indirectly acting sympathomimetic amines having both central and peripheral effects. They exert clinical effects by increasing extracellular catecholamine levels in condition where it is deficit and thereby improving motivation, attention, wakefulness and also stimulate the cardiovascular system. Benzedrine, marketed in 1933 as decongestant, was the first pharmaceutical drug that contained Amphetamine. Bradley, in 1937, reported that the drug also improved behavior problems in children. Dextroamphetamine was also available in 1937, and Methylphenidate became available in 1954 *(Lange, Reichl, Lange, Tucha 2010)*. Since these 70 years, Psychostimulants have been popular and standard treatment for ADHD; however their high efficacy has been challenged with concerns of dependence and growth retardation. A study researching into trends in ADHD medication use in five countries found that its use was highest in 10-14yrs group, with highest use in US and Netherlands, further Amphetamines were being used more in US than Europe, where, Methylphenidate predominated. *(Bachmanna et al 2017)*

The two groups of stimulant medication that have received U.S. Food and Drug Administration (FDA) approval for the treatment of ADHD are Amphetamines and Methylphenidate (MPH). Both are schedule X drug in India, and controlled by the Drugs and Cosmetic Rule, 1945. In US they are schedule II controlled substances. Stimulants are first line drugs in ADHD in children, adolescent and adults and have a legacy of decades of proven efficacy and research (*NICE 2018)*. Both of these have a high effect size relative to non-stimulant medication (>0.8 vs 0.6) and amphetamine has a moderately greater effect size then methylphenidate. Meta-analysis comparing stimulants to non-stimulants found the effect sizes of long-acting stimulants to be significantly higher for stimulants than non-stimulants. *(Faraone, Buitelaar 2010)*

MECHANISM OF ACTION

ADHD is associated with lower levels of Dopamine and Norepinephrine (DA and NA) in prefrontal cortex (PFC) and both of these stimulants act by increasing concentration of DA and NA in the synaptic cleft; MPH acts on the reuptake channels allosterically, blocks both NA and DA reuptake, thus their levels increase in the synaptic cleft and these then engage dopamine (D1) receptors, improving neurotransmission. Amphetamines, on the other hand are competitive inhibitor and pseudosubstrate for reuptake channels of NE and DA and additionally also facilitates the release of DA via reverse transport.

FMRI study shows that MPH improves the response inhibition, frontal activation and increases striatal activity in ADHD children. The striatal activity is decreased if MPH is given to healthy controls *(Vaidya et al, 1998)*. It also shows improvement in working memory and is related to reduction in rCBF in the dorsolateral prefrontal cortex and posterior parietal cortex.*(Mehta et al 2006)*

	Stimulants available in India (Shah, Grover, Avasthi, 2019)	**FORMULATION**	**DOSAGE**
1	Methylphenidate Immediate Release	Tab 10 mg	5 mg OD or BD to 60 mg
2	Methylphenidate Intermediate Release	Tab 10mg,18mg,20mg	10 mg to 60 mg
3	Methylphenidate Long acting (OROS)	Tab 18mg,36mg,54mg	18mg to 72 mg

FORMULATIONS

Methylphenidate, is the only stimulant medication available in India. There are four stereoisomers of MPH (dextro and levo forms of both *threo* and *erythro* isomers), however pharmacologically useful are the *threo-racemate.* In the latter, d-threo is the more active enantiomer. Formulations of MPH use either racemic mixtures of both enantiomers in equal ratios, or only *d-threo* enantiomer. *(Dinis-Oliveira 2017)*

Immediate release(IR) is available in tablet, chewable and liquid form, with short lasting effects of a few hours and thus two or three times dosing is required, this causes fluctuation and unpredictable variance in concentration of the drug in plasma reducing the expected efficacy and also increasing the side-effects. Sustained release (SR) preparations were devised to overcome some of these side effects of IR preparations but at the cost of compromising the desired efficacy, as in these there is development of acute tolerance due to lack of steep absorption phase and a plateau of delivery phase following the achievement of peak levels (*Swanson et al 2013).* Extended release formulations, using beaded technology, have been developed which simulate two-three times daily administration of immediate release formulations. An orally disintegrating tablet has also been developed using osmotic release oral system (*Concerta*) and also a transdermal patch is available to be worn for upto 9hrs a day. SR preparations remain the first line treatment options for ADHD in adults owing to their lower abuse potential and steady state concentrations.

Immediate releasc MPH is completely absorbed after oral administration and reaches peak concentration in one to three hours and is rapidly distributed due to its high lipid solubility and a lesser degree of protein-binding. The dextro enantiomer owes it better action due to better penetration *of* the blood brain barrier. 60-80% of dose elimination occurs in 40-60hrs, primarily in the urine. *(Wolraich, Doffing; 2004)*

Amphetamine is available in Immediate-release and Extended-release beaded formulations. More than 90% of the immediate release, dose is absorbed in the GI tract and the Tmax is 2-4hrs. It is rapidly distributed and readily crosses the Blood Brain Barrier. Immediate release formulations are available as mixed salts (mixture of d- and l- isomers) or as d-amphetamine. The latter reaches a higher concentration in the brain. Lisdexamfetamine is a 'prodrug' in which the dexamfetamine is complexed with the aminoacid lysine and in this form is inactive. It becomes active only after lyses in the red blood cells which makes the dexamfetamine available. It is thus similar to extended-release preparations of methylphenidate; but, unlike them has a much lesser abuse potential. Amphetamine is excreted out mainly through kidneys and is influence by the urinary pH; reportedly the $t_{1/2}$ increases by about seven hours with every unit increase in the urinary pH *(Markowitz, Patrick 2017).* Thus the package warning states changes in the plasma concentration of the drug with consumption of foods with acidic content.

BEHAVIORAL AND COGNITIVE EFFECTS

Stimulants reduce overactivity, and increase concentration in ADHD patients, thereby improving school performance and academics. Although long-term benefits still require evidence, on a daily basis, interruptive behaviours, fidgeting, interactions and compliance shows definitive improvement. Socially these patients show improved compliance to compatible behaviour with medication and improve problem solving during games and sustained attention during play. In terms of Cognitive ability there is decreased response variability and reduced impulsive responses, along with increased precision and improved reaction time and computation ability. *(Richters et al 1995; Tannock, Schachar, Logan 1995)*

ADVERSE EFFECTS

Most of the adverse effects associated with these drugs are generally mild or for short duration and slow titration, dose and timing adjustment alleviates them considerably. Initially autonomic side effects like tremors, raised Blood Pressure and cardiac rhythm disturbances along with sleep disturbances and agitation, feeling nervous might occur due to increase in norepinephrine peripherally and dopamine centrally which can also cause certain psychotic features (1-2%). Less common side effects include: exacerbation of motor and vocal tics, aggressiveness/hostility. Other rare effects include Seizures and rare activation of hypomania or suicidal ideation; priapism and tactile hallucinations are also reported in a few cases taking these drugs. *(Kratochvil CJ, et al 2008)*

The two Cochrane systematic reviews on MPH found 29% increase in risk of any non-serious side-effects. The most common among these were sleep problems (60% greater risk) and decreased appetite (266% greater risk*). (Storebø et al 2015 ; Storebø et al 2018)*

Although the data on usage during pregnancy and lactation is low, no general increase in congenital anomalies have been shown, secretion in human milk is low except for amphetamines which should be avoided. Therefore, due to paucity of data need during pregnancy should be reconsidered and if required the above should be kept in mind.

Effects on Growth

Stimulants have been shown to effect the growth in children although conclusive data is still awaited, monitoring of growth is must in patients being treated with these drugs. Height should be measured every six months in children and young and weight to be monitored every 3 month in patients till 10yrs of age. If on monitoring, height is found to be less than that expected for age then, consider a planned break in treatment (drug holiday). Change of medication can also be considered. *(Poulton 2005)*

NONSTIMULANT MEDICATIONS

Although the stimulant drugs have remained the first line of treatment and choice, the other class of drugs are equally important as they are useful in many a case where stimulants cannot be used as in face of non-response or severe adverse effects. Apart from these indications they are also used as the initial choice on case to case basis.

Atomoxetine

It has been approved by FDA in 2002 for adults and children over 6yrs of age and is licensed in Europe for children and adults if their treatment has started in childhood. The American academy of Child and Adolescent Psychiatry Practise lists it as a first line option.

It is available in capsules of 10mg to 100mg in various strengths (*Strattera® US prescribing information. 2015.)* and acts through inhibition of the pre-synaptic nor-epinephrine transporter. It is a selective norepinephrine reuptake inhibitor, and since Pre-frontal cortex has low concentration of Dopamine-Transporter, inhibiting the NE transporter (which deactivates DA in pre-frontal cortex) increases both NE and DA in this area. Since the Nucleus Acumbens has a few NE transporter, the action of Atomoxetine is not replicated here, making it safe against abuse potential. Thus other drugs acting on the same transporter have also been used with varying results like, Reboxetine, Bupropion, and TCA. *(Stephen M. Stahl Fourth Edition.)*

It is well absorbed after oral dosing with bio-availability ranging 63%-90% and the blood levels are not affected much by food. It has peak plasma concentration in 1-2hrs and has a half life of approximately 5hrs. However in slow metabolisers it may be as high as 20hrs. (*Saue, Ring, Witcher 2005)*

The max daily dose in children and adolescent as per FDA is 1.4mg/kg/day in those with <70kg weight and in those with higher, it is 100mg/day. Studies which used higher doses have not shown any significant advantage. The effect size from various studies is 0.6 to 0.71.

Atomoxetine generally shows improvement in ADHD symptoms within 6 weeks, while some studies show even an earlier effect, with around 25% improvement of symptoms in 3.7 weeks. There is improvement in emotional lability, executive function and quality of life measures. With Atomoxetine children report better sleep, shorter sleep latency and easy to get up in morning, when compared to Methylphenidate, also parents reported less irritability and that children tend to get up and get ready easily in the morning The clinical trials have reported improvement in symptoms of ADHD in patients with comorbid anxiety and tic disorders, without worsening of these comorbid symptoms. A systematic review also supports this claim stating that presence of co-morbidity did not lessen Atomoxetine efficacy of treating ADHD symptoms. The drug has no deleterious effect on growth or sexual development. Partial responders to Atomoxetine may benefit from addition of MPH to regime. *(Wilens et al. 2009; Ann C Childress, 2016)*

Common side effects include sedation, day time somnolescence, fatigue, dry mouth, nausea, decrease in appetite, constipation, abdominal pain and sometimes rise of mean systolic pressure in adults and diastolic pressure in children.

Atomoxetine has a black box warning pertaining to potential suicide attempts. Although the number is small, children and adolescents taking Atomoxetine experience suicidal thoughts or behaviours, compared with none of those taking placebo. Although the literature is divided, but certain studies showing this as a potential issue, caution and information needs to be conveyed to the care-givers. (*Kratochvil et al 2009)*

Guanfecine and Clonidine

α-adrenergic agents, Clonidine ER and Guanfacine ER have been approved by the FDA for ADHD treatment for ages 6 to 17yrs, however these are not available in India (plain Clonidine available in India). Guanfacine is relatively more selective for the α-2A receptors while Clonidine is non-selective with additional actions on various alpha-receptors and also on imidazoline receptors which might explain its sedating action. Thus, Guanfacine will exhibit efficacy with reduced adverse effects, compared to Clonidine. Clonidine is given at 0.1mg to 0.4mg/day in divided doses and Guanfacine, 1-4mg per day. Guanfacine due to its mode of action combats symptoms of oppositional defiance, disobedience, aggression and temper tantrums better than Clonidine. Clonidine is commonly used to treat stimulant-induced tics and insomnia. Full effects may not be seen for 4 to 6 weeks. Common side effects include orthostatic hypotension, dry-mouth, and dizziness. Patients may also complain of weakness or fatigue and sedation. Some may have serious effects like sinus bradycardia and AV block. Slow titration is recommended when Clonidine is discontinued to avoid rebound hypertension.

Other Medications

A lot more of antipsychotics are used as off-label for ADHD patients particularly to control behaviour abnormalities and the percentage of youths with a new ADHD diagnosis treated with these was greater than the overall antipsychotics treatment among youths in general population of US. Aggression, which is common in ADHD and not always responsive to stimulant medications, has been hypothesized to account for much of the off-label use of antipsychotics in youths with ADHD. (*Olfson, King, Schoenbaum. 2015 ; Sultan et al 2019).* Tricyclic antidepressants have also been shown to benefit in ADHD symptoms, however problem with side effects limit their use.

Bupropion is used particularly in adolescent and not recommended for children. It is less effective then stimulants or Atomoxetine. It is used as off-label drug and is FDA approved for depression and smoking cessation.

DIETARY SUPPLEMENTS

Some studies present evidence for the role of nutritional PUFA, zinc, magnesium, iron supplements in the treatment. Pol-unsaturated Fatty acids, various vitamins etc, being prescribed and advertised as supplements are commonly the interventions suggested. The evidence at best, points to a marginal beneficial effect. Zinc, iron and magnesium supplements may reduce symptoms in those with deficiencies or at risk of these deficiencies *(Lange et al 2017).* Reviewing the evidence about artiðcial colors suggest a positive but small effect size. NICE guidelines however state that there is no evidence about the effectiveness or potential harm of a new diet and only limited evidence of short-term benefits are seen.

TRANSCRANIAL DIRECT CURRENT STIMULATION

This mode of treatment has been suggested by a number of studies and the initial results appear to be beneficial. The site of application has been right inferior pre-frontal cortex which is consistently underactive in ADHD and also upregulated with use of stimulants; also left dorsolateral prefrontal cortex and right inferior frontal gyrus has been suggested. Studies have shown, reduced inattention, improved performance in attention, improvement in working memory, improvement both in inhibitory control and interference control. (*Westwood, Radua & Rubia 2019 ; Mirzaiyan et al 2108)*

NEUROFEEDBACK

Through this, the participant can learn to self-regulate his own brain activity to directly alter the underlying neural mechanism of cognition and behavior, based on principles of operant conditioning and procedural skills learning. Proposed that neurofeedback strives to decrease theta and/or increase beta power in central and frontal locations *(Barry, Clarke, Johnstone, 2003).* A recent meta-analysis looking at long term effects of this procedure showed that the effects, after six-month follow-up were no different from the active treatment group which included methylphenidate and the effects of neurofeedback increases with time. Thus the procedure is at least as beneficial as active pharmacological treatment. *(Van Doren et al 2018)*

RECOMMENDATIONS FOR TREATMENT

For children below 5yrs, the NICE guidelines recommend management with ADHD –focussed group parent-training programme, so as to train the parents or caregivers as the first-line of management. They also recommend that medication should be offered in this age-group only after second specialist opinion.

In the age-group over 5yrs, medication is recommended when the symptoms are causing persistent impairment even after environmental modification, and started after briefing parents/caregiver and getting a baseline assessment done. NICE states Methylphenidate as the first line treatment for 5yrs over and young people. If there is not enough benefit after 6wks of trial switch to lisdexamphetamine is recommended and further shift to dexamphetamine in case of non-response.

If there is difficulty in tolerating the stimulants, or if the response is inadequate even after 6wk trial of adequate dose and alternative preparations then Atomoxetine or Guanfacine is to be offered. Adults who have impairment due to ADHD symptoms can be treated in more or less the same lines with adequate dosages. In India as only Methylphenidate and Atomoxetine are available the recommendations should be thus followed accordingly.

Immediate release medications can be used during initial titration and for deciding the correct dose levels and in cases where flexible dosing regimen is required, but with further continuation of treatment once daily preparations are recommended for convenience of use and improving adherence. Once daily dosing provides usage benefits as they are not required to be used in school, risk of misuse as stimulants is reduced and stigma of medications is also taken care of.

During the initial titration phase the progress is to be reviewed regularly and adverse effects to be noticed. The titration should be slow and the co-morbid conditions should be tackled simultaneously. Specific enquiries should be made regarding the improvement like, as to when does the improvement becomes apparent as per the observed behaviour, and as to when the symptoms restart during the day, eg whether during early afternoon the child becomes disruptive or during early evening hours. This helps in titration of dose and scheduling of drug. Appetite suppression could be an early concern for the parents and should be addressed without fail. The combination with behaviour therapy should be offered from start as it has shown benefits particularly in controlling aggression and in some cases reduction in the final medication dose requirement. The titration in the initial phase in case of Methylphenidate for example can start with 5mg twice or thrice a day, after an initial assessment using a scale like SNAP-IV. The improvement is assessed after a two-week period and also by parent's feedback, and if there is no further scope of improvement then the dose can be continued. However, this needs a careful assessment as commonly the improvement may be so satisfying to the parents that many symptoms or lesser degrees of them may be ignored. So, if there is still scope of improvement, the dosage is increased from 5mg to 10mg and follow up continues, and upward titration till maximum response expected is reached or maximum dose is reached. Further augmentation strategy as stated above can be followed and scales to be used for objective assessment at each meeting during dose scheduling. After optimising dose, the drug can be shifted to a longer acting formulation for ease of administration and better compliance and having a smooth concentration in body. It is recommended that the changes in dose schedules be done over weekend as it facilitates early evaluation by parents.(*NICE. Attention deficit hyperactivity disorder: diagnosis and management 2018)*

MANAGING THE CO-MORBIDITIES

ADHD With Tics

Presence of Tics might be initiated or worsened by use of stimulants, so a correct history is required for planning of management. Tics will also limit further dose increase of stimulants. If these are stimulant related, reducing the dose and shifting to different formulation might help or change to Clonidine/ Atomoxetine (or Guanfacine) is recommended. Combination of stimulant and alpha agonist should be used with caution for possibility of heart rhythm disturbances. If the change to different drug does not alleviate the symptoms then tic reducing medication might be used in conjunction (risperidone, SSRI etc). Behavioral therapy like opposing muscle contraction exercise is also found useful. (*Osland, Steeves, Pringsheim, 2018)*

ADHD With Autism Spectrum Disorder

A multidisciplinary specialist intervention is recommended, and the symptoms of ADHD be targeted with medication, Methylphenidate is recommended. Lowest possible dose and very slow titration should be done as these set of patients are more prone to side-effects. Behavior therapy should be delivered simultaneously.

ADHD With Mood Disorder

A major depressive disorder is more common in children and adolescent with ADHD, and as are the chances of recurrence and suicide. The guidelines recommend combination of medication and behavioural intervention be used for effective management and that the treating physician starts with the target symptom of the more disabling condition and then the second drug be added for the remaining symptoms (*Hughes et al 2007)*. While using drugs their interactions should be kept in mind like, Fluoxetine and Atomoxetine are both metabolised by CYP2D6 and thus the levels of each drug will increase, when used simultaneously.

Stimulant medication can cause low mood as side effect, and can also induce manic episode along with psychotic symptoms.(*Kraemer M, et al. 2010)* One line of research states to use mood stabilisers or antipsychotics to manage bipolar disorder before stimulant treatment is initiated. Bipolar in youth can also be managed with atypical antipsychotics, and stimulants along with antipsychotics in these conditions can be beneficial. *(Kowatch et al 2005)*

Some research shows Atomoxetine to be safer although there are studies which have associated its use with mania, hypomania or irritability in almost one-third of the treated patients. Clonidine has also been reported to be effective in the treatment of manic episodes.*(Girard, & Joober, 2017)*

ADHD With Anxiety Disorder

ADHD with comorbid anxiety may not respond as well to stimulants and may report more side effects; however it does not mean that they are ineffective in this scenario. MTA study reports no adverse effects of anxiety on the response of ADHD symptoms to stimulant treatment. However, it also reported beneficial effects of psychosocial treatment and this is recommended in case of comorbid disorder to achieve remission. Atomoxetine has been found to reduce anxiety symptoms and can be used. Atomoxetine does not improve symptoms of anxiety in patients with anxiety disorders without ADHD; so maybe, the improvements seen in symptoms are actually due to ADHD symptom improvement. (March et al 2000)

Investigational Drugs

Many drugs are under investigation and trial for the treatment of ADHD, these include both stimulant and non-stimulant and each is being investigated with a certain advantage, either in context of adverse effect or tolerability or pharmacokinetics.

These include stimulant-under investigations, labelled as HLD200, formulation of MPH being studied for delayed release and extended release drug delivery platform; or SHP465, a triple bead mixed amphetamine salt. Another amphetamine liquid suspension is being developed using Tris Pharma's LiquiXR TM technology.

Non stimulant under investigation are, Edivoxretine, a selective norepinephrine reuptake inhibitor; Dasotraline, triple reuptake inhibitor; Centanafadine, Metadoxine, Amiloride, L-methylfolate, Droxidopa and Vortioxetine are among others under investigation.*(Childress 2016)*

CONCLUSION

Efficient and evidence-based treatment modalities for ADHD are available readily. Both psychosocial and pharmacological treatments are advised with a bent more towards the latter in cases leading to impairment in functioning. In India only a few of the above formulations are available and the plan has to be drawn in accordingly. The treatment must continue with regular follow-up and objective assessment of the symptoms and the adverse effects. The comorbidities should not be ignored as they possess equal capacity for reducing the quality of life and the holistic treatment plan should incorporate them, as they are more common than not. Finally,the patient and care-givers should be prepared for a long-term treatment and follow-up.

REFERENCES

Ann, C. M. D., & Drugs, C. T. C. I.Treatment of Attention-Deficit/Hyperactivity Disorder. (2016). *Expert Opinion on Investigational Drugs.*

Bachmanna. (2017). Trends in ADHD medication use in children and adolescents in five western countries, 2005–2012. *European Neuropsychopharmacology, 27*(5), 484-493.

Barry, R. J., Clarke, A. R., & Johnstone, S. J. (2003). A review of electrophysiology in attention-deficit/hyperactivity disorder: I. Qualitative and quantitative electroencephalography. *Clinical Neurophysiology*, *114*(2), 171–183. doi:10.1016/S1388-2457(02)00362-0 PMID:12559224

Bradley, C. (1937). The behavior of children receiving benzedrine. *The American Journal of Psychiatry*, *94*(3), 577–585. doi:10.1176/ajp.94.3.577

Childress, A. C. (2015). A critical appraisal of atomoxetine in the management of ADHD. *Therapeutics and Clinical Risk Management*, *12*, 27–39. doi:10.2147/TCRM.S59270 PMID:26730199

Christian, L., & Bachmanna, J. (2017, May). Trends in ADHD medication use in children and adolescents in five western countries, 2005–2012. *European Neuropsychopharmacology*, *27*(5), 484–493. doi:10.1016/j.euroneuro.2017.03.002 PMID:28336088

Clarke, A. R., Barry, R. J., Heaven, P. C. L., McCarthy, R., Selikowitz, M., & Byrne, M. K. (2008). EEG in adults with attention-deficit/hyperactivity disorder. *International Journal of Psychophysiology*, *70*(3), 176–183. doi:10.1016/j.ijpsycho.2008.07.001 PMID:18662727

Dinis-Oliveira, R. J. (2017). Metabolomics of methylphenidate and ethylphenidate: Implications in pharmacological and toxicological effects. *European Journal of Drug Metabolism and Pharmacokinetics*, *42*(1), 11–16. doi:10.100713318-016-0362-1 PMID:27438788

Faraone, S. V., & Buitelaar, J. (2010). Comparing the efficacy of stimulants for ADHD in children and adolescents using meta-analysis. *European Child & Adolescent Psychiatry*, *19*(4), 353–364. doi:10.100700787-009-0054-3 PMID:19763664

Faraone, S. V., & Glatt, S. J. (2010). A comparison of the efficacy of medications for adult attention-deficit/hyperactivity disorder using meta-analysis of effect sizes. *The Journal of Clinical Psychiatry*, *71*(6), 754–763. doi:10.4088/JCP.08m04902pur PMID:20051220

Froehlich, T.E., Lanphear, B.P., Epstein, J.N., Barbaresi, W.J., Katusic, S.K., & Kahn, R.S. (n.d.). Prevalence, recognition, and treatment of attention-deficit/hyperactivity disorder in a national sample of US children. Archives of Pediatrics & Adolescent Medicine, 161(9), 857–864. PubMed doi:10.1001/archpedi.161.9.857

Girard, R., & Joober, R. (2017). Treatment of ADHD in patients with bipolar disorder. *Journal of psychiatry & neuroscience. JPN*, *42*(6), E11–E12. doi:10.1503/jpn.170097 PMID:29083298

Hah, M., & Chang, K. (2005). Atomoxetine for the treatment of attention-deficit/hyperactivity disorder in children and adolescent with bipolar disorders. *Journal of Child and Adolescent Psychopharmacology*, *15*(6), 996–1004. doi:10.1089/cap.2005.15.996 PMID:16379520

Hales, C. M., Kit, B. K., Gu, Q., & Ogden, C. L. (2007). Trends in prescription medication use among children and adolescents—United States, 1999-2014. *Journal of the American Medical Association*, *319*(19), 2009–2020.

Henderson, T. A., & Hartman, K. (2004). Aggression, mania and hypomania induction associated with atomoxetine. *Pediatrics*, *114*(3), 895–896. doi:10.1542/peds.2004-1140 PMID:15342872

Hughes, C. W., Emslie, G. J., Crismon, M. L., Posner, K., Birmaher, B., Ryan, N., Jensen, P., Curry, J., Vitiello, B., Lopez, M., Shon, S. P., Pliszka, S. R., & Trivedi, M. H.Texas Consensus Conference Panel on Medication Treatment of Childhood Major Depressive Disorder. (2007). Texas Children's Medication Algorithm Project. Update from Texas Consensus Conference Panel on Medication Treatment of Childhood Major Depressive Disorder. *Journal of the American Academy of Child and Adolescent Psychiatry*, *46*(6), 667–686. doi:10.1097/chi.0b013e31804a859b PMID:17513980

Hutchison, S. L., Ghuman, J. K., Ghuman, H. S., Karpov, I., & Schuster, J. M. (2016). Efficacy of atomoxetine in the treatment of attention-deficit hyperactivity disorder in patients with common comorbidities in children, adolescents and adults: A review. *Therapeutic Advances in Psychopharmacology*, *6*(5), 317–334. doi:10.1177/2045125316647686 PMID:27721971

Keilow, M., Holm, A., & Fallesen, P. (2018). Medical treatment of Attention Deficit/Hyperactivity Disorder (ADHD) and children's academic performance. *PLoS One*, *13*(11), e0207905. doi:10.1371/journal.pone.0207905 PMID:30496240

Kowatch, R. A., Fristad, M., Birmaher, B., Wagner, K. D., Findling, R. L., & Hellander, M. (2005). Treatment guidelines for children and adolescents with bipolar disorders. *Journal of the American Academy of Child and Adolescent Psychiatry*, *44*(3), 213–235. doi:10.1097/00004583-200503000-00006 PMID:15725966

Kraemer, M., Uekermann, J., Wiltfang, J., & Kis, B. (2010). Methylphenidate-induced psychosis in adult attention-deficit/hyperactivity disorder: Report of 3 new cases and review of the literature. *Clinical Neuropharmacology*, *33*(4), 204–206. doi:10.1097/WNF.0b013e3181e29174 PMID:20571380

Kratochvil, C. J., Michelson, D., Newcorn, J. H., Weiss, M. D., Busner, J., Moore, R. J., Ruff, D. D., Ramsey, J., Dickson, R., Turgay, A., Saylor, K., Luber, S., Vaughan, B., & Allen, A. J. (2007). High-dose atomoxetine treatment of ADHD in youths with limited response to standard doses. *Journal of the American Academy of Child and Adolescent Psychiatry*, *46*(9), 1128–1137. doi:10.1097/chi.0b013e318074eeb3 PMID:17712236

Kratochvil, C. J., Vaughan, B. S., Barker, A., Corr, L., Wheeler, A., & Madaan, V. (2009, March). Review of pediatric attention deficit/hyperactivity disorder for the general psychiatrist. *The Psychiatric Clinics of North America*, *32*(1), 39–56. doi:10.1016/j.psc.2008.10.001 PMID:19248915

Lange, K. W., Hauser, J., Lange, K. M., Makulska-Gertruda, E., Nakamura, Y., Reissmann, A., Sakaue, Y., Takano, T., & Takeuchi, Y. (2017). The Role of Nutritional Supplements in the Treatment of ADHD: What the Evidence Says. *Current Psychiatry Reports*, *19*(2), 8. doi:10.100711920-017-0762-1 PMID:28168597

Lange, K. W., Reichl, S., Lange, K. M., Tucha, L., & Tucha, O. (2010). The history of attention deficit hyperactivity Disorder. *Attention Deficit and Hyperactivity Disorders*, *2*(4), 241–255. doi:10.100712402-010-0045-8 PMID:21258430

Maldonado, R. (2013). Comparison of the pharmacokinetics and clinical efficacy of new extended-release formulations of methylphenidate. *Expert Opinion on Drug Metabolism & Toxicology*, *9*(8), 1001–1014. doi:10.1517/17425255.2013.786041 PMID:23611637

March, J. S., Swanson, J. M., Arnold, L. E., Hoza, B., Conners, C. K., Hinshaw, S. P., Hechtman, L., Kraemer, H. C., Greenhill, L. L., Abikoff, H. B., Elliott, L. G., Jensen, P. S., Newcorn, J. H., Vitiello, B., Severe, J., Wells, K. C., & Pelham, W. E. (2000). Anxiety as a predictor and outcome variable in the multimodal treatment study of children with ADHD (MTA). *Journal of Abnormal Child Psychology, 28*(6), 527–541. doi:10.1023/A:1005179014321 PMID:11104315

Markowitz, J. S., & Patrick, K. S. (2017). The clinical pharmacokinetics of amphetamines utilized in the treatment of attention-deficit/hyperactivity disorder. *Journal of Child and Adolescent Psychopharmacology, 27*(8), 678–689. doi:10.1089/cap.2017.0071 PMID:28910145

Mehta, M.A., Owen, A.M., Sahakain, B.J., Mavaddat, N., Pickard, J.D., & Robbins, T.W. (2000). Methylphenidate enhances working memory by modulating discretefrontal and parietal lobe regions in thehuman brain. *J Neurosci, 20*, 1-6.

Mirzaiyan, M., Kunwar, P. S., Uzayisenga, R., & Rashidi, S. (2018). Transcranial Direct Current Stimulation for Treatment of ADHD: A Review of the Mechanisms of Action. *Current Psychiatry Reviews, 14*(4), 215-220.

NICE. (2018). *Attention deficit hyperactivity disorder: diagnosis and management.* Available from: https://www.nice.org.uk/guidance/ng87

Olfson, M., King, M., & Schoenbaum, M. (2015). Treatment of young people with antipsychotic medications in the United States. *JAMA Psychiatry, 72*(9), 867–874. doi:10.1001/jamapsychiatry.2015.0500 PMID:26132724

Osland, S.T., Steeves, T.D.L., & Pringsheim, T. (2018). Pharmacological treatment for attention deficit hyperactivity disorder (ADHD) in children with comorbid tic disorders. *Cochrane Database of Systematic Reviews, 6*.

Poulton, A. (2005). Growth on stimulant medication; clarifying the confusion: A review. *Archives of Disease in Childhood, 90*(8), 801–806. doi:10.1136/adc.2004.056952 PMID:16040876

Reimherr, F. W., Marchant, B. K., Strong, R. E., Hedges, D. W., Adler, L., Spencer, T. J., West, S. A., & Soni, P. (2005). Emotional dysregulation in adult ADHD and response to atomoxetine. *Biological Psychiatry, 58*(2), 125–131. doi:10.1016/j.biopsych.2005.04.040 PMID:16038683

Richters, J.E., Arnold, L.E., Jensen, P.S., Abikoff, H., & Conners, C.K. (1995). IMH collaborative multisite multi-modal treatment study of children with ADHD: I. Background andrationale. *Journal of the American Academy of Child and Adolescent Psychiatry, 34*, 987-1000.

Sangal, R. B., Owens, J., Allen, A. J., Sutton, V., Schuh, K., & Kelsey, D. (2006). Effects of atomoxetine and methylphenidate on sleep in children with ADHD. *Sleep, 29*(12), 1573–1585. doi:10.1093leep/29.12.1573 PMID:17252888

Sauer, J. M., Ring, B. J., & Witcher, J. W. (2005). Clinical pharmacokinetics of atomoxetine. *Clinical Pharmacokinetics, 44*(6), 571–590. doi:10.2165/00003088-200544060-00002 PMID:15910008

Shah, R., Grover, S., & Avasthi, A. (2019). Clinical practice guidelines for the assessment and management of attention deficit/hyperactivity disorder. *Indian Journal of Psychiatry*, *61*(8), 176–193. doi:10.4103/psychiatry.IndianJPsychiatry_543_18 PMID:30745695

Stahl, S. M. (n.d.). *Stahl's Essential Psychopharmacology Neuroscientific Basis and Practical Application* (4th ed.). Cambridge University Press.

Storebø, O. J., Pedersen, N., Ramstad, E., Kielsholm, M. I., Nielsen, S. S., Krogh, H. B., & … . (2018). Methylpheidate for attention deficit hyperactivity disorder (ADHD) in children and adolescents – assessment of possible adverse events in non-randomised studies. *Cochrane Database of Systematic Reviews*, *5*, CD012069. PMID:29744873

Storebø, O. J., Ramstad, E., Krogh, H. B., Nilausen, T. D., Skoog, M., Holmskov, M., & … . (2015). Methyphenidate for children and adolescents with attention deficit hyperactivity disorder (ADHD). *Cochrane Database of Systematic Reviews*, *1*, CD009885. PMID:26599576

Strattera® (atomoxetine capsules) [strattera summary of product characteristics]. (2015). Eli Lilly and Company Ltd.

Sultan, R. S., Wang, S., Crystal, S., & Olfson, M. (2019). Antipsychotic Treatment Among Youths With Attention-Deficit/Hyperactivity Disorder. *JAMA Network Open*, *2*(7), e197850. doi:10.1001/jamanetworkopen.2019.7850 PMID:31348506

Swanson, J., Gupta, S., Guinta, D., Flynn, D., Agler, D., Lerner, M., Williams, L., Shoulson, I., & Wigal, S. (1999). Acute tolerance to methylphenidate in the treatment of attention deficit hyperactivity disorder in children. *Clinical Pharmacology and Therapeutics*, *66*(3), 295–305. doi:10.1016/S0009-9236(99)70038-X PMID:10511066

Tannock, T., & Schachar, L. G. D. (1995). Methylphenidate and cognitive flexibility: dissociated dose effects in hyperactive children. *Journal of Abnormal Child Psychology, 23*, 235-267.

Vaidya, C.J., Austin, G., Kirkorian, G., Ridlehuber, H.W., Desmond, J.E., Glorer, G.H., & Gabrieli, J.D. (1998). Selective effects of methylphenidate in attention deficit hyperactivity disorder: a functional magnetic resonance study. *Proceedings of the National Academy of Science USA, 95*, 14491-14499.

Van Doren, J., Arns, M., Heinrich, H., Vollebregt, M. A., Strehl, U., & Loo, S. K. (2018). Sustained effects of neurofeedback in ADHD: A systematic review and meta-analysis. *European Child & Adolescent Psychiatry*, 1–13. PMID:29445867

Wernicke, J. F., Adler, L., Spencer, T., West, S. A., Allen, A. J., Heiligenstein, J., Milton, D., Ruff, D., Brown, W. J., Kelsey, D., & Michelson, D. (2004). Changes in symptoms and adverse events after discontinuation of atomoxetine in children and adults with attention deficit/hyperactivity disorder: A prospective, placebo-controlled assessment. *Journal of Clinical Psychopharmacology*, *24*(1), 30–35. doi:10.1097/01.jcp.0000104907.75206.c2 PMID:14709944

Westwood, S., Radua, J., & Rubia, K. (2019). Non-invasive brain stimulation as an alternative treatment for ADHD: A systematic review and meta-analysis. *Brain Stimulation*, *12*(2), 502. doi:10.1016/j.brs.2018.12.644

Wilens, T. E., Hammerness, P., Utzinger, L., Schillinger, M., Georgiopoulous, A., Doyle, R. L., Martelon, M. K., & Brodziak, K. (2009). An open study of adjunct OROS-methylphenidate in children and adolescents who are atomoxetine partial responders: I. Effectiveness. *Journal of Child and Adolescent Psychopharmacology*, *19*(5), 485–492. doi:10.1089/cap.2008.0125 PMID:19877972

Wolraich, M. L., & Doffing, M. A. (2004). Pharmacokinetic considerations in the treatment of attention-deficit hyperactivity disorder with methylphenidate. *CNS Drugs*, *18*(4), 243–250. doi:10.2165/00023210-200418040-00004 PMID:15015904

Chapter 9
Living Well With ADHD Across the Lifespan:
How a Multi-Modal Treatment Approach Can Support Its Management

Tsuyoshi Imasaka
Sunrise Behavioural Health, Australia

Jahirul Mullick
RMIT University, Australia

Rajesh Jay Sharma
Sunrise Behavioural Health, Australia

ABSTRACT

Children with attention deficit/hyperactivity disorder (ADHD) are drawn against a number of challenges including staying on task or taking extended time to complete, having trouble listening attentively, or difficulty sitting still. In the past, it was thought that children with ADHD would eventually outgrow the symptoms of the disorder. However, children generally continue to show symptoms of the disorder well into adulthood. The presence of ADHD transforms over the course of a person's lifespan, and the way in which the disorder affects children also changes dramatically when they are older. In adults, one of the core difficulties is executive functioning, which results in restlessness, disorganisation, deviating attention, procrastination, impulsive decision making, and more. In order to prevent the development and escalation of more deviant behaviours, early assessment and treatment program for ADHD should be considered from young age. A highly effective treatment practice for ADHD is a multi-modal approach that combines both pharmacological and behavioural interventions.

DOI: 10.4018/978-1-7998-5495-1.ch009

INTRODUCTION

Attention deficit/hyperactivity disorder (ADHD), a chronic neurodevelopmental disorder, has adverse effect on many aspects of life of a person. It was considered earlier that ADHD is a condition which children could have, and then grow out of it before they reach adulthood. However, recent studies revealed that around 6% to 66% of affected individuals continue to show symptoms of the disorder in their adulthood (Kessler et al., 2006; Rasmussen & Gillberg, 2000). It is also evident in research literature that children with the disorder are at greater risk for adverse outcomes, such as lower academic and employment attainment, and higher criminality and mortality (Barbaresi et al 2013; Frazier et al., 2007). This is because children with ADHD, in general, are easily distracted, often fail to comply with instructions, and unsuccessful to respond to demands placed on them (Wender, 2000). They often perform lower on intelligence tests, which is usually about 7 to 15 IQ points below average, compare to their typically developing peers (Barkley, 1997). Additionally, many children with ADHD show deficits on neuropsychological functions that are related to poor performance in school (Biederman et al., 2004; Butcher et al., 2013). Maintaining

ADHD not only affects children, but also school (approximately 4% to 12%) and college-aged students (estimated 4% to 5%) and adults, because it is often lifelong "with prominent symptoms and impairment spanning into adulthood" (Wilens & Spencer, 2010, p. 97). When children with ADHD get older, the symptoms can be more varied and may be less visible. For example, adults with ADHD can face restlessness, disorganization, deviating attention, procrastination, impulsive decision making and more. The possible consequences of not receiving treatment have multiple dimensions including – a) managing time and task difficult at work, b) controlling impulsivity while responding to others opinion challenging, c) maintaining long-term friendship and romantic-relationships intricate, d) following driving safety hard, e) supporting mental wellbeing without depression and anxiety impossible (Geffen & Forster, 2018). The following sections discusses the impact of ADHD across the lifespan including pre-school years, primary school years, adolescence years, and adulthood.

Pre-School Years

During the preschool years, poor concentration, hyperactivity, and impulsiveness are the common characteristics of typically developing children. Consequently, a high level of supervision is the norm. Even so, children with ADHD may still stand out from their typically developing peers. Pre-school ADHD children will often show an unusually poor intensity of play behaviour and display excessive motor restlessness. In addition, delayed development, oppositional behaviour, and poor social skills may also be present. Even at this early stage of development, the parents of children with ADHD may experience high stress level as their child does not often comply with ordinary parental requests and advice (DuPaul, McGoey, Eckert & VanBrakle, 2001; Sonuga-Barke, Daley, Thompson, Laver-Bradbury & Weeks, 2001). Additionally, parents have less time for themselves as they need to provide high level of supervision and behaviour management for the children.

Having a child with ADHD was found to be associated with many other difficulties for the family members such as strained family relationships, marital problems, and financial and social difficulties (Johnston & Mash, 2001). Siblings of children with ADHD were also found to be negatively affected as they are at increased risk of developing conduct and emotional disorders (Kendall, 1999).

Primary School Years

During the primary school years, functioning becomes more impaired in children with ADHD, where poor level of attention becomes more prominent (American Psychiatric Association, 2013). Children with ADHD frequently begin to be seen as being different as their typically developing peers start to develop the skills and maturity necessary to enable them to learn and attain optimal academic performance and social skill. Due to these differences, children with ADHD may experience a myriad of difficulties in both school and home settings. Although experienced teachers may be able to adjust their classroom to allow an able child with ADHD to succeed, more often, the children may experience a poor academic performance. Furthermore, children with ADHD generally have many social problems with their peers due to their impulsiveness and overactivity. Comorbid problems, such as specific learning difficulties, may also start to emerge, further compounding and complicating diagnosis and management (Harpin, 2005).

Similar to the school setting, difficulties in home setting also become more apparent at this stage of development. Parents may find that family members often refuse to care for their child and that their child is experiencing peer rejection as they fail to get along with their peers. In addition, many children with ADHD have poor sleep patterns, and although they appear not to need much sleep, daytime behaviour is often adversely impacted when children do not have enough sleep. As a result, parents may have to spend more time supervising and managing their child's behaviour. Not surprisingly, parent-child and family relationships may be severely strained, and in some cases break down (Johnston&Mash, 2001). Such adversities may complicate the already difficult situation, bringing additional social and financial difficulties to all parties involved.

Adolescence Years

Adolescence years may bring about a reduction in the hyperactivity, but inattentiveness, impulsiveness, and restlessness remain a major impairment in functioning. During this stage of development, an individual with ADHD may also display increased aggressive and antisocial behaviour adding further problems. Studies have indicated that adolescents with ADHD and aggressive behaviours have a more strained parent-child relationship compared to typically developing adolescents (Robin, Koepke, Moye & Gerhardstein, 2009). Furthermore, adolescents with ADHD have lower grades and class placements, are more likely to be suspended or expelled, have higher level of absenteeism, and are less likely to graduate high school than their typically developing peers (Barbaresi, Katusic, Colligan, Weaver, & Jacobsen, 2007; Harpin, 2005; Molina et al., 2009). In addition to academic difficulties, adolescents with ADHD are at increased risk of teenage pregnancy and criminal behaviours (Butcher et al., 2013; Harpin, 2005). Studies have noted that driving poses an additional risk. Individuals with ADHD are easily distracted from concentrating on driving when going slowly, but may also be dangerous while driving fast (Barkley, 2004; Harpin, 2005). It has been shown that compared with similarly aged cohorts, drivers with ADHD are at increased risk of traffic violations, especially speeding, and are considered to be at fault in more traffic accidents including accidents with fatalities (Barkley, 2004).

Adulthood

As previously mentioned, more than 60% of individuals with ADHD continue to experience residual effect of ADHD in adult life (Kessler et al., 2006; Rasmussen & Gillberg, 2000). Adults with ADHD frequently experience difficulties in both employment and social aspects of their lives. Adults with ADHD are more likely to be dismissed from employment due to interpersonal difficulties, tardiness, excessive errors, inability to produce quality work, and high level of absenteeism (Mannuzza, Klein, Bessler, Malloy & LaPadula, 1993). These adults may also have difficulties finding suitable employment as they often have to try out numerous jobs before being able to find one at which they can succeed in an optimal degree. They may need to choose specific types of jobs and are frequently self-employed. The risk of drug and substance abuse are significantly higher in adults with ADHD compared to typically developing adults (Biederman, Wilens, Mick, Faraone, & Spencer, 1998).

Difficulties in an interpersonal relationship may also lead to relationship difficulties, poor marital quality and break-up (Biederman, Wilens, Mick, Faraone, & Spencer, 1998; Harpin, 2005). The genetic aspects of ADHD mean that parents with ADHD are more likely to pass down genes for this disorder onto their child (Butcher et al., 2013). Meaning, children of parents who are diagnosed or show a symptom of ADHD are more likely to inherit the condition. This, in turn, may cause further problems as the success of a parenting program for parents of children with ADHD is highly influenced by the presence of parental ADHD. Therefore, ADHD in parents and children can lead to a cycle of difficulties (Harpin, 2005).

As discussed above, the ADHD manifest differently throughout the life stages which necessitate the treatment plan to adapt to the individual's developmental, social and personal variables. Long term prognosis review has indicated that individuals with ADHD can attain high educational and vocational success (Mannuzza & Klein, 2000). To prevent the development and escalation of more deviant behaviour, early assessment and treatment program for ADHD should be considered. The most effective treatment for ADHD follows a multi-modal approach that combines both pharmacological and behavioural intervention (Jensen et al., 2001).

This is widely common that when children are diagnosed with ADHD, the parents get concerned about their treatment. This has two aspects including – i) the availability of treatment choices, and ii) appropriateness of the treatments for their children. In most cases, they prefer pharmacological remedies over any other available treatments. Occasionally parents want to believe, mostly at the initial stage, that medication can solve the challenge offering a cure to ADHD. As it is already known to pediatricians, special education teachers, disability workers and other allied health professionals that there is no cure for ADHD and there is no quick solution to the absolute management of ADHD, they often suggest behavior support as the first line of treatment before pharmacological remedies. The following sections present three treatment approaches including pharmacological, behavioural and others.

Pharmacological Treatments for ADHD

Pharmacological approaches to treatment are the most common method of treatment for ADHD. Although disagreement over the use of drugs to treat the symptom of ADHD among children continues, this approach enjoys great appeal in the medical community. A survey study conducted by Runnheim, Frankenberger, & Hazelkorn (1996) has found that 15% to 40% of school children with emotional and behavioural problems associated with ADHD are prescribed medication, mostly Ritalin (methylphenidate), a form of amphetamine.

Ritalin has been shown to be effective in the short-term treatment of ADHD (Butcher et al., 2013; Goldstein, 2009). Interestingly, studies have indicated that amphetamines have a calming effect on children, whereas the opposite effect was observed on adults. Although amphetamines do not cure ADHD, they have reduced the behavioural symptoms. For children with ADHD, such stimulant medication decreases hyperactivity while improving their on-task performance at the same time (Konrad,Gunther, Hanisch, & Herpertz-Dahlmann, 2004). Not surprisingly, children with ADHD prescribed with this type of medication are often able to function much better in school setting (Hazell, 2007). The possible side effects of amphetamines, however, are numerous. The side effects can include impaired thinking ability and memory loss due to disruption of blood flow to the brain, suppression of growth in the body and brain due to disruption of growth hormone, insomnia, and others.

There are newer variants of the drug referred to as extended-release methylphenidate that have similar beneficial effects, but with available doses which was found more suitable to adolescents with ADHD (Butcher et al., 2013). Other medications for treating ADHD have received scholarly attention in recent years. Pemoline is one such medication. Pemoline is chemically different from Ritalin and was found to have a beneficial effect on classroom behaviour by improving cognitive function but with fewer adverse side effects of Ritalin (Bostic et al., 2000).

Although the short-term pharmacological benefits on the symptoms of ADHD on children are well established, their long-term effects are not promising (Safer, 1997). For instance, a study conducted by Carlson and Bunner (1993) found that academic achievement over long periods of time failed to show that the medication has beneficial impact on child's functioning. In addition, the pharmacological similarity of Ritalin and cocaine has raised important ethical and health concerns on its use in the treatment of ADHD (Volkow et al., 1995). Some studies have even reported recreational use of Ritalin, particularly among young adults (Kapner, 2003). As a result, some practitioners/scholars prefer using non-pharmacological interventions program in treating the symptom of ADHD. The majority of non-pharmacological intervention programmes designed to treat symptom of ADHD are primarily based on the principles of behavioural psychology and applied behaviour analysis (ABA). These interventions are concerned with the manipulation of antecedent and consequent behavioural stimuli to facilitate the acquisition of adaptive behaviour (Cooper, Heron, & Heward, 2007). In practice, this usually involves a presentation of reinforcement for desirable behaviour (Cooper et al., 2007; Shapiro & Derr, 1987).

Behavioural Treatment

The American Academy of Pediatrics (AAP) recommends behavior support training for parents of children younger than 6 years of age with ADHD (CDC, 2020). According to Verma et al. (2011), behavior support is also necessary because some children do not display satisfactory outcomes, or show intolerable adverse effects after getting pharmacological remedies; also, some parents do not prefer medication for their young children.

Behavioral support strategies widely known as behavior modifications have been exhibited to be a very successful treatment for children with ADHD, because it reinforces desired behaviors through rewards and praise. The primary goal of behavior treatment is to change the identified challenging behaviors into positive ones, and there are four basic techniques that are widely used to support people with ADHD. **Table 1** presents the four basic techniques which are effective in changing challenging behaviors.

Behavioral support treatments are based on the theories of classical conditioning and operant conditioning (the basic principles of behaviorism) and social learning theory of Bandura (Cooper et al., 2007). Kerr and Nelson (2010) explained that the techniques applied as behaviour support follows a few principles including –

Figure 1. Treatment approach for children younger than six-year of age and older

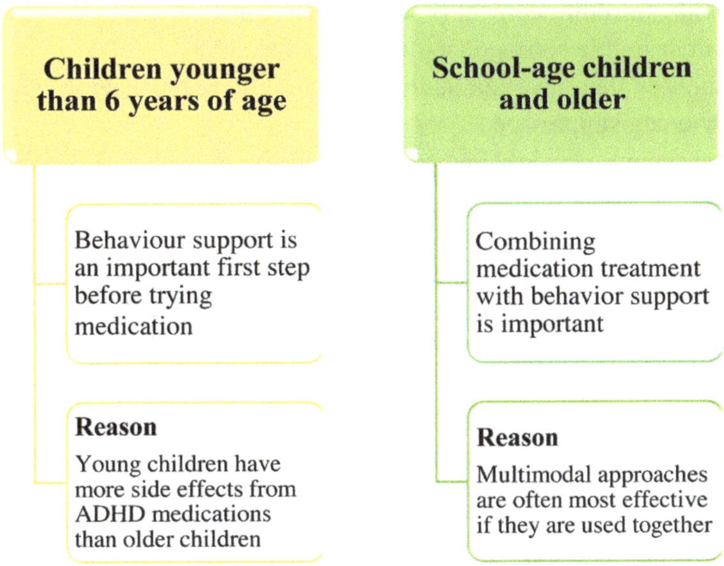

Table 1. Behaviour support techniques with examples

Technique	Description	Example
Token Economies	• Token economy usually applies **reinforcement technique** to modify behaviour. • Clients are allowed to earn tokens that can be **exchanged for** special privileges or desired items. • The basic principle employed in token economy is that – it **provides** compliments or any preferred materials as rewards and offers privileges in response to desired behaviour. It also **removes** access to preferred activity or **withdraws** rewards or privileges because of unwanted behaviour	Child with ADHD earn tokens (e.g., star or points) for engaging in preferred behaviors (e.g., on-task) and may even lose tokens for displaying undesirable behaviors (e.g., non-compliance). These tokens can then be traded for things such as candy, toys, or extra time playing with iPad or a favorite toy.
Contingency Management	• Contingency Management relies on a formal **written contract** between the client and the behaviour professional (it could be parents or teacher) that outlines the behavior contacts (e.g., change goals, reinforcements, and rewards that will be given and the penalties for failing to meet the demands of the agreement.) • In contingency management, behaviour **contracts spell out** the rules clearly in black-and-white, preventing both parties from backing down on **their promises**.	The behaviour professional, parents or teacher reward (e.g., candy) a child who has ADHD for taking small steps toward raising a hand before talking. It was written on the contract that s/he would get a candy each time s/he follows the hand raising procedure before talking.
Modeling	• Modeling technique applies Albert Bandura's social learning theory, which emphasizes the social components of the learning process. • This strategy allows client **watching someone** else perform a desired behaviour or **reading about** how someone else is performing the desired behaviour. It involves **learning through observation and modeling** the behavior of others to learn new skills.	The behaviour professional, parents or teacher model that how to complete a task before moving to do other activities. A social story about on-task behaviour is also effective.
Extinction	• Extinction strategy is a process that **stop reinforcing** a behavior in order to eliminate the response. This gradual weakening of a **conditioned response** results in the behavior decreasing or disappearing. • In extinction, unwanted behavior is eventually extinguished (the conditioned behavior eventually stops) by **taking away the attention** that the child found rewarding.	A child with ADHD who starts yelling or striking other children would be removed from the play activity and required to sit quietly in a corner or another room where there are no opportunities for attention and reinforcement.

Source: (Cherry, 2020)

- Behavior is controlled by consequences (e.g., desirable or undesirable)
- To strengthen a behavior reinforcement (i.e., desirable consequence) is essential
- Punishment (i.e., undesirable consequence) weakens behavior
- Desirable consequences that have maintained or strengthened behavior can also weaken or decrease behavior by being suppressed
- Offering consequences immediately and consistently after occurrence of a target behavior establish contingencies

Modeling is another principle used as behavioral support treatment to strengthen, weaken, or maintain behavior. According to Bandura (1977) there are three types of modeling – a) live model, b) verbal instructional model, and c) symbolic model.

Figure 2. Three types of modelling for behavioral support treatment

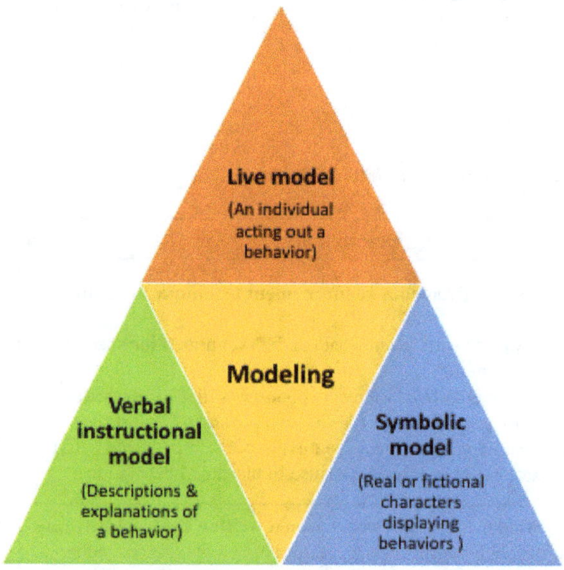

Patience is essential while applying behaviour techniques, because people with ADHD are highly variable in their symptoms. One day, they may demonstrate the expected behaviour, but the next day everything might look different as they could fall back into old patterns. The family members, at times, may feel that the techniques are not effective. Nevertheless, behavioural techniques actually work and parents need to provide more time to allow these to come into regular practice.

Executive Functioning

In general, the primary problem for most people with ADHD is attention. Sometimes people perceive attention as not listening when someone is talking to you, but it is a much larger challenge that affects the management system of the brain known as executive functions. Although it has not as yet been deter-

Tips for Parents
Establishing routines: Having simple, predictable routines throughout the day means necessary tasks get done without last-minute panics. A healthy morning, afternoon, and evening routine may outline the necessary steps to accomplish tasks.
Creating checklists: A checklist can be made for any multi-step process that seems complicated or stressful. It acts as a memory aid and helps you or your child feel organized. For example, you might tape a checklist to the front door listing all the things you or your child needs for the day.
Using timers: To help you or your child pay attention to homework or a work project, set a timer for 15 minutes (indicating a dedicated time of focus). When it rings, have a mini-break and then set your timer again.
Setting alarms: You can set alarms to remind you or your child to take medication or leave the house. Alarms can be empowering because it reduces the need for reminders from others.
Creating charts: If there is a behaviour or habit you want to include in your day, make a chart with the days of the week. Every time you do the behaviour, for example, clean your teeth, you get a star. Both children and adults find this rewarding, and it acts as a reminder and a motivator to do the task.
Using planners: Using a planner helps with understanding the passage of time such as what is planned for the day, and marks deadlines, like when assignments need to be handed in.
Establishing routines: Having simple, predictable routines throughout the day means necessary tasks get done without last-minute panics. A healthy morning, afternoon, and evening routine may outline the necessary steps to accomplish tasks.
Creating checklists: A checklist can be made for any multi-step process that seems complicated or stressful. It acts as a memory aid and helps you or your child feel organized. For example, you might tape a checklist to the front door listing all the things you or your child needs for the day.
Using timers: To help you or your child pay attention to homework or a work project, set a timer for 15 minutes (indicating a dedicated time of focus). When it rings, have a mini-break and then set your timer again.

Source: (Sinfield, 2019)

mined exactly what constitutes all of the executive functions, the following aspects are widely discussed by experts (Rief, 2016, p. 22-23).

- **Inhibition** - controlling impulses
- **Working memory** - holding information in mind long enough to act on it
- **Planning and prioritizing** - thinking through what needs to be done
- **Organization** - imposing order and structure to manage information
- **Arousal and activation**- being able to arouse effort and motivation to start or initiate tasks
- **Sustaining attention** - maintaining alertness and focus and resisting distractions
- **Emotional self-control** - modulating or self-regulating one's frustrations and emotions
- **Time awareness** - keeping track of time
- **Goal-directed persistence** - persevering, maintaining the effort and motivation
- **Shifting and flexibility**- being adaptable and making adjustments when needed
- **Self-monitoring and metacognition**- self-checking one's own behaviour
- **Self-talk and private speech**- using one's inner voice for mentally talking

Brown (2005) identified six clusters of cognitive functions which constitute executive functions including activation (organizing, prioritizing and getting started on tasks), focus (focusing, maintaining, and shifting attention), effort (regulating alertness, sustaining effort, processing speed), emotion (managing frustrations and regulating emotions), memory (using working memory and accessing recall), and action (monitoring and self-regulating action). The following strategies can support people with ADHD to improve their executive functioning.

Figure 3. Behavioural techniques to treat executive functioning

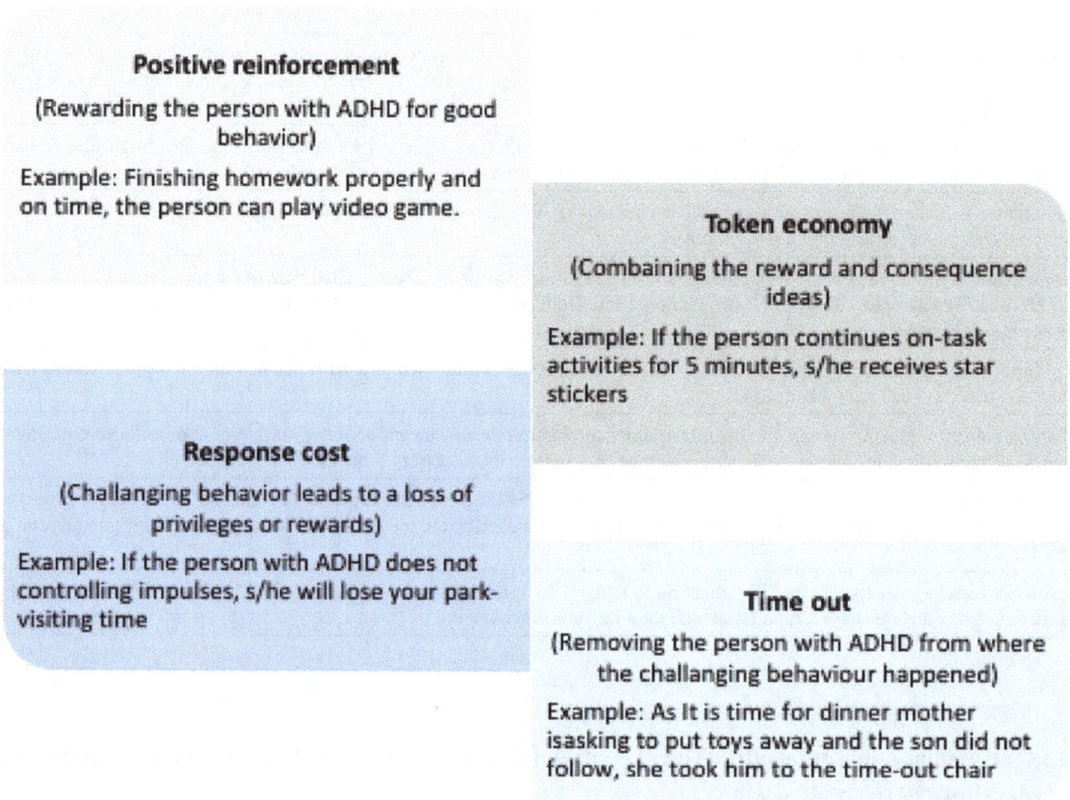

Figure 4. Other treatment approaches

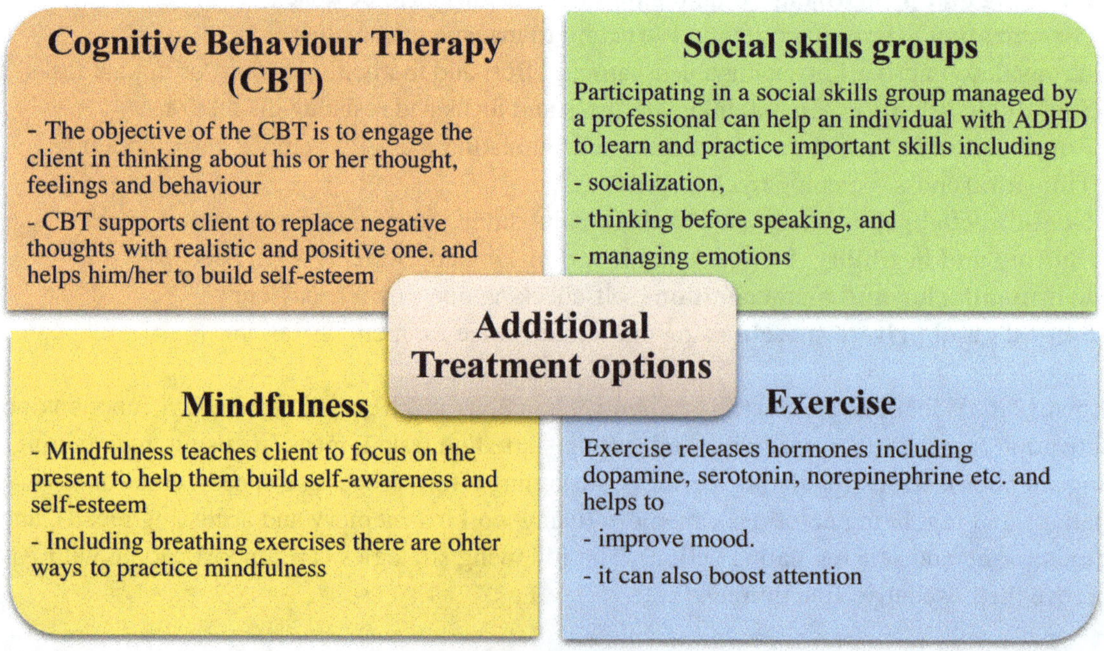

Other Treatment approaches

Parents of children with ADHD often find other non-medical treatments also effective in dealing difficulties in everyday life. The following are some examples of treatments.

It is evident from the above discussion that there are a number of treatment options, but what works best usually depend on the individual and his or her family. In order to identify the effective treatment options, families should work closely with others involved in their children's life including healthcare professionals, psychologist, behaviour specialists, therapists, teachers, and other family members. According to Verma et al. (2011), "ADHD management must be multimodal, with best treatment outcome achieved by appropriate dosing and titration of medications as well as by a combination of pharmacotherapy and psychosocial intervention" (p.16). ADHD symptoms can change over time (i.e., pre-school to adulthood); therefore, maintaining a close communication with all the professionals regularly is inevitable for a right treatment design. In addition, as symptoms of ADHD emerge in young age, early intervention is typically effective in reducing the symptoms and prevent the significant impairment in academic and other functioning.

REFERENCES

American Psychiatric Association. (2013). Diagnostic and statistical manual of mental disorders (5th ed.). Arlington, VA: American Psychiatric Publishing.

Bandura, A. (1977). *Social Learning Theory*. Prentice-Hall.

Barbaresi, W. J., Colligan, R., Weaver, A., Voigt, R., Killian, J., & Katusic, S. (2013). Mortality, ADHD, and psychosocial adversity in adults with childhood ADHD: A prospective study. *Pediatrics*, *131*(4), 637–644. doi:10.1542/peds.2012-2354 PMID:23460687

Barbaresi, W. J., Katusic, S. K., Colligan, R. C., Weaver, A. L., & Jacobsen, S. J. (2007). Long-term school outcomes for children with attention-deficit/hyperactivity disorder: A population-based perspective. *Journal of Developmental and Behavioral Pediatrics*, *28*(4), 265–273. doi:10.1097/DBP.0b013e31811ff87d PMID:17700078

Barkley, R. (1997). Behavioral inhibition, sustained attention, and executive functions: Constructing a unifying theory of ADHD. *Psychological Bulletin*, *121*(1), 65–94. doi:10.1037/0033-2909.121.1.65 PMID:9000892

Barkley, R. (2004). Driving impairments in teens and adults with attention-deficit/hyperactivity disorder. *The Psychiatric Clinics of North America*, *27*(2), 233–260. doi:10.1016/S0193-953X(03)00091-1 PMID:15063996

Biederman, J., Monuteaux, M., Doyle, A., Seidman, L., Wilens, T., Ferrero, F., Morgan, C. L., & Faraone, S. V. (2004). Impact of executive function deficits and attention-deficit/hyperactivity disorder (ADHD) on academic outcomes in children. *Journal of Consulting and Clinical Psychology*, *72*(5), 757–766. doi:10.1037/0022-006X.72.5.757 PMID:15482034

Biederman, J., Wilens, T. E., Mick, E., Faraone, S. V., & Spencer, T. (1998). Does attention-deficit hyperactivity disorder impact the developmental course of drug and alcohol abuse and dependence? *Biological Psychiatry*, *44*(4), 269–273. doi:10.1016/S0006-3223(97)00406-X PMID:9715358

Bostic, J. Q., Biederman, J., Spencer, T. J., Wilens, T. E., Prince, J. B., Monuteaux, M. C., Sienna, M., Polisner, D. A., & Hatch, M. (2000). Pemoline treatment of adolescents with attention deficit hyperactivity disorder: A short-term controlled trial. *Journal of Child and Adolescent Psychopharmacology*, *10*(3), 205–216. doi:10.1089/10445460050167313 PMID:11052410

Brown, T. (2005). *Attention deficit disorder: The unfocused mind in children and adults*. Yale University Press.

Butcher, J., Mineka, S., & Hooley, J. (2013). *Abnormal psychology* (15th ed.). Pearson.

Carlson, C. L., & Bunner, M. R. (1993). Effects of methylphenidate on the academic performance of children with attention deficit hyperactivity disorder and learning disabilities. *School Psychology Review*, *22*(2), 184–198.

Centers for Disease Control and Prevention (CDC). (2019, October 8). *Treatment of ADHD*. https://www.cdc.gov/ncbddd/adhd/treatment.html

Cherry, K. (2020, March 13). *How Behavioral Therapy Is Used in Psychology*. Verywell Mind. https://www.verywellmind.com/what-is-behavioral-therapy-2795998

Cooper, J. O., Heron, T. E., & Heward, W. L. (2007). *Applied behavior analysis* (2nd ed.). Pearson Merrill Prentice Hall.

DuPaul, G., McGoey, K., Eckert, T., & VanBrakle, J. (2001). Preschool children with attention-deficit/hyperactivity disorder: Impairments in behavioral, social, and school functioning. *Journal of the American Academy of Child and Adolescent Psychiatry*, *40*(5), 508–515. doi:10.1097/00004583-200105000-00009 PMID:11349694

Frazier, T., Youngstrom, E., Glutting, J., & Watkins, M. (2007). ADHD and achievement: Meta-analysis of the child, adolescent, and adult literatures and a concomitant study with college students. *Journal of Learning Disabilities*, *40*(1), 49–65. doi:10.1177/00222194070400010401 PMID:17274547

Geffen, J. & Forster, K. (2018). Treatment of adult ADHD: A clinical perspective. *Therapeutic Advances in Psychopharmacology*, *8*(1), 25-32. doi: / doi:10.1177/2045125317734977

Goldstein, S. (2009). Current literature in ADHD summarized by Sam Goldstein. *Journal of Attention Disorders*, *12*(4), 386–388. doi:10.1177/1087054708328266

Harpin, V. (2005). The effect of ADHD on the life of an individual, their family, and community from preschool to adult life. *Archives of Disease in Childhood*, *90*(Suppl1), i2–i7. doi:10.1136/adc.2004.059006 PMID:15665153

Hazell, P. (2007). Pharmacological management of attention-deficit hyper activity disorder in adolescents. *CNS Drugs*, *21*(1), 37–46. doi:10.2165/00023210-200721010-00004 PMID:17190528

Jensen, P. S., Hinshaw, S. P., Swanson, J. M., Greenhill, L. L., Conners, C. K., Arnold, L. E., Abikoff, H. B., Elliott, G., Hechtman, L., Hoza, B., March, J. S., Newcorn, J. H., Severe, J. B., Vitiello, B., Wells, K., & Wigal, T. (2001). Findings from the NIMH multimodal treatment study of ADHD (MTA): Implications and applications for primary care providers. *Journal of Developmental and Behavioral Pediatrics*, *22*(1), 60–73. doi:10.1097/00004703-200102000-00008 PMID:11265923

Johnston, C., & Mash, E. J. (2001). Families of children with attention-deficit/hyperactivity disorder: Review and recommendations for future research. *Clinical Child and Family Psychology Review*, *4*(3), 183–207. doi:10.1023/A:1017592030434 PMID:11783738

Kapner, D. A. (2003). *Recreational use of Ritalin on college campuses. Info Fact Resources*. U.S. Department of Justice.

Kendall, J. (1999). Sibling accounts of attention deficit hyperactivity disorder (ADHD). *Family Process*, *38*(1), 117–136. doi:10.1111/j.1545-5300.1999.00117.x PMID:10207714

Kerr, M. M., & Nelson, C. M. (2010). *Strategies for addressing behavior problems in the classroom* (6th ed.). Pearson.

Kessler, R., Adler, L., Barkley, R., Biederman, J., Conners, C., Demler, O., Faraone, S. V., Greenhill, L. L., Howes, M. J., Secnik, K., Spencer, T., Ustun, T. B., Walters, E. E., & Zaslavsky, A. M. (2006). The prevalence and correlates of adult ADHD in the United States: Results from the national comorbidity survey replication. *The American Journal of Psychiatry*, *163*(4), 716–723. doi:10.1176/ajp.2006.163.4.716 PMID:16585449

Konrad, K., Gunther, T., Hanisch, C., & Herpertz-Dahlmann, B. (2004). Differential effects of methylphenidate on attentional functions in children with attention-deficit /hyperactivity disorder. *Journal of the American Academy of Child and Adolescent Psychiatry*, *43*(2), 191–198. doi:10.1097/00004583-200402000-00015 PMID:14726726

Mannuzza, S., & Klein, R. (2000). Long-term prognosis in attention-deficit/hyperactivity disorder. *Child and Adolescent Psychiatric Clinics of North America*, *9*(3), 711–726. doi:10.1016/S1056-4993(18)30114-7 PMID:10944664

Mannuzza, S., Klein, R. G., Bessler, A., Malloy, P., & LaPadula, M. (1993). Adult outcome of hyperactive boys. Educational achievement, occupational rank, and psychiatric status. *Archives of General Psychiatry*, *50*(7), 565–576. doi:10.1001/archpsyc.1993.01820190067007 PMID:8317950

Molina, B., Hinshaw, S., Swanson, J., Arnold, L., Vitiello, B., Jensen, P., Epstein, J. N., Hoza, B., Hechtman, L., Abikoff, H. B., Elliott, G. R., Greenhill, L. L., Newcorn, J. H., Wells, K. C., Wigal, T., Gibbons, R. D., Hur, K., & Houck, P. R.MTA Cooperative Group. (2009). The MTA at 8 years: Prospective follow-up of children treated for combined-type ADHD in a multi-site study. *Journal of the American Academy of Child and Adolescent Psychiatry*, *48*(5), 484–500. doi:10.1097/CHI.0b013e31819c23d0 PMID:19318991

Rasmussen, P., & Gillberg, C. (2000). Natural outcome of ADHD with developmental coordination disorder at age 22 years: A controlled, longitudinal, community-based study. *Journal of the American Academy of Child and Adolescent Psychiatry, 39*(11), 1424–1431. doi:10.1097/00004583-200011000-00017 PMID:11068898

Rief, S. F. (2016). *How to reach and teach children and teens with ADD/ADHD*. Jossey-Bass.

Robin, A., Koepke, T., Moye, A., & Gerhardstein, R. (2009). Assessment of the parent-adolescent relationship in teens with ADHD. *The ADHD Report, 17*(5), 1–6. doi:10.1521/adhd.2009.17.5.1

Runnheim, V. A., Frankenberger, W. R., & Hazelkorn, M. N. (1996). Medicating students with emotional and behavioral disorders and ADHD: A state survey. *Behavioral Disorders, 21*(4), 306–314. doi:10.1177/019874299602100405

Safer, D. (1997). Central stimulant treatment of childhood attention deficit hyperactivity disorder: Issues and recommendations from a US perspective. *CNS Drugs, 7*(4), 264–272. doi:10.2165/00023210-199707040-00002 PMID:27520752

Shapiro, E., & Derr, T. (1987). School Interventions for Aggression. *Special Services in the Schools, 3*(4), 5-19. doi: / doi:10.1300/j008v03n03_02

Sinfield, J. (2019, August 11). *How Is ADHD Treated for Children and Adults?* Verywell Mind. https://www.verywellmind.com/adhd-treatment-4157278

Sonuga-Barke, E., Daley, D., Thompson, M., Laver-Bradbury, C., & Weeks, A. (2001). Parent-based therapies for preschool attention-deficit/hyperactivity disorder: A randomized, controlled trial with a community sample. *Journal of the American Academy of Child and Adolescent Psychiatry, 40*(4), 402–408. doi:10.1097/00004583-200104000-00008 PMID:11314565

Verma, R., Balhara, Y. P., & Mathur, S. (2011). Management of attention-deficit hyperactivity disorder. *Journal of Pediatric Neurosciences, 6*(1), 13–18. doi:10.4103/1817-1745.84400

Volkow, N. D., Ding, Y.S., Fowler, J. S., Wang, G.J., Logan, J., Gatley, J. S., Dewey, S., Ashby, C., Liebermann, J., &Hitzemann, R. (1995). Is methylphenidate like cocaine? Studies on their pharmacokinetics and distribution in the human brain. *Archives of General Psychiatry, 52*(6), 456-463. doi: / doi:10.1001/archpsyc.1995.03950180042006

Wilens, T. E. & Spencer, T. J. (2010). Understanding attention-deficit/hyperactivity disorder from childhood to adulthood. *Postgraduate Medicine, 122*(5), 97-109. doi: / doi:10.3810/pgm.2010.09.2206

Chapter 10
Parenting Children With Attention Deficit Hyperactivity Disorder

Dorothy Bhandari Deka
Sarvodaya Healthcare, India

ABSTRACT

The prevalence of ADHD is estimated at 5–7% worldwide, which makes it one of the most common psychiatric disorders in children and adolescents. Children with Attention deficit hyperactivity disorder can become difficult if the child is not monitored using correct strategies and techniques. Parents play an integral role in shaping a child. Parenting involves biological as well as the legal aspects and other equally if not more important dimensions of care, protection, nurturance, understanding, guidance, mutual interaction, and partnership occurring within the protective environment of a family. Parenting a differently abled child is very demanding and challenging and the role of family and parents in caring for a child is very crucial, especially development, socializing, and protecting the child.

ATTENTION DEFICIT HYPERACTIVITY DISORDER (ADHD)

Attention deficit hyperactivity disorder is characterized by a brain difference and specific behavioural symptoms, is considered one of the most frequent and globally debilitating of childhood disorders (Barkley, 1981; Linden et.al., 1989, Amen et. al., 1993). The disorder was first described as a cluster of behavioural symptoms thatcomprisedof hyperactivity, poor attention; conduct disorders, and learning problems (Still, 1902). Earlier medication was used to treat thedisorder; it was labelled as Minimal Brain Dysfunction (MBD) (Bradley, 1937). It is neurodevelopmental disorder categorised by high levels of inattention, hyperactivity and impulsivity that are present before the age of seven years, seen in a range of situations, inconsistent with the child's developmental level and causing social or academic impairment (APA 1994).

According to International Classification of Diseases (ICD-10) (WHO 1992), hyperkinetic disorder (HKD) is similar to ADHD but the criteria seems to be more restrictive. Diagnostic and Statistical

DOI: 10.4018/978-1-7998-5495-1.ch010

Manual of Mental Disorders V (DSM-5)has revised the diagnostic criteria for ADHD. To be identified with ADHD, the population needs to meet six out of nine possible inattentive symptoms and/or six out of nine possible hyperactivity/impulsivity symptoms. Also, symptoms need to be present for at least 6 months, occur in at least two different settings, be present before 12 years of age, and not be better explained by another disorder.ADHD is often associated with extreme temperamental characteristics such as negative mood, short persistence, low frustration tolerance and excitability (Linden et.al., 1989). Other characteristics describing the disorder includes minimal brain damage syndrome, developmental hyperactivity, hyperkinetic impulse disorder, hyperkinetic reaction of childhood, attention deficit disorder with or without hyperactivity, and attention deficit hyperactivity disorder (Weiss &Hechtman, 1986).

According to Diagnostic and Statistical Manual of Mental Disorders, Fifth Edition diagnostic criteria for Attention-Deficit/Hyperactivity Disorder (ADHD) are as follows:

A. A persistent pattern of inattention and/or hyperactivity-impulsivity that interferes with functioning or development, as characterized by inattention and/or hyperactivity and impulsivity:
   Inattention: Six (or more) of the following symptoms have persisted for at least 6 months to a degree that is inconsistent with developmental level and that negatively impacts directly on social andacademic/occupational activities: (Note: The symptoms are not solely a manifestation of oppositional behavior, defiance, hostility, or failure to understand tasks or instructions. For older adolescents and adults (age 17 and older), at least five symptoms are required.)
   - Often fails to give close attention to details or makes careless mistakes in schoolwork, at work, or during other activities (e.g., overlooks or misses details, work is inaccurate).
   - Often has difficulty sustaining attention in tasks or play activities (e.g., has difficulty remaining focused during lectures, conversations, or lengthy reading).
   - Often does not seem to listen when spoken to directly (e.g., mind seems elsewhere, even in the absence of any obvious distraction).
   - Often does not follow through on instructions and fails to finish schoolwork, chores, or duties in the workplace (e.g., starts tasks but quickly loses focus and is easily side tracked).
   - Often has difficulty organizing tasks and activities (e.g., difficulty managing sequential tasks; difficulty keeping materials and belongings in order; messy, disorganized work; has poor time management; fails to meet deadlines).
   - Often avoids, dislikes, or is reluctant to engage in tasks that require sustained mental effort (e.g., schoolwork or homework; for older adolescents and adults, preparing reports, completing forms, reviewing lengthy papers).
   - Often loses things necessary for tasks or activities (e.g., school materials, pencils, books, tools, wallets, keys, paperwork, eyeglasses, mobile telephones).
   - Is often easily distracted by extraneous stimuli (for older adolescents and adults, may include unrelated thoughts).
   - Is often forgetful in daily activities (e.g., doing chores, running errands; for older adolescents and adults, returning calls, paying bills, keeping appointments).

   Hyperactivity and impulsivity: Six (or more) of the following symptoms have persisted for at least 6 months to a degree that is inconsistent with developmental level and that negatively impacts directly on social and academic/occupational activities. (Note: The symptoms are not solely a manifestation of oppositional behaviour, defiance, hostility, or a failure to understand tasks or instructions. For older adolescents and adults (age 17 and older), at least five symptoms are required.

- ◦ Often fidgets with or taps hands or feet or squirms in seat.
- ◦ Often leaves seat in situations when remaining seated is expected (e.g., leaves his or her place in the classroom, in the office or other workplace, or in other situations that require remaining in place).
- ◦ Often runs about or climbs in situations where it is inappropriate. (Note: In adolescents or adults, may be limited to feeling restless.)
- ◦ Often unable to play or engage in leisure activities quietly.
- ◦ Is often "on the go," acting as if "driven by a motor" (e.g., is unable to be or uncomfortable being still for extended time, as in restaurants, meetings; may be experienced by others as being restless or difficult to keep up with).
- ◦ Often talks excessively.
- ◦ Often blurts out an answer before a question has been completed (e.g., completes people's sentences; cannot wait for turn in conversation).
- ◦ Often has difficulty waiting his or her turn (e.g., while waiting in line).
- ◦ Often interrupts or intrudes on others (e.g., butts into conversations, games, or activities; may start using other people's things without asking or receiving permission; for adolescents and adults, may intrude into or take over what others are doing).

B. Several inattentive or hyperactive-impulsive symptoms were present prior to age 12 years.

C. Several inattentive or hyperactive-impulsive symptoms are present in two or more settings (e.g., at home, school, or work; with friends or relatives; in other activities).

D. There is clear evidence that the symptoms interfere with, or reduce the quality of, social, academic, or occupational functioning.

E. The symptoms do not occur exclusively during the course of schizophrenia or another psychotic disorder and are not better explained by another mental disorder (e.g., mood disorder, anxiety disorder, dissociative disorder, personality disorder, substance intoxication or withdrawal).

Specification required whether:

- Combined presentation: If both inattention and hyperactivity-impulsivity are met for the past 6 months.
- Predominantly inattentive presentation: If inattention is met but hyperactivity-impulsivity is not met for the past 6 months.
- Predominantly hyperactive/impulsive presentation: If hyperactivity impulsivity is met but Criterion A1 (inattention) is not met over the past 6 months.

Specification required if:

- In partial remission: When full criteria were previously met, fewer than the full criteria have been met for the past 6 months, and the symptoms still result in impairment in social, academic, or occupational functioning.

Specification for current severity required:

- Mild: Few, if any, symptoms in excess of those required to make the diagnosis are present, and symptoms result in only minor functional impairments.
- Moderate: Symptoms or functional impairment between "mild" and "severe" are present.
- Severe: Many symptoms in excess of those required to make the diagnosis, or several symptoms that are particularly severe, are present, or the symptoms result in marked impairment in social or occupational functioning.

Early conduct problems appear to precede antisocial behaviour in later life. The precise relationship between conduct disorder or oppositional defiant disorder and ADHD, especially the mechanism of development of antisocial behaviour in children with ADHD, is not, however, fully understood (Farrington, 1995).

Prevalence, Aetiology and Comorbidity

Attention deficit hyperactivity disorder affects around 1–3% of children in India (Thapar, 2012). The prevalence for ADHD usually varies and depends on various features of the population, sampling methods and the nature of the assessment (Sciutto 2007). The significant geographical variations in the rate of diagnosis and treatment and the prevalence have increased over time.The Centre for Disease Control and Prevention (2005) reports based on a survey conducted in the USA on 102,353 parents with children aged 4 to 17 years and found a lifetime childhood diagnosis of 7.8% (2.5 times as many boys as girls) of whom 4.3% had received medication as treatment.Similarly a review of 50 prevalence studies (including 20 US and 30 non-US sample populations) revealed that the prevalence is similar in US and non-US populations (Faraone 2003). Study by Catherine et.al. (2019) revealed that a high prevalence of ADHD was found among primary school children. Overall prevalence of ADHD was found to be 8.8% and subtypes of ADHD were categorized as 124 for inattentive type and hyperactive type and 38 for combined type of ADHD.Familiar survey conducted in United Kingdom 10,438 children aged 5 to 15 years also found that 3.62% of boys and 0.85% of girls had a diagnosis of ADHD (Ford 2003). Another study by Magnus et. al, 2019, reports that the prevalence of ADHD has increased over time, as school became more standardized for children. It is also important to diagnose and treat the disorder at a young age so that the symptoms do not persist into adulthood and cause other comorbid conditions.

Comorbidity or coexistence with other disorders such as learning disabilities, depression, and conduct disorder is also common (Biederman et.al., 1991). Studies points out that comorbidity between ADHD and conduct problems, developmental and learning problems as well as with a variety of psychiatric disorders (Thapar,2012). A study by Palaniappan et.al. (2013) tried to understand the pattern of co-morbidities in Indian children & adolescents with ADHD and to compare the degree of functional impairment between ADHD subjects with and without comorbidities. Studies revealed that comorbid disorders like anxiety disorders are not as low as projected by the earlier Indian studies.The analysis of the study revealed that 55% of enlisted subjects had comorbidity. Out of which the most highly prevalent lifetime disorder was found to be Oppositional Defiant disorder followed by conduct disorder, bipolar affective disorder, major depressive disorder, communication disorder, substance use disorder, obsessive compulsive disorder, tic disorder, learning disorder, elimination disorder, separation anxiety disorder and social phobia. Subjects with comorbidities had poorer global functioning when compared to ADHD subjects without comorbidities. Also according to British Child and Adolescent Mental Health Survey, 27% and 26% of those with conduct disorder (CD) and oppositional defiant disorder (ODD) fitsfor a diagnosis of ADHD, and more than 50% of those with ADHD had a comorbid behaviour disorder (Ford, 2003). In a recent nationally representative sample from United States, children diagnosed with ADHD, reported 42% of them had comorbidity with ASD and 17% of learning disability (LD) (Gnanavel et. al, 2019)

Although the aetiology of ADHD is still unclear ADHD is highly heritable, although there is no single causal risk factor and non-inherited factors also contribute to its aetiology. The genetic and environmental risk factors that have been implicated appears to be related with a range of neurodevelopmental and neuropsychiatric outcomes, not just ADHD (Thapar, 2012). Twin studies reported a strong genetic effect in the manifestation of the disorder (Biederman, 2005; Rydell, Taylor, & Larsson, 2017). Also in another twin studies it was seen that ADHD is better viewed as an extreme of a continuous, rather than as one category, as it is defined in clinical use (Larsson, Anckarsater, Råstam, Chang, & Lichtenstein, 2012). The manifestation and prevalence of ADHD are also associated with various non-inherited factors such as pre- and perinatal factors, environmental toxins, dietary factors, and psychosocial adversity (Thapar, Cooper, Eyre, & Langley, 2013). These factors have been conceptualised as nonspecific triggers of an underlying predisposition to ADHD (Biederman, 2005). According to NICE (2008) it was said that genetic and environmental risk factors interact to cause ADHD rather than operate in isolation. The evidence suggests that both rare and multiple common genetic variants are likely to contribute to ADHD and modify its phenotype. The genetic contribution to observable phenotypic ADHD traits has been estimated as being up to 76% (Faraone 2005). ADHD or a similar phenotype also appears to be more common in extreme low birth weight and premature children and those exposed to exceptional early adversity. (Thapar, 2012).No large single gene effect has been identified but the DRD4 and DRD5 genes appear to be involved and a specific haplotype of the dopamine transporter gene has been linked with the combined-type ADHD (Li, 2006; Asherson, 2007). Studies indicated an increased rate of chromosomal deletions and duplications in children with ADHD compared to those without ADHD (Jones 2010; McFadden 2010). Other than genetic causal factors the possible environmental factors that studies suggests include maternal smoking, alcohol consumption, heroin use in pregnancy, foetal hypoxia and perinatal exposure to toxins, injury and zinc deficiency (NICE 2008).

Global impairment in children with ADHD grows with increasing number of coexisting disorders. Attention deficit hyperactivity disorder (ADHD) is considered as the most common neurodevelopmental disorder of childhood and can endure during adolescence and adulthood (Catherine et.al, 2019). ADHD children, their parents, schools, and society feel severe impacts of this disability, causing parents to seek a variety of conventional and unconventional treatments (Weiss & Hechtman, 1986).The presence of ADHD in childhood also increases the possibility of additional difficulties in academic performance, social interactions, and low self-esteem among adolescents and young adults. (Catherine et.al., 2019). All these difficulties present in a child with ADHD can lead to difficulty in parenting.

Parenting

The word "parent" has been coined from the Latin word "parens" meaning a person who has produced the offspring or has the legal status of a father or a mother still defining the word parent can be difficult define from a single point of view (Nair & Russel, 2019). According to Morrison (1978) definition parenting as "the process of developing and utilising the knowledge and skills appropriate to planning for, creating, giving birth to, rearing and/or providing care for offspring". The definition means that parenting starts when there is a plan for it and it involves not just bringing up the child but also providing care and support to the child. Nowadays parenting can be a choice in life with the advancement in medical knowledge and technology. As it is a life-long commitment, it comes with lot ofresponsibilities starting from taking good care of the child not just physically but alsopsychologically. Especially in Indian scenario parenting involves not just the couple but all the family members as birth of a child has an emotional impact in the whole family.

Parenting is a complex activity that includes many specific attitudes and behaviours of both mothers and fathers that work separately and collectively to influence child outcomes and generate an emotional bond in which the parent's behaviours are expressed (Darling & Steinberg, 1993; Darling, 1999). According to Onghena (2004) it is an important determinant which affects the whole life of a child. It is one of the toughest responsibilities to describe as every parent would feel that they have given their best possible efforts and hope to succeed in the area as parents. The responsibility of bringing up the child refers to a privilege or responsibility of mother and father, together or independently to prepare the child for society and culture. The process includes promoting and supporting of the physical, emotional, social and intellectual development of a child from infancy to adulthood (Veenes,1973a). During the first years of life of an infant parent assume special responsibility. As the child reaches the stage of adolescence, the youth is apprehensive about the changes in personality and they try to adjustments with the world in diverse ways (Bornstein et al., 2007). Parent's unique attitude, behaviour, belief, values and family culture differ from parent to parent (Bibi et. al., 2013). Parental acceptance is closely associated with positive outcomes of the child (Khaleque & Rohner, 2002). On the other hand, unreasonable parental expectations and faulty parental behaviour patterns can adversely affect the child's psychological development and wellbeing (Wang, 2002). Therefore Learning about the diagnosis when their child is still young may alter parent's perception so the child's behaviour may give them new perspectives on their child and their own parenting. (Ringer et.al, 2019)

One of the most common behavioural issues related to ADHD can be, *inattention* which includes daydreaming, distractibility, difficulty focusing on a single task, whereas the *hyperactivity* part can be expressed as fidgeting, excessive talking, and restlessness (Biederman, 2005). The disorder's secondary consequences, such as social, emotional and learning impairments and with its high comorbidity with other mental health issues such as disruptive behavioural disorders, depression and anxiety disorders lead to its profound effect on the lives of the children and their families(Wehmeyer, et. al. 2010; Pliszka, 2003). The behaviour of children with ADHD is often perceived by parents as challenging to manage, and research has shown that parents of children with ADHD experience more stress than do those of children without disabilities.

A study by Ringer et. al, 2019, explored parents' meaning-making processes in relation to their child receiving an ADHD diagnosis wherein they found out 5 (five) conceptual categories, which can be also understood as components of a process of adaptation.

- Representing the parents' experiences of the child's behaviour as challenging and difficult to understand and manage, is seen as a starting point for an adaptive meaning-making process
- Having an explanation and understanding child's needs
- Adjusting oneself
- Processing emotions
- Negotiating an integration of ADHD with everyday life.

Parenting Challenges, Stress and Coping

In a meta-analysis of 44 quantitative studies, conducted by Theule, Wiener, Tannockand Jenkins (2012), it was found that parents of children with ADHD experienced significantly more parenting stress than parents of children without ADHD. Children with ADHD and their families face many challenges. There are various difficulties faced by children with ADHD and their families to have an impact and the difficulties in the parents impact the child's ADHD symptoms as well. Children with ADHD are described as less attentive to social cues, not listening to adults, and ignoring parental requests. These difficulties impair their academic and social functioning, use of their recreational time as well as the relationship with their parents (Brook& Boaz, 2005). They are often seen as being less compliant even oppositional towards adults (Wells, 2000; DuPaul, 2001).It makes it hard for the parent of a child who is often annoyed and over-reacting to things around him/ her. Parents with ADHD child also have to listen to numerous negative reports and negative reactions of their child from their teachers in schools. Parents often see the problems in the children as the child misbehaving and being under the influence of their peer group. It is often difficult to sort out what difficulties are caused, what factors add to the difficulties and how. Therefore various studies have tried categorizing difficulties associated with ADHD (Rubia et.al.,2007; Barkley, 1997).The first one found was Emotional component, e.g., which means individuals who are easily frustrated, impatient and emotionally reactive. The pathology can be described as the presence of uncontrolled irritable temperament (Rubiaet.al.,2007).The other aspect of difficulty was found to be Social component, e.g., arguing, defiant. The social component is often linked to learned behaviours and is frequently related to the reaction of significant others to the child's behaviour. Many researchers have emphasized the presence of poor Behavioural Inhibition as the central impairment of the disorder (Barkley, 1997). It is described as being impulsive/ impulsiveness in a child. Behaviours that are uncontrollable, involvement of risk taking behaviours are often annoying and cause disturbances or distress to others especially parents. The poor behaviour inhibition and poor impulse control is evident in people with ADHD as they less effective at regulating their emotional and social components (Barkley, 2010).As a result of their inabilities to delay responds for they make frequent hasty decisions and actions that occur in the moment without them considering the possibility of high potential of harm, failure or disappointment to the individuals well as others (APA,2013). Learning from their mistakes does not often occur or is difficult. They are repeatedly unable to use appropriate self-regulation strategies and social skills (Barkley, 1997). These disruptive behaviours often emerge as early as in the preschool years and in many children persisting into adolescence. Children with ADHD have difficulties in their social and adaptive behaviour which are related to the core symptoms of the disorder (Wehmeier et. al, 2010; Barkley, 2002). The difficulties are felt within and outside the family setting with factors in their environment increasing the risk of impairment. Families of children with ADHD have consistently been shown to experience more burdens including stress (Coghill, 2008; Narkunam; 2012). Various studies on families with ADHD children experience significantly higher stress than families without a special child (Breen & Barkley, 1988; Fisher, 1990; Anastopoulos, et al. 1992). The families with ADHD children seems to score higher on stress inventories, and parents indicate higher divorce rates, more negative parent-child interactions and symptoms of clinical depression (Brown & Pacini, 1989; Barkley et.al, 1990; Anastopoulos, 1992).

According to a study by Anastopoulos, et al. (1992) tried to parental stress for their ADHD children. The study included 87 boys and 17 girls ADHD children under the age of 12 and their mothers. Parent interviews including assessment of the mother's health, depression, overall psychopathology, and psychological stress; assessment of family demographics and socioeconomic status; and assessments of problems exhibited by other family members as well as child's overall behaviour assessment such as depression, peer relations, health status, medication status, and special education status including child demographics; were all examined using a variety of instruments. Overall it was found that the stress levels were higher among 90 of the participants especially mothers who did not work outside, the home reported greater parental stress. Other than that environmental stress included marital status, maternal relationship to the biological father, and number of children in the family. This study was typically done on mothers of ADHD children

Another study by Baker (1994) surveyed both maternal and paternal stress. 20 Twenty married couples with an ADHD child were included where he found no difference between the mother and father in their rating of child behaviour as severe However, when compared to the father, the mother stated that the child's behaviour caused more parental stress. There are other various researches which talks about Maternal and Paternal Pathology in Relation to ADHD. Several studies have also linked ADHD to maternal depression (Sobol, et al. 1989; Cunningham, et al. 1988).The parents also reported that their family environments were unsupportive, stressed, high in conflict, low in autonomy and expressiveness, and lacked cohesiveness due which there was more intense stress. The impact of depression was different among mothers and fathers. Unlike mothers, fathers specified that their depression was due to increased occurrence of family activities and greater parental control over their child. Parental depression also had an impact on the way that parents perceived their children. Those who were depressed experienced greater parenting stress, less acceptance of their child's behaviour, and viewed their child as more demanding (Breen &Barkley, 1988). It was also found that although total problem behaviour of the child was the strongest indicator of stress but interestingly being married for fewer years was also associated with elevated stress. Other than that stress based on gender and socioeconomic status seemed have a limited influence (Baker,1994).

Parenting stress appears to be impacted by sibling interactions. Mash and Johnston (1983a) examined sibling interactions between 46 sibling dyads and found that sibling interactions when one child had ADHD was characterized by four times more negative behaviour when there was no adult supervision and twice as much when supervised by mothers. Positive correlation was observed between the mother's report of self-esteem and stress and the degree of negative behaviour and amount of independent play exhibited by the child (Mash & Johnston, 1983a).Stress is increased with a greater degree of hyperactivity, ADHD child, increased display of aggression and oppositional behaviour by the child, and sibling rivalry. External issues unrelated to the child's hyperactivity such as SES, number of children in the family, and psychiatric and medical conditions in fathers do not seem to have a great impact on the parental stress level. However, single parents and those mothers not working outside the home indicated higher stress than their counterparts with ADHD children.

Parents seek a variety of treatments for their children as a way of coping with ADHD. One of these treatments is the administration of stimulant medications. Medication has a positive impact upon ADHD children in the areas of attention, impulsivity, ability to stay on task, frustration level, and compliance (CHADD, 1993). These changes generally are seen with the first dose of medication and result in an immediate positive change in parent commands and negativity (Barkley, 1989; Barkley et.al., 1985). Other conventional treatments include parental psychoeducation, behaviour management training, self-control training for the ADHD child and communication training. In addition to these more accepted practices and treatments methods are being utilized to treat ADHD. Mental Health Professionals can be of a huge help for the parents and family of the child with ADHD.

Parenting Styles

Parenting style is one of the variables which have been studied extensively for human development. According to Darling & Steinberg (1993) parenting style is a constellation of behaviours and attitudes towards the child and that work as taken together or separately to motivate the child and create an emotional atmosphere in which parental attitudes are expressed. Their styles of care giving can have both immediate and lasting effects on children's moral and social functioning in areas from pro-social development to peer play to academic achievement (Bornstein et al., 2007). Parenting can be defined on the basis of two components responsiveness which means, parental emotional characteristics and demandingness, that means set of parental guidelines and disciplines for the child (Fletcher et. al., 2008). Both parenting responsive and demanding has been linked to secure attachment in children (Karavasiliset. al., 2003).

Psychologist Diana Baumrind (1971, 1991) recognized four patterns of parenting styles based upon two aspects of parenting behaviour: one is control and the other is warmth. Parental control meant the degree to which parents manage their children's behaviour i.e. from being very controlling to setting up little rules and demands. On the other hand parental warmth meant the degree to which parents are accepting and responsive of their child's action as opposed to being unresponsive and rejecting. Combining two aspects of parenting behaviour in different ways four types of primary parenting styles can be concluded:

Authoritative parenting styles are warm but firm. They encourage their children to be independent at the same time they need to maintain limits and controls on their actions (Kopko,2007). This style of parenting maintains equilibrium between the levels of responsiveness and demandingness. The control on their children is based as per the child's age and understanding, they make logical demands, create an atmosphere of attachment and warmth where children can express their feelings, points of views and participate in decision making process within the family itself (Berg et al.,2011).

Authoritarian parenting styles display little warmth and are highly controlling(Kopko,2007). They are highly demanding but less responsive to their children(Gustavo et. al, 2010). According to Baumrind (1966), these parents do not allow the child to express their opinions and needs. They set their own standards and rules which they try impose on the child. These parents follow a very restrictive and disciplinary style and which they insist their child to follow, (Kopko, 2007) as they feel that they know the best for their children. They try to mould and control the child's actions and attitudes. Here the parents expect the child to follow each and rule to be followed without any questions or explanation (Baumrind, 1966).

Permissive parenting styles are responsive but exercise low demands on their children. Baumrind (1971, 1989) found that these parents exercise very little control and authority on the child and often fail to set updefined standards and rules for the child. These parents often fail to define the limits of acceptable response and actions of the child. This type of parenting style is very warm, but at the same time they are undemanding. They are indulgent and passive in their parenting and believe that the way to love their child is to give in to their child to fulfil their wishes without any parental demands (Kopko, 2007).

Neglectful parenting style (or uninvolved parents) this style of parenting exhibits low levels of responsiveness as well as low levels of demandingness. Uninvolved Parents are neither warm nor place any demands on their children. Their interaction time is either minimal or neglectful; in some cases they are not even involved for their child's better development.Uninvolved parents are indifferent to their child's needs, experiences at school or with peers (Kopko, 2007). These parents are often ignoring parental responsibilities. They don't even direct their children's actions (Maccoby & Martin, 1983).

Impact of Parent-Child Interactions

Being a parent of a child with ADHD they have a very important role to play in helping their child gain control over their behaviour. Before helping the child first being a parent one should never feel that he/she is a bad parent because at the initial phase it was difficult for the parent to understand the child.Learning specific ways of talking, playing and working with the child can help improve the child's attention and behaviour (Borrill, 2000). Parent-child interactions can greatly influence ADHD behaviours. Parents with ADHD children indicate they are more socially isolated and have fewer extended family contacts than families without ADHD and that the contacts that they have are less helpful (Mash & Johnston, 1983; Cunningham et.al., 1988). Studies confirm that self-esteem is lower in parents who have an ADHD child, with- parents of ADHD children exhibiting more self-blame (Johnston, 1983b).Various studies on ADHD children also reported that the children seemto be more noncompliant and negative than other similar age group children (Mash & Johnston, 1982).

Studies indicate that mothers, of younger hyperactive children show significantly more negative behaviour than mothers of older hyperactive children or mothers of normal children. It is found in studies that the younger hyperactive children portray the most negative behaviours. Campbell (1975) in his study found that the mothers of the hyperactive boys tried to regulate their child's behaviour by giving significant suggestions about impulse control, more disapproval or praise and urging to complete a task than the mothers with learning disabled or normal children. A hyperactive child was found to be more impulsive, disorganized, and dependent on parental interaction to complete their tasks than either the learning disabled child or the normal controls.

Mothers of ADHD children reported to be more negative, demanding, and controlling than mothers of children who do not have ADHD (Barkley et. al., 1992). Mothers of ADHD children view their child's behaviour as more unstable as compared to others. They feel less controlled over their child's behaviour (Sobol et. al., 1989). Such behaviour was especially evident in task situations where ADHD children were found to be more active, less compliant, and less frequently on task. Similar study by Cunningham & Barkley (1979) supported familiar results saying mothers of hyperactive boys were more controlling than mothers of nondisabled children, giving their childmore commands than required. Some of the studies also revealed that mothers of ADHD children were less responsive to the child's initiations and less involved in social interactions with their child. The mothers of normal children interacted more positively with their child, visiting with them, asking questions, and praising them.Cunningham & Barkley (1979) concluded that the mothers of overexcited boys appear more critical and disapproving and seem to have acquired a comprehensive negative set of prospects which adversely influence their perception of and response to the child. Studies with younger ADHD children also supported similar findings (Barkley et.al., 1985; Mash & Johnston, 1982). A lot of studies have reviewed interactions between the mother-child dyad, whereas Tallmadge and Barkley (1983) studied interactions between the father-child dyad. They found similar results were discovered that even fathers of ADHD children were more controlling and negative than the control group and the children were less compliant with commands and complied for shorter periods. Noncompliant behaviours were found to be more when the child was interacting with the mother.

Barkley & Befera (1985) looked at differences in the way mothers interact with their ADHD child based upon the sex of the child, the results revealed that there were very few differences. They found that hyperactive boys used to receive more praise from their mothers than girls even though there were no significant differences in their behaviour.' In another study by Barkley (1989), found that mothers were more controlling, as well as encouraging to a boy. However, his study also found that the boys were more negative and less compliant than the girls in the study.Various studies examined sibling brothers, one with ADHD and one without ADHD, the findings of the study suggests that mothers did not treat their ADHD child differently from the sibling, even though the ADHD child was less responsive to their mothers and portrayed more noncompliance. Mothers tended to treat both the ADHD child and sibling in similar ways(Barkley, 1985). ADHD children are found to be more active, impulsive, disorganized, and dependent than their peers.They are also more noncompliant and even if they comply with requests it is only for a short duration. Overall, both the parents of a ADHD child were found to be more controlling, commanding, and more negative than parents who do not have a ADHD child.

Parent Training Programmes

Parent Training Programmes are basically psychosocial interventions aimed at training parents in behavioural or cognitive techniques to enable them to manage their child's challenging behaviour. The programmes may vary in its style and content but are generally manual-based and may involve discussion and the use of video and role play (Webster-Stratton, 1998). The ADHD-focused parent training often includes psycho educational awareness elements on ADHD it describes how its presence affects a child's functioning and actions. The programmes are usually delivered to groups of parents and generally comprises of 10 to 20 weekly sessions for one to two hours covering a range of areas that include the nature of ADHD, need and requirement of positive reinforcement skills, reward systems, the use of various activities such as 'time out', cooperation with teachers and planning ahead to anticipate problems and work for preventive measures and management (Pliszka, 2007). The aim of the program is to reduce children's problem behaviour by strengthening parent management skills" (Hartman, 2003).

Parent training interventions are mainly based on behaviour management principles that arise from social-learning theory. Parent training usually comprises of structured programmes that are conveyed in a standardised way by professionals trained in behaviour management theory and practices (Kazdin,1997). Precisely families with children who have ADHD, parent training aims at improving the parent's understanding of ADHD or increasing their behavioural management skills, although enhancing both is the actual motive of the professionals. There are number of programmes run by professionals to help parents. Most of these programmes focus on 'behavioural management' of the child with ADHD and equipping parents to manage the everyday issues with the child. Parents may also learn self-management skills aimed at reducing stress and increasing resilience. Studies and researches have suggested that to improve ADHD symptoms parent training could be designed to work on both areas, through cognitive work on self-regulation and through motivational interventions focusing on improving delay tolerance (Sonuga-Barke 2003b). These programs involve learning how to plan and structure activities, and to praise and encourage children for even very small amounts of progress.

Behaviour management approaches often start by teaching parents and carers the A-B-C approach. The theory programs in three simple steps

- Firstly it identifies the events or a circumstance which seems to lead to difficult behaviour or trigger specific problems. These are known as antecedents (A).
- Then describe the actual behaviour (B) in detail basically child's actions and reactions (what does the child do or don't do).

- Finally observe the consequences (C) of the behaviour (what can happen to the child, how other people can react to such behaviour).

Based on these three simple steps of the theory, parents are then shown how to gradually modify their child's actions. They are also asked to concentrate on small changes at a time and do praise for any small step taken by the child towards a right direction. They are based on the theories where in it is believed that behaviour can be influenced by its antecedents and consequences, which a parent can learn how to intervene with both of these (Kazdin, 1997). If parents are given training and support while their children are young it might be possible to prevent problems at later developmental stages of the child. In order to have early detection awareness about child with signs of ADHD need to be spread during standard health checks (Hughes, 2017).

Based on reports of American Academy of Paediatrics (2007) some of the key principles that can be taught to parents for their child as well as it can benefit the parents from being too stressful from their child's behaviour:

- Importance of making eye contact with the child before trying to talk to them (such as is the eye contact maintained or it is partial or not at all eye contact it maintained).
- Careful about how do they response to your instruction (such as if you call out an instruction from another room he/she will not pay attention).Instructions need to be simple i.e the one sentence rule. It is one of the important principle that the parents need to be aware of as studies suggests that a ADHD child usually found to have problems with short-term memory therefore anything longer than one sentence might be either forgotten or might just go unattained. Specific and clear instruction, suggestion or compliments for the child's behaviour is necessary so that the child understands it better and can react accordingly and in a more acceptable manner. Symbolic representation can also be used for communication (Breiner, 2016).
- Any child does mirror their parent's action, especially during their childhood. Therefore a parent needs to be calm to manage any situation and deal with it tactfully. Using a quiet, calm tone of voice helps both parent and child to stay calm.
- Using techniques like 'time out' or 'quiet time' helps deal with temper tantrums. Encourage the child to sit or stay at a place without exchanging any of verbal and nonverbal cues until calm. Distraction is another technique that can be used for a child for temper tantrum or difficult behaviour.
- Providing clear routines makes an ADHD child tackle day to day issues in a better way, also helpful for a parent to make better assumptions and accordingly work on the child's behaviour.
- If choices have to be given it can be only two choices to keep it simple and non-confusing for the child.
- Spending time with the child is one of most important principle not just to understand the child also help the child grow in a better manner. Playing with the child can be one way of spending time, even if it is for only for a short period of time. Children with ADHD do respond to play well.

Children with Attention Deficit Hyperactivity Disorder can become difficult if the child is not monitored using correct strategies and techniques (Breiner, 2016). Therefore in such cases parents play a very crucial role in the process of growth and development of the child. Parents can manage a child's behavioural issues by using very simple and tactful techniques.

Role of professionals

Helping the parents will significantly aid in the progress of the child. The families of children with ADHD experience difficulties in various areas of functioning. The presence of the difficulties in the child as well as comorbidities signifies risk factors for insecure attachment with impact on the parent child relationship. The existence of the factors and its consequences must be accepted and worked upon it. ADHD creates a huge impact not only on the child alone but also upon the whole family. From the very early stage parental factors such as perception of parents/caregivers, the dynamics within the family, emotional difficulties of parents and their parenting skills needs consideration and work upon to modifications as per the child's requirement. Professionals can provide help with such requirement. The child, his/her parents and the whole family can be benefited by considering various preventive and management methods. In pharmacological treatment of ADHD, the effectiveness of medication has been well established. But studies have reported that medication alone might not be sufficient for the treatment. Of recent, increasing evidence has demonstrated the role of multi-modal treatment for effectively addressing the diverse difficulties of children with ADHD (MTA, 2004)

To be most effective in helping children and their families, it is commended that health care professionals have a good understanding of the individual and their family development. Family difficulties are common as discussed earlier in the chapter such as parental depression, aggression, marital discord, and hostile parent child interactions. Assessment should include family factors that may have an impact on the child and their family functioning alone child's history. Family functioning is often related to the origins of behaviour problems in the child (Roelofs, 2006; Schroeder & Mowen, 2014) Understanding family dynamics is most essential, in order to examine the interactions among family members, and identify factors that are triggering or maintaining undesirable behaviours. The dynamic interactionincludes biological, social and psychological factors of the child which can be a contributing factor in longstanding distress for the child as well as for the family (Woods, 2003)

Positive parenting styles are significantly associated with development of more appropriate behaviour in children including their inhibition capacities (Roskam, 2014). Parents often misunderstand the use of punishment in changing a child's behaviour. Using harsh punishment does not help establish new and wanted behaviours rather reinforcement enhances development of appropriate behaviour. In clinical setting it is parents report their children hitting back their parents when in anger or frustrated unfortunately parents do not realize that children often model their parent's behaviour. Therefore along with individual therapy for children multimodal forms of family therapy or parent training is also important(Carr, 2000). Still further research is necessary for examining the effectiveness of family therapy as an relevant intervention for children with ADHD (Bjornstad& Montgomery, 2005). Many clinicians and researchers emphasize the need to regularly focus on children's attachment and attachment difficulties in clinical settings and to incorporate it in the treatment option (Zeanah et. al., 2011). There is now increasing evidence of the implication of parent training programs, with results showing the improvement of the child's behaviour. Client-centred approach can be useful while initiating parenting or family programs (Carr, 2000).Parents along with mental health professionals together can achieve the best possible support future for their children.

CONCLUSION

Children with ADHD show disability not only in attention and focus but also in decision making and emotional regulation. Children with ADHD can have difficulty with social interactions, can be easily frustrated, and can be impulsive. They are often labelled as "trouble makers." To be diagnosed with ADHD; a child must experience symptoms that are more extreme than what would be expected for his or her age and symptoms must be evident in a variety of settings (Shaywitz & Shaywitz, 1984). Currently, diagnosis for ADHD is a multifaceted process which generally includes: history of physical exam, neurological, medical, educational, and behavioural screening along with social and medical history of parents. Standardized questionnaires for parent and teacher are used to determine current functioning and indicators of ADHD in the child; intelligence testing and assessment of academic, developmental, social, and emotional skills, clinical interviews and observations of the child also used to understand the condition of the child (Hunsucker, 1988).

ADHD is not a new problem, but there are new ways of helping children and their families to cope with it. Parenting is challenging enough and the case demonstrates the reality that parenting children with ADHD is a big challenge to many parents. Symptoms of the disorder such as hyperactivity, impulsivity and inattention make parenting more difficult (Biederman, 2008). Although the presentation may change throughout the developmental years, the difficulties are often on going. It is often more challenging during the adolescent years. Due to the pervasiveness of the disability and the long term outcomes for ADHD children, it is also considered to be one of the most debilitating of childhood disorders (Barkley, 1981; Trites et.al, 1979). Parents attributed their high levels of stress to their children's behaviour and social difficulties, their unmet needs for support, and their experiences of social stigma. Similar quantitative literature by Theule et al., 2013 enriches the large body of indicating that parents of children with ADHD display high levels of parenting stress. The parents' perception and understanding of the ADHD diagnosis appeared as quite a dramatic moment of change to them. However, the importance of the diagnosis in their meaning-making process most likely take place over a long period of time, during which they gradually discover new aspects of distress and life challenges and consequently searched for new ways of understanding their parenthood and responsibility for their child, drawing on new reflections on what the diagnosis could mean (Ringer et.al, 2019). Therefore knowledge (awareness) and training can lead to better coping ability for parents to manage the child as well as themselves.

REFERENCES

Amen, D. G., Paldi, J. H., & Thisted, R. A. (1993). Brain SPECT imaging. *Journal of the American Academy of Child and Adolescent Psychiatry*, *32*(5), 1080–1081. doi:10.1097/00004583-199309000-00036 PMID:8407758

American Psychiatric Association. (1994). Diagnostic and Statistical Manual of Mental Disorders, 4th edition (DSM-IV). Washington DC.

American Psychiatric Association. (2013), Diagnostic and statistical manual of mental disorders (5th ed.; DSM–5). Washington, DC.

Anastopoulos, A. D., Guevremont, D. C., Shelton, T. L., & DuPaul, G. J. (1992). Parenting stress among families of children with attention deficit hyperactivity disorder. *Journal of Abnormal Child Psychology*, *20*(5), 503–520. doi:10.1007/BF00916812 PMID:1487593

Anastopoulos, A. D., Shelton, T. L., DuPaul, G. J., & Guevremont, D. C. (1993). Parent training for attentiondeficit hyperactivity disorder: Its impact' of parent functioning. *Journal of Abnormal Child Psychology*, *21*(5), 581–596. doi:10.1007/BF00916320 PMID:8294653

Barkley, R. A. (1981). *Hyperactive children: A handbook for diagnosis and treatment*. Guilford.

Barkley, R. A. (1997). Behavioural inhibition, sustained attention, and executive functions: Constructing a unifying theory of ADHD. *Psychological Bulletin*, *121*(1), 65–94. doi:10.1037/0033-2909.121.1.65 PMID:9000892

Barkley, R. A. (2002). Major life activity and health outcomes associated with attention-deficit/ hyperactivity disorder. *The Journal of Clinical Psychiatry*, *63*(12), 10–15. PMID:12562056

Barkley, R. A. (2010). Deficient emotional self-regulation: A core component of attention-deficit/ hyperactivity disorder. *Journal of ADHD & Related Disorders*, (1), 1–30.

Barkley, R. A., Fischer, M., Edelbrock, C. S., Smallish, L. (1990). The adolescent outcome of hyperactive children diagnosed by research criteria: I. An 8-year prospective follow-up study. *Journal of the American Academy of Child and Adolescent Psychiatry, 29*(4), 546-557.

Barkley, R. A., Guevremont, D. C., Anastopoulos, A. D., & Fletcher, K. E. (1992). A comparison of three family therapy programs for treating family conflicts in adolescents with attention-deficit hyperactivity disorder. *Journal of Consulting and Clinical Psychology*, *60*(3), 450–462. doi:10.1037/0022-006X.60.3.450 PMID:1619099

Barkley, R. A., Karlsson, J., & Pollard, S. (1985). Effects of age on the mother-child interactions of ADD-H and normal boys. *Journal of Child Psychology and Psychiatry, and Allied Disciplines*, *13*(4), 631–637. PMID:4078191

Baumrind, D.(1971). Current patterns of parental authority. *Developmental Psychology Monographs, 4*(1-2).

Baumrind, D. (1991). Effective parenting during the early adolescent transition. In P. A. Cowan & E. M. Hetherington (Eds.), *Advances in family research* (Vol. 2). Erlbaum.

Biederman, J., Newcorn, J., & Sprich, S. (1991). Comorbidity of attention deficit hyperactivity disorder with conduct, depressive, anxiety, and other disorders. *The American Journal of Psychiatry*, *148*(5), 564–577. doi:10.1176/ajp.148.5.564 PMID:2018156

Biederman, J., Petty, C. R., Dolan, C., Hughes, S., Mick, E., Monuteaux, M. C., & Faraone, S. V. (2008). The long-term longitudinal course of oppositional defiant disorder and conduct disorder in ADHD boys: Findings from a controlled 10-year prospective longitudinal follow-up study. *Psychological Medicine*, *38*(7), 1027–1036. doi:10.1017/S0033291707002668 PMID:18205967

Bjornstad, G., & Montgomery, P. (2005). Family therapy for attention-deficit disorder or attention-deficit/hyperactivity disorder in children and adolescents. *Cochrane Database of Systematic Reviews*, *18*(2). Advance online publication. doi:10.1002/14651858.CD005042.pub2 PMID:15846741

Bradley, C. (1937). The behaviour of children receiving Benzedrine. *The American Journal of Psychiatry*, *94*(3), 577–585. doi:10.1176/ajp.94.3.577

Breen, M. J., & Barkley, R. A. (1988). Child psychopathology and parenting stress in girls and boys having attention deficit disorder with hyperactivity. *Journal of Pediatric Psychology*, *13*(2), 265–280. doi:10.1093/jpepsy/13.2.265 PMID:3171819

Brook, U., & Boaz, M. (2005). Attention deficit and hyperactivity disorder/learning disabilities (ADHD/LD): Parental characterization and perception. *Patient Education and Counseling*, *57*(1), 96–100. doi:10.1016/j.pec.2004.03.018 PMID:15797157

Brown, R. T., & Pacini, J. N. (1989). Perceived family functioning, marital status, and depression in parents of boys with attention deficit disorder. *Journal of Learning Disabilities*, *22*(9), 581–587. doi:10.1177/002221948902200911 PMID:2809411

Campbell, S. B. (1975). Mother-child interaction: A comparison of hyperactive, learning disabled, and normal boys. *The American Journal of Orthopsychiatry*, *45*(1), 51–57. doi:10.1111/j.1939-0025.1975.tb01165.x PMID:1111300

Catherine, T. G., Robert, N. G., Mala, K. K., Kanniammal, C., & Arullapan, J. (2019). Assessment of prevalence of attention deficit hyperactivity disorder among schoolchildren in selected schools. *Indian Journal of Psychiatry*, (61), 232–237. PMID:31142899

Center for Disease Control. (2003). *Mental health in the United States: prevalence of diagnosis and medication treatment for attention-deficit/hyperactivity disorder - United States*. Author.

Coghill, D., Soutullo, C., d'Aubuisson, C., Preuss, U., Lindback, T., Silverberg, M., & Buitelaar, J. (2008). Impact of attention-deficit/hyperactivity disorder on the patient and family: Results from a European survey. *Child and Adolescent Psychiatry and Mental Health*, *2*(31), 31. doi:10.1186/1753-2000-2-31 PMID:18957105

Cunningham, C. E., & Barkley, R. A. (1979). The interactions of normal and hyperactive children with their mothers in free play and structured tasks. *Child Development*, *50*(1), 217–224. doi:10.2307/1129059 PMID:446207

Cunningham, C. E., Benness, B. B., & Siegel, L. S. (1988). Family functioning, time allocation, and parental depression in the families of normal and ADHD children. *Journal of Clinical Child Psychology*, *17*(2), 169–177. doi:10.120715374424jccp1702_10

Cunningham, C. E., & Boyle, M. H. (2002). Pre-schoolers at risk for attention-deficit hyperactivity disorder and oppositional defiant disorder: Family, parenting, and behavioural correlates. *Journal of Abnormal Child Psychology*, *30*(6), 555–569. doi:10.1023/A:1020855429085 PMID:12481971

Diagnostic and Statistical Manual of Mental Disorders. (2013). (5th ed.). American Psychiatric Association.

DuPaul, G. J. (2001). Preschool children with attention-deficit/hyperactivity disorder: impairments in behavioral, social, and school functioning. *Journal of American Academy of Child and Adolescent Psychiatry. 40*(5), 508-515.

Faraone, S., Sergeant, J., Gillberg, C., & Biederman, J. (2005). The worldwide prevalence of ADHD: Is it an American condition? *World Psychiatry; Official Journal of the World Psychiatric Association (WPA), 2*(2), 104–113. PMID:16946911

Farrington, D. P. (1995). The development of offending and antisocial behaviour from childhood: Key findings from the Cambridge study in delinquent development. *Journal of Child Psychology and Psychiatry, and Allied Disciplines, 36*(6), 929–964. doi:10.1111/j.1469-7610.1995.tb01342.x PMID:7593403

Ford, T., Goodman, R., & Meltzer, H. (2003). The British Child and Adolescent Mental Health Survey 1999: The prevalence of DSM-IV disorders. *Journal of the American Academy of Child and Adolescent Psychiatry, 42*(10), 1203–1211. doi:10.1097/00004583-200310000-00011 PMID:14560170

Gillberg, C., Carlstrom, G., & Rasmussen, P. (1983). Hyperkinetic disorders in seven-year-old children with perceptual, motor and attention deficits. *Journal of Child Psychology and Psychiatry, and Allied Disciplines, 24*(2), 233–246. doi:10.1111/j.1469-7610.1983.tb00572.x PMID:6841509

Gnanavel, S., Sharma, P., Kaushal, P., & Hussain, S. (2019). Attention deficit hyperactivity disorder and comorbidity: A review of literature. *World Journal of Clinical Cases, 7*(17), 2420–2426. doi:10.12998/wjcc.v7.i17.2420 PMID:31559278

Hartman, R., Stage, S., & Webster-Stratton, C. A. (2003). Growth curve analysis of parent training outcomes: Examining the influence of child risk factors (inattention, impulsivity, and hyperactivity problems), parental and family risk factors. *Journal of Child Psychology and Psychiatry, and Allied Disciplines, 44*(3), 388–398. doi:10.1111/1469-7610.00129 PMID:12635968

Hughes, S. M. (2017). *Coaching parents of children with ADHD: A Western Australian study*. Retrieved from https://ro.ecu.edu.au/ theses/2031

Hunsucker, G. (1988). *Attention Deficit Disorder: A common but often overlooked disorder of children*. Forrest Publishing.

Kazdin, A. (1997). Parent management training: Evidence, outcomes, and issues. *Journal of the American Academy of Child and Adolescent Psychiatry, 36*(10), 1349–1356. doi:10.1097/00004583-199710000-00016 PMID:9334547

Kopko, K. (2007). *Parenting Styles and Adolescents*. Retrieved from: http://www.parenting.cit.cornell.edu

Linden, C. B., Zalenski, J. R., & Newman, R. L. (1989). *Pay attention*. Transact Health Systems.

Magnus, W., Nazir, S., Arayamparambil, C., Kumar, A., & Shaban, K. (2019). *Attention Deficit Hyperactivity Disorder (ADHD)*. Retrieved from: https://www.ncbi.nlm.nih.gov/books/NBK441838

Mash, E, J., & Johnston, C., (1982). A comparison of the mother-child interactions of younger and older hyperactive and normal children. *Journal of Child Development,* (53), 1371-1381.

Mash, E. J., & Johnston, C. (1983b). Parental perceptions of child behaviour problems, parenting self-esteem, and mothers' reported stress in younger and older hyperactive and normal children. *Journal of Consulting and Clinical Psychology*, *51*(1), 86–99. doi:10.1037/0022-006X.51.1.86 PMID:6826870

Mash, E. J., & Sc Johnston, C. (1983a). Sibling interactions of hyperactive and normal children and their relationship to reports of maternal stress and self-esteem. *Journal of Clinical Child Psychology*, *12*(1), 91–99. doi:10.1080/15374418309533116

Morrison, G. S. & Merrill, E. (1978). *Parent involvement in the home, school and community*. Academic Press.

MTA Cooperative Group. (2004). National Institute of Mental Health Multimodal Treatment study of ADHD follow-up: Changes in effectiveness and growth after the end of treatment. *Pediatrics*, *113*(4), 762–769. doi:10.1542/peds.113.4.762 PMID:15060225

NairM. K. C.RussellP. (2019). *Parenting*. Retrieved from www.noblevision.in

Narkunam, N. (2012). Stress among parents of children with attention deficit hyperactivity disorder, a Malaysian experience. *Journal Asia-Pacific Psychiatry,* 1-10.

Palaniappan, P., Seshadri, S., Girimaji, S., & Srinath, S. (2013). Pattern of comorbidities in indian children and adolescents with attention deficit hyperactivity disorder. *European Psychiatry*, *28*, 1. doi:10.1016/S0924-9338(13)77398-X

Plantation, F. L., (1993). *Children & Adults with Attention Deficit Disorders (CHADD). The disability named ADD*. Academic Press.

Pliszka, S., Bernet, W., Bukstein, O., Walter, H., Arnold, V., & Beitchman, J. (2007). Practice Parameters for the Assessment and Treatment of Children and Adolescents with Attention Deficit Hyperactivity Disorder. *Journal of the American Academy of Child and Adolescent Psychiatry*, *46*(7), 894–921. doi:10.1097/chi.0b013e318054e724 PMID:17581453

Ringer, N., Wilder, J., Scheja, M., & Gustavsson, A. (2019). Managing children with challenging behaviours. Parents' meaning-making processes in relation to their children's ADHD diagnosis. *International Journal of Disability Development and Education*. Advance online publication. doi:10.1080/1034912X.2019.1596228

Roelofs, J., Meesters, C., ter Huurne, M., Bamelis, L., & Muris, P. (2006). On the links between attachment style, parental rearing behaviours, and internalizing and externalizing problems in non-clinical children. *Journal of Child and Family Studies*, *15*(3), 331–345. doi:10.100710826-006-9025-1

Roskam, I., Stievenart, M., Meunier, J.-C., & Noël, M.-P. (2014). The development of children's inhibition: Does parenting matter? *Journal of Experimental Child Psychology*, *122*, 166–182. doi:10.1016/j.jecp.2014.01.003 PMID:24607865

Rubia, K., Smith, A., & Taylor, E. (2007). Performance of children with Attention Deficit Hyperactivity Disorder (ADHD) on a test battery of impulsiveness. *Child Neuropsychology*, *13*(3), 276–304. doi:10.1080/09297040600770761 PMID:17453834

Santosh, P. J., Taylor, E., Swanson, J., Wigal, T., Chuang, S., & Davies, M. (2005). Refining the diagnoses of inattention and over activity syndromes: A reanalysis of the Multimodal Treatment study of attention deficit hyperactivity disorder (ADHD) based on ICD-10 criteria for hyperkinetic disorder. *Clinical Neuroscience Research*, (5), 295–306.

Schroeder, R. D., & Mowen, T. J. (2014). Parenting style transitions and delinquency. *Youth & Society*, *46*(2), 228–254. doi:10.1177/0044118X12469041

Scuitto, M., & Eisenberg, M. (2007). Evaluating the evidence for and against the overdiagnosis of ADHD. *Journal of Attention Disorders*, *11*(2), 106–113. doi:10.1177/1087054707300094 PMID:17709814

Shaywitz, S. E., & Shaywitz, B. A. (1984). (in Review). Evaluation and treatment of children with attention deficit disorders. *Pediatrics*, *6*(4), 99–109.

Sobob, M. P., Ashbourne, D. T., Earn, B. M., & Cunningham, C. E. (1989). ' Parents' attributions for achieving compliance from attention-deficit-disordered children. *Journal of Abnormal Child Psychology*, *17*(3), 359–369. doi:10.1007/BF00917405 PMID:2754118

Solanto, M., Abikoff, H., Sonuga-Barke, E., Schachar, R., Logan, G. D., Wigal, T., Hechtman, L., Hinshaw, S., & Turkel, E. (2001). The ecological validity of delay aversion and response inhibition as measures of impulsivity in ADHD: A supplement to the NIMH multi-modal treatment study of AD/HD. *Journal of Abnormal Child Psychology*, *29*(3), 215–228. doi:10.1023/A:1010329714819 PMID:11411784

Sonuga-Barke, E., Dalen, L., & Remington, B. (2003). Do executive deficits and delay aversion make independent contributions to preschool Attention Deficit/Hyperactivity Disorder symptoms? *Journal of the American Academy of Child & Adolescent Psychiatrists*, *42*(11), 1335–1342. doi:10.1097/01.chi.0000087564.34977.21 PMID:14566171

Still, G. F. (1902). The Coulsonian lectures on some abnormal physical conditions in children. *Lancet*, *I*, 1008–1012, 1077–1082, 1163–1168.

Tallmadge, J., & Barkley, R. A. (1983). The interactions of hyperactive and normal boys' with their fathers and mothers. *Journal of Child Psychology and Psychiatry, and Allied Disciplines*, *11*(4), 565–580. PMID:6655156

Thapar, A., Cooper, M., Jefferies, R., & Stergiakouli, E. (2012). What causes attention deficit hyperactivity disorder? *Archives of Disease in Childhood*, *97*(3), 260–265. doi:10.1136/archdischild-2011-300482 PMID:21903599

Trites, R. L., Dugas, F., Lynch, G., & Ferguson, H. B. (1979). Prevalence of hyperactivity. *Journal of Pediatric Psychology*, *4*(2), 179–188. doi:10.1093/jpepsy/4.2.179

Wehmeier, P. M., Schacht, A., & Barkley, R. A. (2010). Social and emotional impairment in children and adolescents with ADHD and the impact on quality of life. *The Journal of Adolescent Health*, *46*(3), 209–217. doi:10.1016/j.jadohealth.2009.09.009 PMID:20159496

Weiss, G. S., & Hechtman, L. T. (1986). Hyperactive children grown up: Empirical findings and theoretical considerations. New York: Guilford Press.

Wells, K. C., Epstein, J. N., Hinshaw, S. P., Conners, C. K., Klaric, J., Abikoff, H. B., Abramowitz, A., Arnold, L. E., Elliott, G., Greenhill, L. L., Hechtman, L., Hoza, B., Jensen, P. S., March, J. S., Pelham, W. Jr, Pfiffner, L., Severe, J., Swanson, J. M., Vitiello, B., & Wigal, T. (2000). Parenting and family stress treatment outcomes in attention deficit hyperactivity disorder (ADHD): An empirical analysis in the MTA study. *Journal of Abnormal Child Psychology*, *28*(6), 543–553. doi:10.1023/A:1005131131159 PMID:11104316

Wood, J. J., McLeod, B. D., Sigman, M., Hwang, W.-C., & Chu, B. C. (2003). Parenting and childhood anxiety: Theory, empirical findings, and future directions. *Journal of Child Psychology and Psychiatry, and Allied Disciplines*, *44*(1), 134–151. doi:10.1111/1469-7610.00106 PMID:12553416

World Health Organization. (1992). *International Statistical Classification of Diseases and Related Health Problems.10th Revision (ICD-10) edition*. Geneva: World Health Organization.

Zeanah, C. H., Berlin, L. J., & Boris, N. W. (2011). Practitioner Review: Clinical applications of attachment theory and research for infants and young children. *Journal of Child Psychology and Psychiatry, and Allied Disciplines*, *52*(8), 819–833. doi:10.1111/j.1469-7610.2011.02399.x PMID:21554304

Chapter 11
ADHD and Its Impact on Interpersonal Relationships

Ambika Kathju
Independent Researcher, Australia

ABSTRACT

This chapter is an attempt to discuss the interpersonal difficulties encountered by adults with ADHD. ADHD is one of the most common psychiatric disorders, while adult ADHD still remains the most undiagnosed one due to its comorbidity with other psychiatric disorders. It was until recently that the importance of adult ADHD was recognized to have an impact on the interpersonal difficulties faced by them. The core symptoms of ADHD in the form of behavioral and cognitive impairments along with social skill deficits are associated with maladjustments in their social and personal relationships that often lead to marital discord, problems with peers, family dysfunction, and parent-child conflicts.

INTRODUCTION

Attention Deficit and Hyperactivity Disorder (ADHD) was perceived as a childhood disorder until the 1970s when rigorous work on the topic paved the path for a better understanding of the core symptoms of ADHD that were thought to disappear in adulthood (Retz and Klein, 2010). The reason for this bigotry was the focus on only one aspect of the disorder, that was, hyperactivity, which was supposed to dissipate during adolescence. However, unlike the assumption, the child does not outgrow his symptoms, but the symptoms manifest in different ways due to maturation, for instance, hyperactivity is likely to be experienced as tension and restlessness in adulthood (Resnick, 2005).

Many individuals are diagnosed for the first time during their adulthood, making adult ADHD as the most common and undiagnosed psychiatric disorder of adult life. The common symptoms of adult ADHD, like procrastination, low motivation, fluctuating mood, anxiety, low self-esteem, and unpredictable behavior, are shared with other psychiatric disorders that have better awareness (Goldman, Genel, Bezman, and Slanetz, 1998; Wender, 1998). Therefore, when these symptoms are presented without a childhood diagnosis of ADHD, it is mostly diagnosed as either generalized anxiety disorder (GAD), bipolar disorder, or depression (Biederman, 2004; Murphy and Adler, 2004). Also, at times adult ADHD

DOI: 10.4018/978-1-7998-5495-1.ch011

is misdiagnosed because its symptoms are comorbid with other disorders like depression, substance abuse, anxiety, and marital distress. One of the researches by Able, Johnston, Adler, and Swindle (2007), concluded that individuals with undiagnosed ADHD have to undergo higher functional and psychosocial difficulties than the ones who are negatively screened for ADHD, thereby, posing a severe burden to adults even when clinically undiagnosed. Thus, the impaired functioning due to ADHD symptoms and availability of appropriate treatment plans are often not known to them, thereby, leaving them with poor quality of living, disorganized life, substance abuse, interpersonal conflicts, trouble at work, and difficulty in forming and sustaining friendships (Koemans, Vroenhoven, Karrenman and Bekker, 2015).

A vast array of literature on ADHD indicates that people who have ADHD possess deficits in social and emotional domains (Barkley, 1997; American Psychiatric Association, 2013) that create obstacles in having healthy interpersonal interactions. Barkely (1997), one of the pioneers in the field of ADHD, predicted that many socially relevant behaviors in ADHD individuals are affected by deficits in behavioral inhibitions, which are ultimately linked to executive functioning. He further predicted that ADHD individuals have a precise perceptual awareness of interpersonal cues but are unable to act on it because of impaired inhibition. The decreased ability to delay their response to the cues heightens their emotional reactivity, diminishes the frustration tolerance, and mars their ability to consider and implement appropriate behaviors; thus, disrupting interpersonal interaction. Some researchers suggest that a range of other emotional and social disruptions are related to non-executive functions like inattention and inability to recognize facial affect. Inattention can cause the ADHD individual to miss a crucial emotional cue that causes them to disregard the information necessary for a meaningful conversation. Also, the subtle visuospatial deficits may cause them to distort the interpersonal cues of others. Moreover, the inability to recognize other's facial affect incapacitates them to respond appropriately; as a result, their interpersonal skills may be doubly hindered due to inaccurate reading and interpretation of the available cues (Rapport, Friedman, Tzelepis, and Voorhis, 2002).

Therefore, the lack of social skills, executive dysfunctions, and the typical ADHD symptoms makes it even more difficult for them to form a significant interpersonal relationship. Their impulsivity, distractibility, impaired self-regulation often comes in their way to clearly express themselves, leaving them misunderstood and socially neglected. Females tend to be more negatively impacted by this deficit as they typically have a greater need for affiliation than males (Nadeau, 1999). This chapter discusses the ADHD symptoms and its impact on interpersonal relationships in the form of marital discords, parenting capabilities, dating, and sexual behavior.

FRIENDSHIP, DATING, AND SEXUAL BEHAVIOR

Friendship and Peer Issues

Friendship is a dyadic relationship based on reciprocity and mutual affection (Berndt, 1999). Friendship provides a companionship; feeling of self-validation and ego support; emotional security; a context of self- disclosure, help, and guidance; and they are reliable allies (Marton, Wiener, Rogers, and Moore, 2015, p. 872). Having close friends act as a buffer against the consequences of peer rejection and adjustment problems (Parker and Asher, 1993; Lauren, Bukowski, and Nurmi, 2007). According to Rose and

Asher (2000), friendship problems can be defined in various ways, like having no friends, poor quality of friendship, and having short and unstable friendships that eventually affect the social-emotional functioning of the person. There is enough literature to prove that children with ADHD have to suffer from peer rejection and isolation because of their poorly developed skills to negotiate, cooperate and resolve conflicts (Hoza, 2007; Molina, 2005). However, given the recency of the inclusion of adult ADHD as a psychiatric disorder, there is still a dearth of research pertaining to adult friendships. Although, studies have linked the predictability of persistence of peer problems into adolescence and young adulthood (Bagwell, Molina, Pelham and Hoza, 2001; Mrug et al., 2012).The empirical evidence suggests that, for ADHD individuals, maintaining friendships is tougher in adulthood than it is in childhood. As adults have fewer enforced obligations to maintain friendships, unlike in childhood, when children are obligated to have school play friends (Bramham and Young, 2007).

The existing literature on ADHD posits that adults with ADHD suffer from social skill deficits. Social skills can be defined as our ability to communicate and interact effectively (Riggio, 1986; Spitzberg, 1987). The absence of accurately reading and interpreting the social cues hinders the development and sustenance of a meaningful relationship and results in frequent rejections and bitter separations. Constant relationship failures and persistent efforts in search of a significant relationship further reduce the self-esteem of the ADHD adult (Robbins, 2005). Decreased self-worth, along with constant efforts to affiliate with a peer group, often makes them vulnerable to fall preyto a bad company (Marshal, Mollina, and Pelham, 2003).

According to Barkley (1997;2007), adults with ADHD either have fewer friends or their friendships do not last long. He reasons these failures to impaired emotional functioning, self-regulation, and working memory that impacts the friendship in various ways. For instance, a fine modulation of one's own emotional reaction is needed to connect with a friend emotionally. The ability to correspond to the affect and arousal of a friend promote intimacy, which is both missing in adults with ADHD. Also, poor organizational skills and working memory makes it difficult to manipulate the pieces of information required to understand a friend's perspective. Further, he mentions that perspective-taking has acritical role to play in being supportive of a friend's needs, to resolve the conflicts with consideration of their feelings, and to be trustworthy to their friend. In his other work, Barkely (2005) mentions that ADHD adults are described as rude, inconsiderate, irresponsible, and unpleasant by their peers and are not preferred in any friend-circle. Additionally, he noticed that the hyperactive subtype has significantly fewer social acquaintances and close friends, and they have more difficulty in maintaining friendships. In another research, it was found that adults with ADHD are not considered friend worthy, and are negatively appraised by their peers because of two reasons. Firstly, the adult symptoms of ADHD, like, inattention, impulsivity, and anti-sociality, are considered to generate aversion in others. Secondly, a cognitive route to rejection which is, the stigma attached to the disorder that discourages others from form a friendship with an ADHD person (Canu, Newman, Morrow, and Pope, 2007). Brod and Adler (2005), describes how the symptoms of impulsivity, social inappropriateness, difficulty following through a task or being attentive during an interaction results in poor social relationships of ADHD adults. In their study, the ADHD participants described their symptoms in a slogan as "Ready, Fire, Aim," explaining how they verbalize their thoughts and took impulsive actions. The study elucidates that the blurting-out of comments at the wrong time or impulsively acting out causes them to lose their friendships, and hinders the prospects of finding new friends.

Dating and Romance

Romantic relationships are an essential characteristic of adolescence, and by late adolescence, more than 70% of teens are engaged in romantic relationships (Carver, Joyner, and Udry, 2003; Furman, Low, and Ho, 2009). These relationships not only play a significant role in adolescent development and but have an impact later on adult functioning (Giordano, Manning, and Longmore, 2006). However, the symptoms of ADHD like, inattention, impulsivity, hyperactivity, social skill deficits, executive dysfunction like poor self-regulation, are said to negatively affect romantic relationships. These features interfere in forming a close relationship that includes the virtue of reciprocity, sensitivity, intimacy, acceptance, and trust. Consequently, a lower level of trust and reciprocity in ADHD adults ultimately manifests in their fear of commitment, and a perpetual thought of rejection and abandonment (Marsh, Norvilitis, Ingersoll, and Li, 2015). Novotni (1999), conducted a research on understanding the impact of social skill deficit in interpersonal relationships and identified the issues related to attribution and misattribution. According to her, individuals who suffer from constant rejections are misattributed to their ADHD symptoms of being egoist, low in warmth, reckless, and self-centered. For instance, when an individual is late on his date, his partner would attribute his delay to him being selfish and careless, instead attributing it to his ADHD symptoms of poor time management.

Researches on ADHD and its impact on relationships reveals that the symptoms of ADHD affect the onset, duration, and quality of the relationships. According to Canu and Carlson (2003), in their study on college students found that college students who are high on attentional deficit achieve dating milestones later, as compared to the group with no ADHD, and have fewer steady relationships than the non-ADHD group. Also, the extraverted, non-ADHD males are attracted to ADHD females assuming that a woman with ADHD will be more talkative, energetic, and outgoing than the rest of the females. The study also examined the effects of ADHD subtypes on the behaviors and perception in an interactive task with the opposite sex. They concluded that non-ADHD females preferred to continue their interaction and considered to date ADHD males with combined subtype, rather than the inattentive type. The passivity, unassertiveness, disinterest, and inexperience make the inattentive type less desirable than the combined subtype. Furthermore, the passivity of the inattentive type is seen as an obstacle in the initiation of the romantic relationship, but while they are in a relationship, they are less likely to react negatively over a disagreement, and may consequently cause less relational disruptions.

Similarly, Salvatore, Kuo, Steele, Simpson, and Collins (2011), in their research, noted that the metacognitive skills required to disengage from conflict and regulate anger are both missing in the individuals with ADHD combined type. This lack of skill may stimulate the negative emotions from the past arguments to undermine the effectiveness of the dyadic tasks, like decision making, and providing emotional support, that are essential for easing-out the conflict. Marsh, Norvilitis, Ingersoll, and Li (2012), in their study, also made comparisons regarding the ADHD subtype and its impact on romantic relations. They found that the partners of the inattentive subtype report their relationship to be unsatisfactory, and they lack an intimate connection with their ADHD partner. They further concluded that individuals with more symptoms and lower levels of social skills feel less competent to make their relationship last.

Study on ADHD and the nature of romantic relationship indicates that these individuals have a pattern of short and fast fluctuating relationships due to their typical symptoms. The previous studies on romantic involvement establish that young adults with ADHD are more involved in verbally aggressive and violent romantic relationships (Wymbs et al., 2012). The quality of the romantic relationship deteriorates with the involvement of an ADHD partner. Also, the necessary skills that are required to form and successfully maintain peer relations in childhood serve to predict the quality of romantic relationships in adulthood (Collins, Hennighausen, Schmit, and Sroufe, 1997). For instance, children with ADHD symptoms do not view peer rejection as more negative or report a higher level of loneliness than the other non-ADHD students. This lack of self-awareness related to peer rejection in childhood can also be witnessed in adulthood when they are rejected for their romantic advances. But, as the ADHD adults underestimate their likelihood of being rejected, they may not be vigilant enough to attune their behavior with their partners. As a result of this lack of self-awareness, a break-up with their partner often comes as a surprise to them (Canu and Carlson, 2007; Diamantopoulou, Henricsson, and Rydell, 2005; Heiman, 2005).

Sexual Behavior

The symptoms of ADHD that affect peer relations and romantic relationships have a subsequent effect on the sexual relationship as well. The landmark longitudinal study by Weiss and Hechtman (1993) was the first to evaluate the sexual activities of hyperactive children in adulthood. It was determined that 20% of adults from the study experienced problems in sexual adjustment (versus 2.4% for the controlled group). However, the nature of sexual adjustment was not mentioned by the researchers. In its follow-up Milwaukee study (Barkley, Fischer, and Fletcher, 2006), it was concluded that the hyperactive group experienced intercourse earlier than the controlled group (15 vs. 16 years), they had more sexual partners (19 vs. 7), the hyperactive young adults were more likely to have unprotected sex, were more likely to have unwanted teenage pregnancies (38% vs. 4%), and were more likely to have contracted sexually transmitted diseases (17% vs. 4%). The later researches on this topic have also highlighted similar trends, according to them,constant rejection and humiliation by their partners, along with the ADHD symptoms lead to risky sexual behaviors, such as early coitus, increased likelihood of casual sex, multiple sexual partners, and having unprotected sex that causes unwanted pregnancies and sexually transmitted diseases (Flory, Molina, Pelham, Gnangy and Smith, 2006).Interaction of the core ADHD symptoms, especially impulsivity and family factors like poor monitoring and trust, conflicting parent-child relationships, have been linked to such risky sexual behaviors (Barkley, 2006; Borawski, Ievers-Landis, Lovegreen, and Trapl, 2003).

Further, a symptom subtype difference has been observed in the ADHD adults, where the combined subtype is found to have a greater urge for sex, frequently masturbate to release their inner unrest, and have diverse sexual experiences, than the inattentive types (Canu and Carlson, 2003 and 2007).Some of the researches have also linked ADHD symptoms with sexual disorders. According to these researches, certain sexual disorders are commonly seen in ADHD adults like hypersexuality, sadomasochistic desires, pedophilic desire, and ambivalent gender identity (Bijlenga et al., 2018; Strang et al., 2014).

In one of the researches by Kooij (2012), she found that ADHD adults face sexual problems more than the general population with no ADHD symptoms. These problems are related to sexual aversion, negative emotions during sex, too little excitement, and difficulty reaching orgasm. She attributed these problems to the ADHD symptoms of inattention, distractibility, and impulsivity. Sleep pattern in ADHD adults is another contributor for sexual problems, poor planning and delayed sleep phase found in most of the adults with ADHD cause them to sleep on different timings, which further reduces the chances to indulge sexually (Veen, Kooij, Boonstra, Gordijin, and Someren, 2010). A Dutch research on adult ADHD and sexual problems report that more than half of the male participants experienced sexual problems, out of which the common concern was either too much sex drive or too little sex drive. The gender difference revealed that the majority of the sexual problems were related to either 'too much sex drive', was faced by the male participants or 'too little sex drive' experienced by the female participants (Kooij, 2002). The other problems associated with the symptoms of ADHD that lead to risky sexual behavior are more alcohol use before sex, intercourse with uncommitted partners, more impulsive anal sex, and less use of contraceptives (Marsh et al., 2015).

Lastly, gender differences found in the sexual behaviors reveal that females are more susceptible to compensate for their impaired social skills by engaging in risky sexual behaviors, as compared to men. These women were observed to be inclined towards more promiscuous behaviors, were less consistent in contraceptive use, and more likely to have contracepted sexually transmitted diseases (Bramham, Young, Morris, Asherson and, Toone, 2005).

MARRIAGE AND ADHD

Marriage is an institution, a bond that requires love, caring, and sharing of equal responsibilities. However, for people with ADHD symptoms, it can be a challenging task, compared to the other individuals without the symptoms. According to clinicians, marital conflict is one of the most common complaints by ADHD adults seeking treatment (Dixon, 1995; Weiss, Hechtman, and Weiss, 1999). The complaint often consists of the ADHD adult losing interest in their partner. During the courtship period, the ADHD partner is highly stimulated due to the newness of this experience. He goes overboard to make their partner feel special and centre of attention. But as soon as the newness of this period wears-off and everything becomes a commonplace experience, the stimulation also diminishes. Thereby, it leaving the non-ADHD partner confused and hurt, thinking that it must be their fault (Orlov, 2010).

It has been observed that poor communication skills, procrastination, emotional sensitivity, over-reactivity, and unequal share of responsibilities are some of the chief complaints of spouses with ADHD partners that lead to either separation or divorce (Robbins, 2005; Resnick, 2005; Biederman et al., 1993;Biederman, Faraone, Spencer, Wilens, Mick and Lapey, 1994).

Communication

Communication is an integral component of social and interpersonal skills. It is represented in the form of both verbal and non-verbal abilities. We tend to communicate not only through words but also through our gestures, postures, facial expressions, and eye contact. However, for an individual with ADHD who lack in this particular social skill, along with their typical ADHD symptoms, interfere with forming and maintaining a healthy relationship (Robbins, 2005). The core symptoms of impulsivity and inattention negatively affect individual's conversational and listening skills. The tendency to dominate a conversation by having their last word, wandering-off from the topic of discussion due to distractibility, forgetting what was being said, not acknowledging the other person in conversation and having little regard for taking-turns are some of the deterring factors in a healthy relationship, that leave the non-ADHD partner feeling frustrated and agitated (Wender and Tomb, 2017). According to Orlov (2010), sometimes it is not just the distractibility of the ADHD partner that is destructible, but the misinterpretation of the ADHD symptoms by their non-ADHD partner that amplifies the conflicts.

Moreover, the listening skills that are part of the communication abilities are also affected by the core symptoms of ADHD. Individuals with ADHD only listen to parts of a conversation and let go of the other information because of their distractibility. Thus, unknowingly are disconnected by the real meaning of what was being said. Their inattention and lack of acknowledgement often result in being misinterpreted by their spouse as uninterested in the conversation. This inattention is sometimes misunderstood by the non-ADHD partner as feeling unloved and neglected. According to researchers, the reason for such poor listening skills was, firstly because they do not give their partner an opportunity to speak and appear to be uninterested in their point of view. Secondly, because they get distracted by their surroundings or are perhaps disturbed by their internal dialogue, consequently leading to a failure to communicate effectively results in them to believe they have already conveyed their message by saying, I thought I told you. This lag in communication is followed by a further misunderstanding between the partners; subsequently, one of them or both of them being emotionally hurt. (Bramham & Young, 2007; Robbins, 2005)

Emotional Sensitivity and Overreaction

Individuals with ADHD have a low boiling point and are hypersensitive to even the slightest trigger in their surroundings. They are irritated or offended easily by even the smallest inconvenience. During childhood, these symptoms are displayed as temper tantrums and frequent fights in school, but when they grow-up, this sensitivity and over-reactivity are exhibited as full-blown outburst causing severing of relationships. The inability to control their anger and impulsivity results in an unstable relationship with their partner, as it gets difficult for the non-ADHD partner to frequently go through such emotional turmoil alone. The non-ADHD partner often describes their struggle to deal with their ADHD partner's emotional sensitivity and overreaction, as 'walking on eggshells,' not knowing what might come next. The unpredictability of anger outbursts, irritability, and rude behavior of the ADHD partner always keeps their spouse on vigilant (Orlov, 2010). Hypersensitivity, as one of the symptoms of the ADHD partner, is often criticized by the non-ADHD partner as being thin-skinned, making mountains out of a molehill, and overreacting to a normal situation. Their overreaction to stress also increases their difficulty in solving a problem, which further leads to worsening the situation, producing a vicious cycle of failure to solve a problem and increasing the tension. Situations like these intensify the friction between the couple as the responsibility to solve the situation falls on the already burdened non-ADHD partner (Wender and Tomb, 2017). The symptoms of hypersensitivity and impulsivity may also act as an impediment in the intimate relationships, as the romantic gestures of cuddling and caressing can be perceived as unpleasant by the ADHD partner, while impulsivity and predisposition to boredom may lead them to have an extra-marital affair and risky sexual behaviors (Betchen, 2003).

Adults with ADHD may often feel under-stimulated and may try to stimulate themselves by provoking their partner to start an argument over an unimportant matter as a way to excite themselves both physically and emotionally. Once starting an argument, they would want to have the last word and then are unable to hold themselves from arguing further even after knowing that it was a futile argument (Barkely, 2010). Unfortunately, this need for stimulation results in a breakdown or major conflict. Since this need for self-stimulation is brief, the conflict raised from such arguments is also short-lived but intense, leaving their non-ADHD partner feeling bitter for long (Betchen, 2003; Resnick, 2005). For instance, an ADHD man who is in the middle of an argument may hit his wife but will be astonished to find that she was not romantically inclined later in the evening (Wender, 1995).

Executive Dysfunction

Executive functioning is an umbrella term to describe a variety of cognitive processes, including planning, working memory, attention, inhibition, self-monitoring, self-regulation, and initiation carried out by the prefrontal areas of the frontal lobes (Goldstein, Naglieri, Princoitta and Otero, 2014). As children with ADHD mature, their hyperactivity declines, but impulsivity and impairments related to executive functioning become more distinct due to higher demand for self-control and organizational abilities required in adulthood. It is not uncommon for the ADHD adult to be attracted to a partner who is good at organizing and planning. During the courtship period, the organizational ability of the non-ADHD partner and the easy-going nature of the ADHD partner keeps their relationship lively. However, after marriage, the easy-going nature of the ADHD partner is now negatively seen by the non-ADHD spouse, due to a higher demand for organizational abilities (Orlov, 2010). Disorganization and forgetfulness can be seen on the part of the ADHD partner as unfinished laundry, cluttered desk, chronic lateness in the form of unpaid bills, frequently losing keys, and missing events. These behaviors decay the non-ADHD partner's trust in long run that contributes to an impaired sense of intimacy and feeling of being loved, crucial for a loving relationship (Halverstadt, 1998; Robbins, 2005; Bilkey, Surman, and Weintraub, 2014).

Organizational and memory problems particularly can be off-putting for the non-ADHD partner as the onus of finishing their partner's chores also falls on to them. ADHD individuals find it difficult to stimulate themselves to do things that are of low-interest value, like doing chores. Therefore, an unbalanced share of responsibilities creates friction between the couple, as the dysfunction around the chores increases. It eventually shadows the future of the relationship as the non-ADHD partner loses trust in their ability to cope together (Orlov, 2010).

Thus, ADHD has an important role to play when it comes to marital discord, with a growing body of research on adult ADHD, it can be held responsible for a high rate of separation or divorce among these individuals. Notable gender differences were found by Robin and Payson (2000), in their research on adult ADHD, they found that there were significant gender differences in the behaviors that affected the marriage of spouses with ADHD. They found a more significant marital disruption when the wife had ADHD. They postulated this difference to ADHD, as it interferes with women's abilities to fulfill the societal gender-role expectations more than it does to men. Similarly, in another study by Minde et al. (2003), it was found that men married to ADHD women were more distressed and critical, while the women who were married to ADHD men were more supportive and willing to compromise for their husband's limitations.

PARENTING CHALLENGES

Taking into account the heritability and persistence of ADHD across the life span and its related functional impairments, families with ADHD parents are the most overlooked group. More than half of the parents with ADHD have a child with ADHD, and a quarter of the children diagnosed with ADHD have at least one ADHD parent (Faraone, 1997).Since many individuals are diagnosed for the first time during their adulthood, following their children's ADHD diagnosis. A lot of times, the other spectrum of the group, i.e., families with no ADHD children, the parent's symptoms remain undiagnosed, causing dysfunction in the family. Most of the older studies on ADHD focused on studying the relationship between ADHD children and non-ADHD parents, and the effect it had on parenting. However, with the recent recognition of adult ADHD, the focus shifted to understanding the effect parent's ADHD had on their ADHD/ non-ADHD children (Resnick, 2005; Koeman et al., 2015).

Parenting is a complex task, and it involves a higher level of emotional and cognitive capabilities, which makes parenting tougher for adults with ADHD. The problems encountered by parents with ADHD typically revolves around their own difficulties, which is poor memory and planning, impulsivity, and inconsistency in emotional responsiveness. According to Rutter and Quinton (1984), more negative effect was seen in children, when the same-sexed parent had ADHD. Also, children of ADHD adults exhibited a higher rate of behavioral disorders (Biederman, Newcorn, and Spritch, 1991).The parenting behavior can be characterized as two inter-related dimensions, i.e., effective behavioral control and emotional responsiveness to a child (Darling & Steinberg, 1993; Rothbaum & Weisz, 1994). Both of these characteristics are seen to be impaired with ADHD parents. The behavioral control is demonstrated as inconsistency in the behavior of the parent, in the form of either over-controlled or lax parenting, while emotional responsiveness can be observed as a parent's expression of warmth and affection, which can be either a cold or a hostile stance towards the child or being too involved with the child(Collins, Maccoby, Steinberg, Hetherington, & Bornstein, 2003; Kendziora & O'Leary,1993).

Self-regulation

Over the years, researches have consistently indicated a deficit in self-regulation in adults with ADHD. Self-regulation plays a crucial part to play in parenting as it involves the parent's ability to show ideal parenting along the dimensions of emotional responsiveness and behavioral control, as aforementioned. It helps the parents to monitor and make decisions according to the situations. For example, a mother may recognize her frustration with her child's repeated interruptions and use this as a cue for her emotional modulation to successfully come out of that situation. Deficits in self-regulation often lead to the failure on the part of the parent to detect their own failure to meet their child's needs. For instance, a parent will be unable to detect their child's need for increased empathy when their child fails at a task. Since, parents are the first role models for their children, their ability to cope with their own emotions and the way they respond to their child's expressions, have an impact on the development of the child's emotional and social competence (Eisenberg, Cumberland, and Spinrad, 1998). For example, a mother who was intolerant of her child's negative emotions, is more likely to have children who will develop difficulties in regulating their own emotions and exhibit aggressive behaviors (Ramsden and Hubbard, 2002).

One of the researches that linked self-regulation with working memory revealed that working memory is an essential factor in self-regulation of emotions, and in encouraging the best possible response to challenge the child's behavior. Working memory helps in reappraisal of the parenting actions of the past and to decide the future course of action. When working memory is impaired, parenting is poorly regulated and is a mere reaction to situations rather than a controlled parental action (Deater-Decard, Sewell, Petrill, and Thompson, 2010). In a research by Barkley, Murphy, and Fischer (2008), impatience, low tolerance, and hot temper were the characteristics of emotional impulsiveness or poor self-regulation that result in severe reactions to misbehavior by their children, and an increase in overall parental stress. Also, mothers with ADHD were seen to be less effective at problem-solving with their child's behavioral issues. Previous studies that assess parents with ADHD, display clear associations between the ADHD symptoms and ineffective parenting. For instance, when at least one of the parents is diagnosed with ADHD, parenting is found to be lax and inconsistent in enforcing limits with their children. This is possibly due to a higher attentional demand required to monitor the child's behavior and provide consistent consequences (Murray and Johnston, 2006). Also, ADHD parents who suffer from mood lability may find it difficult to handle their child's tantrum, as they would 'react' to the tantrum and escalate the situation instead of disengaging (Weiss et al., 2000).

Further, studies done on parents with ADHD, indicate that mothers with higher levels of ADHD were more inconsistent in imposing limits with their children, were easily distressed and showed a non-supportive response to their children's negative emotions, while fathers with ADHD who were highly involved with their children, were harsher in their parenting style as compared to non-ADHD parents. The inconsistencies observed in parenting were caused due to the deficiencies in inhibiting negative responses (Arnold, O'Leary, & Edwards,1997; Mokrova, O'Brien, Calkins, & Keane, 2010).

Organizational and Memory Deficits

Individuals with ADHD have shown to have working memory deficits, poor planning, and organizational skills. As a result, they are always worked-up, in a hurry, and often overscheduled. These overcommitments and its related stress leave them with no time to be emotionally available to their children. Poor execution of plans and mismanagement are frequent occurrences for them. For example, an ADHD mother decided to celebrate her son's birthday party at home. While cleaning the dishes that morning, she realizes she has to arrange her son's party, so she leaves her dishes and heads straight to buy party decorations. After returning home, she finds that she has forgotten the cake mix that was needed. After she returns, she struggles to complete her morning dishes, do her laundry, and bake the birthday cake; thus, failing to prioritize her work. Therefore, by the time children began to arrive, she was so worn-out that she could hardly enjoy the birthday party or be involved with her son (Wender & Tomb, 2017).

Working memory has a significant role in parenting, and its impairment leads to several inconsistencies in the parent's behavior. Working memory helps in making important parental decisions by assessing the inputs from the child, its context, and similar past experiences to make future decision (Barrett and Fleming, 2011). An adequate level of working memory is therefore required to reach a correct decision, especially when the child is misbehaving. For instance, an ADHD father who ignored his child's tantrum, on one occasion, loses his temper on the second occasion for the same tantrum that leaves the child confused due to the inconsistency of his behavior. Difficulties in sustained attention and procrastination can also be a hindrance to the parenting tasks. Parents with ADHD often report that they find it difficult to supervise and monitor their children, for example, a mother would find it difficult to supervise her child playing on monkey bars while sitting with other mothers. In the process, she would lose track of either supervision or conversation. The challenge to perform the instrumental and organizational tasks of parenting like helping with their child's homework, carpools, and birthday parties become more challenging with planning deficits, and even simple tasks of bath and bed time are procrastinated. The organizational deficit of these parents can also be observed from their problem in prioritizing the parental tasks, for example, a parent who has difficulty in holding time limits in his mind or withholding strong, ongoing responses may be unable to stop playing the video games in order to respond to their child's potentially dangerous play near the stairs (Johnston, Mash, Miller, & Ninowski, 2012; Barkey, Fischer, Smallish, & Fletcher, 2004). Thus, planning failures along with procrastination further exacerbate the anxiety of the ADHD parent, which affects not only their own well-being but also the mood of all the family members (Weiss, Hechtman, and Weiss, 2000).

Motivational Deficits

Motivational deficit includes an aversion to delays in rewards, altered sensitivity to rewards, or deficits in the extinction of reinforced behavior (Sagvolden, Aase, Johansen, & Russell, 2005; Sonuga-Barke, 2003). Motivational impairments in adults with ADHD result in reduced efforts to perform or respond to a task. As a parent with ADHD, the impairment reduces their sensitivity to receive positive feedback from their child, which results in their cold emotional responsiveness. For example, the parent would be less likely to be involved with their toddler to play peek-a-boo because of its repetitive and boring nature. Considering the impulsivity and motivational deficits, it is also difficult for the ADHD parents to enjoy the rewarding aspect of childrearing, and may hold less incentive value in guiding such parenting efforts. Moreover, such parents experience problems with their impulsivity as they may be at risk of indulging in permissive or inconsistent parenting due to administering inconsistent reinforcements (Johnston et al., 2012).

Thus, parents with ADHD symptoms experience a range of cognitive and affective difficulties that influence the quality of their parenting and the support required for adequate parenting.

Parenting Styles

The current researches on adult ADHD have examined the effect of parent's ADHD symptoms on the parenting styles. The construct, 'parenting styles' used in the ADHD literature is based on Baumrind's work. Baumrind identified three parenting styles, namely authoritarian, authoritative, and permissive, that affected the child's social and emotional development. The authoritarian style was characterized as high control and low emotional responsiveness; the authoritative style, as opposed to an authoritarian style, had high control and high emotional responsiveness. And, the permissive style was characterized by low control and high responsiveness (Baumrind, 1991; Steijn, Oerlemans, Ruiter, Aken, Buitelaar, and Rommelse, 2013).

The studies demonstrate that parents with a high level of ADHD symptoms display a permissive style of parenting. The reason for using this form of parenting style can be traced back to their lack of effective monitoring skills, low warmth and, an inconsistent discipline approach; while, fathers with higher ADHD symptoms are seen to use an authoritarian parenting style. The ADHD parents who use the authoritarian style of parenting exhibit dominance on the child, are insensitive to their child's need, and are inconsistent in their response to the non-compliance of the child (Rogers, Wiener, Marton, and Tannock, 2009; Murray and Johnston, 2006). Therefore, as both permissive and authoritarian styles are ineffective parenting styles, it can be concluded that the presence of ADHD symptoms in parents will have a detrimental effect on the parenting style.

CONCLUSION

ADHD is one of the most common psychiatric disorders, while adult ADHD remains the most underdiagnosed one due to its comorbidity with other psychiatric disorders. It was until recently that the importance of adult ADHD was recognized to have an impact on the interpersonal difficulties faced by them. The core symptoms of ADHD in the form of behavioral and cognitive impairments are associated with maladjustments in social and personal relationships that lead to peer problems, sexual difficulties, marital discords, family dysfunctions, and parenting struggles. Peer relations developed during childhood and adolescence are the foundation to predict the nature of relationships that develop in the future. Therefore, the rejection and isolation faced by ADHD children due to their impaired social skills and typical ADHD symptoms are also seen during adulthood in the form of their strained interpersonal relationships. Studies have established that ADHD symptoms correlated with a poor relationship with peers, they were less likely chosen in the peer groups, they were regarded as self-centered, hostile, dominating, and women were less likely to date or are in a steady relationship with an ADHD partner (Zambo, 2008; Kim et al., 2015; Canu et al., 2008). Also, sexual behavior of ADHD adults was seen to be adversely affected by their impulsivity and inattention that leads them to have early coitus, multiple sexual partners, indulgence in risky sexual behavior, less use of contraceptives, unwanted pregnancies, and difficulty to reach orgasm (Florey et al., 2006; Kooji 2012).When it comes to marital arrangement, marital discords are the most common complaints of the couples having at least one ADHD partner. Marital discords arise from the ADHD adult's deficits in social skills and executive functioning. Their poor communication abilities, hypersensitivity, inattention, need for stimulation, and organizational failures leave their non-ADHD partner emotionally distant, resentful, and burdened with extra work. While on the other hand, parenting capabilities are also affected when at least one of the partners is diagnosed with ADHD. Parenting struggles can be seen in the form of inconsistency in reinforcement, inability to supervise and monitor their children, low motivation due to boredom, inability to plan and organize, procrastinate important work and lower emotional sensitivity to their children's need (Johnston, Mash, Miller,& Ninowski, 2012; Weiss, Hechtman and Weiss, 2000).

REFERENCES

Able, S. L., Johnston, A. J., Adler, L. A., & Swindle, R. W. (2006). Functional and Psychological Impairment in Adults with Undiagnosed ADHD. *Psychological Medicine*, *37*(1), 97–107. doi:10.1017/S0033291706008713

Arnold, E. H., O'Leary, S. G., & Edwards, G. H. (1997). Father involvement and self-report parenting of children with attention deficit-hyperactivity disorder. *Journal of Consulting and Clinical Psychology*, *65*(2), 337–342. doi:10.1037/0022-006X.65.2.337

Bagwell, C. L., Molina, B. S., Pelham, W. E. Jr, & Hoza, B. (2001). Attention-deficit hyperactivity disorder and problems in peer relations: Predictions from childhood to adolescence. *Journal of the American Academy of Child and Adolescent Psychiatry*, *40*(11), 1285–1292. doi:10.1097/00004583-200111000-00008

Barkley, R. A. (2006). *Attention-deficit hyperactivity disorder: A handbook for diagnosis and treatment* (3rd ed.). Guilford.

Barkley, R. A., Fischer, M., Smallish, L., & Fletcher, K. (2004). Young adult follow-up of hyperactive children: Antisocial activities and drug use. *Journal of Child Psychology and Psychiatry, and Allied Disciplines*, *45*(2), 195–211. doi:10.1111/j.1469-7610.2004.00214.x

Barkley, R. A., Murphy, K. R., & Fischer, M. (2008). ADHD in adults: What the science says. New York: Guildford.

Barrett, J., & Fleming, A. S. (2011). Annual research review: All mothers are not created equal: Neural and psychobiological perspectives on mothering and the importance of individual differences. *Journal of Child Psychology and Psychiatry, and Allied Disciplines*, *52*(4), 368–397. doi:10.1111/j.1469-7610.2010.02306.x

Baumrind, D. (1991). Effective parenting during the early adolescent transition. In P. A. Cowan & E. M. Hetherington (Eds.), *Family transitions* (pp. 111–163). Lawrence Erlbaum Associates.

Biederman, J., Faraone, S. V., Spencer, T., Wilens, T., Mick, E., & Lapey, K. A. (1994). Gender differences in a sample of adults with Attention Deficit Hyperactivity Disorder. *Psychiatry Research*, *53*(1), 13–29. doi:10.1016/0165-1781(94)90092-2

Biederman, J., Faroane, S. V., Spencer, T., Wilens, T., Norman, D., Lapey, K. A., & .... (1993). Patterns of psychiatric comorbidity, cognition, and psychosocial functioning in adults with Attention Deficit Hyperactivity Disorder. *The American Journal of Psychiatry*, *150*(12), 1792–1798. doi:10.1176/ajp.150.12.1792

Biederman, J., Newcorn, J., & Sprich, S. (1991). Comorbidity of attention deficit hyperactivity disorder with conduct, depressive, anxiety, and other disorders. *The American Journal of Psychiatry*, *148*(5), 564–577. doi:10.1176/ajp.148.5.564

Biederman, J., Petty, C. R., Woodworth, K. Y., Lomedico, A., Hyder, L. L., & Faraone, S. V. (2012). Adult outcome of attention-deficit/hyperactivity disorder: A controlled 16-year follow-up study. *The Journal of Clinical Psychiatry*, *73*(7), 941–950. doi:10.4088/JCP.11m07529

Bijlenga, D., van der Heijden, K. B., Breuk, M., van Someren, E. J., Lie, M. E., Boonstra, A. M., Swaab, H. J., & Kooij, J. J. (2013). Associations between sleep characteristics, seasonal depressive symptoms, lifestyle, and ADHD symptoms in adults. *Journal of Attention Disorders*, *17*(3), 261–275. doi:10.1177/1087054711428965

Bilkey, T., Surman, C., & Weintraub, K. (2014). ADHD grows up. *Scientific American Mind*, *25*(1), 64–69. doi:10.1038cientificamericanmind0114-64

Borawski, E. A., Ievers-Landis, C. E., Lovegreen, L. D., & Trapl, E. S. (2003). Parental monitoring, negotiated unsupervised time, and parental trust: The role of perceived parenting practices in adolescent health risk behaviors. *The Journal of Adolescent Health*, *33*(2), 60–70. doi:10.1016/S1054-139X(03)00100-9

Bramham, J., Young, S. J., Morris, R. G., Asherson, P., & Toone, B. K. (2005). *Behavioural symptoms and cognitive deficits in adults with ADHD: do they improve with age?* Paper presented at the Division of Clinical Psychology, British Psychological Society Conference.

Canu, W., & Carlson, C. (2007). Rejection sensitivity and social outcomes of young adult men with ADHD. *Journal of Attention Disorders*, *10*(3), 261–275. doi:10.1177/1087054706288106

Canu, W., Newman, M., Morrow, T., & Pope, D. (2008). Social appraisal of adult ADHD: Stigma and influences of the beholder's big five personality traits. *Journal of Attention Disorders*, *11*(6), 700–710. doi:10.1177/1087054707305090

Canu, W. H., & Carlson, C. L. (2003). Differences in heterosocial behavior and outcomes of ADHD- symptomatic subtypes in a college sample. *Journal of Attention Disorders*, *6*(3), 123–133. doi:10.1177/108705470300600304

Collins, W. A., Hennighausen, K. C., Schmit, D. T., & Sroufe, L. A. (1997). Developmental precursors of romantic relationships: A longitudinal analysis. *New Directions for Child and Adolescent Development*, *78*(78), 69–84. doi:10.1002/cd.23219977807

Darling, N., & Steinberg, L. (1993). Parenting style as context: An integrative model. *Psychological Bulletin*, *113*(3), 487–496. doi:10.1037/0033-2909.113.3.487

Deater-Deckard, K., Sewell, M. D., Petrill, S. A., & Thompson, L. A. (2010). Maternal working memory and reactive negativity in parenting. *Psychological Science*, *21*(1), 75–79. doi:10.1177/0956797609354073

Diamantopoulou, S., Henricsson, L., & Rydell, A. (2005). ADHD symptoms and peer relations of children in a community sample: Examining associated problems, self-perceptions, and gender differences. *International Journal of Behavioral Development*, *29*(5), 388–398. doi:10.1177/01650250500172756

Dixon, E. B. (1995). Impact of adult ADD on the family. In K. Nadeau (Ed.), *A comprehensive guide to attention deficit disorder in adults: Research, diagnosis, and treatment* (pp. 236–259). Bruner/Mazel.

Flory, K., Molina, B., Pelham, W. Jr, Gnagy, E., & Smith, B. (2006). Childhood ADHD predicts risky sexual behavior in young adulthood. *Journal of Clinical Child and Adolescent Psychology*, *35*(4), 571–577. doi:10.120715374424jccp3504_8

Goldstein, S., Naglieri, J. A., Princoitta, D., & Otero, T. M. (2014). Introduction: A History of executive functioning as a theoretical and clinical construct. In S. Goldstein & J. A. Naglieri (Eds.), *Handbook of executive functioning* (pp. 3–12). Springer. doi:10.1007/978-1-4614-8106-5_1

Halverstadt, J. (1998). *A.D.D. and romance: Finding fulfilment in love, sex, and relationships*. Taylor Publishing Company.

Heiman, T. (2005). An examination of peer relationships of children with and without attention deficit hyperactivity disorder. *School Psychology International*, *26*(3), 330–339. doi:10.1177/0143034305055977

Johnston, C., Mash, E. J., Miller, N., & Ninowski, J. E. (2012). Parenting in adults with attention-deficit/hyperactivity disorder (ADHD). *Clinical Psychology Review*, *32*(4), 215–228. doi:10.1016/j.cpr.2012.01.007

Jokela, M., Power, C., & Kivimäki, M. (2009). Childhood problem behaviors and injury risk over the life course. *Journal of Child Psychology and Psychiatry, and Allied Disciplines*, *50*(12), 1541–1549. doi:10.1111/j.1469-7610.2009.02122.x

Koemans, R. G., van Vroenhoven, S., Karreman, A., & Bekker, M. H. J. (2015). Attachment and autonomy problems in adults with ADHD. *Journal of Attention Disorders*, *19*(5), 435–446. doi:10.1177/1087054712453170

Kooij, J. J. S. (2012). *Adult ADHD: Diagnostic assessment and Treatment* (3rd ed.). Springer.

Manuzza, S., Klein, R. G., Bessler, A., Malloy, P., & LaPadula, M. (1998). Adult psychiatric status of hyperactive boys grown up. *The American Journal of Psychiatry*, *155*(4), 493–498. doi:10.1176/ajp.155.4.493

Marsh, L. E., Norvilitis, J. M., Ingersoll, T. S., & Li, B. (2015). ADHD symptomatology, fear of intimacy, and sexual anxiety and behavior among college students in China and the Unites States. *Journal of Attention Disorders*, *19*(3), 211–221. doi:10.1177/1087054712453483

McLean, A., Dawson, J., Toone, B., Young, S., Bazanis, E., Robbins, T. W., & Sahakian, B. J. (2004). Characteristic neurocognitive profile associated with adult attention-deficit/hyperactivity disorder. *Psychological Medicine*, *34*(4), 681–692. doi:10.1017/S0033291703001296

Mikami, A. Y. (2010). The importance of friendship for youth with attention-deficit/hyperactivity disorder. *Clinical Child and Family Psychology Review*, *13*(2), 181–198. doi:10.100710567-010-0067-y

Mokrova, I., O'Brien, M., Calkins, S., & Keane, S. (2010). Parental ADHD symptomology and ineffective parenting: The connecting link of home chaos. *Parenting, Science and Practice*, *10*(2), 119–135. doi:10.1080/15295190903212844

Mrug, S., Molina, B. S., Hoza, B., Gerdes, A. C., Hinshaw, S. P., Hechtman, L., & Arnold, L. E. (2012). Peer rejection and friendships in children with attention-deficit/hyperactivity disorder: Contributions to long-term outcomes. *Journal of Abnormal Child Psychology*, *40*(6), 1013–1026. doi:10.100710802-012-9610-2

Murphy, K. R., & Barkley, R. A. (1996). Attention Deficit Hyperactivity Disorder in adults. *Comprehensive Psychiatry*, *37*(6), 393–401. doi:10.1016/S0010-440X(96)90022-X

Murray, C., & Johnston, C. (2006). Parenting in mothers with and without attention-deficit/ hyperactivity disorder. *Journal of Abnormal Psychology*, *115*(1), 52–61. doi:10.1037/0021-843X.115.1.52

Nadeau, K. (1999). *Understanding girls with ADHD*. Advantage Books.

Novotni, M. (1999). *What does everybody else know that I don't? Social skills help for adults with attention-deficit hyperactivity disorder (ADHD)*. Speciality Press.

Ramsay, J. R., & Rostain, A. L. (2005). Adapting psychotherapy to meet the needs of adults with attention-deficit/hyperactivity disorder. *Psychotherapy (Chicago, Ill.)*, *42*(1), 72–84. doi:10.1037/0033-3204.42.1.72

Resnick, R. J. (2005). Attention deficit hyperactivity disorder in teens and adults: They don't all outgrow it. *Journal of Clinical Psychology*, *61*(5), 529–533. doi:10.1002/jclp.20117

Robbins, C. A. (2005). ADHD couple and family relationships: Enhancing communication and understanding through imago relationship therapy. *Journal of Clinical Psychology*, *61*(5), 567–577. doi:10.1002/jclp.20120

Robin, A., & Payson, E. (2000). Can your marriage survive ADHD? Presented at the *Children and Adults with ADD (CHADD) National Conference*, Chicago, IL.

Rogers, M. A., Wiener, J., Marton, I., & Tannock, R. (2009). Supportive and controlling parental involvement as predictors of children' academic achievement: Relations to children's ADHD symptoms and parenting stress. *School Mental Health, 1*(2), 89–102. doi:10.100712310-009-9010-0

Rokeach, A., & Wiener, J. (2014). The romantic relationships of adolescents with ADHD. *Journal of Attention Disorders*, 1–11.

Rothbaum, F., & Weisz, J. R. (1994). Parental caregiving and child externalizing behaviour in nonclinical samples: A meta-analysis. *Psychological Bulletin, 116*(1), 55–74. doi:10.1037/0033-2909.116.1.55

Sagvolden, T., Johansen, E. B., Aase, H., & Russell, V. A. (2005). A dynamic developmental theory of attention-deficit/hyperactivity disorder (ADHD) predominantly hyperactive/impulsive and combined subtypes. *Behavioral and Brain Sciences, 28*(3), 397–419. doi:10.1017/S0140525X05000075

Salvatore, J. E., Kuo, S., Steele, R. D., Simpson, J. A., & Collins, W. (2011). Recovering from conflict in romantic relationships: A developmental perspective. *Psychological Science, 22*(3), 376–383. doi:10.1177/0956797610397055

Seiffge-Krenke, I. (2003). Testing theories of romantic development from adolescence to young adulthood: Evidence of a developmental sequence. *International Journal of Behavioral Development, 27*(6), 519–531. doi:10.1080/01650250344000145

Strang, J. F., Kenworthy, L., Dominska, A., Sokoloff, J., Kenealy, L. E., Berl, M., Walsh, K., Menvielle, E., Slesaransky-Poe, G., Kim, K.-E., Luong-Tran, C., Meagher, H., & Wallace, G. L. (2014). Increased gender variance in autism spectrum disorders and attention deficit hyperactivity disorder. *Archives of Sexual Behavior, 43*(8), 1525–1533. doi:10.100710508-014-0285-3

Thapar, A., van den Bree, M., Fowler, T., Langley, K., & Whittinger, N. (2006). Predictors of antisocial behaviour in children with attention deficit hyperactivity disorder. *European Child & Adolescent Psychiatry, 15*(2), 118–125. doi:10.100700787-006-0511-1

Theriault, S. W., & Holmberg, D. (2001). Impulsive, but violent? Are components of the attention deficit-hyperactivity syndrome associated with aggression in relationship? *Violence Against Women, 7*(12), 1464–1489. doi:10.1177/10778010122183946

Van Steijn, D. J., Oerlemans, A. M., de Ruiter, S. W., van Aken, M. A., Buitelaar, J. K., & Rommelse, N. N. (2013). Are parental autism spectrum disorder and/or attention-deficit/Hyperactivity disorder symptoms related to parenting stylesin families with ASD (+ADHD) affected children? *European Child & Adolescent Psychiatry, 22*(11), 671–681. doi:10.100700787-013-0408-8

Van Veen, M. M., Kooij, J. J., Boonstra, A. M., Gordijn, M. C., & van Someren, E. J. (2010). Delayed circadian rhythm in adults with attention-deficit/hyperactivity disorder and chronic sleep-onset insomnia. *Biological Psychiatry, 67*(11), 1091–1096. doi:10.1016/j.biopsych.2009.12.032

Weiss, M., Hechtman, L., & Weiss, G. (1999). *ADHD in adulthood: A guide to current theory, diagnosis, and treatment*. The John Hopkins University Press.

Wender, P. H. (1995). *Attention-deficit hyperactivity disorders in adulthood*. Oxford University Press.

Wymbs, B., Molina, B., Pelham, W., Cheong, J., Gnagy, E., Belendiuk, K., Walther, C., Babinski, D., & Waschbusch, D. (2012). Risk of intimate partner violence among young adult males with childhood ADHD. *Journal of Attention Disorders*, *16*(5), 373–383. doi:10.1177/1087054710389987

Chapter 12
Social Functioning, Interpersonal Difficulties, Social Deficits, and Social Skills Training in ADHD

Vaishali S. Chaudhari
General Hospital, Bharuch, India

ABSTRACT

Attention-deficit/hyperactivity disorder (ADHD) is one of the most common behavioral disorders of childhood. Children with ADHD exhibit developmentally inappropriate levels of inattention, impulsivity, and/or motor activity. Attention-deficit/hyperactivity disorder (ADHD) is one of the most frequent mental disorders affecting children. ADHD also affects many adults. Symptoms of ADHD include inattention, hyperactivity, and impulsivity. ADHD may also negatively affect the learning environment in children's homes. This chapter talks about social functioning, social deficits, interpersonal difficulties, and social skills training in ADHD. Individuals with ADHD have problems in the areas of peer interaction, emotional regulation, and pro-social behaviours. These social problems are associated with a greater risk for developing problems later in life.

WHAT IS ADHD?

Attention deficit hyperactivity disorder (ADHD), which is one of the most common childhood psychiatric disorders, is a neuropsychiatric disorder characterized by developmentally Inappropriate levels of activity, distractibility, and impulsivity (APA,2000) Behavioral problems in children with ADHD include acting without adequate consideration as to the cost of their actions and inability to postpone performance with impulsive decisions and behaviors. ADHD negatively influence social communications with peers, interpersonal relationships with parents, teachers and peers as well as academic success and social functions (Barkley, 2006) and (Dulcan, 1997), Children with attention-deficit/hyperactivity disorder APA, (1994) firmly display levels of activity that are far in excess of their age group; they are

DOI: 10.4018/978-1-7998-5495-1.ch012

not capable to sustain attention, interest, and persistence to tasks as well as to connections with peers, and their self-regulation lag far behind expectations for their developmental level. Children with ADHD repeatedly suffer from co morbid disorders, such as oppositional-defiant disorder, conduct disorder and internalizing disorders (Barkley, 2003).Children with ADHD are very likely to be impaired in the social, academic, familial, and, later, occupational domains of life (Barkley, 2003). Among the different symptom pictures evidenced by children with ADHD, severe social incompetence and peer relationship difficulties play a important role (Kolko, Loar, &Sturnick 1990; Landau & Moore, 1991; Pelham & Bender, 1982; Van der Oord et al., 2005). According to these researches individual with ADHD have more difficult behaviours then without ADHD children.

A diagnosis of ADHD is made through credit of excessive inattention, hyperactivity, and impulsivity in a child, before 12 years of age that causes impairment to them functioning or development (DSM-5; ICD-10). The principal classification systems for diagnosing ADHD are: International Classification of Diseases - 10th version (ICD-10); and the Diagnostic and Statistical Manual of Mental Disorders (DSM) Fourth Edition (DSM-IV), Fourth Edition - Text Revision (DSM-IV-TR), and a fifth Edition (DSM-5).In the DSM-IV and DSM-5, there are three different sub diagnoses, where exacting symptoms are identified and classified: the 'predominantly inattentive type'; the 'predominantly hyperactive impulsive type'; and the 'combined' type, which presents with both hyperactive-impulsive and inattentive symptoms Willcut(2012). Co morbid disorders, like behavioural disorders, depression, anxiety, bipolar disorder, tics, motor skill development disturbance, learning difficulties, and verbal and cognitive difficulties are common in ADHD (Newcorn 2008; Schmidt 2009; Yoshimasu 2012; Czamara 2013; Perroud 2014). Thus, they have symptoms of ADHD and many co morbid disorders can be present.

Prevalence

ADHD seem to enlarge premature mortality by 50%, compared to persons without ADHD, in a 24.9 million person-years (Dalsgaard 2015).Children with attention deficit hyperactivity disorder (ADHD) experience determined interpersonal difficulties and peer dissatisfaction that go beyond the diagnostic criteria. ADHD occurs in approx 3–5% of the school-aged population, with male to female ratios ranging from 4:1 to 9:1, depending on the setting (APA,1994). The disorder persist into adolescence in about 50–80% of cases clinically diagnosed in childhood (Weiss, & Hechtman,1993).Attention-deficit/hyperactivity disorder (ADHD) is a common, early-onset neuropsychiatric disorder that affects an estimated 3% to 7% of school-aged children (APA, 2000) and 4%of adults (Barkley, 1998). An estimated 8.4 percent of children by Danielson et al.(2016) and 2.5 percent of adults have ADHD (Simon, Czobor, Bálint et al., 2009).The problems of children with ADHD in their social interactions and peer relations are a elementary object for intervention Hinshawet al.(2001). Attention deficit hyperactivity disorder (ADHD) affects 3% to 5% of all children (Polanczyk 2007; Thomas 2015). The main symptoms of ADHD include problems with attention, impulsiveness, and hyperactivity (Sergeant 2003; Pasini 2007). Prevalence estimates for ADHD vary across the international literature. A large survey in the UK found that 3.6% of boys aged five to 15 years had ADHD; for girls of the same age, this study reported a prevalence of 0.9% (Ford 2003). In one study from Columbia, the reported prevalence was considerably higher: 19.9% for boys and 12.3% for girls (Pineda 2003). A systematic review on the prevalence of ADHD reported a mean proportion of 5.3% children and adolescents having ADHD overall, and concluded that much of the variation is derived from differences in methods used to diagnose the condition (Polanczyk, 2007). Among US children and adolescents, the estimated prevalence of diagnosed attention deficit hyperactivity disorder increased from 6.1% in 1997-1998 to 10.2% in 2015-2016 (Xu, 2018).The etiology of ADHD involves genetic, environmental, and social factors that are not clearly understood. Environmental risk factors include prenatal substance exposures, heavy metal and chemical exposures, nutritional factors, and lifestyle and psychosocial factors (Froehlich, 2011).

ADHD in Adulthood

ADHD is often first identified in school-aged children when it leads to interruption in the classroom or problems with schoolwork. It can also affect adults and more common among boys than girls. They have problems in the areas of peer interaction, emotional regulation, and pro-social behaviours. These social problems are associated with a greater risk for developing problems later in life (Biederman, Faraone, Keenan et al, 1992). Studies have shown a high heritability and with no sex differences of heritability. Genetic factors also involved in determining the perseverance of ADHD into adulthood (Neale 2010; Franke 2012; Faraone 2000). ADHD is associated with negative social outcomes such as severe social incompetence, and displays of task, disruptive and rule violating behaviour (Kolko, 1990; Landau, 1991), health problems such as abuse of drugs or alcohol, and criminality later in life (Barkley, 2002; Dalsgaard, 2002; Storebø, 2014; Koisaari, 2015).

Adult inattentive symptoms as opposed to hyperactive/ impulsive symptoms may be most associated with social problems (Knouse et al., 2008), ADHD is associated with both early-onset tobacco and alcohol use (Chang, 2012). In the same way, ADHD comorbidity with conduct disorder can lead to adverse outcomes in failure to complete high school academic achievement, criminality, substance use disorder, and unemployment (Erskine, 2016). Adolescents who do not find acceptance during these years report high levels of internalizing problems and emotional distress (Prinstein& La Greca, 2002; Rubin et al., 1995) The significant symptoms of ADHD (i.e., inattention, hyperactivity, and impulsivity) can be expected to interfere with the child's social functioning and social adjustment. These difficulties are directly related to the condition and are the primary basis for these children's problems with social skills (Whalen, 1985; Landau, 1991). Mothers with ADHD, relative to mothers without ADHD, self-report greater difficulties with involvement (Chronis-Tuscano et al., 2008), as well as with consistent discipline and monitoring (Murray & Johnston, 2006). Adult ADHD and Parenting Behaviors ADHD in children has been associated with nervous parent–child relationships (Johnston & Mash, 2001), research also suggests a negative impact of adult ADHD on parenting. Compared to mothers with less severe symptoms, mothers with more severe ADHD symptoms self-report less confidence in their parenting ability, decreased parenting satisfaction, and more lax and overreactive disciplinary styles (Banks et al., 2008). Some studies indicate a negative relationship between motherly ADHD and positive parenting practices such as admiring and satisfying (Chronis-Tuscano et al., 2008), whereas others suggest no relationship (Murray & Johnston, 2006). Adolescents who do not find acceptance during these years report high levels of internalizing problems and emotional distress (Prinstein& La Greca, 2002; Rubin et al., 1995) and these effects are larger than those found in childhood (Rose, 2002). These negative peer interactions may relate to the high co morbidity between ADHD and depressive symptoms that emerges around adolescence and remains stable into adulthood (Wolraich et al., 2005) or the increase in ADHD symptom severity that appears at the transition to middle school (Langberg et al., 2008). Compounding these issues is the fact that many youth who cannot gain admission to friendly peer groups often find acceptance with unusual peers. Adolescents with ADHD frequently follow this course, reporting deviant peer affiliation at higher rates than demographically-matched controls (Marshal et al., 2003). These interactions are especially concerning as they can lead to substance abuse, delinquent behavior, and academic failure (Marshal et al., 2003; Moffitt &Caspi, 2001). Because social dynamics change dramatically at the transition to middle school, traditional childhood treatments for the social impairment associated with ADHD (Pelham &Hoza, 1996) may not appropriately address the difficulties experienced by adolescents with the disorder. Unfortunately, the field still lacks an efficacious intervention targeting impaired social functioning in these adolescents. Currently, most assumptions about the interpersonal problems experienced by these youth derive from upward extensions of findings in the childhood literature, but few studies have been published that test these findings in an adolescent sample (Bagwell et al., 2001). In fact, evidence suggests that some of the assumptions derived from the literature on elementary-school aged children may be potentially inaccurate for adolescents. For example, young children with ADHD exhibit disruptive behaviors that have been shown to be insensitive to peers (Erhardt&Hinshaw, 1994); however, by some accounts, disruptive behavior is associated with peer acceptance in adolescence (Bukowski et al., 2000; Salmivalli et al., 2000). In addition to developmental changes in behavior, it is uncertain how qualitative cognitive changes at the cusp of adolescence might alterfindings from childhood samples (Keating, 2004). Hence ADHD in adulthood creates so many problems with family members and also in society.

SOCIAL FUNCTIONING IN ADHD

This topic is reviews relevant to the social functioning with ADHD including social status, social interactions with peers, social skills and behavior problems, and social–cognitive skills. Children with ADHD experience serious difficulties in the social domain (Frederick et al., 1994). The social functioning of ADHD subgroups and controls without ADHD revealed that children with ADHD-combined type were judged by parents and teachers to be less popular than controls, whereas children with ADHD-inattentive type were not rated as evidencing impaired social status. Despite of group, social performance, emotional regulation, and to a lesser extent, social knowledge appeared to be predictive of social status. On the whole, the results of these studies highlight the complexity of the concomitants and the underlying bases for social status difficulties of children with ADHD. Children with ADHD are described by peer as annoying, boisterous, irritating, and intrusive (Whalen & Henker, 1985) when compared to boys with learning disabilities or low-achieving comparisons, boys with ADHD were seen by peers as disruptive and by teachers as oppositional/defiant, and as deficient on cooperation and self-control (Flicek,1992). Children's social functioning, parents who have ADHD may also be more concerned towards the social struggles of their children with ADHD, and this supportiveness may cover the peer problems naturally experienced by these children. A further option, consistent with similarity in shape is that the negative impact of parental ADHD will be greater for normally developing children than for children with ADHD. This is because parents with ADHD symptoms are hypothesized to have bargain abilities to coach their children socially, but children with ADHD may already be maximally impaired so that parental behaviors have little effect. (Biederman et al., 2002).Adequate social functioning and healthy peer relationships are considered a primary condition for children's optimaldevelopment (Parker & Asher, 1987).

Interpersonal Difficulties

This topic is reviews relevant to the interpersonal difficulties with ADHD. Parents with ADHD may struggle to provide proper training in socially skilled behavior to their children, if the findings about interpersonal difficulties amongst adults with ADHD are correct. Parents with ADHD who have difficulty socially networking with other parents may also be less expected to arrange playdates for their children. This effect was mainly leading for children with ADHD; emphasize the important role parents can play in the social success of these children. Children with ADHD, previously at risk socially, may fall additional behind their peers without very helpful parent. The peer relationships of characteristically developing children may be less affected by parental ADHD, because these children may as expected make friends without parental education. Reliable with this statement, (Minde et al. 2003) reported that parental ADHD was related with less fortunate parent-evaluated social modification if the youngster additionally had ADHD and not if the kid was typically creating. Parents with ADHD may be more liberal than are parents without ADHD regarding the behaviors of their children with ADHD, and as a result show more positivity towards these children. Research by Alessandri (1992) the interpersonal problems of children with ADHD visible during early childhood, evenbefore the children enter school. For instance, preschool children with ADHD were found to be less skillful with peers than without ADHD preschoolers, and were less attentive and cooperative during group actions. Crick and Dodge's (1994) children's motivations to respond in firm ways to resolve everyday situations they come upon were examined. Students with ADHD displayed lower social information-processing skills in comparison to controls, in both the response building and the response decision processes. Age differences in social information processing skills were established across the two groups, while group differences remained. Children with ADHD were likely to be determined by a will tocontrol and to exercise power in their social interactions with peers. Murphy et al. (1992) study unsuccessful to find significant differences between subgroups of high-aggressive and low-aggressive boys with ADHD on several social information processing measures like encoding, attribution bias, and response decision bias. Interpersonal problems have been shown to be well represented by the IPC (e.g., Alden, Wiggins, &Pincus, 1990; Sodano& Tracey, 2011), which has its roots in Interpersonal theory (Sullivan, 1953). Interpersonal problems generally take the form of behaviors one does too much (e.g., disagreeing) or are difficult for one to start (e.g., be assertive; Horowitz, Rosenberg, Baer, Ureno, &Villasenor, 1988). The Wiggins Interpersonal Behavior Circle and the Type A behavior pattern consists of the two main interpersonal personality dimensions of Dominance and Affiliation (Wiggins, 1982), representing preferences for both control and communion, correspondingly, in interpersonal relationships (Leary, 1957). Children with ADHD begin having problems with social skills at an early age. Researchers Milich, Landau, Kilby,Whitten et al. (1982) have assessed whether preschool children can successfully identify externalizing indicative behaviors (i.e., hyperactivity and aggression) in their male classmates, and whether these perceptions were associated with peer-rated popularity and rejection. Results indicated that preschool children's nominations of externalizing behavior correlated significantly with teacher ratings of the same behavior. Merrell and Wolfe (1998) examined the relationship of teacher-rated social skills deficits and ADHD characteristics among nursery school-aged (5–6 yr) children. Result shows that young children with ADHD individuality were rated as having especially poorer social skills than matched children with no ADHD. Even if young children with ADHD exhibit comparative deficits in close to all areas of social skill, they were especially lacking in social cooperation skills. Children in the ADHD group were between five and six times as likely as children in the non-ADHD group to be rated by their teachers as having significant deficit in mainly social skills. The fact that more than half of the participants in the ADHD group showed significant social skills deficits indicates a strong co-occurrence of these problems.Social skills deficits of children with ADHD have been found to persist from early childhood into the basic school years and adolescence and to have negative effects on social and emotional adjustment (Barkley

RA, 1998). Hubbard and Newcomb (1991) found that children with ADHD timely a more controlling, less cooperative pattern of responses from without ADHD peers. One of the most invasive social problems for children with ADHD is the development of aggressive behavior (Stormont, 2001). Research by Vitaro, Tremblay, Gagnon &Pelletier (1994) has recognized that young children who had high ratings in kindergarten of hyperactivity and aggression were more likely than children who had average or low ratings of these measures to have third- and fourth-grade outcomes of peer-ratings of aggression and self-reports of misbehavior. Tur-Kaspa and Michal (2003) examined two social information-processing skills; response access or construction, and response decision of diagnosed children and adolescents with ADHD compared to those children without ADHD. Bagwell, Molina, Pelham, and Hoza (2001) found that the social problems in children with ADHD are still highly salient in adolescence. In common, social impairment is a significant interpreter of an adverse long-termoutcome in adolescence (Greene, Biederman, Faraone, Sienna, & Garcia-Jetton, 1997; Greene et al., 1999). Hence social incompetence is a serious debilitating condition. Children with ADHD display high rates of off-task, disruptive, noisy and rule-violating behavior (Landau & Moore, 1991) making them vulnerable to social rejection (Guevremont& Dumas, 1994). It takes normal children about 30min and a few social exchanges to categorize the child with ADHD as disruptive, unpredictable, and often also aggressive and to react to themwith criticism, rejection and withdrawal (Milich& Landau, 1982; Pelham & Bender, 1982; Pelham &Milich, 1984). Thus, can shows there are so many interpersonal difficulties in ADHD then without ADHD.

Social Deficits

Children with ADHD are at bigger risk for poor school performance, poor peer relations, anxiety and depression, aggression, conduct problems and delinquency, early substance use, as well as difficulties in social and personal relations during adulthood (Barkley, 1998).Individuals with ADHD also there with difficulties in the domains of attention and cognitive functions, such as problem-solving, planning,orienting, flexibility, sustained attention, response inhibition, and working memory (Sergeant,2003; Pasini, 2007). Guardians with ADHD may battle to show or give justifiable guidance in socially capable conduct to their kids, if the discoveries in regards to relational challenges among grown-ups with ADHD are right. For instance, guardians with ADHD who experience issues socially connecting with different guardians may similarly more averse to organizer play dates for their youngsters. In an ongoing examination including the present investigation members, guardians' practices toward their kids, including assistance of their kid's companion communications, medicinal guidance, analysis, warmth, and applause showed during lab-based playgroups, anticipated youngsters' friend connections (Mikami, et al., 2010). This effect was particularly leading for children with ADHD, underscore the important role parents can play in the social success of these children. Children are expected to take over ADHD symptomatology from parents with ADHD, and it sounds as if ADHD-related social problems. Parental ADHD may predict poorer child social functioning beyond the supposition resulting from common genetics. Adult ADHD and Social Functioning among Parents and their children even if peer problems in children with ADHD have been well recognized (Hoza, 2007), observed (Canu& Carlson, 2003) a example in compare to findings regarding children with ADHD, whereby hyperactivity/ impulsivity is more injurious to peer relationships than is inattention (Mikami et al., 2007; Milich et al., 2001). Parental ADHD absolutely impacted children with ADHD, though negatively impinge on the scholastic functioning of children without ADHD. There are several social-cognitive deficits that have been found in basic school-aged children with ADHD (Lorch et al., 2000; Milich& Dodge 1984; Zentall et al., 2001) but have not been tested in an adolescent sample. Research suggests that younger children with ADHD have deficits in found causal relationships in stories about social situations and it is hypothesized that these deficits may create an incomplete understanding of one's social environment (van den Broek, 1997). The relative contributions of low achievement, learning disabilities, and ADHD to problems in social status and social behavior among second through sixth grade boys revealed that the combination of ADHD and learning disabilities was associated with the greatest risk of social status problems and of social behavior problems (Flicek, 1992).

Social Skill Training

Social skills training were developed in the early 1970s. According to Jacobs (2002), its aim is to teach the micro skills of social interaction such as eye contact, smiling and body posture and behaviours of ADHD. Children and young people who have ADHD often present with difficult family relationships and may have poor social skills and peer relationships. Social skills are described as the behaviours and skills necessary to engage in developing and maintaining practical social relationships. Social skills training use techniques from cognitive and behavioural approaches and are conducted within groups. Kavale et al. (1997) and Van der Oord, S. et al. (2008) identified four meta-analyses on social skills training for children with ADHD. Two of them affirm that social skills training for children with ADHD has no effect and two of them affirm that social skills training for children with ADHD has a significant helpful treatment effect De Boo and Prins (2007) and Majewicz-Hefley and Carlson (2007).ADHD are still extremely salient in adolescence. Sufficient social functioning and healthy peer relationships are considered a primary condition for children's optimal development (Parker & Asher, 1987). In common, social impairment is a important interpreter of an adverse long-term outcome in adolescence (Greene, Biederman, Faraone, Sienna, & Garcia-Jetton, 1997; Greene et al., 1999). Hence, social incompetence is a serious unbearable condition. In answer to the pressing need for intervention, social skills training (SST) has become a widely accepted treatment in clinical practice (Mrug, Hoza, &Gerdes, 2001; Nixon, 2001). SST has been demonstrated to be effective inimproving social functioning for aggressive and antisocial children (Webster Stratton, Reid, & Hammond, 2001). However, for children with learning disabilities, children with ADHD and children with internalizing disorders results were less positive and mixed (Forness&Kavale, 1996; Kolko et al., 1990; Tiffen & Spence, 1986). Researchers have not found convincing proof that social skills learned in treatment, generalize to the home and the classroom (DuPaul& Eckert, 1994), and long-term effects have not been established (Beelman, Pfingsten, &Lösel, 1994). Pfiffner andMcBurnett (1997) stated that for children with ADHD. There is a lack of controlled outcome studies and that it is doubtful whether SST is an effective treatment for their social difficulties. There is evidence on the effect of behavioural treatment on children with ADHD. (Shmueli-Goetz, Target, Fonagy, &Datta, 2008) For cognitive treatment, on the other hand, Wood, Egger, Gluud, Schulz, Jüni,et al. (2008) found there is no clear evidence, so it cannot be suggested either as an independent treatment nor in combination with medical treatment . A Cochrane review by Zwi et al. (2001) found that parental training might have a positive effect on the behaviour of children with ADHD, but the ADHD symptom data are unclear and all the included studies were of poor methodological quality. Also found that there is currently no evidence of parent training for children that could form practice recommendations.Social skills training try to teach children how to standardize their behaviour according to normal social rules. This is a method of intervention, which can help children improve their social competences. Learning occur using role-play exercises and games as well as homework involving parents and teachers. The main element of social skills training focuses on to change an individual's cognitive assessment of other people and social situations. The training focuses on the understated cuts in social interaction and on being able to recognize the emotional expressions of others (Liberman et al., 1988 &Abikoff et al., 2004).The often include training parents and teachers. The management time is often relatively short, lasting from eight to ten weeks, but it can last up to two years (Abikoff et al., 2004 & Antshel, 2003). Thus more of these researches suggest social skill training helps to improvement in ADHD.

This chapter reviews the research relevant to the social functioning, interpersonal difficulties, social deficits and social skill training in children with ADHD including social status, social interactions with peers, social skills and behavior problems, and social–cognitive skills.

REFERENCES

Abikoff, H., Hechtman, L., Klein, R. G., Weiss, G., Fleiss, K., Etcovitch, J., Cousins, L., Greenfield, B., Martin, D., & Pollack, S. (2004). Symptomatic improvement inchildren with ADHD treated with long-term methylphenidate and multimodal psychosocial treatment. *Journal of the American Academy of Child and Adolescent Psychiatry*, *43*(7), 802–811. doi:10.1097/01.chi.0000128791.10014.ac PMID:15213581

Alessandri, S. M. (1992). Attention, play, and social behavior in ADHD preschoolers. *Journal of Abnormal Child Psychology*, *20*(3), 289–302. doi:10.1007/BF00916693 PMID:1619135

Andrade, B. F., Brodeur, D. A., Waschbusch, D. A., Stewart, S. H., & McGee, R. (2009). Selective and sustained attention as predictors of social problems in children with typical and disordered attention abilities. *Journal of Attention Disorders*, *12*(4), 341–352. doi:10.1177/1087054708320440 PMID:18596299

Antshel, K. M., & Remer, R. (2003). Social skills training in children with attention deficit hyperactivity disorder: Arandomized- controlled clinical trial. *Journal of Clinical Child and Adolescent Psychology*, *32*(1), 153–165. doi:10.1207/S15374424JCCP3201_14 PMID:12611031

Asherson, P. J., Levy, F., &Faraone, S. V. (2011). Quantitative and moleculer genetic studies of attention-deficit hyperactivity disorder in adults. *ADHD in Adults*, 25.

Bagwell, C. L., Molina, B. S., Pelham, W. E. Jr, & Hoza, B. (2001). Attention-deficit hyperactivity disorder and problems in peer relations: Predictions from childhood to adolescence. *Journal of the American Academy of Child and Adolescent Psychiatry*, *40*(11), 1285–1292. doi:10.1097/00004583-200111000-00008 PMID:11699802

Bagwell, C. L., Molina, B. S., Pelham, W. E. Jr, & Hoza, B. (2001). Attention-deficit hyperactivity disorder and problems in peer relations: Predictions from childhood to adolescence. *Journal of the American Academy of Child and Adolescent Psychiatry*, *40*(11), 1285–1292. doi:10.1097/00004583-200111000-00008 PMID:11699802

Banks, T., Ninowski, J. E., Mash, E. J., & Semple, D. L. (2008). Parenting behavior and cognitions in a community sample of mothers with and without symptoms of attention-deficit/hyperactivity disorder. *Journal of Child and Family Studies*, *17*(1), 28–43. doi:10.100710826-007-9139-0

Barkley, R. A. (1998). Attention-deficit hyperactivity disorder. *Scientific American*, *279*(3), 66–71. do i:10.1038cientificamerican0998-66 PMID:9725940

Barkley, R. A. (2002). *ADHD--Long-term course, adult outcome, and comorbid disorders*. Academic Press.

Barkley, R. A. (2006). Attention-deficit hyperactivity disorder: A handbook for diagnosis and treatment (3rd ed.). New York: Guilford.

Biederman, J., Faraone, S. V., & Monuteaux, M. C. (2002). Impact of exposure to parental attention-deficit hyperactivity disorder on clinical features and dysfunction in the offspring. *Psychological Medicine*, *32*(5), 817–827. doi:10.1017/S0033291702005652 PMID:12171376

Canu, W. H., & Carlson, G. L. (2003). Differences in heterosocial behavior and outcomes of ADHD-symptomatic subtypes in a college sample. *Journal of Attention Disorders*, *6*(3), 123–133. doi:10.1177/108705470300600304 PMID:12821877

Chang, Y. K., Liu, S., Yu, H. H., & Lee, Y. H. (2012). Effect of acute exercise on executive function in children with attention deficit hyperactivity disorder. *Archives of Clinical Neuropsychology*, *27*(2), 225–237. doi:10.1093/arclin/acr094 PMID:22306962

Cheng, X., & Qi, Y. (2010). Variations of eddy kinetic energy in the South China Sea. *Journal of Oceanography*, *66*(1), 85–94. doi:10.100710872-010-0007-y

Chronis-Tuscano, A., Raggi, V. L., Clarke, T. L., Rooney, M. E., Diaz, Y., & Pian, J. (2008). Associations between maternal attention-deficit/hyperactivity disorder symptoms and parenting. *Journal of Abnormal Child Psychology*, *36*(8), 1237–1250. doi:10.100710802-008-9246-4 PMID:18553132

Crick, N. R., & Dodge, K. A. (1994). A review and reformulation of social information-processing mechanisms in children's social adjustment. *Psychological Bulletin*, *115*(1), 74–101. doi:10.1037/0033-2909.115.1.74

Dalsgaard, S., Mortensen, P. B., Frydenberg, M., & Thomsen, P. H. (2002). Conduct problems, gender and adult psychiatric outcome of children with attention-deficit hyperactivity disorder. *The British Journal of Psychiatry*, *181*(5), 416–421. doi:10.1192/bjp.181.5.416 PMID:12411268

Dalsgaard, S., Østergaard, S. D., Leckman, J. F., Mortensen, P. B., & Pedersen, M. G. (2015). stergaard SD, Leckman JF, Mortensen PB, Pedersen MG. Mortality in children, adolescents, and adults with attention deficit hyperactivity disorder: A nationwide cohort study. *Lancet*, *385*(9983), 2190–2196. doi:10.1016/S0140-6736(14)61684-6 PMID:25726514

Dalsgaard, S., Østergaard, S. D., Leckman, J. F., Mortensen, P. B., & Pedersen, M. G. (2015). Mortality in children, adolescents, and adults with attention deficit hyperactivity disorder: A nationwide cohort study. *Lancet*, *385*(9983), 2190–2196. doi:10.1016/S0140-6736(14)61684-6 PMID:25726514

De Boo, G. M., & Prins, P. J. (2007). Social incompetence in children with ADHD: Possible moderators and mediators in social-skills training. *Clinical Psychology Review*, *27*(1), 78–97. doi:10.1016/j.cpr.2006.03.006 PMID:16814435

Dulcan, M. (1997). Practice parameters for the assessment and treatment of children, adolescents, and adults with attention-deficit/hyperactivity disorder. *Journal of the American Academy of Child and Adolescent Psychiatry*, *36*(10), 85S–121S. doi:10.1097/00004583-199710001-00007 PMID:9334567

Dumas, M. C. (1998). The risk of social interaction problems among adolescents with ADHD. *Education & Treatment of Children*, 447–460.

Erhardt, D., & Hinshaw, S. P. (1994). Initial sociometric impressions of attention-deficit hyperactivity disorder and comparison boys: Predictions from social behaviors and from nonbehavioral variables. *Journal of Consulting and Clinical Psychology*, *62*(4), 833–842. doi:10.1037/0022-006X.62.4.833 PMID:7962888

Erskine, H. E., Norman, R. E., Ferrari, A. J., Chan, G. C., Copeland, W. E., Whiteford, H. A., & Scott, J. G. (2016). Long-term outcomes of attention-deficit/hyperactivity disorder and conduct disorder: A systematic review and meta-analysis. *Journal of the American Academy of Child and Adolescent Psychiatry*, *55*(10), 841–850. doi:10.1016/j.jaac.2016.06.016 PMID:27663939

Ervin, R. A., Kern, L., Clarke, S., DuPaul, G. J., Dunlap, G., & Friman, P. C. (2000). Evaluating assessment-based intervention strategies for students with ADHD and comorbid disorders within the natural classroom context. *Behavioral Disorders*, *25*(4), 344–358. doi:10.1177/019874290002500403

Faraone, S. V., Biederman, J., Spencer, T., Wilens, T., Seidman, L. J., Mick, E., & Doyle, A. E. (2000). Attention-deficit/hyperactivity disorder in adults: An overview. *Biological Psychiatry*, *48*(1), 9–20. doi:10.1016/S0006-3223(00)00889-1 PMID:10913503

Flicek, M. (1992). Social status of boys with both academic problems and attention-deficit hyperactivity disorder. *Journal of Abnormal Child Psychology*, *20*(4), 353–366. doi:10.1007/BF00918981 PMID:1527277

Franke, B., Faraone, S. V., Asherson, P., Buitelaar, J., Bau, C. H., Ramos-Quiroga, J. A., ... Lesch, K. P. (2012). International Multicentre persistent ADHD CollaboraTion. The genetics of attention deficit/hyperactivity disorder in adults, a review. *Molecular Psychiatry*, *17*(10), 960–987. doi:10.1038/mp.2011.138 PMID:22105624

Froehlich, T. E., Anixt, J. S., Loe, I. M., Chirdkiatgumchai, V., Kuan, L., & Gilman, R. C. (2011). Update on environmental risk factors for attention-deficit/hyperactivity disorder. *Current Psychiatry Reports*, *13*(5), 333–344. doi:10.100711920-011-0221-3 PMID:21779823

Gentschel, D. A., & McLaughlin, T. F. (2000). Attention deficit hyperactivity disorder as a social disability: Characteristics and suggested methods of treatment. *Journal of Developmental and Physical Disabilities*, *12*(4), 333–347. doi:10.1023/A:1009432130076

Gomez, K. M., & Cole, C. L. (1991). Attention deficit hyperactivity disorder: A review of treatment alternatives. *Elementary School Guidance & Counseling*, *26*(2), 106–114.

Greene, R. W., Biederman, J., Faraone, S. V., Wilens, T. E., Mick, E., & Blier, H. K. (1999). Further validation of social impairment as a predictor of substance use disorders: Findings from a sample of siblings of boys with and without ADHD. *Journal of Clinical Child Psychology*, *28*(3), 349–354. doi:10.1207/S15374424jccp280307 PMID:10446684

Griggs, M. S., & Mikami, A. Y. (2011). The role of maternal and child ADHD symptoms in shaping interpersonal relationships. *Journal of Abnormal Child Psychology*, *39*(3), 437–449. doi:10.100710802-010-9464-4 PMID:20931275

Harstad, E. B., Weaver, A. L., Katusic, S. K., Colligan, R. C., Kumar, S., Chan, E., Voigt, R. G., & Barbaresi, W. J. (2014). ADHD, stimulant treatment, and growth: A longitudinal study. *Pediatrics, 134*(4), e935–e944. doi:10.1542/peds.2014-0428 PMID:25180281

Hennig, T., Schramm, S. A., Linderkamp, F., & Koglin, U. (2016). Mediation and moderation of outcome in a training intervention for adolescents with attention-deficit/hyperactivity disorder. *Journal of Cognitive Education and Psychology, 15*(3), 412–427. doi:10.1891/1945-8959.15.3.412

Hinshaw, S. P., Zupan, B. A., Simmel, C., Nigg, J. T., & Melnick, S. (1997). Peer status in boys with and without attention-deficit hyperactivity disorder: Predictions from overt and covert antisocial behavior, social isolation, and authoritative parenting beliefs. *Child Development, 68*(5), 880–896. doi:10.2307/1132039 PMID:29106718

Hoza, B. (2007). Peer functioning in children with ADHD. *Journal of Pediatric Psychology, 32*(6), 655–663. doi:10.1093/jpepsy/jsm024 PMID:17556400

Hubbard, J. A., & Newcomb, A. F. (1991). Initial dyadic peer interaction of attention deficit-hyperactivity disorder and normal boys. *Journal of Abnormal Child Psychology, 19*(2), 179–195. doi:10.1007/BF00909977 PMID:2056162

Johnston, C., & Mash, E. J. (2001). Families of children with attention-deficit/hyperactivity disorder: Review and recommendations for future research. *Clinical Child and Family Psychology Review, 4*(3), 183–207. doi:10.1023/A:1017592030434 PMID:11783738

Kavale, K. A., Mathur, S. R., Forness, S. R., Rutherford, R. B., & Quinn, M. M. (1997). Effectiveness of social skills training for students with behavior disorders: A meta-analysis. *Advances in Learning and Behavioral Disabilities, 11*, 1–26.

Klimowicz, A., Janicic, A., & IsHak, W. W. (2017). Sex and chronic psychiatric illness. In *The Textbook of Clinical Sexual Medicine* (pp. 507-524). Springer.

Koisaari, T., Michelsson, K., Holopainen, J. M., Maksimainen, R., Päivänsalo, J., Rantala, K., & Tervo, T. (2015). Traffic and criminal behavior of adults with attention deficit–hyperactivity with a prospective follow-up from birth to the age of 40 years. *Traffic Injury Prevention, 16*(8), 824–830. doi:10.1080/15389588.2015.1029068 PMID:25837647

Landau, S., & Moore, L. A. (1991). Social skill deficits in children with attention-deficit hyperactivity disorder. *School Psychology Review, 20*(2), 235–251.

Langberg, J. M., Epstein, J. N., Altaye, M., Molina, B. S., Arnold, L. E., & Vitiello, B. (2008). The transition to middle school is associated with changes in the developmental trajectory of ADHD symptomatology in young adolescents with ADHD. *Journal of Clinical Child and Adolescent Psychology, 37*(3), 651–663. doi:10.1080/15374410802148095 PMID:18645755

Liberman, R. P. (Ed.). (1988). *Psychiatric rehabilitation of chronic mental patients*. American Psychiatric Pub.

Lopez-Williams, A., Chacko, A., Wymbs, B. T., Fabiano, G. A., Seymour, K. E., Gnagy, E. M., Chronis, A. M., Burrows-Maclean, L., Pelham, W. E. Jr, & Morris, T. L. (2005). Athletic performance and social behavior as predictors of peer acceptance in children diagnosed with attention-deficit/hyperactivity disorder. *Journal of Emotional and Behavioral Disorders, 13*(3), 173–180. doi:10.1177/10634266050130030501

Lorch, E. P., Milich, R., Sanchez, R. P., van den Broek, P., Baer, S., Hooks, K., Hartung, C., & Welsh, R. (2000). Comprehension of televised stories in boys with attention deficit/hyperactivity disorder and nonreferred boys. *Journal of Abnormal Psychology, 109*(2), 321–330. doi:10.1037/0021-843X.109.2.321 PMID:10895570

Mangle, L., Phillips, P., Pitts, M., & Laver-Bradbury, C. (2014). Implementation of independent nurse prescribing in UK mental health settings: Focus on attention-deficit/hyperactivity disorder. *ADHD Attention Deficit and Hyperactivity Disorders, 6*(4), 269–279. doi:10.100712402-014-0138-x PMID:24744052

Marshal, M. P., Molina, B. S., & Pelham, W. E. Jr. (2003). Childhood ADHD and adolescent substance use: An examination of deviant peer group affiliation as a risk factor. *Psychology of Addictive Behaviors, 17*(4), 293–302. doi:10.1037/0893-164X.17.4.293 PMID:14640825

Merrell, K. W., & Wolfe, T. M. (1998). The relationship of teacher-rated social skills deficits and ADHD characteristics among kindergarten-age children. *Psychology in the Schools, 35*(2), 101–110. doi:10.1002/(SICI)1520-6807(199804)35:2<101::AID-PITS1>3.0.CO;2-S

Mikami, A. Y., Huang-Pollock, C. L., Pfiffner, L. J., McBurnett, K., & Hangai, D. (2007). Social skills differences among attention-deficit/hyperactivity disorder types in a chat room assessment task. *Journal of Abnormal Child Psychology, 35*(4), 509–521. doi:10.100710802-007-9108-5 PMID:17354064

Milich, R., & Dodge, K. A. (1984). Social information processing in child psychiatric populations. *Journal of Abnormal Child Psychology, 12*(3), 471–489. doi:10.1007/BF00910660 PMID:6747124

Milich, R., Whitten, P., Landau, S., & Kilby, G. (1982). Preschool peer perceptions of the behavior of hyperactive and aggressive children. *Journal of Abnormal Child Psychology, 10*(4), 497–510. doi:10.1007/BF00920750 PMID:7161441

Murphy, D. A., Pelham, W. E., & Lang, A. R. (1992). Aggression in boys with attention deficit-hyperactivity disorder: Methylphenidate effects on naturalistically observed aggression, response to provocation, and social information processing. *Journal of Abnormal Child Psychology, 20*(5), 451–466. doi:10.1007/BF00916809 PMID:1487590

Murray, C., & Johnston, C. (2006). Parenting in mothers with and without attention-deficit/hyperactivity disorder. *Journal of Abnormal Psychology, 115*(1), 52–61. doi:10.1037/0021-843X.115.1.52 PMID:16492095

Newcorn, J. H., Kratochvil, C. J., Allen, A. J., Casat, C. D., Ruff, D. D., Moore, R. J., & Michelson, D. (2008). Atomoxetine/Methylphenidate Comparative Study Group: Atomoxetine and osmotically released methylphenidate for the treatment of attention deficit hyperactivity disorder: acute comparison and differential response. *The American Journal of Psychiatry, 165*(6), 721–730. doi:10.1176/appi.ajp.2007.05091676 PMID:18281409

Newton-Howes, G. (2004). What happens when children with attention deficit/hyperactivity disorder grow up? *Journal of the Royal Society of Medicine*, *97*(11), 531–535. PMID:15520147

Normand, S., Schneider, B. H., Lee, M. D., Maisonneuve, M. F., Kuehn, S. M., & Robaey, P. (2011). How do children with ADHD (mis) manage their real-life dyadic friendships? A multi-method investigation. *Journal of Abnormal Child Psychology*, *39*(2), 293–305. doi:10.100710802-010-9450-x PMID:20824323

O'Leary, P. A. (1957). Dermatohistopathology of various types of scleroderma. *A.M.A. Archives of Dermatology*, *75*(1), 78–87. doi:10.1001/archderm.1957.01550130080008 PMID:13381197

Parker, J. G., & Asher, S. R. (1987). Peer relations and later personal adjustment: Are low-accepted children at risk? *Psychological Bulletin*, *102*(3), 357–389. doi:10.1037/0033-2909.102.3.357 PMID:3317467

Pasini, A., Paloscia, C., Alessandrelli, R., Porfirio, M. C., & Curatolo, P. (2007). Attention and executive functions profile in drug naive ADHD subtypes. *Brain & Development*, *29*(7), 400–408. doi:10.1016/j.braindev.2006.11.010 PMID:17207595

Pelham, W. E., Jr., &Hoza, B. (1996). *Intensive treatment: A summer treatment program for children with ADHD*. Academic Press.

Polanczyk, G., De Lima, M. S., Horta, B. L., Biederman, J., & Rohde, L. A. (2007). The worldwide prevalence of ADHD: A systematic review and metaregression analysis. *The American Journal of Psychiatry*, *164*(6), 942–948. doi:10.1176/ajp.2007.164.6.942 PMID:17541055

Prinstein, M. J., Boergers, J., & Vernberg, E. M. (2001). Overt and relational aggression in adolescents: Social-psychological adjustment of aggressors and victims. *Journal of Clinical Child Psychology*, *30*(4), 479–491. doi:10.1207/S15374424JCCP3004_05 PMID:11708236

Ros, R., & Graziano, P. A. (2018). Social functioning in children with or at risk for attention deficit/hyperactivity disorder: A meta-analytic review. *Journal of Clinical Child and Adolescent Psychology*, *47*(2), 213–235. doi:10.1080/15374416.2016.1266644 PMID:28128989

Rubin, K. H., Chen, X., McDougall, P., Bowker, A., & McKinnon, J. (1995). The Waterloo Longitudinal Project: Predicting internalizing and externalizing problems in adolescence. *Development and Psychopathology*, *7*(4), 751–764. doi:10.1017/S0954579400006829

Salehinejad, M. A., & Nejati, V. (2019). Cognition-engaging physical exercise for improving cognitive impairments in attention-deficit hyperactivity disorder: A behavioral medicine approach. *Heart and Mind*, *3*(2), 73. doi:10.4103/hm.hm_54_19

Salmivalli, C., Kaukiainen, A., & Lagerspetz, K. (2000). Aggression and sociometric status among peers: Do gender and type of aggression matter? *Scandinavian Journal of Psychology*, *41*(1), 17–24. doi:10.1111/1467-9450.00166 PMID:10731839

Saylor, K. E., & Amann, B. H. (2016). Impulsive aggression as a comorbidity of attention-deficit/hyperactivity disorder in children and adolescents. *Journal of Child and Adolescent Psychopharmacology*, *26*(1), 19–25. doi:10.1089/cap.2015.0126 PMID:26744906

Schmidt, S., & Petermann, F. (2009). Developmental psychopathology: Attention deficit hyperactivity disorder (ADHD). *BMC Psychiatry*, *9*(1), 58. doi:10.1186/1471-244X-9-58 PMID:19761584

Sergeant, J. A., Geurts, H., Huijbregts, S., Scheres, A., & Oosterlaan, J. (2003). The top and the bottom of ADHD: A neuropsychological perspective. *Neuroscience and Biobehavioral Reviews*, *27*(7), 583–592. doi:10.1016/j.neubiorev.2003.08.004 PMID:14624803

Sharp, C. (2002). Sex Differences in Antisocial Behaviour: Conduct Disorder, Delinquency and Violence in the Dunedin Longitudinal Study. By T. Moffitt, A. Caspi, M. Rutter and P. Silva.(Pp. 278;£ 14.95/$21.95.) Cambridge University Press: Cambridge. 2001. *Psychological Medicine*, *32*(8), 1475–1478. doi:10.1017/S0033291702216670

Shmueli-Goetz, Y., Target, M., Fonagy, P., & Datta, A. (2008). The Child Attachment Interview: A psychometric study of reliability and discriminant validity. *Developmental Psychology*, *44*(4), 939–956. doi:10.1037/0012-1649.44.4.939 PMID:18605826

Sibley, M. H., Evans, S. W., & Serpell, Z. N. (2010). Social cognition and interpersonal impairment in young adolescents with ADHD. *Journal of Psychopathology and Behavioral Assessment*, *32*(2), 193–202. doi:10.100710862-009-9152-2

Simon, V., Czobor, P., Bálint, S., Mészáros, A., & Bitter, I. (2009). Prevalence and correlates of adult attention-deficit hyperactivity disorder: Meta-analysis. *The British Journal of Psychiatry*, *194*(3), 204–211. doi:10.1192/bjp.bp.107.048827 PMID:19252145

Sodano, S. M., Tamulonis, J. P., Fabiano, G. A., Caserta, A. M., Hulme, K. F., Hulme, K. L., Stephan, G. R., & Tronci, F. (2019). Interpersonal Problems of Young Adults With and Without Attention-Deficit/ Hyperactivity Disorder. *Journal of Attention Disorders*. doi:10.1177/1087054718821728 PMID:30614417

Sontag, T. A., Tucha, O., Walitza, S., & Lange, K. W. (2010). Animal models of attention deficit/hyperactivity disorder (ADHD): A critical review. *ADHD Attention Deficit and Hyperactivity Disorders*, *2*(1), 1–20. doi:10.100712402-010-0019-x PMID:21432586

Storebø, O. J., Gluud, C., Winkel, P., & Simonsen, E. (2012). Social-skills and parental training plus standard treatment versus standard treatment for children with ADHD–the randomised SOSTRA trial. *PLoS One*, *7*(6), e37280. doi:10.1371/journal.pone.0037280 PMID:22745657

Stormont, M. (2001). Social outcomes of children with AD/HD: Contributing factors and implications for practice. *Psychology in the Schools*, *38*(6), 521–531. doi:10.1002/pits.1040

Tur-Kaspa, H., & Michal, Y. (2003). *Social information-processing skills of students with ADHD*. Poster presented at the Society for Research in Child Development Conference, Tampa, FL.

Van der Oord, S., Prins, P. J., Oosterlaan, J., & Emmelkamp, P. M. (2008). Efficacy of methylphenidate, psychosocial treatments and their combination in school-aged children with ADHD: A meta-analysis. *Clinical Psychology Review*, *28*(5), 783–800. doi:10.1016/j.cpr.2007.10.007 PMID:18068284

Vitaro, F., Tremblay, R. E., Gagnon, C., & Pelletier, D. (1994). Predictive accuracy of behavioral and sociometric assessments of high-risk kindergarten children. *Journal of Clinical Child Psychology*, *23*(3), 272–282. doi:10.120715374424jccp2303_5

Vokina, V. A., & Sosedova, L. M. (2018). Correlation between behavioural and eeg components of prenatal hypoxed rats. *GISAP: Medical Science Pharmacology*, (11), 30–32.

Wang, C. H., Mazursky-Horowitz, H., & Chronis-Tuscano, A. (2014). Delivering evidence-based treatments for child attention-deficit/hyperactivity disorder (ADHD) in the context of parental ADHD. *Current Psychiatry Reports, 16*(10), 474. doi:10.100711920-014-0474-8 PMID:25135774

Warner, D. O., Zaccariello, M. J., Katusic, S. K., Schroeder, D. R., Hanson, A. C., Schulte, P. J., ... Hu, D. (2018). Neuropsychological and behavioral outcomes after exposure of young children to procedures requiring general anesthesia: The MASK study. *Anesthesiology, 129*(1), 89–105. doi:10.1097/ALN.0000000000002232 PMID:29672337

Webster-Stratton, C., Reid, M. J., & Hammond, M. (2001). Preventing conduct problems, promoting social competence: A parent and teacher training partnership in Head Start. *Journal of Clinical Child Psychology, 30*(3), 283–302. doi:10.1207/S15374424JCCP3003_2 PMID:11501247

Weiss, G., & Hechtman, L. T. (1993). *Hyperactive children grown up: ADHD in children, adolescents, and adults*. Guilford Press.

Whalen, C. K., & Henker, B. (1985). The social worlds of hyperactive (ADDH) children. *Clinical Psychology Review, 5*(5), 447–478. doi:10.1016/0272-7358(85)90004-2

Wolraich, M. L., Wibbelsman, C. J., Brown, T. E., Evans, S. W., Gotlieb, E. M., Knight, J. R., ... Wilens, T. (2005). Attention-deficit/hyperactivity disorder among adolescents: A review of the diagnosis, treatment, and clinical implications. *Pediatrics, 115*(6), 1734–1746. doi:10.1542/peds.2004-1959 PMID:15930238

Wood, L., Egger, M., Gluud, L. L., Schulz, K. F., Jüni, P., Altman, D. G., Gluud, C., Martin, R. M., Wood, A. J. G., & Sterne, J. A. (2008). Empirical evidence of bias in treatment effect estimates in controlled trials with different interventions and outcomes: Meta-epidemiological study. *BMJ (Clinical Research Ed.), 336*(7644), 601–605. doi:10.1136/bmj.39465.451748.AD PMID:18316340

Xu, G., Strathearn, L., Liu, B., Yang, B., & Bao, W. (2018). Twenty-year trends in diagnosed attention-deficit/hyperactivity disorder among US children and adolescents, 1997-2016. *JAMA Network Open, 1*(4), e181471–e181471. doi:10.1001/jamanetworkopen.2018.1471 PMID:30646132

Yoshimasu, K., Barbaresi, W. J., Colligan, R. C., Voigt, R. G., Killian, J. M., Weaver, A. L., & Katusic, S. K. (2012). Childhood ADHD is strongly associated with a broad range of psychiatric disorders during adolescence: A population-based birth cohort study. *Journal of Child Psychology and Psychiatry, and Allied Disciplines, 53*(10), 1036–1043. doi:10.1111/j.1469-7610.2012.02567.x PMID:22647074

Zentall, S. S., Cassady, J. C., & Javorsky, J. (2001). Social comprehension of children with hyperactivity. *Journal of Attention Disorders, 5*(1), 11–24. doi:10.1177/108705470100500102

Zwi, M., Jones, H., Thorgaard, C., York, A., & Dennis, J. A. (2011). Parent training interventions for Attention Deficit Hyperactivity Disorder (ADHD) in children aged 5 to 18 years. *Cochrane Database of Systematic Reviews*, 12. doi:10.1002/14651858.CD003018.pub3 PMID:22161373

Chapter 13
Executive Function Deficits Among ADHD Students in Classroom Learning:
Issues and Strategies

Ashwini Deshpande Nagarhalli
Little Pods, India

ABSTRACT

Attention deficit hyperactivity disorder (ADHD) is one of the widely prevalent externalizing disorders from the category of neurodevelopmental disorders. With the constant rise in the diagnosis of a number of cases presenting ADHD or ADHD-like symptoms, the need to understand issues as experienced by the student requires the right interventions for effective management. The core challenges in the area of academics and overall presentation lie with the executive function deficits that the child has. Hence, addressing those and working on skills like attention, working memory, response inhibition, goal setting, planning, problem solving, and organization has to be considered as part of the management plan. The current chapter explores evidence-based issues and strategies to be targeted in the classroom set up for students with ADHD. It also highlights some classroom-specific strategies, which can be focused by the teachers and remedial therapists.

INTRODUCTION

Attention Deficit Hyperactivity Disorder (ADHD) presents with a challenge for a developing child with regard to all his chronological milestones. ADHD has a prevalence rate of about 3.55%, according to DSM-V. Population surveys suggest that ADHD occurs in most cultures in about 5% of children and about 2.5% of adults (DSM V, 2013) Hence, a diagnosis of ADHD entails myriad issues with an impact on a number of areas of routine functioning. The impact for a child attending mainstream and an inclusive school requires further emphasis as every situation becomes challenging for the child. The child is forever stuck solving puzzles, where all the pieces of different puzzles are mixed up, leading to ultimate chaos for the child.

DOI: 10.4018/978-1-7998-5495-1.ch013

EXECUTIVE FUNCTIONS AND ADHD

The role of executive functions assumes maximum significance and importance for children diagnosed with Learning Disabilities and ADHD. The cause of academic difficulties with ADHD is unknown, however, the problems in executive functions come across as one of the contributory causes (Johnson et al, 2011). Executive Functions involve the metacognitive knowledge regarding strategies and tasks, attention and memory systems that support these processes like the working memory, and the self-regulatory processes like planning and self-monitoring (Meltzer,2007). According to Biedermann et al, (2004) students with ADHD have executive function deficits.

Executive functions involve planning, organizing, maintaining effort and monitoring activities that are necessary for academic success (Johnson et al,2011), clearly which a child with ADHD is often found struggling vis-a-vis the symptoms and their clinical presentation at school and home. Thus, executive function deficits can negatively affect academic performance (Clark, Prior& Kinsella, 2002).

A number of theoretical models have added executive function deficits as their primary characteristics (e.g. Barkley,2006), so it goes without any argument that the executive deficits play a significant role in academics for students with ADHD (Johnson et al,2011) and hence the approaches to intervention planning and management need to weigh heavily in targeting these deficits. The students who were identified with comorbid LD and ADHD had more executive dysfunction (Watson et al, 2016).

The researches also found a significant correlation among IQ, executive functions and achievement. Additionally, students with impaired executive functions were found to be at a risk for engaging in impulsive or hostile responses to stressful situations (Ricco et al 2011) (Santor et al, 2003) and repeated academic failure can trigger either student withdrawal, acting-out behaviors. To sum it up poor executive functioning skills can place students with ADHD on a slippery slope that all too often leads to significant social and/ or academic problems (Watson et al, 2016).

The Challenge of Executive Deficits In The Classroom

The executive dysfunctions pose a serious challenge to students with ADHD due to the restless and fidgety presentation, the child already finds it very difficult to engage himself at the pace of the class. Additionally, at the same time his/ her inherent metacognitive structures do not make the process of learning very smooth.

To register every instruction that is conveyed in the classroom, sustaining the attention to register the instruction and execute all parts of the same requires every ounce of focus and attentional process by the student at that point of time. Hence for execution of an instruction simultaneous and successive processing could pose a challenge for a student with ADHD.

The central axiom of the Dual Pathway Model explains that ADHD can be caused by both bottom-up and top-down mechanisms (Sonuga-Barke, 2002). While the former is associated with inhibitory dysregulation the latter accounts to the motivational style and reward mechanisms associated with it. According to this view, inattention, overactive and impulsive behaviors can be functional expressions of delay aversions.

When faced with a choice between immediacy and delay, children with ADHD will choose the former (Sonuga-Barke, et al,1992). When neither of the choices is available, they will reduce the perception of time by engaging in task-irrelevant or incompatible (hyperactive) behavior or being inattentive. In this model, the cognitive deficits such as impaired planning and working memory, are seen as secondary to the bottom-up effects of delay aversion for some subjects with ADHD (Egeland,2012). The same seems to apply to the classroom set up.

The multidimensional nature of executive functions includes attention control, working memory, cognitive flexibility, planning, initiating of activity. Hoffman et al (2012) synthesized into three basic executive functions: working memory operations (updating), inhibitions of impulses (inhibiting), and mental set or task shifting (shifting). Thus, executive functions play an important role in determining the successful cognitive, academic, and social functioning of students with and without disabilities (Watson et al, 2016).

Working Memory

Working memory is comprised of distinct but interacting cognitive and neural systems that coordinate higher-level attentional control and the temporary storage of information, providing vital ongoing support for complex cognitive activities (Baddeley,2000).Poor Working memory during development has begun to be investigated in its own right rather than as a secondary symptom of another disorder, and has been found to be closely associated both with low academic achievement (Gathercole & Alloway, 2008; Alloway et al., 2009) and with some of the attention problems typical of children with ADHD (Gathercole et al.2008).Warner-Rogers and colleagues suggest that children who find it hard to pay attention, but who are not disruptive in the classroom are at risk for being neglected in educational settings (Warner-Rogers et al., 2000). The direct implication of these deficits are observed in mathematics and reading where part of the information is expected to be in temporary storage and part of it needs to be manipulated becomes cognitively challenging for a child with ADHD. Hence, classroom instructions, maintaining a flow of information and successively engaging into problem solving is difficult for students with ADHD.

Response Inhibition

Inhibitory control has been defined as the ability to deliberately suppress or interrupt the expression of cognitive, emotional, or behavioral responses (Schacher et al,2000). Barkley further elaborates that such inhibition is composed of three separated and overlapping processes, responsible for: a) inhibiting a certain unwanted behavior, creating a delay in the final answer; b) stopping an answer in progress, being sensitive to error and changing the course of an answer which will prove unsatisfactory; c)resisting the distraction that can occur during the delayed response, allowing oneself to carry the decision of changing the strategy until the end (Schacher et al,2000)

According to Johnson& Reid (2011), there are three executive function problems which may be directly associated with academic success: a) Adopting a planful, strategic approach to the academic tasks; b) goal setting; and c) persistence or sustaining efforts on a task and completing the same. The teachers however should be focused to address these as part of the strategies (Johnson et al, 2011).

Planning

The problems of impulsivity among students with ADHD are synonymous with their lack of ability to plan and organize themselves. They rarely take the time to plan an activity and seldom analyze a task to determine the behaviors needed to complete the task, and also may be unable to effectively combine the behaviors needed to accomplish a task (Barkley, 2006).

Goal Setting

According to Barkley (2006), goal setting is also a common area of challenge for students with ADHD. Students with ADHD may be unaware of the goal associated with an academic task or may also have difficulty remembering goals (Barkley, 2006).

Adding on to their difficulties is the fact that they are unable to focus on task-specific goals. Their orientation may lean on goals that are less adaptive to the situation at hand and also inhibiting performance. Some students with ADHD actually exhibit performance-avoidance goals, namely to avoid demonstrating incompetence (Barron, Evans, Baranik, Serpell & Buyinger, 2006). If student's goals are to avoid showing what they cannot do, they are not concerned with accomplishing tasks (Johnson& Reid, 2011)

Persistence

According to various studies documented, a consistent finding has been related to the lack of persistence in students with ADHD. They lack persistence and quit the task significantly more than their non-ADHD peers, especially when they encounter difficulties with a task. They tend to give up easily even when the task is less challenging in nature. According to Walcott & Landau (2004), this may be as a result of problems with regulation of emotion caused by frustration. They do not try to overcome or resolve these feelings which may compel them to give up on the task as soon as they get frustrated (Scime & Norvilitis, 2006).

Studies by Barkley (2006) have identified the source of frustration could be due to lack of progress monitoring. It is possible that students with ADHD may not be completely aware of their progress on a task. Such lack of progress may lead to unrealistic appraisals which could be positive or negative regarding their performance and may result in frustration which consequently has a negative effect on persistence.

For every child, the challenge in accomplishing an academic task requires the use of executive functions. Academic tasks involve reading comprehension, written expression and note taking which all become very challenging as it involves the use of executive functions like planning, organizing, self-regulation, shifting strategies and metacognition (Denckla et al,2013); (Labuan et al, 2010). This poses a problem to lack of conceptual clarity at each grade level and unable to cope up with the curriculum with progressive grade level. As they grow older, the curriculum may reflect more complex task demands that expect a student to possess strong executive function skills.

In addition to written language and reading comprehension, executive functions negatively impact a student's mathematical skills. Along with LD, there is compelling evidence that students with ADHD also exhibit difficulty in acquiring mathematics conceptual understanding (e.g number sense) and skills like computational facts and have multiple cognitive deficits that include executive functions (Kolkman et al, 2013 & LeFevre et al, 2012)

Implications and Strategies for the Classroom

Researches by Hawley and Newman (2010) have emphasized that teaching of executive function skills should follow a systematic approach of stages, which should be sequential and consistent as the student begins to develop these skills. They have suggested five stages for teaching executive function skills: 1) engagement (i.e. attention and motivation), 2) awareness of strengths and needs, 3) goal setting (i.e. identifying realistic and measurable goals), 4) skill mastery and 5) generalization.

This is mainly necessary because of the cognitive processes that coordinate, integrate and control processes, strategies to promote executive functions generally address three main areas, self-regulation, working memory and metacognition all of which allow students to engage in problem-solving and goal-directed behavior (Watson et al,2016).

Environmental Modifications

For the students with executive dysfunctions and ADHD, there is a need for a highly structured and well-organized classroom, an environment that circumvents the difficulties related to poor inhibition. Any potential distractions should be carefully controlled to restrict the amount of irrelevant stimuli students that they must deal with. Especially for test-taking and writing tasks, the child can be provided with an independent workstation to minimize the surrounding distraction and help him/her focus better.

Environmentally-based interventions (e.g cueing, providing concrete information) may evade inhibition and facilitate student behavior self-regulation. The use of compensatory strategies and externally generated structures like checklists, computerized reminder systems, limit the number of tasks that require updating at both encoding and retrieval stages can facilitate student self-regulation during complex task performance (Dawson et al, 2010) Ferney et al 2006). A classmate, a buddy, or even a support teacher can aid this process by breaking down the complex tasks to smaller parts and assist the child with ADHD in attempting each level.

Planning and Organizing

Teachers can help students with ADHD overcome their deficits with planning and strategy use by providing direct instruction in planning and using strategies. Many strategies actually combine planning and task-related strategies, and all strategies provide step-by-step algorithms for accomplishing academic tasks (Reid & Lienemann, 2006). Effective strategy instruction for students with ADHD should: (a) directly and explicitly teach the steps in the strategy, (b) provide students with information on the value of the strategy (e.g., why use the strategy, how the strategy helps), and (c) continue until the student has mastered the strategy and can use it independently.

A study by Reid and Lienemann (2006) demonstrates how these steps can be accomplished in practice. The study included elementary students with ADHD who were taught the POW+WWW, What=2, How=2 strategy for narrative writing.POW, which refers to pick your own ideas, organize your thoughts and write and say more serves as a planning strategy to be used before beginning to write.WWW, What=2, How=2(Who,Where, When, What do the main characters do? What happens next? How does the story end? And How do the characters feel?) is used to help students organize their story and ensures that the students include all parts of the story (Johnson & Reid et al, 2011).

Working Memory

To offset the problem of working memory, teachers can support a student's working memory by presenting concepts and ideas that are limited in number. Miller's (1956) notion of the "magic number seven" (minus or plus two) can be helpful when planning how much information to convey at one time. For example, it is easier to remember a five-to seven-word sentence than a longer one; by the same token, it is much easier to remember five new concepts than nine (Watson et al, 2016).

Chunking is another way of grouping information to avoid an overload of a student's working memory. Organizing visual or verbal information according to specific categories is one way of grouping or chunking information. Be it numbers or spellings it is easier to remember spelling words chunked by word families than a list of random words. The method has been of utmost significance especially for students for whom the working memory withholding and updating difficulties are prominent (Watson et al, 2016).

Goal Setting

According to studies by Konrad, Fowler, Walker, Test, and Wood in 2007, goal setting has been evidenced to improve the academic productivity of students with ADHD.

Hence, like the other areas students with ADHD can also be trained to work on their goal-setting skills. The intervention begins when the teacher or the counselor is able to explain the importance and need to set goals, requires that the students set goals, and also provides means of tracking or monitoring progress. According to Bandura (1988), the most effective goals would be the ones that are specific, proximal and moderately challenging. Proximal goals are quite critical for students with ADHD as the students need frequent reinforcements and challenge should help the child acknowledge that the goal has to be achieved (Johnson & Reid 2011).

Persistence

Apart from goal setting, the methods to persist at academic tasks are also essential. The teachers can attempt to reduce frustration and ensure that students have sufficient instructions and opportunities. This will help the students to successfully master the skills needed to perform on a task. The teachers also need to constantly model the 'Can do it' attitude to the students. Additionally, it has been evidenced that by teaching students self-monitoring strategies, increases their academic performance (Reid, Trout, & Schartz, 2005). According to Johnson& Reid, self-monitoring involves self-assessing academic performance or behavior (e.g number of correct answers, whether the student was attending to the task) and self-recording the results.

Mnemonic Keyword

The mnemonic keyword method is another evidenced strategy that improves the paired-associate learning such as learning vocabulary words. According to studies by Atkinson and Rugh in1975 using the keyword method. A keyword is a concrete, associated word that is acoustically similar to the information to be learned (e.g vocabulary words, places) that can be associated with the information to be remembered. An interactive visual image or a drawing of the associated word is then created and/ or sentence that shows the definition of doing something with the keyword can be added (Johnson et al, 2016). Strategies similar to these like mind maps, tree diagrams and concept bubbles can help in developing a child's ability to visually organize all the elements, making them proficient in note-taking and subsequently not only helps the encoding process but also supports the retrieval.

Sustaining Attention

Another strategy used in the management of younger children with ADHD is by giving them cues in mnemonic forms for how to behave in certain situations to sustain attention and alertness. An example of such cue could be "SLANT", where S means "Sit up Straight", L means "Lean Forward", A means " Activate thinking and Ask questions", N means "Name the key information and Nod your head to validate the teacher/speaker" and T means "Track the teacher/ speaker" (Mercer, 2011). It is also helpful for the child if the instruction is made to recall and repeat in terms if "Say it back to me" is employed parallel by the teacher.

The additional strategy emphasized by Diane Dempster and Elaine Klaus (2016), for a number of children is "conscious fidgeting". They recommend that the child can be given a small "fidget" like a mood stone, or squeeze ball or a piece of modeling clay. You can set an agreement with the child and the teacher to make sure that the fidget doesn't become an object of hyper-focus, but helps him engage his fingers so that the brain also remains engaged. Fidgets can be helpful outside of school or when standing or waiting or even in situations where larger movements cannot be accommodated. Every child can select what works for him or her like rubik's cube in concert, crayons in church or even squishy toys to help him/her wait at the clinics or airports. When the fidgeting is planned just like a planned movement break then there is not much redirection and the child can be trained to assume responsibility to manage his hyperactivity. The embodied cognition literature emphasizes the central role the body plays in mediating cognition (Wilson, 2002). In this context one potentially fruitful way to view fidgeting is as an "embodiment" of the act of sustaining attention.

CONCLUSION

The number and type of challenges as experienced by a child with ADHD in the classroom is difficult to generalize. However, some of the popular and well-researched strategies can be worked and trained with the child from the beginning to ensure he/she understands his strengths and weaknesses and adopt strategies. Once the child learns to adapt and inherit these strategies then the avoidance and aversion to academic performance can also be observed to decrease. The child becomes more motivated and finds goals achievable. however, if children with ADHD are not supported by a multimodal model and consistent efforts by teachers and parents, they may continue to underperform despite high IQs and exceptional abilities. The executive functions also help in honing up the child's overall development as learning problem solving and self regulation skills are of significance throughout the trajectory of the child's development.

REFERENCES

Barkley, R. (2008). Classroom Accommodations for Children with ADHD. *The ADHD Report, 16*(4), 7–10. doi:10.1521/adhd.2008.16.4.7

Barkley, R. A. (1998). *Attention Deficit Hyperactivity Disorder: A Handbook for Diagnosis and Treatment.* The Guilford Press.

Brown, T. (2009, March). ADD/ADHD and impaired executive function in clinical practice. *Current Attention Disorders Reports, 1*(1), 37–41. doi:10.100712618-009-0006-3

Dawson, P., & Guare, R. (2010). *Executive skills in children and adolescents: A practical guide to assessment and intervention (2nd ed.).* Guilford.

Denckla, M. B., Barquero, L. A., Lindstrom, E. R., Benedict, S. L., & Wilson, L. M. (2013). Attention-deficit/hyperactivity disorder, executive function and reading comprehension: Different but related. In Handbook of learning disabilities (2nd ed.). New York, NY: Guilford.

Diagnostic and Statistical Manual of Mental Disorders. (2013). *American Psychiatric Association* (5th ed.). American Psychiatric Publishing.

Egeland, J. (2012). Cutting Corners: Neuropsychological Research into the Energetics of ADHD. In *Contemporary Trends in ADHD Research.* InTech. Available from: http://www.intechopen.com/books/contemporary-trends-in-adhd-research/cutting-corners- neuropsychological-research-into-the-energetics-of-adhd

Elaine Klaus-Taylor & Dempster Diane. (2016). *Parenting ADHD Now! Easy Intervention Strategies to Empower Kids with ADHD* (1st ed.). Althea Press.

Farley, J., Risko, E., & Kingstone, A. (2013). Everyday attention and lecture retention: The effects of time,fidgeting and mind wandering. *Frontiers in Psychology, 4*, 619. PMID:24065933

Feeney, T., & Ylvisaker, M. (2006). Context-sensitive cognitive-behavioural supports for young children with TBI: A replication study. *Brain Injury, 20*(6), 629–645. doi:10.1080/02699050600744194 PMID:16754288

Harris, K. R., Graham, S., & Mason, L. H. (2003). Self-regulated strategy development in the classroom: Part of a balanced approach to writing instruction for students with disabilities. *Focus on Exceptional Children, 35*, 1–16.

Holmes, J., Hilton, K. A., Place, M., Alloway, T. P., Elliott, J. G., & Gathercole, S. E. (2014). Children with low working memory and children with ADHD: Same or different? *Frontiers in Human Neuroscience, 8*, 976. doi:10.3389/fnhum.2014.00976 PMID:25538599

Joseph, J., & Robert, R. (2011). Overcoming Executive Function Deficits With Students With ADHD. *Theory into Practice, 50*(1), 61–67. doi:10.1080/00405841.2010.534942

Kolkman, M., Hoijtink, H. J. A., Kroesbergen, E. H., & Leseman, P. P. M. (2013). The role of executive functions in numerical magnitude skills. *Learning and Individual Differences, 24*, 145–151. doi:10.1016/j.lindif.2013.01.004

Labuhn, A. S., Zimmerman, B. J., & Hasselhorn, M. (2010). Enhancing students' self-regulation and mathematics performance: The influence of feedback and self-evaluative standards. *Metacognition and Learning, 5*(2), 173–194. doi:10.100711409-010-9056-2

LeFevre, J.-A., Berrigan, L., Vendetti, C., Kamawar, D., Bisanz, J., Skwarchuk, S.-L., & Smith-Chant, B. L. (2012). The role of executive attention in the acquisition of mathematical skills for children in grades 2 through 4. *Journal of Experimental Child Psychology*, *114*(2), 243–261. doi:10.1016/j.jecp.2012.10.005 PMID:23168083

Meltzer, L. (2007). Executive function difficulties and learning disabilities: Understandings and misunderstandings. In L. Meltzer (Ed.), *Executive function in education: From theory to practice* (pp. 77–105). Guilford.

Meltzer, L., Pollica, L., & Barzillai, M. (2007). Executive function in the classroom: Embedding strategy instruction into daily teaching practice. In L. Meltzer (Ed.), *Executive function in education: From theory to practice* (pp. 165–193).

Mercer, C. M. (2011). *Teaching Students With Learning Problems* (8th ed.). Pearson.

Reardon & Naglieri. (1992). PASS cognitive processing characteristics of normal and ADHD males. *Journal of School Psychology*, *30*(2).

Reid, R. (1996). Self-monitoring for students with learning disabilities: The present, the prospects, the pitfalls. *Journal of Learning Disabilities*, *29*(3), 317–331. doi:10.1177/002221949602900311 PMID:8732894

Reid, R., & Lienemann, T. O. (2006a). *Strategy in- struction for students with learning disabilities*. Guilford.

Schachar, R., Mota, V. L., Logan, G. D., Tannock, R., & Klim, P. (2000). Confirmation of an inhibitory control deficit in attention-deficit/hyperactivity disorder. *Journal of Abnormal Child Psychology*, *28*(3), 227–235. doi:10.1023/A:1005140103162 PMID:10885681

Schunk, D. (1990). Goal setting and self-efficacy dur- ing self-regulated learning. *Educational Psychologist*, *25*(1), 71–86. doi:10.120715326985ep2501_6

Scime, M., & Norvilitis, J. M. (2006). Task perfor- mance and response to frustration in children with attention deficit hyperactivity disorder. *Psychology in the Schools*, *43*(3), 377–386. doi:10.1002/pits.20151

Watson, G.R.A., & Morin, L.L. (2016). The Role of Executive Functions in Classroom Instruction of Students with Learning Disabilities. *International Journal of School Cognitive Psychology, 3*, 167. doi:10.4172/2469-9837.1000167

Wilhelm, H., Brandon, S., & Alan, B. (2012, March). Executive functions and self-regulation. *Trends in Cognitive Sciences*, *16*(3). PMID:22336729

Wilson, M. (2002). Six views of embodied cognition. *Psychonomic Bulletin & Review*, *9*(4), 625–636. doi:10.3758/BF03196322 PMID:12613670

Chapter 14
ADHD and Substance Abuse in Children and Adolescents

Mohd Altaf Paul
Government Degree College, Kulgam, India

Bilal Ahmad Teli
SKIMS Medical College and Hospital, India

ABSTRACT

Children and adolescents with ADHD are at an increased risk for various substance use disorders and developing early-onset substance abuse. Both ADHD and substance abuse are said to be disorders of disinhibition, which suggests that both share an underlying vulnerability and have more chances to co-occur. The substance abuse in children and adolescents with ADHD is growing, and many factors accumulate to heighten the risk for such problem. The symptoms of ADHD and their secondary problems, availability of drugs, poor coping mechanisms, and the need for adventure and excitement lead them into substance abuse easily. Once they are trapped into substance abuse, it becomes difficult for them to quit, and the tolerance for drugs and risk taking behaviours makes them experiment with new drugs with more quantity. This in turn results in severe consequences and affects them physically, psychologically, and socially, as well as their overall quality of life.

INTRODUCTION

Attention Deficit Hyperactivity Disorder is a grave problem because children with the ADHD may develop a wide range of secondary problems. Difficulties in attention may result in poor academic achievement in schools.Impulsivity and aggression can lead to relationship issues and difficulties in making supportive peer group.Impulsivity may result in excessive risk taking behaviours with consequent complications such as substance abuse. These risk taking behaviours compromise later adjustment and give rise to many other problems (Carr, 2015)

DOI: 10.4018/978-1-7998-5495-1.ch014

ADHD has comorbidity with many other learning and psychiatric problems (Wilens & Spencer, 2010) However, substance abuse is the most problematic co-occurring disorders with ADHD (Wilens et al, 2011). Children with ADHD have high risk for substance abuse in their adolescence as compared to general population (Galera et al, 2013; Mochrie, et al. 2020).Van Emmerik (2012) in his international met-analysis reported that 23% of treatment-seeking young adult for substance abuse had ADHD as well. Researchers report that the risk of substance abuse is twice as high among people with ADHD (Wilens et al., 2011). Cigarette smoking is one of the important antecedents for substance abuse in ADHD adolescents. Studies have found more than half of adolescents who smoke have ADHD.Apart from tobacco, such people are at higher risk for early use of alcohol as well (Chang et al., 2012).

Previously, ADHD was thought to be only childhood disorder however, long-term controlled follow-up studies have reported that it continuing into adolescence for approximately three-quarters of cases and into adulthood for half of cases (Wilens & Spencer, 2010).

There are many studies which shows modest correlation between ADHD and substance abuse and many reasons behind such correlation has been explored. Some of the symptoms and issues in ADHD itself along with its consequences can result in substance abuse in adolescence. It is quite common that high stress levels, poor academic performance in school, lack of social support and risk taking behavior are linked with substance abuse. Apart from this, adolescents with ADHD abuse substances to attenuate their moods and to help them sleep. Risk taking behaviours along with easy availability of drugs and exposure to friend circle who abuse such drugs increase the risk of substance abuse.Studies have also reported neurobiological connection between ADHD and substance abuse. Deficits have been seen in anterior cingulate activation and the fronto-subcortical systems, in both individuals with ADHD and SUD (Casey & Jones, 2010). Furthermore, dopamine systems and striatal involvement are similar for the two disorders (Frodl, 2010). The same dopamine system is targeted in ADHD medication as well. Hence researches have been conducted to study the link between ADHD treatment by stimulant therapy and substance abuse. There are no conclusive evidence supporting that stimulant therapy can lead to substance abuse. However it is found that some abuse the same ADHD medication which further enhance their risk for other substances as well.Some other explanations for the link between ADHD and substance abuse include genetic loading and parental exposure to substance abuse. Exposure to nicotine or alcohol during pregnancy and in early developmental stages of child results in increased risk for ADHD in offspring (Zulauf, et al. 2014).

While comparing adolescents with and without ADHD, it has been found that adolescents with ADHD has higher risk for substance abuse as well as have an earlier onset and more chronic path. Kousha et al. (2012) found that adolescents with ADHD had a younger age of onset for substance abuse, a shorter period for developing a fulminate substance abuse and severe functional impairment.

DIAGNOSTIC CRITERIA

ADHD has been already discussed in this book and the criteria for diagnosing ADHD need not to be discussed again here. However it is very important to understand when to say that a person with ADHD has comorbid substance abuse. Generally many substances like cigarette, alcohol etc are being used and are not treated as any problem. It is even served in some social and cultural functions. However the repeated use of substance becomes a problem and abuse when it interferes with normal functioning of an individual. It is then considered a psychological problem that demands treatment. The problem becomes worse when it is found comorbid in children and adolescents with ADHD and thus becomes a major public health issue because of its serious long term consequences. The earlier a child abuses substances, the higher is the risk for other health problems and adult substance addiction. Moreover the earlier abuse of substances in formative years interferes with acquisition of various life skills. Here it becomes necessary to understand when a substance use becomes abuse and thus a psychological problem. American Psychiatric Association has given detailed description of criteria of substance abuse in its diagnostic and statistical manual (DSM). As per DSM-5 (American Psychiatric Association, 2013) there are some criteria of substance abuse which are as follows:

Impaired Control Over Substance use (Criteria 1–4).

1) Taking substance in larger amounts or over a longer period than was originally intended.
2) Multiple unsuccessful efforts to decrease or discontinue use of substance despite persistent desire to cut down or regulate substance use.
3) Spending a great deal of time obtaining the substance, using the substance, or recovering from its effects.
4) Craving which is manifested by an intense desire or urge for the drug

Social Impairment (Criteria 5–7).

5) Failure to fulfill major role obligations at work, school, or home due to recurrent substance use.
6) Continuous substance use despite having persistent or recurrent social or interpersonal problems.
7) Giving up or reducing important social, occupational, or recreational activities.

Risky use of the Substance (Criteria 8–9).

8) Recurrent substance use in situations in which it is physically hazardous
9) Continuous substance use despite knowledge of having a persistent or recurrent physical or psychological problem caused or exacerbated by the substance.

Pharmacological Criteria (Criteria 10 and 11).

10) Tolerance or requiring a markedly increased dose of the substance to achieve the desired effect.
11) Withdrawal which is a syndrome that occurs when blood or tissue concentrations of a substance decline in an individual who had maintained prolonged heavy use of the substance.

Consumption of licit and illicit substances has increased all over the world and the age of initiation of abuse is progressively falling. In India, the mean age-at-first-use of the primary substance is 12.3 years (Dhawan et al., 2017). The common drugs of abuse amongst children and adolescents in India are tobacco and alcohol. Uses of illicit drugs like cannabis and heroin have also been reported. Inhalant abuse, correction fluid and glue are also common among children and adolescents. A high prevalence of drug use and even intravenous use among street children and working children is a matter of concern in India (Tripathi & Lal, 1999). Generally the pattern of substance abuse involves initiation with tobacco which is followed by inhalants, cannabis, alcohol, opioids, pharmaceutical drugs and finally injectable (Dhawan et al., 2017).

RISK FACTORS

Certain factors that put children with ADHD at risk for development of substance abuse and dependence include following factors:

Genetic factor: Genetic factors are estimated to contribute 40–60 percent of vulnerability to drug abuse. Probands reported higher levels of alcohol, tobacco, and illicit drug use than did controls. Within probands, severity of childhood inattention symptoms predicted multiple substance use outcomes (Brooke & William, 2003). Children whose parents abuse drugs have high risk of substance abuse.

Constitutional and Psychological Factors

- Having history of physical, sexual or emotional abuse and psychiatric comorbidity can increase the risk for substance abuse.
- Difficult temperament during childhood can have negative impact on self-regulation, parent child relation which can in turn increase the risk for substance abuse.
- Problems in attachment like insecure attachment during childhood can make a child to be aggressive or withdrawn which increases the risk.
- Impulsive and aggressive behaviour can lead to problems in school which can increase the chances for substance abuse. Hyperactivity in children also imparts high risk for later substance abuse.
- Chronic, intense and prolonged stress during childhood can diminish a child's ability to cope and increase the chance for substance abuse.

(Whitesell, et al. 2013; Carr, 2015)

Sociocultural Factors

- **Parental substance use**: Parental substance use affects children directly as well as indirectly. Substance abuse by mothers can affect a developing foetus by crossing the placenta and directly expose the foetus to drugs. It can also pass to child through breast feeding. It also affects indirectly when parents smoke in the home and expose children to second hand smoke and increase the chances of substance abuse (Ningombamety al., 2011).
- **Family:** Parental experience and attitude towards drug use, history of parental divorce or separation, low expectation for the child, childhood abuse especially in girls are some risk factors for substance abuse.
- **Peers:** Peer pressure is important factor both in initiation as well as abstinence of substance abuse. Friends who use drugs and their attitude towards drug use pose a great risk for a child or adolescent to engage in such behaviours.
- **School Failure:** School failure and dropping out can be a factor for substance abuse as well as consequence of it. Bullying in school can also lead to substance abuse.

- **Community:** Community attitude towards drug use, economic and social deprivation, availability of drugs and alcohol are some significant risk factors for substance abuse.

(Whitesell, et al. 2013; Carr, 2015)

CONSEQUENCES

The substance abuse has both short term and long term consequences. In the case of children and adolescents with ADHD, substance abuse can prove fatal for its ill effects get more strengthened with the passage of time and have more severe consequences in the formative years of such children and adolescents. Its effects can be summarised below in main two categories:

Physical effects:

- Substance abuse affects the functioning of the brain and the way the body feels pleasure.
- It has links with Heart problems like heart attack or heart failure
- Respiratory problems such as lung cancer, emphysema and breathing problems are also associated with substance abuse.
- Abdominal pain, vomiting, constipation and diarrheais common.
- Damage of kidney and liver is also reported.
- Disturbances in appetite and sleep.
- It can also result indirectly to AIDS, due to sharing of syringes which injecting drugs.
- Deliberate self harm, sexual disinhibition and teenage pregnancy are common in adolescents who abuse drugs.

(Carr, 2015; Geddes, 2020)

Psycho-social effects:

- Long-term substance abuse can result in increased stress
- Substance abuse can result in mood swings, anxiety and depression.
- Decrease in pleasure in everyday life
- Substance abuse can lead to paranoia and violence
- It can complicate the already existing mental illness
- It can result in hallucinations and confusion.
- Substance abuse can result in psychological tolerance
- Such people can engage in risky behaviour
- It can decline academic performance
- It can worsen interpersonal relationships
- It can lead to financial complications as lot of money is wasted in it.

(Carr, 2015; Geddes, 2020)

EVALUATION AND TREATMENT

For effective treatment, evaluation of the problem is compulsory because the effective treatment depends largely on proper evaluation. Wilens (2004) has given some guidelines for proper evaluation and effective treatment of comorbid ADHD and SUD patients as follows:

- Careful evaluation of the patient involving assessment of social, cognitive, psychiatric, addiction, educational, and family characteristics should be done before intervention..
- History of substance use should be obtained.
- Differential diagnoses, including medical and neurologic conditions whose symptoms may overlap with ADHD should be done.
- Current psychosocial factors need to be explored.
- For accurate and reliable assessment of ADHD symptoms in a patient with active SUD requires at least 1 month of abstinence.
- Semi-structured psychiatric interviews or validated rating scales of ADHD should be used for proper diagnostic assessment.

Generally pharmacotherapy in patients with ADHD involve psychostimulants, however in patients with comorbid substance abuse, it has remain controversial for its potential risk of abusing the drug. In such cases, nonstimulant drugs have also been recommended, however they have reported comparatively less efficacy than stimulant drugs (Biederman, Spencer, & Wilens, 2004)). For the patients with comorbid ADHD and SUD, Psychotherapy is always recommended along with or without medication. Psycho-education is also an important element of treatment. The specific psychosocial treatments such as cognitive behavioral therapy (CBT) or dynamic psychotherapies are used to treat concomitant ADHD and SUD. Research suggests that modifications of CBT such as structured skills training or cognitive remediation for ADHD with SUD in adolescents is effective. Antshel, Faraone and Gordon (2014) recently examined a modified CBT intervention demonstrating the success of CBT for reducing ADHD symptoms and SUD.

There is a well-developed literature showing that specific family interventions are often an effective component of adolescent substance abuse treatment programs, and the efficacy and effectiveness of family therapy models as well as cognitive-behavior therapy are widely reported in the literature (Slesnick, Kaminer, & Kelly, 2008). Therapeutic approaches that address motivation using cognitive-behavioral strategies, and that facilitate 12-step involvement, have all been shown to be effective for adults with substance use disorders.

Additional behavioral strategies for ADHD that are used clinically but not studied in controlled trials in adults include coaching and behavior modification (Safren et al. 2005). Coaching is a collaborative relationship between the patient and a professional to develop strategies for managing problems such as procrastination, time-management, and organization. Behavior modification is a technique used mainly for children where desired behaviors are positively reinforced to increase their frequency (Stevenson et al., 2002).

CONCLUSION

A convincing literature shows that children and adolescents with ADHD are at an increased risk for various substance use disorders and developing early-onset substance abuse. Both ADHD and substance abuse are said to be disorders of disinhibition, which suggests that both share an underlying vulnerability and has more chances to co-occur.The substance abuse in children and adolescents with ADHD is growing and many factors accumulate to heighten the risk for such problem. It generally starts,as a result of their impulsivity and risk taking behaviour, with licit drugs and finally ends with substance abuse and then substance addiction. Unfortunately such children are more concerned about their ADHD symptoms and do not seek treatment in the beginning phase which makes them later more resistant to treatment. The symptoms of ADHD and their secondary problems, availability of drugs, poor coping mechanisms and the need for adventure and excitement lead them into substance abuse easily. Once they are trapped into substance abuse, it becomes difficult for them to quit and the tolerance for drugs and risk taking behaviours makes them to experiment new drugs with more quantity. This in turn results in severe consequences and affects them physically, psychologically and socially as well and affects their overall quality of life. So proper assessment needs to be done for effective treatment which can involve both pharmacotherapy as well as nonpharmacotherapy methods.

REFERENCES

American Psychiatric Association. (2013). *Diagnostic and statistical manual of mental disorders* (5th ed.). Author.

Antshel, K. M., Faraone, S. V., & Gordon, M. (2014). Cognitive behavioral treatment outcomes in adolescent ADHD. *Journal of Attention Disorders, 18*(6), 483–495. doi:10.1177/1087054712443155 PMID:22628140

Biederman, J., Spencer, T., & Wilens, T. (2004). Evidence based pharmacotherapy for attention deficit hyperactivity disorder. *International Journal of Neuropharmocotherapy, 7*, 77-97

Carr, A. (2015). *The handbook of child and adolescent clinical psychology: a contextual approach* (3rd ed.). Routledge. doi:10.4324/9781315744230

Casey, B. J., & Jones, R. M. (2010). Neurobiology of the adolescent brain and behavior: Implications for substance use disorders. *Journal of the American Academy of Child and Adolescent Psychiatry, 49*(12), 1189–1201. doi:10.1097/00004583-201012000-00005 PMID:21093769

Chang, Z., Lichtenstein, P., & Larsson, H. (2012). The effects of childhood ADHD symptoms on early-onset substance Use: A Swedish twin study. *Journal of Abnormal Child Psychology, 40*(3), 425–435. doi:10.100710802-011-9575-6 PMID:21947618

Dhawan, A., Pattanayak, R. D., Chpra, A., Tikko, V. K., & Kumar, R. (2017). Pattern and profile of children using substances in India: Insights and recommendations. *The National Medical Journal of India, 30*(4), 224–229. doi:10.4103/0970-258X.218679 PMID:29162759

Dongre, A., Deshmukh, P., Murali, N., & Garg, B. (2008). Tobacco consumption among adolescents in rural Wardha: Where and how tobacco control should focus its attention? *Indian Journal of Cancer*, *45*(3), 100–106. doi:10.4103/0019-509X.44065 PMID:19018113

Frodl, T. (2010). Comorbidity of ADHD and Substance Use Disorder (SUD): A neuroimaging perspective. *Journal of Attention Disorders*, *14*(2), 109–120. doi:10.1177/1087054710365054 PMID:20495160

Galera, C., Pingault, J., Fombonne, E., Michel, G., Lagarde, E., Bouvard, M.-P., & Melchior, M. (2013). Attention problems in childhood and adult substance use. *The Journal of Pediatrics*, *163*(6), 1677–1683.e1. Advance online publication. doi:10.1016/j.jpeds.2013.07.008 PMID:23972646

Geddes, J. R., & Andreasen, N. C. (2020). *New Oxford Textbook of Psychiatry* (3rd ed.). Oxford University Press. doi:10.1093/med/9780198713005.001.0001

Kilpatrick, D. G., Ruggiero, K. J., Acierno, R., Saunders, B. E., Resnick, H. S., & Best, C. L. (2003). Violence and risk of PTSD, major depression, substance abuse/dependence, and comorbidity: Results from the National Survey of Adolescents. *Journal of Consulting and Clinical Psychology*, *71*(4), 692–700. doi:10.1037/0022-006X.71.4.692 PMID:12924674

Kousha, M., Shahrivar, Z., & Alaghband-Rad, J. (2012). Substance use disorder and ADHD: Is ADHD a particularly "specific" risk factor? *Journal of Attention Disorders*, *16*(4), 325–332. doi:10.1177/1087054710387265 PMID:22127397

Mochrie, K. D., Whited, M. C., Cellucci, T., Freeman, T., & Corson, A. T. (2020). ADHD, Depression and substance abuse risk among beginning college students. *Journal of American College Health*, *68*(1), 6–10. doi:10.1080/07448481.2018.1515754 PMID:30257141

Molina, B. S. G., & Pelham, W. E. (2003). Childhood predictors of adolescent substance use in a longitudinal study of children with ADHD. *Journal of Abnormal Psychology*, *112*(3), 497–507. doi:10.1037/0021-843X.112.3.497 PMID:12943028

Nabors, L. (2020). Substance abuse and anxiety in children. In Anxiety management in children with Mental and Physical health problems. Springer. doi:10.1007/978-3-030-35606-4_4

Ningombam, S., Hutin, Y., & Murhekar, M. V. (2011). Prevalence and pattern of substance use among the higher secondary school students of Imphal, Manipur, India. *The National Medical Journal of India*, *24*(1), 11–15. PMID:21608351

Safren, S. A., Otto, M. W., Sprich, S., Winett, C. L., Wilens, T. E., & Biederman, J. (2005). Cognitive-behavioral therapy for ADHD in medication-treated adults with continued symptoms. *Behaviour Research and Therapy*, *43*(7), 831–842. doi:10.1016/j.brat.2004.07.001 PMID:15896281

Saluja, B. S., Grover, S., Irpati, S. R., Mattoo, S. K., & Basu, D. (2004). Drug dependence in adolescents 1978-2003: A clinical –based observation from north India. *Indian Journal of Pediatrics*, *74*(5), 455–458. doi:10.100712098-007-0077-z PMID:17526956

Schnabel, W. (2005). Nicotine use in suicides: A case–control study Barbara Schneider Axel. *European Psychiatry*, *20*(2), 129–136. doi:10.1016/j.eurpsy.2004.04.016 PMID:15797697

Sinha, R., & O'Malley, S. S. (2000). Alcohol and Eating Disorders: Implications for Alcohol Treatment and Health Services Research. *Alcoholism, Clinical and Experimental Research, 24*(8), 1312–1319. doi:10.1111/j.1530-0277.2000.tb02097.x PMID:10968671

Slesnick, N., Kaminer, Y., & Kelly, J. (2008). Most common psychosocial intervention for adolescent use disorder. In Y. Kaminer & O. G. Bukstien (Eds.), *Adolescent substance abuse: psychiatric comorbidity and high risk behaviors*. Routledge, Taylor, and Francis Group.

Stevenson, C. S., Whitmont, S., Bornholt, L., Livesey, D., & Stevenson, R. J. (2002). A cognitive remediation programme for adults with Attention Deficit Hyperactivity Disorder. *The Australian and New Zealand Journal of Psychiatry, 36*(5), 610–616. doi:10.1046/j.1440-1614.2002.01052.x PMID:12225443

Swendsen, J. D., & Merikangas, K. R. (2000). The comorbidity of depression and substance use disorders. *Clinical Psychology Review, 20*(2), 173–189. doi:10.1016/S0272-7358(99)00026-4 PMID:10721496

Thirthalli, J., & Benegal, V. (2006). Addictive disorders Psychosis among substance users. *Current Opinion in Psychiatry, 19*(3), 239–245. doi:10.1097/01.yco.0000218593.08313.fd PMID:16612208

Triparthi, B. M., & Lal, R. (1999). Substance abuse in children and adolescents. *Indian Journal of Pediatrics, 66*(4), 269–575. PMID:10798113

VanEmmerik-van Oortmerssen, K., van de Glind, G., van den Brink, W., Smit, F., Crunelle, C. L., Swets, M., & Schoevers, R. A. (2012). Prevalence of attention-deficit hyperactivity disorder in substance use disorder patients: A meta-analysis and meta-regression analysis. *Drug and Alcohol Dependence, 122*(1–2), 11–19. doi:10.1016/j.drugalcdep.2011.12.007 PMID:22209385

Whitesell, M., Bachand, A., Peel, J., & Brown, M. (2013). Familial, social, and individual factors contributing to risk for adolescent substance abuse. *Journal of Addiction, 2013*, 1–9. Advance online publication. doi:10.1155/2013/579310 PMID:24826363

Wilens, T. E. (2004). Attention deficit/hyperactivity disorder and the substance use disorders: The nature of the relationship, subtypes at risk, and treatment issues. *The Psychiatric Clinics of North America, 27*(2), 283–301. doi:10.1016/S0193-953X(03)00113-8 PMID:15063998

Wilens, T. E., Martelon, M., Joshi, G., Bateman, C., Fried, R., Petty, C., & Biederman, J. (2011). Does ADHD predict substance-use disorders? A 10-year follow-up study of young adults with ADHD. *Journal of the American Academy of Child and Adolescent Psychiatry, 50*(6), 543–553. doi:10.1016/j.jaac.2011.01.021 PMID:21621138

Wilens, T. E., & Spencer, T. J. (2010). Understanding attention-deficit/hyperactivity disorder from childhood to adulthood. *Postgraduate Medical Journal, 122*(5), 97–109. doi:10.3810/pgm.2010.09.2206 PMID:20861593

Zulauf, C. A., Sprich, S. E., Safren, S. A., & Wilens, T. E. (2014). The Complicated Relationship Between Attention Deficit/Hyperactivity Disorder and Substance Use Disorders. *Current Psychiatry Reports, 16*(3), 436. doi:10.100711920-013-0436-6 PMID:24526271

Chapter 15
ADHD and Addiction:
A Story of Complex Interaction and Interphase

Tanay Maiti
All India Institute of Medical Sciences, Bhubaneswar, India

Aastha Dhingra Hasija
Faculty of Behavioural Sciences, Shree Guru Gobind Singh Tricentenary University (SGT University), Gurgaon, India

ABSTRACT

ADHD or attention deficit hyperactivity disorder has gained immense importance both among the clinicians and researchers because of its early onset, variable clinical presentations, and prominent heritability. Along with the established symptom clusters of attention deficit and hyperactivity, a load of comorbidities have been found hugely prevalent for this population, increasing the morbidity and distress level and turning the management more complex. The early childhood and adolescent onset of this externalizing behavior-based disorder also makes the individual more prone to other externalizing behavioral problems, like addiction to variable psychoactive substances. Adolescent, being a natural age towards risk taking and novelty seeking, addiction proneness itself is a major individual and public health challenge to which ADHD works as potential fuel. In recent times, the upsurge of various behavioral addictions has also been seen prominently in the ADHD population increasing the morbidity and complexity. Treatment options need to be researched in detail.

INTRODUCTION

Comorbidity is almost a rule in case of ADHD in both children and adults as it impacts their ability to function successfully. However the conditions could be both comorbid disorders and differential diagnoses (with behaviours similar to that of ADHD), to be recognised in their individual capacity. Multiple comorbidities have been correlated with ADHD, some of them are Bipolar affective disorder, Obsessive compulsive disorder (OCD), Sensory Integration Disorder, Early Speech/Communication problems,

DOI: 10.4018/978-1-7998-5495-1.ch015

substance abuse disorder, conduct disorder (CD), Major depressive disorder, Communication disorder, Social phobia and Separation anxiety disorder, etc.

Substance Use Disorder (SUD) and ADHD seem to have bidirectional relationship. Study of their comorbidity is pertinent to research and clinical practice in developmental pediatrics, psychology and psychiatry. The study is useful for diagnosis, prognosis, treatment and healthcare delivery. Based on available facts, about a quarter to half of adolescents and adults with SUD have ADHD.

ADHD is a chronic condition which is often correlated with demoralization and failure. An improvement in attention and executive functions has been identified by adults with addiction to nicotine, similar to a literature recommendation in the treatment of ADHD. There has also been reports of emotional ease and help with falling asleep by adolescents with active SUD, stated as a reason of their substance use. Based on this, "self-medication" hypothesis has gained limelight.

Prevalence of Substance Abuse in ADHD

A number of studies with clinical as well as population samples show that the probability of receiving a diagnosis of SUD is high in adolescents and adults with ADHD. Thus, it may be summed up that each of these comorbidities as an individual diagnosis already has its numerous negative effects and it becomes the most problematic conditions when it is seen together with ADHD. Many studies and reviews have documented that individuals with ADHD are at risk for increased substance use, abuse, and experimentation (Barkley, Fischer, Smallish, & Fletcher, 2004; Burke, Loeber, & Lahey, 2001; Charach, Yeung, Climans, & Lillie, 2011; Faraone et al., 2007; Gittelman, Mannuzza, Shenker, & Bonagura, 1985; Hartsough & Lambert, 1987; Lee, Humphreys, Flory, Liu, & Glass, 2011; Molina & Pelham, 2014; Molina, Flory et al., 2007; Molina & Pelham, 2003; Molina, Smith, & Pelham, 1999; Sibley, Pelham, Molina, Kipp, Gnagy, Meinzer, Ross & Lahey, 2014a; Wilson & Levin, 2005).

In a meta-analysis and meta-regression study by Dennis (2004) including 29 international studies it was reported that 23.1% of young adults diagnosed with ADHD were also seeking treatment for SUD. The cross-sectional International ADHD in Substance Use Disorders Prevalence (IASP) study on a sample of 3,558, among 10 countries, a prevalence of 40.0% for ADHD in patients seeking treatment for SUD was reported. In a screening study carried out in Istanbul with 4,938 10th-grade students from 45 schools in 15 districts by Evren, Dalbudak, Evren, Can, Umut (2014), the severity of ADHD symptoms were found to be higher in students with a lifetime history of smoking and alcohol/substance use.

Behavioural Addiction in ADHD

Various researches indicate lower levels of Dopamine in people with ADHD. While involving in risky behaviours increases the dopamine level, therefore some individuals with ADHD are drawn towards risky behaviours. Nonetheless, certain genetic traits may also make and ADHD child or adult prone to risky or impulsive actions.

Some of the difficult or risky behaviors related to ADHD include: (Pagán nd)

- Trouble getting motivated or finishing tasks (either at work or at home)
- Being late or not following through on commitments, appointments, or responsibilities
- Impulsive spending or overspending
- Starting fights or arguing

- Trouble maintaining friendships and romantic relationships
- Speeding and dangerous driving
- Substance abuse
- Risky sexual behaviours, such as having unprotected sex

ADHD and SUD both are correlated with high levels of drug-related and sexual risk-taking. However in a study by Darke et al.(1992) it has been highlighted that likelihood of risky drug-related and sexual practices is similar is no higher in case of screening positive for ADHD symptoms, than in case of SUD alone. The levels of HIV risk-taking were found of clinical significance, among those that had engaged in injecting drug use and sexual activity in the month preceding interview.

It is clearly indicated in various research findings that even after controlling potential confounders, symptoms of adult ADHD were associated with a larger extent and severity of driving-related risk behaviour than that related to SUD alone.

Comorbidity of ADHD with SUD tends to increase the risk-taking behaviour in those with SUD symptoms, with adult ADHD symptoms independently predicting the increased levels of driving-related risk behaviours. Maintenance of the SUD treatment and outcomes are certainly compromised by ADHD, even though adult ADHD is not typically screened by many SUD treatment service providers (McAweeney et al., 2010). Those with SUD experience higher risk-taking and consequent harm in case of comorbidity with ADHD. In such cases, interventions to manage risk-taking are strongly recommended along with routine screening for ADHD at treatment intake and further assessment if ADHD is indicated.

ADHD is a biological, neurological, and genetic disorder. It's real, and it can have real consequences for the people who have it, so it's essential to acknowledge that the individual is not blamed for his/her acts, rather corrected with right measures like by being a partner in their planning process, making them do exercises, etc.

Gul,Yurumez Solmaz, Gul, & Oner (2018) reported in their study that there exists positive relationship between impulsivity, ADHD, externalisation factors and addictive behaviours. The relationship between internalising and externalizing symptoms and Facebook overuse can also be seen in many literatures available.

Adult ADHD and Addiction

It was initially believed that childhood condition resulting in delayed impulse control development that would be turned into hindrance in adolescents is adult ADHD. Approximately four percent prevalence of ADHD in the population was suggested by various evidences. There is an increase of dopamine transporter binding densities in the striatum of the brain and decreased prefrontal glucose metabolism on PET compared with adults without ADHD. The methylphendiate treatment of ADHD decreases and blocks DAT activity to normalise the patient of ADHD. In adult ADHD five additional symptoms were included they are ongoing difficulties with inattentiveness, hyperactivity and three other symptoms such as mood lability, irritability and hot temper, impaired stress tolerance, disorganisation. Compared with general people adult ADHD people demonstrate higher rates of anxiety, mood and learning disorders along with substance abuse. Adult ADHD people meet the criteria of inattentive type rather than showing impulsive hyperactive symptoms. Standard ways to monitor drug response and patience compliance should be used by psychiatrist and clinical psychologists. Only long-acting stimulants are FDA approved in the treatment of ADHD.

Cultural Variation

Some regions which are key to psychological well-being like language, feeling, consideration, connection, horrible encounters, social desires and resilience, setting limits and different parts of child rearing and youngster raising, etc., are certainly impacted by culture. Social setting in which an individual is comprehended and treated, assume a significant ground, without a doubt.

Members of different cultural groups understand and respond differently to challenging behavior in their children, based on their respective culturally appropriate factors. Factors could be beliefs, values, perceptions, limited knowledge, fear of stigmatization, norms, medical approaches, language difficulties, limited insurance coverage,, mistrust in school or health care institution, limited healthcare facilities, and higher threshold for behavioral tolerance before seeking assessment, etc.

Various Cross-cultural studies, from the U.S, Europe and Israel have shown that ethnic minority children are less likely to be recognized and treated for ADHD than their counterparts. In some cultures, for example, the Muslim and Christian Lebanese, hyperactivity and/or impulsivity in boys can be recognized as characteristic by parents and viewed as gender specific behaviour (Slobodin & Crunelle, 2019).

According to the American National Institute of Mental Health, adults of an ethnic minority background are less likely to be diagnosed with ADHD than non-minority groups. However, the efficacy of ADHD treatment in reducing psychiatric morbidity, transport accidents and criminality emphasizes the academic and clinical imperative of studying ethnic diversity in ADHD care among various ethnic and cultural groups.

Neurobiology

ADHD is believed to be a highly genetic condition beta heritability up to 77% as seen in multiple twin studies (Polanczyk, 2007).Two approaches has been taken see the genetic basis of ADHD 1)The genome scan and 2)candidate gene approach. Among various genetic locus Regions 16p13 And 17 p11 Has been linked persistently with a ADHD (Fernandez, Gupta, & Hoffman, 2017).

Biological Adversity

Several Biological factors has been Associated with ADHD from diet of food additive pregnancy factors to environmental toxin Exposure to alcohol or tobacco. Among the pregnancy factors toxemia preeclampsia, Duration of labour fetal distress, low birth weight, and antepartum haemorrhage happen thought to have a predisposing role into child's ADHD (Reinhardt, 2013).

Increased genetic liability of ADHD carries a high risk for substance abuse in the population. The Association of substance abuse with ADHD has been found more for females suggesting more genetic predisposition for them (Kelly,2004). Significant linkages at 4q13.1 - 13.2 and 5q31 - 33 for ADHD have been implicated in alcohol dependence and nicotine dependence (Carroll, 1993). Also, genetic association studies have suggested several genes which are responsible for both ADHD and alcohol dependence. For example, it has been reported associations between the dopamine transporter (DAT) gene polymorphisms and human disorders including ADHD and alcohol dependence (Kelly, 2004). There is consistent evidence of association between ADHD and a dopamine D4 receptor gene VNTR and a dopamine D5 receptor gene microsatellite marker. The association of D2 receptor that is DR D2 has been found to have common linkage in between alcoholism, smoking along with the risk factors like obesity, Pathological gambling and other compulsive behaviours. Dopamine D2 receptor gene variants: association and linkage studies in impulsive-addictive-compulsive behaviour.

Specific neurotransmitter dopamine have been strongly associated with ADHD. Expected the medications also act mostly on dopaminergic system. However involvement of multiple other mono amines like serotonin nor epinephrine has been found to have contributing role in the population of ADHD and SUD.

Risk Factors

A recent large-scale population-based twin study found a strong correlation between ADHD and AUD with a 3.58 times increased risk. Twin analyses showed that shared genetic factors explain 64.0% of the overlap between ADHD and AUD, while the remaining 36.0% are explained by non-shared environmental factors; the contribution of shared environmental factors was found to be very small.

A. **Pregnancy:** smoking in pregnancy is a known and established risk factor.
B. **Mental health conditions:** Various studies have shown that parental psychiatric disorder was significantly associated with ADHD in children. Parental history of antisocial personality disorder, alcohol use disorder or conversion disorder (specifically, paternal anxiety-mood disorder) has also been shown to be related to higher risk of ADHD and its persistence into adulthood. Parental addiction has also been postulated as contributory for adolescent ADHD symptoms.

MANAGEMENT

Pharmacotherapy

On multiple evidences, pharmacotherapy has been considered as first line of treatment for Attention Deficit and Hyperactivity Disorder. Medicines, which stimulate the central nervous system, popularly known as stimulants are the first choice with greatest efficacy shown over multiple researches and randomised controlled trials. The stimulants are Methylphenidate, dextroamphetamine and dextroamphetamine plus amphetamine combinations available in various oral forms including chewable forms, also wait skin patches (Daytrana, a methylphenidate patch). Other than stimulants, Non stimulant medication like Atomoxetine is approved by US food and drug administration for the treatment of ADHD. Other psychopharmacological agents light Alpha agonists (like Clonidine and Guanafacine) Antidepressant, like Bupropion have shown some efficacy for ADHD too (Konstenius, JayaramLindstrom, Beck, & Franck, 2010).

In short, stimulants are dopamine agonists, which have shown very good efficacy in children with ADHD with tolerable side effects. Stimulants should be given in the morning or daytime as its effect stays mostly 12 hrs, and late administration might cause insomnia or sleep disturbance. Its available in 5mg, 10 mg, 18 mg dosage and can be given up to 1-1.5 mg/kg/day. Side effects like nausea, appetite loss and growth restriction has been mentioned in some of adolescent population. Among non stimulants atomoxetine have a half life of 5 hours and administered twice a day. Its relatively safer and works on presynaptic nor epinephrine transporter. Side effects are diminished appetite, irritability and dizziness. For the population of ADHD with co morbid substance abuse, stimulants carry extra risk for abuse and misuse. Antidepressants like bupropion have been shown to efficacious to this particular population in multiple studies. (Kaplan and Saddock,2007).

Psychotherapy

Although pharmacotherapy lays the foundation of treatment for ADHD with SUD, a multimodal intervention plan can be employed in combination with medication to enhance the long-term management of this chronic disorder and to stabilize the substance use prior to initiating pharmacotherapy.

Psychoeducation: An imperative element of the treatment of ADHD is Psychoeducation. Having the patient and the family learn about the disorder, its etiology and its pervasive effects on their functioning, its impact on the family members and caregivers, etc can help to set the stage for developing an effective therapeutic alliance. Providing authentic educational literature or referrals to different support groups can prove be very useful for patients and families in becoming considerate towards the patient.

Cognitive behaviour therapy: Studies show that CBT and integrated CBT are effective in adolescents and adults with ADHD and SUD. Initially each disorder needs to be assessed in detail and both familial and individual support are crucial. In cases with active substance used, management of SUD and controlling the condition, becomes necessary before therapy. Subsequently, re-evaluation of the individual is required. It is necessary to establish if continuing symptoms are related to SUD or to comorbid ADHD or anxiety or mood disorders. Despite dearth of literature available CBT has proved to be effective in ADHD comorbid with SUD.

Multi systematic therapy (MST) is the family and community-based treatment. This therapy targets various particular factors such as attitudes peer pressure neighbourhood culture and associated problems such as serious antisocial behaviour in children and adolescents with ADHD who abuses drugs. Multi systematic therapy is based on nine principles that guide the assessment and intervention process. MST team aims to enhance the capacity of family members to track the behaviour of the patient and accordingly provide rewards for positive behaviour and punishments for negative or irresponsible behaviour. Therapists purely concentrate on parental skills and building natural support systems of families, friends, and community members. While working on strengths, therapists also address the obstructions to therapy (if any) such as parental substance use and conflict within family etc.

Brief strategic family therapy (BSFT) targets basically on family interactions that are thought to sustain or aggravate adolescent drug abuse and other problem behaviors that co-occur like oppositional behavior, law-breaking behaviour, associating with disruptive peers, antagonistic and violent behavior, and risky sexual behaviors etc. The main therapeutic techniques fall into 3 categories:

- The therapist initially joins the family by encouraging family members to behave as they normally would while the therapist is present
- Repetitive patterns of family interactions are determined
- Family dynamics are restructured to promote new, more adaptive patterns of interaction.

The primary goals of BSFT are to eliminate or reduce the adolescent' use of drugs and associated problem behaviours (symptom focus) and to change the family interactions that are associated with the adolescent' drug abuse (system focus). In addition to proven efficacy for drug abuse treatment for youths, BSFT is associated with high levels of engagement of family members and with improving conduct problems, delinquency, and family functioning.

Training Mindfulness

Mindfulness training is designed to improve mindful attention to one's own thoughts and actions, training individuals to focus on present and to inhibit distracting thoughts and stimuli. It usually includes mindful meditation, it's a cognitive-based therapy. Mindfulness training seems to be connected with increased grey matter volume in the hippocampus and changes in the structure of amygdala, as shown by neuroimaging studies. ADHD symptoms like hyperactivity/impulsivity and attention problems, emotional dis-regulation, etc. have been found to be reduced by this training, while boosting self-directedness and self-regulation. Children, adolescents and adults with ADHD have been reported to benefit, in terms of starting and maintaining improvements in mood, anxiety, and social behavior due to its practice. Parents may also benefit from mindfulness by using it to improve their interactions with their children with ADHD.

What can be Done at Home?

Development of planning and organizational skills may be required to improve functioning within unstructured environments like social situations, extracurricular activities, home life, etc., which is generally found to be sub-optimal in individuals with ADHD. Lacking these skills can lead to feeling overwhelmed, followed by stress, anger, panic, frustration, losing self-esteem, dysfunction and significant relationship conflicts, etc. Encouraging a structured lifestyle can promote organized, predictable, consistent and calm relationships, leading to positive outcomes. Introducing an external structure and modelling expected behaviors is crucial for improved self-esteem, self-control and harmonious relationships. An important point to note is that some families may create such a structural environment easier than others as ADHD can be multi-generational.

Inspire Hope

Informing families about existence of evidence-based treatments and interventions, will fetch a positive response. Hence eventually promoting a concrete therapeutic alliance and generating favourable results.

Motivate, Guide and Encourage

The process of assessment may turn out to be excessively negative experience for some, as areas of difficulties are the primary focus in it. This can be alleviated by identifying strengths and following up during the assessment process. Families and individuals can be encouraged to promote strengths and talents like creative skills in the field of music, drama, arts, etc. Encouragement can be in the form of attending their games, performance, recitals, hanging their art or trophies, basically expressing interest in their children's achievements. Therapeutic intervention could use leveraging of their existing strengths and talents for preventing the process from becoming negative.

Express sensitivity to all cultures and genders

ADHD and its treatment is perceived differently among different ethnicities, cultures and genders. For example, ADHD has stigma associated with it in certain cultures and is seen in a negative light. Clarifying and explaining ADHD with sensitivity, in such circumstances is especially pivotal.

Encourage a Balanced lifestyle

Individuals with ADHD comorbid SUD need encouragement towards a balanced and healthy lifestyle as they tend to struggle with their basic needs like eating, personal hygiene, sleep, etc. Healthy habits and routines like regular exercise, consistent sleep hygiene, nutritious food consumption, etc. can be advised by the clinician, leading patients to prioritize "self-care". Regular exercise specifically decreases stress and frustration, increases endorphins, uplifts mood, improves focus and cognitive clarity and leads to an overall sense of well-being. Core symptoms of ADHD commonly comorbid with anxiety/ SUD have been proven to be reduced with aerobic exercises.

FUTURE DIRECTION

The problem of substance abuse in the ADHD population is rising and tendency to use newer psychoactive substances including inhalants and synthetically produced substances. The need for novel kick or high is worrisome and needs further research with appropriate intervention strategies. The uniqueness of this population with special needs considering their externalizing behaviour and traits needs to be addressed accordingly.

REFERENCES

ADHD Resource Center. (n.d.). *American Academy of Child & Adolescent Psychiatry website.* Available at http://www.aacap.org/AACAP/Families%5Fand%5FYouth/Resource%5FCenters/ADHD%5FResource%5FCenter/Home.aspx

Anker, E., Bendiksen, B., & Heir, T. (2018). Comorbid psychiatric disorders in a clinical sample of adults with ADHD, and associations with education, work and social characteristics: A cross-sectional study. *BMJ Open*, *8*(3), e019700. doi:10.1136/bmjopen-2017-019700 PMID:29500213

Assessing adults with ADHD and comorbidities. (2009). *Primary care companion to the Journal of Clinical Psychiatry, 11*(1), 25. doi:10.4088/pcc.7129bs4c

Attention-deficit hyperactivity disorder (ADHD) in children and adolescents. (n.d.). EBSCO DynaMed Plus website. Available at: https://www.dynamed.com/topics/dmp~AN~T113926/Attention-deficit-hyperactivity-disorder-ADHD-in-children-and-adolescents

Banerjee, T. D., Middleton, F., & Faraone, S. V. (2007). Environmental risk factors for attention-deficit hyperactivity disorder. *Acta Paediatrica (Oslo, Norway), 296*(9), 1269–1274. doi:10.1111/j.1651-2227.2007.00430.x PMID:17718779

Besag, F., Gobbi, G., Aldenkamp, A., Caplan, R., Dunn, D. W., & Sillanpää, M. (2016). Psychiatric and Behavioural Disorders in Children with Epilepsy (ILAE Task Force Report): Behavioural and psychiatric disorders associated with childhood epilepsy syndromes. *Epileptic Disorders*. Advance online publication. doi:10.1684/epd.2016.0815 PMID:27184676

Biederman, J., Newcorn, J., & Sprich, S. (1991). Comorbidity of attention deficit hyperactivity disorder with conduct, depressive, anxiety, and other disorders. *The American Journal of Psychiatry*, *148*(5), 564–577. doi:10.1176/ajp.148.5.564 PMID:2018156

Bögels, S., Hoogstad, B., van Dun, L., de Schutter, S., & Restifo, K. (2008). Mindfulness training for adolescents with externalizing disorders and their parents. *Behavioural and Cognitive Psychotherapy*, *36*(2), 193–209. doi:10.1017/S1352465808004190

Brikell, I., Ghirardi, L., D'Onofrio, B. M., Dunn, D. W., Almqvist, C., Dalsgaard, S., Kuja-Halkola, R., & Larsson, H. (2018). Familial Liability to Epilepsy and Attention-Deficit/Hyperactivity Disorder: A Nationwide Cohort Study. *Biological Psychiatry*, *83*(2), 173–180. doi:10.1016/j.biopsych.2017.08.006 PMID:28950988

Brookes, K. J., Mill, J., Guindalini, C., Curran, S., Xu, X., Knight, J., Chen, C.-K., Huang, Y.-S., Sethna, V., Taylor, E., Chen, W., Breen, G., & Asherson, P. (2006). A common haplotype of the dopamine transporter gene associated with attention-deficit/hyperactivity disorder and interacting with maternal use of alcohol during pregnancy. *Archives of General Psychiatry*, *63*(1), 74–81. doi:10.1001/archpsyc.63.1.74 PMID:16389200

Bukstein, O. G. (2012). Attention Deficit Hyperactivity Disorder and Substance Use Disorders. In C. Stanford & R. Tannock (Eds.), *Behavioral Neuroscience of Attention Deficit Hyperactivity Disorder and Its Treatment, Current Topics in Behavioral Neurosciences 9* (pp. 145–172). Springer-Verlag Berlin Heidelberg.

Burton, K., Rogathe, J., Hunter, E., Burton, M., Swai, M., Todd, J., Neville, B., Walker, R., & Newton, C. (2011). Behavioural comorbidity in Tanzanian children with epilepsy: A community-based case-control study. *Developmental Medicine and Child Neurology*, *53*(12), 1135–1142. doi:10.1111/j.1469-8749.2011.04109.x PMID:22092080

Cantwell, D. P. (1996). Attention deficit disorder: A review of the past 10 years. *Journal of the American Academy of Child and Adolescent Psychiatry*, *35*(8), 978–987. doi:10.1097/00004583-199608000-00008 PMID:8755794

Capusan, A. J., Bendtsen, P., Marteinsdottir, I., Kuja-Halkola, R., & Larsson, H. (2015). Genetic and environmental contributions to the association between attention deficit hyperactivity disorder and alcohol dependence in adulthood: A large population-based twin study. *Neuropsychiatric Genetics*, Part *B* of the *American Journal* of Medical. *Genetics*, *168*, 414–422. PMID:25711682

Carroll, K. M., & Rounsaville, B. J. (1993). History and significance of childhood attention deficit disorder in treatment-seeking cocaine abusers. *Comprehensive Psychiatry*, *34*(2), 75–82. doi:10.1016/0010-440X(93)90050-E PMID:8485984

Charach, A., Yeung, E., Climans, T., & Lillie, E. (2011). Childhood attention-deficit/hyperactivity disorder and future substance-use disorders: Comparative meta-analyses. *Journal of the American Academy of Child and Adolescent Psychiatry*, *50*(1), 9–21. doi:10.1016/j.jaac.2010.09.019 PMID:21156266

Chidi, I. R., Chidi, N. A., Ebele, A. A., & Chinyelu, O. N. (2014). Co-Morbidity of attention deficit Hyperactivity Disorder (ADHD) and epilepsy In children seen In University of Nigeria Teaching Hospital Enugu: Prevalence, Clinical and social correlates. *The Nigerian Postgraduate Medical Journal*, *21*, 273–278. PMID:25633443

Chiodo, L. M., Jacobson, S. W., & Jacobson, J. L. (2004). Neurodevelopmental effects of postnatal lead exposure at very low levels. *Neurotoxicology and Teratology*, *26*(3), 359–371. doi:10.1016/j.ntt.2004.01.010 PMID:15113598

D'Agati, E., Curatolo, P., & Mazzone, L. (2019). Comorbidity between ADHD and anxiety disorders across the lifespan. *International Journal of Psychiatry in Clinical Practice*, *23*(4), 238–244. doi:10.1080/13651501.2019.1628277 PMID:31232613

Darke, S., Baker, A., Dixon, J., Wodak, A., & Heather, N. (1992). Drug use and HIV risk taking behaviour among clients in methadone maintenance treatment. *Drug and Alcohol Dependence*, *29*(3), 263–268. doi:10.1016/0376-8716(92)90101-H PMID:1559433

Datta, S. S., Premkumar, T. S., Fielding, S., Chandy, S., Kumar, S., Eagles, J., & Cherian, A. (2006). Impact of pediatric epilepsy on Indian families: Influence of psychopathology and seizure related variables. *Epilepsy & Behavior*, *9*(1), 145–151. doi:10.1016/j.yebeh.2006.04.011 PMID:16725375

Dennis, M., Godley, S. H., Diamond, G., Tims, F. M., Babor, T., Donaldson, J., Liddle, H., Titus, J. C., Kaminer, Y., Webb, C., Hamilton, N., & Funk, R. (2004). The Cannabis Youth Treatment (CYT) Study: Main findings from two randomized trials. *Journal of Substance Abuse Treatment*, *27*(3), 197–213. doi:10.1016/j.jsat.2003.09.005 PMID:15501373

Dunn, D. W., & Kronenberger, W. G. (2005). Childhood epilepsy, attention problems, and ADHD: Review and practical considerations. *Seminars in Pediatric Neurology*, *12*(4), 222–228. doi:10.1016/j.spen.2005.12.004 PMID:16780293

Evren, C. (2018). Comorbidity of attention deficit-hyperactivity disorder and substance use disorder. *Dusunen Adam The Journal of Psychiatry and Neurological Sciences*, *31*, 115–124. doi:10.5350/DAJPN20183102001

Evren, C., Dalbudak, E., Evren, B., Can, Y., & Umut, G. (2014). The severity of attention deficit hyperactivity symptoms and its relationship with lifetime substance use and psychological variables among 10th grade students in Istanbul. *Comprehensive Psychiatry*, *55*(7), 1665–1670. doi:10.1016/j.comppsych.2014.06.002 PMID:25015303

Faraone, S. V., & Biederman, J. (1997). Do attention deficit hyperactivity disorder and major depression share familial risk factors? *The Journal of Nervous and Mental Disease*, *185*(9), 533–541. doi:10.1097/00005053-199709000-00001 PMID:9307614

Fernandez, T. V., Gupta, A., & Hoffman, E. H. (2017). Assessing risk: gene discovery. In A. Martin, F. R. Volkmar, & M. H. Bloch (Eds.), *Lewis's Child and Adolescent Psychiatry: A Comprehensive Textbook* (pp. 246–261). Wolters Kluwer Health.

Friedrichs, B., Igl, W., Larsson, H., & Larsson, J.-O. (2012). Coexisting psychiatric problems and stressful life events in adults with symptoms of ADHD–a large Swedish population-based study of twins. *Journal of Attention Disorders, 16*(1), 13–22. doi:10.1177/1087054710376909 PMID:20686099

Frodl, T. (2012). Comorbidity of ADHD and Substance Use Disorder (SUD): A neuroimaging perspective. *Journal of Attention Disorders, 14*(2), 109–120. doi:10.1177/1087054710365054 PMID:20495160

Froehlich, T. E., Lanphear, B. P., Auinger, P., Hornung, R., Epstein, J. N., Braun, J., & Kahn, R. S. (2009). Association of tobacco and lead exposures with attention-deficit/hyperactivity disorder. *Pediatrics, 124*(6), e1054–e1063. doi:10.1542/peds.2009-0738 PMID:19933729

Galéra, C., Côté, S. M., & Bouvard, M. P. (2011). Early risk factors for hyperactivity-impulsivity and inattention trajectories from age 17 months to 8 years. *Archives of General Psychiatry, 68*(12), 1267–1275. doi:10.1001/archgenpsychiatry.2011.138 PMID:22147844

Grizenko, N., Fortier, M. E., & Zadorozny, C. (2012). Maternal stress during pregnancy, ADHD symptomatology in children and genotype: Gene-environment interaction. *Journal of the Canadian Academy of Child and Adolescent Psychiatry, 21*, 9–15. PMID:22299010

Grohol, J. (2020). Causes & Risk Factors of Childhood ADHD. *Psych Central*. Retrieved on May 3, 2020, from https://psychcentral.com/childhood-adhd/causes-risk-factors-of-childhood-adhd/

Gul, H., Solmaz, Y. Y., Gul, E., & Oner, O. (2018). Facebook overuse and addiction among Turkish adolescents: Are ADHD and ADHD-related problems risk factors? *Psychiatry and Clinical Psychopharmacology, 28*(1), 80–90. doi:10.1080/24750573.2017.1383706

Haworth, C. M. A., Wright, M. J., Luciano, M., Martin, N. G., de Geus, E. J. C., van Beijsterveldt, C. E. M., Bartels, M., Posthuma, D., Boomsma, D. I., Davis, O. S. P., Kovas, Y., Corley, R. P., DeFries, J. C., Hewitt, J. K., Olson, R. K., Rhea, S.-A., Wadsworth, S. J., Iacono, W. G., McGue, M., ... Plomin, R. (2010). The herita- bility of general cognitive ability increases linearly from childhood to young adulthood. *Molecular Psychiatry, 15*(11), 1112–1120. doi:10.1038/mp.2009.55 PMID:19488046

Heinonen, K., Räikkönen, K., Pesonen, A. K., Andersson, S., Kajantie, E., Eriksson, J. G., Wolke, D., & Lano, A. (2010). Behavioural symptoms of attention deficit/hyperactivity disorder in preterm and term children born small and appropriate for gestational age: A longitudinal study. *BMC Pediatrics, 10*(1), 91. doi:10.1186/1471-2431-10-91 PMID:21159164

Hjern, A., Weitoft, G. R., & Lindblad, F. (2010). Social adversity predicts ADHD-medication in school children–a national cohort study. *Acta Paediatrica (Oslo, Norway), 99*(6), 920–924. doi:10.1111/j.1651-2227.2009.01638.x PMID:20002622

Hultman, C. M., Torrång, A., Tuvblad, C., Cnattingius, S., Larsson, J. O., & Lichtenstein, P. (2007). Birth weight and attention-deficit/hyperactivity symptoms in childhood and early adolescence: A prospective Swedish twin study. *Journal of the American Academy of Child and Adolescent Psychiatry, 46*(3), 370–377. doi:10.1097/01.chi.0000246059.62706.22 PMID:17314723

Jacob, C. P., Nguyen, T. T., Dempfle, A., Heine, M., Windemuth-Kieselbach, C., Baumann, K., Jacob, F., Prechtl, J., Wittlich, M., Herrmann, M. J., Gross-Lesch, S., Lesch, K.-P., & Reif, A. (2010). A gene-environment investigation on personality traits in two independent clinical sets of adult patients with personality disorder and attention deficit/hyperactive disorder. *European Archives of Psychiatry and Clinical Neuroscience*, *260*(4), 317–326. doi:10.100700406-009-0079-0 PMID:19894072

Kahn, R. S., Khoury, J., Nichols, W. C., & Lanphear, B. P. (2003). Role of dopamine transporter genotype and maternal prenatal smoking in childhood hyperactive-impulsive, inattentive, and oppositional behaviors. *The Journal of Pediatrics*, *143*(1), 104–110. doi:10.1016/S0022-3476(03)00208-7 PMID:12915833

Kaplan & Sadock. (2007). *Kaplan & Sadock's Synopsis of Psychiatry: Behavioral Sciences/clinical Psychiatry* (10th ed.). Wolter Kluwer/Lippincott Williams & Wilkins.

Katzman, M. A., Bilkey, T. S., Chokka, P. R., Fallu, A., & Klassen, L. J. (2017). Adult ADHD and comorbid disorders: Clinical implications of a dimensional approach. *BMC Psychiatry*, *17*(1), 302. doi:10.118612888-017-1463-3 PMID:28830387

Kelly, T. M., Cornelius, J. R., & Clark, D. B. (2004). Psychiatric disorders and attempted suicide among adolescents with substance use disorders. *Drug and Alcohol Dependence*, *73*(1), 87–97. doi:10.1016/j.drugalcdep.2003.10.004 PMID:14687963

Kelly, T. M., Cornelius, J. R., & Clark, D. B. (2004). Psychiatric disorders and attempted suicide among adolescents with substance use disorders. *Drug and Alcohol Dependence*, *73*(1), 87–97. doi:10.1016/j.drugalcdep.2003.10.004 PMID:14687963

Kessler, R. C., Adler, L., Barkley, R., Biederman, J., Conners, C. K., Demler, O., Faraone, S. V., Greenhill, L. L., Howes, M. J., Secnik, K., Spencer, T., Ustun, T. B., Walters, E. E., & Zaslavsky, A. M. (2006). The prevalence and correlates of adult ADHD in the United States: Results from the National Comorbidity Survey Replication. *The American Journal of Psychiatry*, *163*(4), 716–723. doi:10.1176/ajp.2006.163.4.716 PMID:16585449

Kim, H. W., Cho, S. C., Kim, B. N., Kim, J. W., Shin, M. S., & Kim, Y. (2009). Perinatal and familial risk factors are associated with full syndrome and subthreshold attention-deficit hyperactivity disorder in a Korean community sample. *Psychiatry Investigation*, *6*(4), 278–285. doi:10.4306/pi.2009.6.4.278 PMID:20140126

Konstenius, M., Jayaram-Lindström, N., Beck, O., & Franck, J. (2010). Sustained release methylphenidate for the treatment of ADHD in amphetamine abusers: A pilot study. *Drug and Alcohol Dependence*, *108*(1-2), 130–133. doi:10.1016/j.drugalcdep.2009.11.006 PMID:20015599

Krisanaprakornkit, T., Ngamjarus, C., Witoonchart, C., & Piyavhatkul, N. (2010). Meditation therapies for attention-deficit/hyperactivity disorder (ADHD). *Cochrane Database of Systematic Reviews*, (6), CD006507. doi:10.1002/14651858.CD006507.pub2 PMID:20556767

Langer, N., Benjamin, C., Becker, B. L., & Gaab, N. (2019). Comorbidity of reading disabilities and ADHD: Structural and functional brain characteristics. *Human Brain Mapping*, *40*(9), 2677–2698. doi:10.1002/hbm.24552 PMID:30784139

Langley, K., Holmans, P. A., van den Bree, M. B., & Thapar, A. (2007). Effects of low birth weight, maternal smoking in pregnancy and social class on the phenotypic manifestation of attention deficit hyperactivity disorder and associated antisocial behaviour: Investigation in a clinical sample. *BMC Psychiatry*, *7*(1), 26. doi:10.1186/1471-244X-7-26 PMID:17584500

Lara, C., Fayyad, J., De Graaf, R., Kessler, R. C., Aguilar-Gaxiola, S., Angermeyer, M., Demytteneare, K., de Girolamo, G., Haro, J. M., Jin, R., Karam, E. G., Lépine, J.-P., Mora, M. E. M., Ormel, J., Posada-Villa, J., & Sampson, N. (2009). Childhood predictors of adult attention-deficit/hyperactivity disorder: Results from the World Health Organization World Mental Health Survey Initiative. *Biological Psychiatry*, *65*(1), 46–54. doi:10.1016/j.biopsych.2008.10.005 PMID:19006789

Levin, F. R., & Kleber, H. D. (1995). Attention-deficit hyperactivity disorder and substance abuse: Relationships and implications for treatment. *Harvard Review of Psychiatry*, *2*(5), 246–258. doi:10.3109/10673229509017144 PMID:9384909

Lewis, M. (2002). *Child and Adolescent Psychiatry: A Comprehensive Textbook* (3rd ed.). Lippincott Williams & Wilkins.

Mandal, A. M. (2019, February 26). *ADHD Causes and Risk factors. News-Medical.* Retrieved on May 03, 2020 from https://www.news-medical.net/health/ADHD-Causes-and-Risk-factors.aspx

Martel, M. M., Nikolas, M., Jernigan, K., Friderici, K., Waldman, I., & Nigg, J. T. (2011). The dopamine receptor D4 gene (DRD4) moderates family environmental effects on ADHD. *Journal of Abnormal Child Psychology*, *39*(1), 1–10. doi:10.100710802-010-9439-5 PMID:20644990

Mikami, A. Y., Cox, D. J., Davis, M. T., Wilson, H. K., Merkel, R. L., & Burket, R. (2009). Sex differences in effectiveness of extended-release stimulant medication among adolescents with attention-deficit/hyperactivity disorder. *Journal of Clinical Psychology in Medical Settings*, *16*(3), 233–242. doi:10.100710880-009-9165-8 PMID:19418208

Mongia, M., & Hechtman, L. (2016). Attention-deficit hyperactivity disorder across the lifespan: Review of literature on cognitive behavior therapy. *Current Developmental Disorders Reports*, *3*(1), 7–14. doi:10.100740474-016-0072-z

Neuman, R. J., Lobos, E., Reich, W., Henderson, C. A., Sun, L.-W., & Todd, R. D. (2007). Prenatal smoking exposure and dopaminergic genotypes interact to cause a severe ADHD subtype. *Biological Psychiatry*, *61*(12), 1320–1328. doi:10.1016/j.biopsych.2006.08.049 PMID:17157268

Nikolas, M., Friderici, K., Waldman, I., Jernigan, K., & Nigg, J. T. (2010). Gene x environment interactions for ADHD: Synergistic effect of 5HTTLPR genotype and youth appraisals of inter-parental conflict. *Behavioral and Brain Functions*, *6*(1), 23. doi:10.1186/1744-9081-6-23 PMID:20398347

Pagán, C. N. (n.d.). *ADHD and Risky Behavior in Adults*. https://www.webmd.com/add-adhd/features/adhd-dangerous-risky-behavior#1

Palaniappan, P., Seshadri, S., Girimaji, S. C., & Srinath, S. (2013). Pattern of comorbidities in Indian children and adolescents with attention deficit hyperactivity disorder. *European Psychiatry*, *28*, 1. doi:10.1016/S0924-9338(13)77398-X

Philip, J., Patil, N. M., & Kamate, M. (2016). Attention-deficit hyperactivity disorder in children with idiopathic epilepsy: A cross-sectional study. *Indian Journal of Health Sciences and Biomedical Research, 9*(1), 31–34. doi:10.4103/2349-5006.183682

Pingali, S., & Sunderajan, J. (2014). A study of comorbidities in attention deficit hyperactivity disorder: A retrospective analysis of case records. *Andhra Pradesh Journal of Psychological Medicine, 15*(2), 206–210.

Polanczy, G., de Lima, M. S., Horta, B. L., Biederman, J., & Rohde, L. A. (2007). The worldwide prevalence of ADHD: A sys- tematic review and metaregression analysis. *The American Journal of Psychiatry, 164*(6), 942–948. doi:10.1176/ajp.2007.164.6.942 PMID:17541055

Reale, L., Bartoli, B., Cartabia, M., Zanetti, M., Costantino, M. A., Canevini, M. P., Termine, C., & Bonati, M. (2017). Comorbidity prevalence and treatment outcome in children and adolescents with ADHD. *European Child & Adolescent Psychiatry, 26*(12), 1443–1457. doi:10.100700787-017-1005-z PMID:28527021

Reinhardt, M. C., & Reinhardt, C. A. (2013). Attention deficit-hyperactivity disorder, comorbidities, and risk situations. *The Journal of Pediatrics, 89*(2), 124–130. doi:10.1016/j.jped.2013.03.015 PMID:23642421

Retz, W., Freitag, C. M., Retz-Junginger, P., Wenzler, D., Schneider, M., Kissling, C., Thome, J., & Rösler, M. (2008). A functional serotonin transporter promoter gene polymorphism increases ADHD symptoms in delinquents: Interaction with adverse childhood environment. *Psychiatry Research, 158*(2), 123–131. doi:10.1016/j.psychres.2007.05.004 PMID:18155777

Riggs, P. D., Winhusen, T., Davies, R. D., Leimberger, J. D., Mikulich-Gilbertson, S., Klein, C., Macdonald, M., Lohman, M., Bailey, G. L., Haynes, L., Jaffee, W. B., Haminton, N., Hodgkins, C., Whitmore, E., Trello-Rishel, K., Tamm, L., Acosta, M. C., Royer-Malvestuto, C., Subramaniam, G., ... Liu, D. (2011). Randomized controlled trial of osmotic-release methylphenidate with cognitive-behavioral therapy in adolescents with attention-deficit/ hyperactivity disorder and substance-use disorders. *Journal of the American Academy of Child and Adolescent Psychiatry, 50*(9), 903–914. doi:10.1016/j.jaac.2011.06.010 PMID:21871372

Rowland, A. S., Skipper, B. J., Rabiner, D. L., Qeadan, F., Campbell, R. A., Naftel, A. J., & Umbach, D. M. (2018). Attention-deficit/hyperactivity disorder (ADHD): Interaction between socioeconomic status and parental history of ADHD determines prevalence. *Journal of Child Psychology and Psychiatry, and Allied Disciplines, 59*(3), 213–222. doi:10.1111/jcpp.12775 PMID:28801917

Safren, S. A., Sprich, S., & Mimiaga, M. J. (2010). Cognitive behavioral therapy vs relaxation with educational support for medicationtreated adults with ADHD and persistent symptoms: A randomized controlled trial. *Journal of the American Medical Association, 304*(8), 875–880. doi:10.1001/jama.2010.1192 PMID:20736471

Sánchez-Mora, C., Richarte, V., & Garcia-Martínez, I. (2015). Dopamine receptor DRD4 gene and stressful life events in persistent attention deficit hyperactivity disorder. *Neuropsychiatric Genetics, Part B of the American Journal of Medical Genetics, 168*, 480-491.

Sander, J. W., & Shorvon, S. D. (1996). Epidemiology of the epilepsies. *Journal of Neurology, Neurosurgery, and Psychiatry, 61*(5), 433–443. doi:10.1136/jnnp.61.5.433 PMID:8965090

Slobodin, O., & Crunelle, C. L. (2019). Mini Review: Socio-Cultural Influences on the Link Between ADHD and SUD. *Frontiers in Public Health, 7*, 173. doi:10.3389/fpubh.2019.00173 PMID:31294015

Solanto, M. (2011). *Cognitive-Behavioral Therapy for Adult ADHD: Targeting Executive Dysfunction*. Guilford Press.

Spencer, T. J. (2006). ADHD and comorbidity in childhood. *The Journal of Clinical Psychiatry, 67*(8), 27–31. PMID:16961427

Srinivasaraghavan, R., Mahadevan, S., & Kattimani, S. (2013). Impact of Comorbidity on Three Month Follow-up Outcome of Children with ADHD in a Child Guidance Clinic: Preliminary Report. *Indian Journal of Psychological Medicine, 35*(4), 346–351. doi:10.4103/0253-7176.122223 PMID:24379493

Stormont-Spurgin, M., & Zentall, S. S. (1996). Child-rearing practices associated with aggression in youth with and without ADHD: An Exploratory Study. *International Journal of Disability Development and Education, 43*(2), 135–146. doi:10.1080/0156655960430204

Surkan, P. J., Zhang, A., Trachtenberg, F., Daniel, D., McKinlay, S., & Bellinger, D. (2007). Neuropsychological function in children with blood lead levels <10 microg/dL. *Neurotoxicology, 28*(6), 1170–1177. doi:10.1016/j.neuro.2007.07.007 PMID:17868887

Takahashi, K., Miyawaki, D., Suzuki, F., Mamoto, A., Matsushima, N., Tsuji, H., Horino, A., Ballas, P. A., & Kiriike, N. (2007). Hyperactivity and comorbidity in Japanese children with attention-deficit/hyperactivity disorder. *Psychiatry and Clinical Neurosciences, 61*(3), 255–262. doi:10.1111/j.1440-1819.2007.01651.x PMID:17472593

Thapar, A., Fowler, T., Rice, F., Scourfield, J., van den Bree, M., Thomas, H., Harold, G., & Hay, D. (2003). Maternal smoking during pregnancy and attention deficit hyperactivity disorder symptoms in offspring. *The American Journal of Psychiatry, 160*(11), 1985–1989. doi:10.1176/appi.ajp.160.11.1985 PMID:14594745

Understanding, A. D. H. D. (n.d.). *Information for parents. Healthy Children—American Academy of Pediatrics website*. Available at: https://www.healthychildren.org/English/health-issues/conditions/adhd/Pages/Understanding-ADHD.aspx

Van Emmerik-van Oortmerssen, K., van de Glind, G., van den Brink, W., Smit, F., Crunelle, C. L., Swets, M., & Schoevers, R. A. (2012). Prevalence of attention-deficit hyperactivity disorder in substance use disorder patients: A meta-analysis and meta-regression analysis. *Drug and Alcohol Dependence, 122*(1-2), 11–19. doi:10.1016/j.drugalcdep.2011.12.007 PMID:22209385

Van Emmerik-van Oortmerssen, K., Vedel, E., van den Brink, W., & Schoevers, R. A. (2015). Integrated cognitive behavioral therapy for patients with substance use disorder and comorbid ADHD: Two case presentations. *Addictive Behaviors, 45*, 214–217. doi:10.1016/j.addbeh.2015.01.040 PMID:25706067

Venkatesh, C., Ravikumar, T., Andal, A., & Virudhagirinathan, B. S. (2012). Attention-deficit/ Hyperactivity Disorder in Children: Clinical Profile and Co-morbidity. *Indian Journal of Psychological Medicine*, *34*(1), 34–38. doi:10.4103/0253-7176.96155 PMID:22661805

Wilens, T. E., & Morrison, N. R. (2012). Substance-use disorders in adolescents and adults with ADHD: Focus on treatment. *Neuropsychiatry*, *2*(4), 301–312. doi:10.2217/npy.12.39 PMID:23105949

Chapter 16
An Exploration of ADHD and Comorbidity With Substance Abuse and Brain Development:
Long-Term Impact of Methylphenidate on Adolescents

York Williams
West Chester University, USA

ABSTRACT

Methylphenidate (MPH) is the most commonly used drug to treat attention deficit/hyperactivity disorder (ADHD) in children effectively and safely. However, in spite of its widespread application throughout what is considered one of the most plastic and sensitive phases of brain development in children, very little is known to date about its long-term effects on brain structure and function leading well into later adolescence and adulthood. Additionally, there is scant information available to parents, clinicians, and clients with ADD/ADHD about the influence of MPH on brain development. More importantly, recent human and animal studies suggest that MPH alters the dopaminergic system with long-term effects beyond the termination of treatment. As such, a multimodal treatment with psychodynamic therapies can assist the treatment team to support the development of the client's pro-social skills in addition to medication treatment, thus reducing full reliance on MPH as the primary treatment for ADD/ADHD.

INTRODUCTION

Beiderman et al. (1995) maintains that the co-occurrence of attention deficit hyperactivity disorder (ADHD) and psychoactive substance use disorder has been reported in a variety of clinical and research settings and continues to be a focus of attention and controversy. Accordingly, studies have documented a higher than normal risk for psychoactive substance use disorders in adults who had ADHD as children (Hesson & Fowler, 2018; Kessler et al., 2006; Kooij, 2012; Mao & Findling, 2014; Moore, Sunjic, Kaye,

DOI: 10.4018/978-1-7998-5495-1.ch016

Archer, & Indig, 2016; Newcorn, Weiss, & Stein, 2007; Rucklidge, Downs-Woolley, Taylor, Brown, & Harrow, 2016). Similarly, studies of referred and non-referred adults with ADHD of childhood onset have documented the high risk for substance use disorders in these children becoming adults. Whether ADHD on comorbid disorders are risk factors for substance use disorders raises important clinical and scientific questions awaiting clarification given the use of one strong drug used to treat ADHD known as Methylphenidate (MPH). Another concern is raised in that MPH has been identified as the preferred treatment for youth and young adults with an ADHD, but more importantly impacts youth from culturally and linguistically diverse (CLD) backgrounds such African American and Latino males (DuPaul, Barklay & McMurray, 1994) who are already often over-identified in special education with this disability under the Individual Disability Education Act (IDEA, 2004). The use of MPH as the primary treatment for ADHD in children has also led to a concern about its impact on brain development in adolescents during this very critical stage of development (Breggin, 2001; Fitzgerald, 2009; Madhiraju, 2001).

This chapter examines various arguments around the use of MPH as these empirical based accounts provide both pros and cons that can assist the consumer (parent, therapist, teacher, medical doctor) in making informed decisions about the use of MPH in children, particularly adolescents during one of the most critical developmental periods of brain development which occurs between the ages of 12-21 years of age (Gaviria & Smith, 2001). Next, a comparative summary of the primary research utilized in this analysis is laid out so as provide an internal polemical argument. Following the summary, the author critiques the primary arguments provided by the authors of the studies with a conclusive summary based on the overall analysis.

Neurodevelopmental Disorders, ADHD and DSM-V

Neurodevelopmental disorders are disabilities associated primarily with the functioning of the neurological system and brain. Examples of neurodevelopmental disorders in children include attention-deficit/hyperactivity disorder (ADHD), autism, learning disabilities, intellectual disability (also formerly known as mental retardation), conduct disorders, cerebral palsy, and impairments in vision and hearing. Children with neurodevelopmental disorders can experience difficulties with language and speech, motor skills, behavior, memory, learning, or other neurological functions (America's Children and the Environment (ACE), 2015; Seligman & Reichenberg, 2016).

Neurodevelopmental disorders are disabilities associated primarily with the functioning of the neurological system and brain. Examples of neurodevelopmental disorders in children include attention-deficit/hyperactivity disorder (ADHD), autism, learning disabilities, intellectual disability (also known as mental retardation), conduct disorders, cerebral palsy, and impairments in vision and hearing. Children with neurodevelopmental disorders can experience difficulties with language and speech, motor skills, behavior, memory, learning, or other neurological functions.

Other disorders, including anxiety disorders, depression, and learning disabilities, can be expressed with signs and symptoms that resemble those of ADHD. A diagnosis of ADHD requires a certain amount of judgment on the part of a doctor, similar to diagnosis of other mental disorders. Despite the variability among children diagnosed with the disorder and the challenges involved in diagnosis, ADHD has good clinical validity, meaning that impaired children share similarities, exhibit symptoms, respond to treatment, and are recognized with general consistency across clinicians.

A great deal of research on ADHD has focused on aspects of brain functioning that are related to the behaviors associated with ADHD. Although this research is not definitive, it has found that children with

ADHD generally have trouble with certain skills involved in problem-solving (referred to collectively as executive function). These skills include working memory (keeping information in mind while briefly doing something else), planning (organizing a sequence of activities to complete a task), response inhibition (suppressing immediate responses when they are inappropriate), and cognitive flexibility (changing an approach when a situation changes). Children with ADHD also generally have problems in maintaining sustained attention to a task (referred to as vigilance), and/or maintaining readiness to respond to new information (referred to as alertness) (ACE, 2015; Seligman & Reichenberg, 2016).

Based on the types of symptoms, three kinds (presentations) of ADHD can occur: *Combined Presentation*: if enough symptoms of both criteria inattention and hyperactivity-impulsivity were present for the past 6 months; *Predominantly Inattentive Presentation*: if enough symptoms of inattention, but not hyperactivity-impulsivity, were present for the past six months and; *Predominantly Hyperactive-Impulsive Presentation*: if enough symptoms of hyperactivity-impulsivity but not inattention were present for the past six months. Because symptoms can change over time, the presentation may change over time as well. Seligman & Reichenberg (2016) note the special considerations for educators, parents and clinicians to consider when working with or evaluating students identified with an ADHD (Figure 1).

Figure 1. Illustrates the number of additional considerations for understanding ADHD

In Children must be distinguished from typical developmental milestones p. 50 (Symptoms often occur in pre-school)	DSM has expanded the setting requirements that require these symptoms to occur in two or more settings.	The symptoms may range from Mild, Moderate or Severe	If symptoms of ADHD cause clinically significant distress but do not meet the full criteria for a diagnosis, clinicians may use the "other" criteria for a diagnosis.	Co-Occurring disorders are found in as many as 50% of children
A Primary diagnosis of ASD or IDD can obscure or mask the diagnosis of ADHD (p.50).	Emotional problems and conduct problems are likely to be present in students with ADHD but should not construed to be interrelated to or a major part of behaviors exhibited by all students with an ADHD.	ADHD can also be distinguished from bipolar disorder or depressive disorder – based on the length of time of the major characteristics such as impulsive behavior, excessive movement and energy commonly associated with ADHD which are more continuous.	Children with an ADHD who may also have a SLD can be distinguished by the presence of ADHD symptoms and behavior outside of the presence of classroom instruction and learning. Untreated, ADHD may transition into behaviors associated with conduct disorder and ODD and in children can result in poor school outcomes, failures and drop-out.	Adults with ADHD are likely to exhibit poor work performance, multiple job changes, difficult taking direction from others, punctuality and failure to sustain efforts at work. An Adult diagnosis must contain at least five symptoms that manifested before the age of 12. Relationships also suffer due to one's poor self-regulation and self-discipline.

Since MPH is the most commonly used drug to treat attention deficit/hyperactivity disorder ADHD in children with a record of the most effective treatment to reduce the impact of executive dysfunction that accompanies this disease; most consumers seem to have very little regards for its safety and health risks in children's brain development (Breggin, 2001; Fitzgerald, 2009; Madhiraju, 2001). Additionally, the field of psychopharmacology and psychiatric medicine report limited studies regarding the long-term safety and health risks of such a powerful stimulant/drug on the minds and soma of youth (Fitzgerald, 2009). A case in point, very little seems to be known about the long term effects of treating children during adolescence with MPH and its long term effects on brain development and co-morbid substance abuse disorder (Gill at al., 2012). Studies note that in spite of its widespread application throughout one of the most plastic and sensitive phases of brain development, very little is known to date about how and to what degree MPH effects brain structure and function (Barbesi et al., 2002; Done and Nutt, 2005; Loureiro-Vieira, et al., 2017; Songura-Barke, 2005; Van der Marel et al., 2015). The author examined what long-term impact does the use of MPH have on overall brain development and substance abuse for children using the drug into adult-hood? This chapter outlines the use of MPH as the primary treatment in children identified with an ADHD that can lead to a substance abuse disorder and brain development problems (dual diagnosis) if not properly understood by the general educational, behavior health community.

MPH and Substance Abuse Linkages

Guevara et al. (2005) suggests that Attention-deficit/hyperactivity disorder (ADHD) is among the most prevalent behavioral conditions affecting school-age children in the U.S. Clinical practice guidelines endorsed by the American Academy of Pediatrics have recommended that practitioners collaborate with schools and mental health agencies to coordinate the care of children with ADHD. However, primary care practitioners may experience difficulty communicating with schools to obtain academic information or to solicit input on the effects of treatment regimens. Additionally, primary care practitioners may encounter problems making referrals to mental health providers or making contact with mental health providers to obtain consultation or to discuss treatment plans. Finally, managed care policies may contribute to this fragmentation by creating carve-out plans that limit communication between primary care practices and mental health agencies. To this end, the use of MPH is often prescribed for treating ADHD where parents, schools and pediatricians are not communicating about its short-term or long term effects on the health of children and without full knowledge that MPH is a strong drug with addictive qualities (Fitzgerald, 2009).

Amphetamine (MPH) is known to have many detrimental effects on users, including the potential for addictive behaviors. In the UK, widespread abuse of 'speed' in the 1960s prompted legislative changes to restrict its availability. More recently, the Health Education Authority has published a guide to drugs in which many adverse effects of amphetamines are listed. These adverse effects include lethargy, panic, tension and hyper-arousal (Anderson & Baldwin, 2000). The authors maintain that substance-related disorders (e.g. amphetamine addiction) was once located on Axis 1 under the previous DSM-IV. The addictive behaviors associated with MPH misuse can be damaging to the mental health of an individual (APA 1994). Ironically, childhood disorders such as ADD/ADHD are also considered a medical diagnosis in both DSM's (IV and V) previously located on Axis 1. According to the psychiatric orthodoxy, MPH is highly likely to be prescribed for ADD/ADHD, despite its known addictive properties. The use of MPH has also been used as the primary treatment for inattention and executive dysfunction which is a large part of the disorder in children that impacts learning under the IDEA (2004).

According to Scott (2011), attention and concentration appear to be simple concepts on the surface, but these appear to become more complex when one has to assess or differentiate among capacities (p. 149). The range of attention is related to behaviors that includes everything from autonomic and reflexive auditory and visual orientation, to sound and movement, in addition to being able to several stimuli simultaneously while alternating back and forth between competing stimuli (Scott, 2011; p. 149). As such, while broad in scope, the central components of attention entail orienting, selecting stimuli and maintenance for a necessary time for successful completion of a task (p. 149). Overall, the capacity to sustain and ignore competing stimuli is essential towards understanding what is central to this disorder. Scott maintains that attention is a prerequisite skill for accurate assessment of more complex neuropsychological functions. Damage to the frontal lobes may be most detrimental to attention skills. Finally, Scott maintains that attention should be assessed at multiple levels, from voluntary to alternating. Furthermore, attention and concentration deficits may compromise from virtually any region of the brain, but certain regions contribute different aspects of the attentional process (p. 150). Common features of this disease include inattention, hyperactivity and impulsivity, distractibility, over a period of at least six months and under the IDEA (part B), has an adverse impact on educational performance (ages 3-21). The clinical assessment of attention ranges from tasks requiring simple attentional capacities to complex attentional ones involving selecting, sustaining and alternating attention as well as inhibiting distraction or avoiding unwanted attentional switching to autonomic or overlearned processes (p. 154). There are challenges in assessment especially with respect to their occurrence during the assessment.

Substance Abuse Risks

Anderson and Baldwin argue that professionals disregard the fact that MPH is an amphetamine-like substance. Instead they continue to prescribe MPH, despite the obvious risks and dangers. Further, researchers have established that amphetamine users experience tolerance and dependence (Hesson & Fowler, 2018; Kessler et al., 2006; Kooij, 2012; Mao & Findling, 2014; Moore, Sunjic, Kaye, Archer, & Indig, 2016; Newcorn, Weiss, & Stein, 2007; Rucklidge, Downs-Woolley, Taylor, Brown, & Harrow, 2016). Overall, MPH is as addictive as amphetamine; it has essentially the same biochemical and physio logical properties. The authors contend that this drug choice used to treat ADHD in children is based on a conceptually weak and scientifically inconsistent basis and is overused as a prescription as a substance to minors that is likely to promote addiction as well as subsequent misuse. In conclusion, the biochemical properties of dextroamphetamine, amphetamine and methylphenidate are very similar, as all have high potential for addiction and subsequent misuse.

Morton and Stockton (2000) argue that as ADHD is more accurately diagnosed and treated appropriately with stimulant medication, there will be a continued increase in the amount of MPH prescribed and dispensed. Given this increasing number of patients receiving MPH and the increase of its availability, there is an increased potential for this medication to be abused by both adolescents and young adults (2000). Further, when MPH and cocaine are administered intravenously, their pharmacokinetics are quite similar. The authors noted that in a study referenced by Volkow, Wang & Gatley (1995) they found that the percentage of each drug taken up by the brain and their rates of uptake were parallel. However, the clearance from the brain of cocaine was faster than that of MPH. In addition, the receptor-binding affinities for cocaine and methylphenidate were reportedly similar at the dopamine transporter in the basal ganglia and the striatum. Intravenous methylphenidate reached peak concentrations in the basal ganglia in 8 to 15 minutes, whereas the associated "high" feeling peaked in 1 to 3 minutes.

MPH and Brain Development in Adolescents

Methylphenidate has been recognized as one of the most commonly used drug to treat attention deficit/hyperactivity disorder (ADHD) in children effectively and safely. However, Grund et al., (2006) suggest that despite its widespread application and use given research on its safety, very little remains to be known about its long term effects on the brain development, in particular that of children. However, the authors resolve that MPH is only given to children with clear ADHD symptomatology leading to psychosocial impairment. Grund et al., maintain that childhood and adolescence are a highly plastic and sensitive period of brain maturation, during which environmental and pharmacological influences exert strong effects on neural structure and function (p. 2). During this period of development, cognitive, motivational and emotional functions mature intensively. Such functions are sub served by brain areas that are characterized by a selective innervation of dopamine (DA), i.e. the prefrontal cortex (PFC), nucleus accumbens (NAc) and amygdala (p. 2). Grund et al., suggests that it is known that neurotransmitters and their agonists exert a strong morphogenetic influence on single neurons and nervous tissues.

The authors studied long-term plastic effects of MPH in a model of hyperkinetic behavior that bears some resemblance to ADHD, i.e. gerbils after an early traumatic experience. A single dose of MPH was administered to young adult gerbils in the study. Two control groups were taken, one being left undisturbed, whereas the other received water. The increased DA fiber density found in the basolateral amygdala of MPH-treated MA-intoxicated gerbils is a first hint that MPH affects neural systems beyond PFC and NAc. It corresponds to further results from the above mentioned behavior study showing that MPH-treated rats respond stronger to aversive situations and show more anxiety-like behavior. Orally taken, MPH has no abuse potential because of its slow increase of the plasma level, while a "high. The authors note that the results demonstrate that by i.p. application, MPH can indeed impair the postnatal maturation of DA fibers in the ventral striatum (p. 10). Accordingly, the study noted that in patients with ADHD, MPH simultaneously compensates a prefrontal DA hypofunction and probably restrains an accumbal DA hyperfunction in the long run. Grund et al., concluded that what must be deduced from the study with caution is that both the DA innervation and the behavioral function of the amygdala are altered by MPH, making animals more fearful and sensitive to stressful stimuli, but also resolve that more investigation is warranted since this study focused on animals and not humans.

According to dela Pena at al., (2013), brain development-associated genes mediate the reinforcing effects of MPH, amphetamine, and methylphenidate and that these transcripts may underlie susceptibility to psychostimulant addiction. This may have implications for long-term use in adolescents undergoing rapid brain development during the middle stages of adolescent development (McMahan, 2009). Drug treatment (twice daily, intraperitoneal [i.p.]) commenced when rats in this study were 6 weeks old and lasted for7days. The rats were divided into two groups: (cohort 1) four groups of rats (n=12 rats per group) administered saline only (1 mg/kg, i.p., "drugnaive" rats) and (cohort 2) three groups of rats administered either methamphetamine, amphetamine, or MPH (5 mg/kg, i.p., "drug-pretreated"). Conditioned Placed Preference ("CPP") tests were conducted a day after the last drug or saline administration and the tests were performed in a two-compartment place preference apparatus. Animal movement and behavior were video recorded and analyzed using the Ethovision (Noldus, Netherlands) system. According to Ike et al., (2013), the rats that demonstrated robust CPP to the drugs were used for further tests (n=6–8 rats per group). The authors reported that a meta-analysis was conducted to identify similar gene expression profiles influencing behavioral responses to psychostimulants and other drugs of abuse (p. 403).

The reported results demonstrated that enhanced MPH and MPH-induced CPP in rats pre-exposed to psychostimulants. The two-way ANOVA conducted on these data revealed significant effects of pretreatment (p. 403). Six rats from the saline-treated groups were also used as controls and results demonstrated enhanced methamphetamine and amphetamine self-administration in rats pre-exposed to psychostimulants. The rats acquired stable stimulant self-administration based on more numerous responses made on the active vs. the inactive lever. The responses of saline-treated rats via self-administered saline also showed as a control for general activity. A two-way ANOVA indicated that the MPH pretreated rats obtained more MPH infusions than the drugnaïve rats. In conclusion, stimulant pretreatment increased CPP and/or enhanced self-administration of these drugs, indicating the occurrence of behavioral sensitization, a phenomenon associated with enhanced behavioral response to repeated treatment of addictive drugs.

Critical Analysis

Upadhyaya (2008) maintains that ADHD is frequently comorbid with substance use disorder (SUD) associated with alcohol, tobacco, and other drugs. Most drug use and SUD originate in adolescence or even in childhood. Substance use disorder is thus being increasingly conceptualized as a developmental disorder, as is ADHD, indicating that the earlier in the course of these disorders that treatment is initiated, the more successful the outcome, but there needs to be more understanding of treating this disorder with MPH (2008).

Grund et al., concluded that both the DA innervation and the behavioral function of the amygdala are altered by MPH which makes the case that in lab rat studies, conclusively, there is some impact on brain functioning. This is important since the amygdala is a part of the limbic system within the brain, which is responsible for emotions, survival instincts, and memory. Memory and emotionality are important developmental milestones in children, in which, if not fully developed will have implications on overall functioning into adulthood. However, Grund et al., report multiple contradictions in their research that require additional follow up, especially the impact they note around neurotoxicity using MPH as one treatment option for ADHD in teens.

Similarly, dela Pena et. al., (2013) noted that increased CPP and/or enhanced self-administration of stimulants used in the study increased the behavioral sensitization - a phenomenon associated with enhanced behavioral response to repeated treatment of addictive drugs. This is important since prolonged use of the medication is noted to have deleterious effects on overall functioning of youth, but if during the developmental period youth are exposed to this drug, their developing organs may yearn for more of it and as a result, act as a gateway drug making them vulnerable to addiction or a search for harder drugs. This is a call for observation and mixed treatments including the use of self-regulation and therapy (Preston et al., 2017).

Finally, Bethancourt et al. (2009) noted that although there was no significant effect of MPH treatment on body weight and reaction to various measures under treatment in their study; that the effects of MPH vary across hippocampal-sensitive tasks. This means that instead of the research academy looking for one-way effects, that there may be a need for more study to determine how and to what degree MPH effects hippocampal sensitive tasks which are associated mainly with memory, in particular long-term memory and its addictive risks in teens leading to adulthood. Youth who develop with memory issues have a hard time in learning new material and retrieving what does make it to LTM so that it can be utilized in future learning tasks (Preston et al., 2017). What must be reconciled however, is the various tasks that are impacted by MPH and as the authors note, the MPH associated effects on cognitive processes and the consequences of conducting extensive drug treatment during particular developmental stages that make youth more vulnerable than others under the use of this drug used to treat ADHD. The authors do resolve that understanding these effects may lead to better practices related to stimulant treatment in children (Bethancourt, 2009; p. 56).

Dual Treatment Options:

Behavior Therapy, Cognitive Behavioral Therapy (CBT) and Client Centered Therapy (CCT)

According to Corey (2017), contemporary behavior therapy can be understood by considering four major areas of development: (1) classical conditioning, (2) operant conditioning, (3) social learning theory, and (4) cognitive behavior therapy.

Classical conditioning refers to what happens prior to learning that creates a response through pairing. Operant conditioning involves a type of learning in which behaviors are influenced mainly by the consequences that follow them. Social learning and cognitive theory involves a triadic reciprocal interaction among the environment, personal factors (beliefs, preferences, expectations, self-perceptions, and interpretations), and individual behavior. Finally, CBT encompasses a number of techniques, particularly those developed within the last three decades that emphasize cognitive processes that involve private events such as the client's self-talk as mediators of behavior change (Corey, 2017).

The basic process within the functional assessment model entails behavioral analysis used to identify the phenomenon that is maintaining conditions by systematically gathering information about situational antecedents, the dimensions of the problem behavior, and the consequences of the problem. This is known as the ABC model, which addresses antecedents, behaviors, and consequences. Corey notes that this model of behavior suggests that behavior (B) is influenced by some particular events that precede it, called antecedents (A), and by certain events that follow it called consequences (C). Antecedent events are ones that cue or elicit a certain behavior. Additionally, an assessment interview allows the therapist's to identify the particular antecedent and consequent events that influence or are functionally related to an individual's behavior.

Self-modification strategies include self-monitoring, self-reward, self-contracting, stimulus control, and self-as-model. The basic idea of self-modification assessments and interventions is that change can be brought about by teaching people to use coping skills in problematic situations. Generalization and maintenance of the outcomes are enhanced by encouraging clients to accept the responsibility for carrying out these strategies in daily life. To generalize means to practice those same skills learned in a different setting in all appropriate ones. Maintenance means to tune-up and manage how those skills are being utilized. These tools can support the learner with inattention, self-regulation deficits and clinical depression while at the same time balancing out the medication treatments that go along with supporting clients with an ADD or ADHD. Cognitive Behavior Therapy has also become a popular therapeutic intervention used as a part of a multi-modal treatment for clients experiencing ADD/ADHD.

Cognitive Behavior Therapy ("CBT") has become one of the most widely used psychological interventions used to treat children who exhibit social emotional and behavior disorders. Additionally, CBT has become one of the better researched alternatives to psychotherapy for treating school aged youth who present with disturbances that impact their schooling and major life activities (Seligman and Ollendick, 2011). According to Hofman et al. (2012) years of research confirm the positive effects of CBT and demonstrate significant reductions in a variety of child and adolescent emotional and behavioral problems. However, the Client Centered Therapeutic ("CCT") approach has been regarded as one of the most effective forms of client to therapist interventions because it is only in trust and reciprocity that clients, especially children, can open up and learn.

In contrast, from a Rogerian perspective, humans have an innate ability to know what they need and what is essential for a fulfilling life (Joseph & Linley, 2004). In a more cohesive sense, it is the fully functioning person that can obtain balance and happiness. For students who present with cognitive and behavior needs, self-actualization and efficacy become critical to their development. The good life, the good student is based on the schema of a fully functioning child who feels secure and understands how his or her environment supports their development (Patterson and Joseph, 2007). As a special education professional I maintain that both CBT and CCT can be utilized as one combined theoretical tool to assist students that I work with to make meaning of their behavior and learning challenges and to develop the tools required to engage more fully in life, school and with family.

The framework for CBT is broad and comprehensive. According to Herbert and Foreman (2012), various theories, principles, models, and techniques fall under the general rubric of CBT, and these approaches have been applied to the full range of human experience, from the assessment and treatment of severe psychopathology and profound developmental delays to primary prevention efforts to enhancing peak performance among athletes. More contemporary CBT therapists often focus on the present rather than the past in order to emphasize continuity with a theoretical explanation interwoven with a strategy to ground the persons' experiences and concerns into a more manageable program based on basic learning principles.

However, clinicians working with clients with an ADD/ADHD need to understand the variables that impact executive functioning and the importance of developing an internal lens that can assist them with better understanding how they engage and learn which is an integral part of the CCT approach. Additionally, coupled with a Rogerian lens clinicians can assist clients to know themselves in order to apply

Figure 2. above illustrates the use clinical therapeutic approaches as a multimodal treatment with any medication utilizing MPH

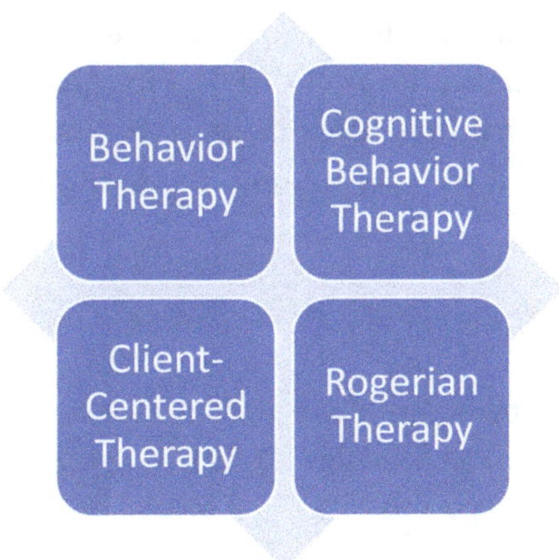

self-help strategies. Based on the primary tenets of CCT, the narrow goals focus on increasing one's self-esteem and openness to diverse experiences. Rogers posits that the congruent therapist is one who provides unconditional positive regard and empathy that can stimulate change in a vulnerable person to become a creative, responsible, developing individual. In the Rogerian tradition (Rogers, 1940) this framework entails important elements of leading the client to the point of positionality which focuses on his or her ability to develop the skills necessary to address their inner feelings, growing tensions, anxieties and struggles through self-acceptance. Here, given a more paradigmatic shift, the two therapies can be integrated with the focus on helping clients with an ADD/ADHD to help themselves in addition to any medication so as to reduce the dependence on same, and to avoid the vicious cycle associated with risks of drug dependency on associated MPH.

CONCLUSION

In conclusion, the research confirms the importance of my research question: *what long-term impact does the use of MPH have on overall brain development and substance abuse for children using the drug into adult-hood?* The primary studies cited here maintain impacts on: (a) the brain functioning; (b) emotions; (c) memory; (d) behavior sensitization related to drug addiction and; (e) various hippocampal sensitive tasks (STM and LTM). As such, it is critical as noted within the articles cited herein that more study is necessary in order to better treat children under the care of stimulants since these drugs appear to have serious implications for dual diagnosis that impact the brain during this developmental period in their lives; one of the most important periods of brain development overall (Gavaria & Smith, 2001) and a period of time when youth are most vulnerable to drug experimentation and here, to replace the high experienced with their treatment of MPH if already predisposed. With better research, precaution, awareness and treatment, schools, clinicians, parents and medical doctors can provide the safest and most appropriate amount of stimulant medication with careful oversight in partnership with therapists and clinicians. A limitation here is the age of some of the research since substantive data on the topic within the last five years was not readily available to answer the initial research question inquiry. Additionally, the sources here were more focused on lab animals, and so there was very little inference given to the effect of MPH on adolescents leading to a dual diagnosis and addiction well into adulthood with a narrow focus (Hesson & Fowler, 2018; Kessler et al., 2006; Kooij, 2012; Mao & Findling, 2016; Moore, Sunjic, Kaye, Archer, & Indig, 2013; Newcorn, Weiss, & Stein, 2007; Rucklidge, Downs-Woolley, Taylor, Brown, & Harrow, 2016). However, we now have enough data to determine that ongoing and long-term use of MPH as the only primary treatment for ADD/ADHD may have questionable implications on the health of children into adulthood. A multimodal treatment is recommended so as to minimize this causal linkage between MPH and substance abuse, at least until more research is available within the academy.

REFERENCES

America's Children and the Environment. 3rd Ed. (2015). Retrieved from the WWW on Friday August 2, 2019 From file:///E:/Clarion%20Folder/COUN %20591/ace3_neurodevelopmental.pdf

American Psychiatric Association. (2013). *Diagnostic and Statistical Manual of Mental Disorders* (Fifth Edition, Text Revision). American Psychiatric Association.

Anderson, R., & Baldwin, S. (2000). What's in a name? Amphetamine and methylphenidate. *Journal of Substance Use*, *5*(2), 89–91. doi:10.3109/14659890009053070

Bethancourt, J. A., Camarena, Z. Z., & Britton, G. B. (2009). Exposure to oral methylphenidate from adolescence through young adulthood produces transient effects on hippocampal-sensitive memory in rats. *Behavioural Brain Research*, *202*(1), 50–57. doi:10.1016/j.bbr.2009.03.015 PMID:19447280

Biederman, J., Wilens, T., Mick, E., Milberger, S., Spencer, T. J., & Faraone, S. V. (1995, November). Psychoactive substance use disorders in adults with attention deficit hyperactivity disorder (ADHD): Effects of ADHD and psychiatric comorbidity. *The American Journal of Psychiatry*, *152*(11), 1652–1658. doi:10.1176/ajp.152.11.1652 PMID:7485630

Breggin, P. (2001). *Talking back to Ritalin: What doctors aren't telling you about stimulants and ADHD*. Perseus Books Group.

Cohen, J. A., & Mannarino, A. P. (2008). Trauma-focused cognitive behavioral therapy for children and parents. *Child and Adolescent Mental Health*, *13*(4), 158–162. doi:10.1111/j.1475-3588.2008.00502.x

Cohen, J. A., Mannarino, A. P., & Deblinger, E. (2006). *Treating trauma and traumatic grief in children and adolescents*. Guilford Press.

Corey, G. (2017). *Theory and practice of counseling and psychotherapy*. Nelson Education.

dela Peña, I., Jeon, S. J., Lee, E., Ryu, J. H., Shin, C. Y., Noh, M., & Cheong, J. H. (2013). Neuronal development genes are key elements mediating the reinforcing effects of methamphetamine, amphetamine, and methylphenidate. *Psychopharmacology*, *230*(3), 399–413. doi:10.100700213-013-3168-8 PMID:23783774

DuPaul, G. J., Barkley, R. A., & McMurray, M. B. (1994). Response of children with ADHD to methylphenidate: Interaction with internalizing symptoms. *Journal of the American Academy of Child and Adolescent Psychiatry*, *33*(6), 894–903. doi:10.1097/00004583-199407000-00016 PMID:8083147

Education for All Handicapped Children Act of 1975, Pub. L. No. 94-142.

Fitzgerald, M. M., & Cohen, J. A. (2012). Trauma-focused cognitive behavior therapy for school psychologists. *Journal of Applied School Psychology*, *28*(3), 294–315. doi:10.1080/15377903.2012.696037

Fone, K. C., & Nutt, D. J. (2005). Stimulants: Use and abuse in the treatment of attention deficit hyperactivity disorder. *Current Opinion in Pharmacology*, *5*(1), 87–93. doi:10.1016/j.coph.2004.10.001 PMID:15661631

Gaviria, M., & Smith, M. (Producers). (2001). Frontline: Medicating kids [Television broadcast]. Alexandria, VA: Public Broadcasting Service.

Gill, K. E., Pierre, P. J., Daunais, J., Bennett, A. J., Martelle, S., Gage, H. D., Swanson, J. M., Nader, M. A., & Porrino, L. J. (2012). Chronic treatment with extended release methylphenidate does not alter dopamine systems or increase vulnerability for cocaine self-administration: A study in nonhuman primates. *Neuropsychopharmacology*, *37*(12), 2555–2565. doi:10.1038/npp.2012.117 PMID:22805600

Grund, T., Lehmann, K., Bock, N., Rothenberger, A., & Teuchert-Noodt, G. (2006). Influence of methylphenidate on brain development–an update of recent animal experiments. *Behavioral and Brain Functions*, *2*(1), 2. doi:10.1186/1744-9081-2-2 PMID:16403217

Hamblen, J. L., Gibson, L. E., Mueser, K. T., & Norris, F. H. (2006). Cognitive behavioral therapy for prolonged postdisaster distress. *Journal of Clinical Psychology*, *62*(8), 1043–1052. doi:10.1002/jclp.20288 PMID:16700022

Herbert, J. D., & Forman, E. M. (2012). Mindfulness and Acceptance Techniques. In D. J. A. Dozois (Ed.), *Cognitive Behavioral Therapy: A Complete Reference Guide*. John Wiley.

Hesson, J., & Fowler, K. (2018). Prevalence and correlates of self-reported ADD/ADHD in a large national sample of Canadian adults. *Journal of Attention Disorders*, *22*(2), 191–200. doi:10.1177/1087054715573992 PMID:25749874

Hofmann, S. G., Asnaani, A., Vonk, I. J., Sawyer, A. T., & Fang, A. (2012). The Efficacy of Cognitive Behavioral Therapy: A Review of Meta-analyses. *Cognitive Therapy and Research*, *36*(5), 427–440. doi:10.100710608-012-9476-1 PMID:23459093

Individuals with Disabilities Education Act, 20 U.S.C. § 1400 (2004).

Joseph, S., & Linley, P. A. (2004). Positive therapy: A positive psychological theory of Therapeutic practice. In P. A. Linley & S. Joseph (Eds.), *Positive psychology in practice* (pp. 354–368). John Wiley. doi:10.1002/9780470939338.ch22

Kessler, R. C., Adler, L., Barkley, R., Biederman, J., Conners, C. K., Demler, O., ... Spencer, T. (2006). The prevalence and correlates of adult ADHD in the United States: Results from the National Comorbidity Survey Replication. *The American Journal of Psychiatry*, *163*(4), 716–723. doi:10.1176/ajp.2006.163.4.716 PMID:16585449

Kooij, J. S. (2012). *Adult ADHD: Diagnostic assessment and treatment*. Springer Science & Business Media.

Loureiro-Vieira, S., Costa, V. M., Lourdes Bastos, M., Carvalho, F., & Capela, J. P. (2017, August). Methylphenidate effects in the young brain: Friend or foe? *International Journal of Developmental Neuroscience*, *60*(1), 34–47. doi:10.1016/j.ijdevneu.2017.04.002 PMID:28412445

Madhiraju, P. (2001). R.I.P. Ritalinin proportion! The Eighth Circuit's restriction on a parent's right to have schools accommodate the needs of their disabled children: Debord and Davis. *Northwestern University Law Review*, *95*, 1661–1697.

Mao, A. R., & Findling, R. L. (2014). Comorbidities in adult attention-deficit/hyperactivity disorder: A practical guide to diagnosis in primary care. *Postgraduate Medicine*, *126*(5), 42–51. doi:10.3810/pgm.2014.09.2799 PMID:25295649

McMahan, I. (2009). *Adolescence*. Pearson Education.

Moore, E., Sunjic, S., Kaye, S., Archer, V., & Indig, D. (2016). Adult ADHD among NSW prisoners: Prevalence and psychiatric comorbidity. *Journal of Attention Disorders*, *20*(11), 958–967. doi:10.1177/1087054713506263 PMID:24134874

Morton, W. A., & Stockton, G. G. (2000). Methylphenidate abuse and psychiatric side effects. *Primary Care Companion to the Journal of Clinical Psychiatry*, *2*(5), 159–164. doi:10.4088/PCC.v02n0502 PMID:15014637

Newcorn, J. H., Weiss, M., & Stein, M. A. (2007). The complexity of ADHD: Diagnosis and treatment of the adult patient with comorbidities. *CNS Spectrums*, *12*(S12), 1–16. doi:10.1017/S1092852900026158 PMID:17667893

Patterson, T. G., & Joseph, S. (2007). Person-centered personality theory: Support from self-determination theory and positive psychology. *Journal of Humanistic Psychology*, *47*(1), 117–139. doi:10.1177/0022167806293008

Preston, J., O'Neal, J. H., & Talaga, M. C. (2017). *Handbook of clinical psychopharmacology for therapists*. New Harbinger Publications.

Rogers, C. R. (1940). The processes of therapy. *Journal of Consulting Psychology*, *4*(5), 161–164. doi:10.1037/h0062536

Rucklidge, J. J., Downs-Woolley, M., Taylor, M., Brown, J. A., & Harrow, S. E. (2016). Psychiatric comorbidities in a New Zealand sample of adults with ADHD. *Journal of Attention Disorders*, *20*(12), 1030–1038. doi:10.1177/1087054714529457 PMID:24743977

Scott, J. G., & Schoenberg, M. R. (2011). Frontal lobe/executive functioning. In The little black book of neuropsychology (pp. 219-248). Springer.

Seligman, L., & Reichenberg, L. W. (2016). *Selecting effective treatments: A comprehensive, systematic guide to treating mental disorders* (5th ed.). John Wiley & Sons.

Seligman, L. D., & Ollendick, T. H. (2011). Cognitive behavioral therapy for anxiety disorders in youth. *Child and Adolescent Psychiatric Clinics of North America*, *20*(2), 217–238. doi:10.1016/j.chc.2011.01.003 PMID:21440852

Turnbull, H. R., & Turnbull, A. (1998). *Free appropriate public education: The law and children with disabilities* (5th ed.). Love.

Upadhyaya, H. P. (2008). Substance use disorders in children and adolescents with attention- deficit/hyperactivity disorder: Implications for treatment and the role of the primary care physician. *Primary Care Companion to the Journal of Clinical Psychiatry*, *10*(3), 211–221. doi:10.4088/PCC.v10n0306 PMID:18615170

Van der Marel, K., Bouet, V., Meerhoff, G. F., Freret, T., Boulouard, M., Dauphin, F., & Reneman, L. (2015). Effects of long-term methylphenidate treatment in adolescent and adult rats on hippocampal shape, functional connectivity and adult neurogenesis. *Neuroscience*, *309*, 243–258. doi:10.1016/j.neuroscience.2015.04.044 PMID:25934041

Volkow, N. D., Wang, G. J., Gatley, S. J., Fowler, J. S., Ding, Y.-S., Logan, J., Volkow, N. D., Hitzemann, R., Angrist, B., & Lieberman, J. (1996). Temporal relationships between the pharmacokinetics of methylphenidate in the human brain and its behavioral and cardiovascular effects. *Psychopharmacology*, *123*(1), 26–33. doi:10.1007/BF02246277 PMID:8741951

Chapter 17
ADHD Symptoms, Comorbidities, Social, and Familial Adversities on Offences

Rejani Thudalikunnil Gopalan
https://orcid.org/0000-0002-5957-8144
Mahatma Gandhi Medical College and Hospital, India

ABSTRACT

Attention deficit hyperactivity (ADHD) manifests with symptoms of inattention, hyperactivity, and impulsivity. The long term consequences of ADHD have been explored on different dimensions such as physical growth, cognitive functions, and other mental health problems. The link between ADHD and criminal activities in adolescents and adulthood were also studied cross sectional and longitudinal methods and many found a relation with criminal activities. But it is important to explore how the disorder, its symptoms, co morbidities including addiction, social and familial adversities affects the relation. This chapter attempted to find the link on these dimensions. Studies have pointed out that ADHD diagnosis poses the increased risk for committing offenses and repetition of acts as well as prone for bullying and victimization, and it is not the symptoms but other environmental and familial factors are also need to be looked in to understand the link between ADHD and crime. Though many studies have shown an association of ADHD with co morbid Addictive disorders to crime, more studies are required to establish exact nature of the relationship.

INTRODUCTION

Attention Deficit Hyperactivity Disorder is one of the most prevalent neurodevelopmental disorder among children and the clinical picture varies with the developmental stage. In pre-school years (3-5 years) the clinical picture is characterized by excessive physical activity, difficulty in cooperation with peers and non-compliance to the recommendations of adults. In school age (6-12 years), apart from the nuclear symptoms of the disorder, as described in the classification systems, i.e. inattention, hyperactivity and impulsivity, oppositional behavior often occurs, conflicts with peers and academic problems. In

DOI: 10.4018/978-1-7998-5495-1.ch017

adolescence hyperactivity lessens, conflicts with parents continue and high risk behaviors often appear. In adults physical activity usually decreases significantly, while inattention and impulsivity still remain. With the passing of time the number of symptoms is usually reduced, however the impact and impairment caused by the disorder remain (Koumoula, 2012).

The long term consequences of ADHD have been explored on different dimensions such as physical growth, cognitive functions, and other mental health problems. The link between ADHD and criminal activities in adolescents and adulthood were also studied by using cross sectional and longitudinal methods and many found a relation with criminal activities. But it is important to explore how the disorder, its symptoms, comorbidities, social and familial adversities affects the relation. This chapter attempted to find the link on these dimensions.

ADHD and Crime

There is growing evidence of an association between ADHD and rule-breaking behaviour and that subjects with ADHD are more likely to be involved in the legal system(Philipp-Wiegmann, Rösler,Clasen,Zinnow, Retz-Junginger, &Retz,2018). Young, González, Mullens, Mutch, Malet-Lambert, & Gudjonsson (2018) reported that 25% of inmates in a prison had a diagnosis of ADHD. Many different types of crimes were reported among individuals with ADHD such as traffic violations and speeding, property theft, carrying a concealed weapon, illegal drug possession, and the rate of performing risky and recidivistic behaviors were also found to be high(Mannuzza&Klein,2000;Biederman,&Faraone,2005;Barkley,Fischer,Smallish,&Fletcher, 2004:Valero,Bosch,Corominas,Barrau,Ramos-Quiroga & Casas,2018).

In a meta-analysis and systematic review of the risks associated with childhood attention-deficit hyperactivity disorder on long-term outcome of arrests, convictions, and incarcerations, Mohr-Jensen & Steinhausen (2016) reported that childhood ADHD was significantly associated with adolescent and adulthood arrests, convictions and incarcerations. Individuals with ADHD had a younger age at onset of antisocial involvement and an increased risk of criminal recidivism. The most frequently committed criminal offenses were theft, assault, drug- and weapon-related crimes. Early antisocial behavior problems, childhood maltreatment, sex, and IQ were identified as potentially relevant predictors for antisocial outcomes. The conclusion was drawn based on a total of 15,442 individuals with childhood ADHD from nine unique samples. The findings support a substantial long-term risk associated with ADHD for later antisocial involvement.

In a fifteen year follow-up study, Philipp-Wiegmann et al. (2018) explored the impact of ADHD on the course of delinquency in a sample of 106 incarcerated young men and reported that offenders with ADHD reoffended 2.5 times faster and showed a higher rate of recidivism and further incarcerations compared to non-ADHD offenders. More or less similar findings were in another study by Román-Ithier, González,Vélez-Pastrana, González-Tejera,& Albizu-García(2017).They found that adult offenders with a history of attention deficit hyperactivity disorder (ADHD) were more likely to re-offend, ADHD was independently associated with being under 15 years of age at first arrest and a number of violent and non-violent offences. Although some associations between ADHD and offending may be accounted for by co-morbidity with substance use disorders, early onset of offending and repeated violent offending appeared to be directly related to ADHD.

ADHD and Types of Offenses

Patients with ADHD often fall into crises of catastrophic life events such as suicide or homicide and substance-related and addictive disorders were found to be played an important role in leading ADHD patients to such events. Because ADHD is characterized by inattentiveness and impulsivity, any kinds of substances, legal or illegal, can deteriorate ADHD symptoms, leading ADHD patients to such catastrophic events. The comorbidity with internalizing and externalizing mental disorders poses the increased risk to lead ADHD patients to substance-related and addictive disorders (SRAD), and once these patients suffer from SRAD, risk of catastrophic life events seems to increase due to the irreversibility of their adverse mentality (Yoshimasu,2016).

ADHD was found to be associated with intimate partner violence (IPV) perpetration and victimization. Greater ADHD symptom severity-particularly inattention, indicated higher rates of psychological IPV perpetration and victimization among college students and ADHD significantly predicted IPV perpetration resulting in injury. The link between ADHD and IPV were explained in terms of deficits in attention and impulsivity. Many established that impulsivity and inattentive symptoms might affect basic processes such as emotional decoding and set-shifting abilities, which are important processes for emotional and behavioral regulation and these symptoms, entail a reduction in sensitivity to key contextual stimuli. IPV perpetrators had higher trait impulsivity and greater attention switching costs and poor ability to recognize facial which increases the risk for intimate partner violence. Other factors like alcohol abuse and illicit drug use and comorbidity with conduct disorder were consistently associated with violence in intimate relationships(Wymbs,Dawson,Suhr, Bunford, &Gidycz,2017;Fang, Massetti, Ouyang,Grosse,Mercy,2010;Romero-Martínez,Lila,& Moya-Albiol,2019).

Many researchers have observed relation between ADHD and bullying victimization and perpetration. Hellström (2019) found an increased risk for violence and victimization for children with ADHD and reported prevalence rate of 7.3% for polyvictimization. Though children with ADHD were severely beating and threatening other people, they were more being the victim of bullying experiences than general students (Huh, Kim, Lee, Jung, Choi, & Kim, 2019). The prevalence rates of the pure victims, pure perpetrators, and victim-perpetrators of bullying in a sample of adolescents with ADHD were found to be 14.6%, 8.4%, and 5.6%, respectively (Chou, Liu, Yang, Yen, & Hu,2018).

The reasons for bullying and victimization were associated with comorbid disorders, medications, and psychosocial factors. Comorbidity such as internalizing behaviors were more strongly related to peer victimization among children with ADHD and internalizing behaviors and peer victimization appeared to share a dynamic relationship; that is, decreases in internalizing behaviors predict similar decreases in peer victimization (Fogleman,Leaberry,Rosen,Walerius,&Slaughter,2018). Deficit in socio-communication increases the risk of being pure victims and victim-perpetrators among adolescence and parent-reported victim-perpetrators had more severe ODD symptoms than did parent-reported pure victims (Chou et al., 2019). Both witnessing and being a victim of violence were associated with significantly increased odds for depressive symptoms in adolescents with ADHD symptoms compared to non-ADHD adolescents who had not experienced community violence and only being a victim of violence continued to be associated with significantly increased odds for depression(Stickley,Koposov, Koyanagi,Inoue & Ruchkin,2019). Adolescents with ADHD and recent stimulant prescription reported more victimization than those without ADHD (Epstein-Ngo,McCabe,Veliz,Stoddard,Austic, &Boyd,2016). Young age, comorbidity with autism spectrum disorders, and low satisfaction with family relationships were linked with severe bullying victimization and a high score of fun seeking and low satisfaction with family relationships were related with severe bullying perpetration (Chou et al., 2018).

The link between sexual offences and ADHD are also well known. The majority of peer-to-peer sexual victimization and perpetration occurred by someone of the opposite sex, however, same-sex victimization and perpetration were not uncommon and Ngo,Veliz, Kusunoki, Stein, &Boyd(2018) have reported that Substance use, depression, Attention Deficit Hyperactivity Disorder (ADHD), and conduct disorder were associated with peer-to-peer sexual violence (victimization or perpetration) for both males and females among adolescence.

Researchers suggested that ADHD diagnosis poses the increased risk for committing offenses and repetition of acts; however they were also prone for bullying and victimization. Studies have reported that the maltreatment in childhood would leads to later substance use disorders (SUDs) and other disorders which is true with ADHD also (Sanctis,Trampush,Harty,Marks,Newcorn, Miller,Halperin,2008).

ADHD Symptoms and Crime

Many studies have indicated strong relation between inattentive symptoms of ADHD and crime or antisocial behaviours. Using latent change models, Giannotta and Rydell (2016) found that initial levels of, as well as increases in, hyperactivity/impulsivity and oppositional behaviors and initial levels of inattention behaviors predicted youth antisocial behaviors. They also reported that child hyperactive/impulsive behaviors predicted youth antisocial behaviors only in children for whom the quality of the parent-child relationship deteriorated from childhood to adolescence. While exploring the risk for adult illegal behaviour or arrest related to ADHD, Gunter, Arndt, Riggins-Caspers, Wenman, & Cadoret (2006) indicated that inattention was the most common domain impaired among those with ADHD, followed closely by hyperactivity, with impulsivity reported least often among those endorsing symptoms of ADHD. Both inattentive and hyperactive symptoms during childhood increase the likelihood of engaging in numerous types of criminal activities. However, there is little evidence that individuals with symptoms of the combined type of ADHD face a multiplicative risk (Freeman, 1996).

Fletcher and Wolfe (2009) have reported that both types of ADHD symptoms were likely to lead to an increase in stealing but more with inattentive type. The increase in selling drugs among those with inattentive symptoms was consistent with a lack of understanding of the consequences of such behavior. The unemployment rate, the percent in poverty, and juvenile crime rates were associated with the chances of reporting stealing. The higher probability of arrest of those with impulsive symptoms might reflect the more "immediate' crime committed without consideration of the probability of being caught by those with such symptoms. Turning to results on type of ADHD, the evidence suggests that persons with the inattentive type symptoms were more likely to commit all of the studied crimes except robbery than individuals with no ADHD symptoms. This group was more likely to engage in crimes that might require some planning such as selling drugs or burglary. Individuals with impulsive symptoms had the highest increase in criminal activities of all the ADHD-types and were more likely to be arrested and convicted of a crime. The impulsive nature of their disorder seemed to lead them to engage in more impulsive crimes such as theft and robbery. Interestingly, individuals with the combined-type of ADHD symptoms had the weakest associations with crime.

There is an argument that not only the symptoms but other environmental and familial factors are also need to be looked in to understand the link between ADHD and crime. Pingault, Côté, Lacourse, Galéra, Vitaro, et al. (2013) reported in a longitudinal study involving more than 2,700 individuals that childhood physical aggression was directly predictive of later criminal behavior. The findings revealed that while less than 10% of the total sample exhibited physical aggression in childhood, this small group represented 30% of the criminal activity in adolescence and young adulthood. Further, these same participants were responsible for almost half of the criminal charges on record and nearly 60% of all the violent criminal charges. Family adversity also increased the risk for criminal behavior in the aggressive participants. Results show that not all children with ADHD are at risk of engaging in criminal behavior. But children with aggressive traits, and especially those with ADHD and family adversity, are more vulnerable to criminal activities.

ADHD, Comorbidities and Crime

Studies among prisoners indicated presence of high prevalence of psychiatric disorders especially conduct disorder, ADHD and antisocial personality disorder. In South Korea, conduct disorder was found to be a common psychiatric disorder among juvenile detainees who tended to commit more violent crimes, had suffered more physical, emotional, and sexual abuse; and showed more psychopathology than detainees who did not have conduct disorder(Choi, Kim, Kim, Kim 2017). Among 105 Juvenile offenders admitted to Malaysian prisons, almost all of the offenders had at least one diagnosable psychiatric disorder and more than half had two or more psychiatric diagnoses. Conduct disorder (CD) was the commonest disorder (59.0 per cent), while substance use disorders (SUD) was the commonest co-morbidity. A significant correlation was found between presence of CD, education level and SUD. Almost all of the detainees with CD, had not completed schooling and detainees with this disorder were more likely to use substances than detainees without CD (Aida, Aili, Manveen, Salwina, Subash, Ng, & Muhsin, 2014). The most common psychiatric disorders among delinquent youths in Turkey were found to be ADHD, oppositional defiant disorder, conduct disorder (CD) and anxiety disorder (Taşkıran, Mutluer, Tufan, & Semerci, 2017). Sibley, Pelham, Molina et al. (2011) examined the association between childhood ADHD and juvenile delinquency by analyzing data from the Pittsburgh ADHD Longitudinal Study (PALS), a follow-up study of individuals diagnosed with ADHD in childhood (ages 5-12) and recontacted in adolescence and young adulthood for yearly follow-up. Participants were 288 males with childhood ADHD and 209 demographically similar males without ADHD who were recruited into the follow-up study. Four childhood diagnostic groups [ADHD-only ADHD + ODD, ADHD + CD and comparison were used to examine group differences on delinquency outcomes across three dimensions of delinquency (i.e., severity, age of initiation, and variety). Individuals with childhood ADHD + CD displayed significantly worse delinquency outcomes than the other three groups, across almost all indices of offending. When compared to comparison participants, boys with ADHD-only and ADHD + ODD in childhood displayed earlier ages of delinquency initiation, a greater variety of offending, and higher prevalence of severe delinquency. These findings suggest that although childhood ADHD + CD creates the greatest risk for delinquency, boys with ADHD-only and ADHD + ODD also appear at a higher risk for later offending.

A total of 80 out of 230 juvenile detainees in Turkey, (34.8%) were found to have substance abuse excluding nicotine and alcohol. The substances abused in preferential order were cannabis (72.5%), volatile substances (21.3% bally and 3.7% thinner; 25%) and sedative hypnotic drugs and biperidents (2.5%). The rate of conduct disorder was 46.3% in substance abusers and 25.3% in the others. The rate of substance abuse was 48.5% in the juveniles who had committed multiple crimes and 14.1% in the others. The study shows that conduct disorder was very high in juvenile detainees and conduct disorder was higher in substance-abusing than in non-abusing juvenile detainees. Substance-abusing juvenile detainees were found to have a higher detention rate than non-abusing juvenile detainees. There was a close relation between conduct disorder and substance abuse and multiple crimes (Copur,Turkcan,&Erdogmus,2005). Kolla,Maas,Erickson,Mann,Seeley,&Vingilis (2018) noted that ADHD did not predict history of arrest, and conduct disorder symptoms and cannabis misuse exerted stronger effects on history of arrest for females than males which suggested that the relative importance and type of clinical risk factors for arrest may differ according to sex.

Bessler, Stiefel, Barra, Plattner,& Aebi (2019) observed that 90.2% of the prisoners suffered from at least one mental illness and four independent psychiatric disorder categories were identified: affective disorders, anxiety disorders, behavioural disorders and substance abuse disorders. Recidivism for violent crime was found more frequently in juveniles with behavioural disorders (especially when suffering from conduct disorder and/or attention deficit and hyperactivity disorder) and/or substance abuse compared to juvenile ex-convicts without psychiatric disorders. In addition, study revealed that the time interval between discharge and the commitment of a new violent crime was shorter for juveniles of a younger age.

Neurodevelopmental disorders (NDD)(Attention-Deficit/Hyperactivity Disorder (ADHD), Autism Spectrum Disorder (ASD), tic disorder, intellectual disability (ID), in prison populations have received increased attention and Billstedt, Anckarsäter, Wallinius, & Hofvander(2017) reported in their study among 270 young adult male that sixty-three percent of the study group met DSM-IV criteria for childhood ADHD, 43% for ADHD in adulthood, 10% met criteria for an ASD, 6% for Tourette syndrome, and 1% for Intellectual Disbaility and twenty-two percent had borderline intellectual functioning. A substantial rate of overlap between the NDDs was found and the combined NDD group had an earlier onset of anti-social behavior, had more aggressive behavior and lower school achievements than the non-NDD group.

Autism spectrum disorders (ASDs) were known to be associated with an increased risk of aggression and challenging behavior and the ASD-offenders had significantly more often been diagnosed with a neurodevelopmental disorder (i.e. ASD or ADHD) and ASD offenders were overrepresented in sex crimes with a child victim(Hofvander, Bering, Tärnhäll, Wallinius, & Billstedt, 2019).

The long term consequences of ADHD were found to be associated with many different psychiatric disorders. Studies found that ADHD youth were at high risk for a wide range of adverse psychiatric outcomes including markedly elevated rates of antisocial, addictive, mood and anxiety disorders and high morbidity associated with ADHD across the life-cycle The comorbidity of conduct disorder was associated with significantly increased risk for psychoactive substance use disorders, smoking, and bipolar disorder(Biederman,Monuteaux,Mick,Spencer,Wilens,Silva,Snyder, & Faraone,2006; Biederman, Petty, Dolan,Hughes,Mick, Monuteaux, &Faraone,2008). Negative outcomes were observed in females with ADHD diagnosis by Owens and Hinshaw (2016) and they tested whether conduct problems predicted young adult functioning and psychiatric symptoms among women diagnosed with attention-deficit/hyperactivity disorder (ADHD) during childhood, in the context of 3 potential adolescent mediators: internalizing problems, peer rejection, and school failure and disciplinary problems. Same like for boys, childhood and adolescent conduct problems were associated with poor adult outcomes among girls with ADHD, with school failure and disciplinary problems, internalizing problems, and peer conflict functioning as mediators of these relations.

Studies have indicated that presence of psychiatric comorbidities increases the risk for crime in individuals with ADHD. It was also determined that the children diagnosed with ADHD were exposed to more physical and emotional abuse, and physical and emotional neglect (Gokten,Duman,Soylu,& Uzun,2016).

In a 3-year follow-up study, Ståhlberg, Boman, Robertsson, Kerekes, Anckarsäter, & Nilsson (2017) compared background variables, extent of criminality and criminal recidivism in the form of all court convictions, the use of inpatient care, and number of early deaths in Swedish institutionalized adolescents and found that substance use disorders(SUD) plus ADHD group displayed a somewhat more negative outcome with regard to criminality, the rate of criminal recidivism was strikingly high in all three groups (with ADHD, with SUD, those with SUD but no ADHD, and those without SUD), and age at first conviction emerged as the only significant predictor of persistence in violent criminality. Regardless of whether SUD, with or without ADHD, is at hand or not, institutionalized adolescents describe a negative course with extensive criminality and frequent episodes of inpatient treatment, and those with comorbid SUD and ADHD have the worst prognosis with regard to criminality, health, and untimely death.

Previous studies strongly pointed out that the prevalence of ADHD in prison populations may vary but remain higher than those found in the general population. Violence committed by a person with ADHD seems to be against other persons rather than property offences and reactive-impulsive violence seems to be more prevalent than pro-active instrumental violence. The existence of ADHD does not appear as a risk factor of recidivism and the violence risk may be increased by the occurrence of comorbidities as conduct disorders and mental deficiency. There may be a preferential association between ADHD and antisocial personality disorder or substance abuse which both increases the risk of violence (Galland, Tisserant, & Notardonato, 2017).

Psychosocial Factors Related with ADHD and Crime

The possible risk factors related to family, social and school has been linked with antisocial behavior of children in their first contact with the judicial authorities. Family history of crime was found to be very strong predictor of severity of crime and ADHD and CD were associated with commitment of more severe crimes in delinquent youths(Carabellese, Tegola,Margari,Craig,Ostuni,Scardaccione,Perrini,& Margari,2016;Taşkıran,Mutluer,Tufan,& Semerci,2017). An association was noticed between inadequate parenting practices, punishment and negligence and behavioral of problems of children and adolescents with ADHD(Teixeira, Marino,& Carreiro, 2015).

Comorbidity with substance use disorder, oppositional-defiant disorder/conduct disorder, low family socioeconomic status, parental incarceration, and parental relationship status all significantly increased the risk of conviction and incarceration among individuals with ADHD. Crime rates increased with the number of associated risks but were reduced during periods of taking ADHD medication. In addition to ADHD, a broad range of individual, familial, and social factors increase the risk of antisocial development (Mohr-Jensen, Bisgaard, Boldsen, & Steinhausen, 2019). Sitnick, Galán, & Shaw (2019) investigated whether individual, family, and community risk factors from 18 to 42 months of age were predictive of violent criminal arrests during late adolescence and early adulthood using a sample of 310 low-income male participants living in an urban community. They reported that early childhood family income, home environment, emotion regulation, oppositional behavior, and minority status were all significant in distinguishing violent offending boys from those with no criminal records. In addition, trajectories of early childhood conduct disorder, but not attention deficit hyperactivity disorder, were significantly related to self-report of violent behavior, depressive symptoms, and anxiety symptoms.

Long-term academic risk was associated with ADHD, particularly inattentive symptoms (Sayal,Washbrook,& Propper,2015). Studies pointed at substantial evidence for a negative association between ADHD symptoms and mathematical ability and this association was particularly marked for the inattentive component of ADHD than for the hyperactive-impulsive component. Evidence from twin studies also showed a significant genetic correlation between mathematics and ADHD, which was greater for the inattentive component of ADHD compared to the hyperactive-impulsive component (Tosto, Momi, Asherson,& Malki, 2015). Patients with greater ADHD symptoms severity were less likely to be employed and had higher rates of unemployment, other co-morbid mental health conditions, and heavy tobacco smoking(Lugoboni,Levin,Pieri,Manfredini,Zamboni,Somaini,Gerra,&Gics,2017).

Prior research has shown that attention deficit/hyperactivity disorder (ADHD) related to various negative outcomes in adolescence, including academic failure, behavioral problems at school, and criminal behavior. Watts (2018) found that a retrospective account of ADHD symptomatology during childhood and early adolescence predicts weakened school attachment, lower grades, and higher risks for both out-of-school suspension and crime. School attachment, grades, and out-of-school suspension had the expected effects on crime among females and males and among females, these school factors mediate the effects of ADHD symptomatology on crime while the effect of ADHD symptomatology on crime among males remains significant when controlling for school factors.

Addiction and ADHD and its Relation with Crime

Attention-deficit hyperactivity disorder (ADHD) and substance-use disorders are related to each other in a variety of ways. Although within the child-psychiatry literature earlier investigations was inconsistent regarding such a link, prospective studies that followed hyperactive children and normal controls into adulthood have found that hyperactive adults with a history of ADHD are more likely than controls to have substance-use disorders (Levin & Kleber, 1995). Literature showed an association between ADHD and addiction with alcohol, drugs, nicotine and gambling. Lee, Humphreys, Flory, Liu, & Glass (2011) meta-analyzed longitudinal studies that prospectively followed children with and without ADHD into adolescence or adulthood to examine the association of childhood attention-deficit/hyperactivity disorder (ADHD) with substance use (nicotine, alcohol, marijuana) and abuse/dependence outcomes (nicotine, alcohol, marijuana, cocaine, other). They reported that children with ADHD were more likely to develop disorders of abuse/dependence for nicotine, alcohol, marijuana, cocaine, and other substances (i.e., unspecified) in adolescence and adulthood. In a meta analysis, Groenman, Janssen, & Oosterlaan (2017) found that childhood ADHD, ODD, CD, and depression increase the risk of developing substance-related disorders and in another meta analysis, Charach, Yeung, Climans, & Lillie(2011) found that childhood ADHD was associated with alcohol and drug use disorders in adulthood and with nicotine use in adolescence. Estévez, Dey, Eich-Höchli, Foster, Gmel, & Mohler-Kuo(2016) found that adult ADHD was significantly associated with a propensity to experiment with licit and illicit substances, especially at earlier ages, to exhibit risky substance use patterns, and to subsequently develop SUDs.

Available studies vary in their estimated prevalence of attention deficit/hyperactivity disorder (ADHD) in substance use disorder (SUD) patients, ranging from 2 to 83%. van de Glind, Konstenius, & Koeter et al.(2014) reported that prevalence of DSM-IV and DSM-5 adult ADHD varied for DSM-IV from 5.4% for Hungary to 31.3% for Norway and for DSM-5 from 7.6%) for Hungary to 32.6% for Norway. Davids and Gastpar (2003) reported up to 50% of patients with on continuing ADHD symptoms from childhood were found to develop a substance-use disorder and suggested that the presence of ADHD may influence adolescent and adult substance-use disorders in different ways: earlier age of onset, higher frequency, longer duration of substance abuse and transition from alcohol-abuse to other substance-use disorders. Dirks, Scherbaum, Kis & Mette (2017) observed that prevalence of comorbid ADHD in substance-use disorder (SUD) patients was high and nearly one quarter of these patients fulfill the DSM IV criteria for ADHD. Review of literature continues to highlight the high risk for comorbid ADHD in patients with Substance Use Disroder; and conversely, the high risk for SUD developing in ADHD across the lifespan, particularly in the context of comorbid conduct disorder (Zulauf, Sprich, Safren, & Wilens, 2014). Comorbid conduct disorder further increases the risk of developing psychoactive substance use disorder and nicotine dependence (Groenman,Oosterlaan,Rommelse et al., 2013).Treatment-seeking substance use disorder patients with attention deficit hyperactivity disorder were at a very high risk for additional externalizing disorders and comorbidity patterns differed between ADHD subtypes and seventy-five per cent of ADHD patients had at least one additional comorbid disorder compared with 37% of SUD patients without ADHD (van Emmerik-van Oortmerssen, van de Glind, & Koeter et al., 2014).

Studies always have shown relationship between ADHD and risk for alcohol abuse but Kuppa and Maysun (2019) reported in a systematic review that several studies put forward the concept of a positive association between alcohol abuse and ADHD symptoms, but a minority of them also showed opposing and contradictory results and the inconsistency observed in studies could be a result of a biased approach in studies and a subjective attempt in interpretations.

Studies have reported strong relation between ADHD and drug abuse and dependence. Levin and Kleber (1995) suggested that persons with a substance-use disorder, and particularly those with a cocaine-use disorder, may be more likely than the general population to have a childhood history of ADHD. Saules, Pomerleau, & Schubiner (2003) reported more severe adult ADHD symptom profile among ADHD smokers with cocaine dependence, accounted for by elevated hyperactive/impulsive but not inattentive features, suggests that cocaine use in smokers with ADHD may be driven by excesses in hyperactivity. Lambert & Hartsough (1998) found high rate of cocaine dependence among participants with ADHD. Szobot, Rohde, Bukstein, Molina, Martins, Ruaro, & Pechansky(2007) screened a total of 968 male adolescents (15-20 years of age) for illicit substance use disorders (SUD) (marijuana, cocaine and inhalants) in their households and found that adolescents with ADHD presented a significantly higher odds ratio (OR) for illicit SUD than youths without ADHD. In the observational follow-up of the Multimodal Treatment Study of Children with ADHD (MTA), Molina, Howard,Swanson, Stehli,Mitchell, Kennedy et al. (2018) reported that in adulthood, weekly marijuana use and daily cigarette smoking were more prevalent in the ADHD group and also the cumulative record revealed more early substance users in adolescence for ADHD than control group including younger first use of alcohol, cigarettes, marijuana, and illicit drugs. Alcohol and nonmarijuana illicit drug use escalated slightly faster in the ADHD group in early adolescence.

Childhood, adolescent and adult ADHD all increase risk for smoking. Childhood ADHD increases risk for early smoking during adolescence, particularly if untreated and in combination with conduct disorder (CD). Attention deficit hyperactivity disorder in adolescence increases the risk of daily smoking in adulthood (Modesto-Lowe, Danforth, Neering, & Easton, 2010). Lambert and Hartsough (1998) found that by age 17, 46% of all participants with ADHD, as contrasted with 24% of the age-mate controls, reported smoking cigarettes daily. In adulthood, the proportion of participants with ADHD who were current smokers (42%) continued to exceed that of the age-mate controls (26%). Among current adult smokers, 35% with ADHD smoked daily as compared to 16% of the age-mate controls. There were significantly different lifetime tobacco dependence rates--40% compared to 19% for age-mate controls. They also reported a significant difference in rates of daily smoking and tobacco dependence for those with ADHD who had used stimulant medication in childhood in contrast to controls. A meta-analysis illustrated a clinically important link between childhood ADHD and tobacco smoking in adolescence but not later in life (Fond, Loundou, Guillaume et al., 2014).

Adolescents who had more severe ADHD symptoms as children were more likely to initiate smoking and to start smoking younger and the association of ADHD symptoms with daily smoking, number of cigarettes per day, and nicotine dependence was greater in females than in males (Elkins, Saunders, Malone, Keyes, Samek,McGue, & Iacono, 2018).ADHD youth who smoked cigarettes were significantly more likely to subsequently use alcohol and illicit drugs as well as to develop abuse and dependence compared to ADHD youth who did not smoke and these results extend the gateway hypothesis to an ADHD sample and provide evidence that this effect may be particularly robust in ADHD youth (Biederman, Monuteaux, Mick, Wilens, Fontanella, Poetzl, Kirk, Masse,& Faraone 2006). Wilens and Biederman (2006) reported ADHD as an antecedent disorder to subsequent SUD. ADHD and its co-occurring comorbid psychopathology increase the risk for cigarette smoking and SUD and are associated with greater SUD severity and chronicity and the treatment of ADHD appears to decrease the risk for cigarette smoking and SUD.

Children of parents with substance use disorders (SUDs) have been shown to demonstrate an increased risk for cigarette smoking in adolescence. In a prospective study, conduct disorder (CD) and parental smoking predicted earlier daily cigarette smoking, and mediated the relationship between risk status and offspring daily cigarette smoking (Clark & Cornelius, 2004). Mick, Biederman, Faraone, Sayer, & Kleinman (2002) suggested that ADHD may be an additional deleterious outcome associated with prenatal exposure to alcohol independently of the association between prenatal exposure to nicotine and smoke products and other familial risk factors for the disorder. They found that ADHD cases were 2.1 times more likely to have been exposed to cigarettes and 2.5 times more likely to have been exposed to alcohol in utero than were the non-ADHD control subjects.

Comorbid gambling disorder symptoms in chronic Alcohol use disorder (AUD) was connected to more severe alcohol-related variables and higher trait impulsivity was also linked with gambling disorder symptoms in patients with chronic AUD (Kovács, Demeter, Janka, Demetrovics, Maraz, & Andó,2020). The prevalence of at-risk and problem gambling was higher in individuals with ADHD symptoms than in those without ADHD symptoms. ADHD symptoms were positively associated with problem gambling (Jacob, Haro, & Koyanagi,2018).

Relation with Crime

Adolescent delinquency and alcohol abuse have become a growing concern. Psychopathology, a dysfunctional family and specific personality factors have all been linked to addictive and antisocial behavior. Alcohol-abusing delinquents scored significantly higher on novelty seeking and maternal emotional warmth and reported higher levels of psychopathology, as compared to nonalcohol-abusing delinquents (Koposov, Ruchkin, Eisemann, & Sidorov, 2005; Hunter, Miles, Pedersen, Ewing, D'Amico.2014). Mason and Windle (2002) revealed in their study that a model of bidirectional effects between polysubstance use and general delinquency was plausible for boys but not for girls. For boys, the effect of delinquency on substance use was small but consistent over time, whereas the effect of substance use on delinquency was larger but restricted to the earlier waves of the study. There is considerable evidence linking substance use and delinquent behavior among adolescents and adolescents with psychiatric concerns. However, the nature and temporal ordering of this relationship remain uncertain, particularly among early adolescents and those with significant psychopathology (Becker,Nargiso,Wolff,Uhl,Simon, Spirito, & Prinstein,2012).

Substance-related and addictive disorders (SRAD) can be a critical risk factor of suicide and homicide among patients with ADHD. In a study on the role of substance-related and addictive disorders (SRAD) that lead patients with attention-deficit hyperactivity disorder (ADHD) to suicide and homicide, Yoshimasu (2016) noted that comorbid psychiatric disorders such as conduct disorder, oppositional defiant disorder and antisocial personality disorder which are characterized by aggressive or antisocial behaviors or emotions towards others are apt to lead ADHD patients to SRAD, and once these patients suffer from SRAD, risk of catastrophic life events seems to increase due to the irreversibility of their adverse mentality.

Among 198 Scottish prisoners, the ADHD symptomatic group had significantly higher rates of total, acquisitive and violent offending than other prisoners, as well as greater regular heroin use. Frequent use of heroin in the year prior to imprisonment was the single most powerful predictor of the extent of total offending, with ADHD symptoms also adding independently to the variance in offending. In contrast, for violent offending, ADHD symptoms were the strongest predictor followed by alcohol dependence. The findings demonstrate the importance of heroin use and ADHD symptoms in the persistence of offending (Young, Wells, & Gudjonsson, 2011).

Self-reported ADHD among 1179 adult sentenced population of Puerto Rico (USA) was associated with age of first arrest, a number of violent and non-violent offences and re-offending. Although some associations between ADHD and offending may be accounted for by co-morbidity with substance use disorders, early onset of offending and repeated violent offending appear to be directly related to ADHD (Román-Ithier, González, Vélez-Pastrana, González-Tejera, Albizu-García, 2017). Though many studies have shown an association of ADHD with comorbid Addictive disorders to crime, more studies are required to establish exact nature of the relationship.

CONCLUSION

ADHD heralds persistence of ADHD and comorbid symptoms into adolescence, as well as significant risks for functional impairment and juvenile justice involvement (Bussing, Mason, Bell, Porter, & Garvan, 2010). In the follow up of Multimodal Treatment Study of Children with ADHD (MTA), it was found that adult functioning after childhood ADHD varies by domain and is generally worse when ADHD symptoms persist. The poor outcomes were noted in post-secondary education, times fired/quit a job, current income, receiving public assistance, and risky sexual behavior, jail time,alcohol use disorder and number of jobs held (Hechtman, Swanson, Sibley et al.,2018). Merrill, Molina, Coxe et al. (2020) found five profiles among young adults with ADHD such as prototypic impairment group (54%), high binge-drinking group (17%), high marijuana use group (10%), high criminal activity group (3%), and high cross-domain impairment group (17%). Young adults with childhood ADHD have differentiable impairment patterns that vary based on substance use, criminal behavior, and number of clinically impaired domains. Use of specific substances was elevated among subgroups of young adults with ADHD histories.

In addition to impairments, ADHD has also been shown to be linked with several measures of criminal activity, although much of this research has used small convenience samples of individuals or assessed the relationship in a cross-sectional data on fewer than 300 individuals (Fletcher& Wolfe,2009). There were studies which indicted ADHD was not directly link with crime. In a 30 years follow-up study using official crime records, Mordre, Groholt, Kjelsberg, Sandstad, Myhre (2011) reported that conduct disorder in childhood was highly associated with later delinquency both alone or in combination with hyperactivity, but less associated when combined with an emotional disorder. ADHD in childhood was no more associated with later delinquency than the rest of the disorders in the study population. The authors argued that the finding strengthens the assumption that there was no direct association between ADHD and criminality. Future studied need to look in to the association of ADHD and crime on symptoms, comorbidity, and psychosocial dimensions with large sample size and robust methodology.

REFERENCES

Aida, S. A., Aili, H. H., Manveen, K. S., Salwina, W. I. W., Subash, K. P., Ng, C. G., & Muhsin, C. G. (2014). Prevalence of psychiatric disorders among juvenile offenders in Malaysian prisons and association with socio-demographic and personal factors. *International Journal of Prisoner Health, 10*(2), 132–143. doi:10.1108/IJPH-06-2013-0029 PMID:25764076

Barkley, R. A., Fischer, M., Smallish, L., & Fletcher, K. (2004). Young adult follow-up of hyperactive children: Antisocial activities and drug use. *Journal of Child Psychology and Psychiatry, and Allied Disciplines*, *45*(2), 195–211. doi:10.1111/j.1469-7610.2004.00214.x PMID:14982236

Becker, S. J., Nargiso, J. E., Wolff, J. C., Uhl, K. M., Simon, V. A., Spirito, A., & Prinstein, M. J. (2012). Temporal relationship between substance use and delinquent behavior among young psychiatrically hospitalized adolescents. *Journal of Substance Abuse Treatment*, *43*(2), 251–259. doi:10.1016/j.jsat.2011.11.005 PMID:22197300

Bessler, C., Stiefel, D., Barra, S., Plattner, B., & Aebi, M. (2019). Mental disorders and criminal recidivism in male juvenile prisoners. *Zeitschrift fur Kinder- und Jugendpsychiatrie und Psychotherapie*, *47*(1), 73–88. doi:10.1024/1422-4917/a000612 PMID:30156463

Biederman, J., & Faraone, S. V. (2005). Attention-deficit hyperactivity disorder. *Lancet*, *366*(9481), 237–248. doi:10.1016/S0140-6736(05)66915-2 PMID:16023516

Biederman, J., Monuteaux, M. C., Mick, E., Spencer, T., Wilens, T. E., Silva, W. J., Snyder, L. E., & Faraone, S. V. (2006). Young adult outcome of attention deficit hyperactivity disorder: A controlled 10-year follow-up study. *Psychological Medicine*, *36*(2), 167–179. doi:10.1017/S0033291705006410 PMID:16420713

Biederman, J., Monuteaux, M. C., Mick, E., Wilens, T. E., Fontanella, J. A., Poetzl, K. M., Kirk, T., Masse, J., & Faraone, S. V. (2006). Is cigarette smoking a gateway to alcohol and illicit drug use disorders? A study of youths with and without attention deficit hyperactivity disorder. *Biological Psychiatry*, *59*(3), 258–264. doi:10.1016/j.biopsych.2005.07.009 PMID:16154546

Biederman, J., Petty, C. R., Dolan, C., Hughes, S., Mick, E., Monuteaux, M. C., & Faraone, S. V. (2008). The long-term longitudinal course of oppositional defiant disorder and conduct disorder in ADHD boys: Findings from a controlled 10-year prospective longitudinal follow-up study. *Psychological Medicine*, *38*(7), 1027–1036. doi:10.1017/S0033291707002668 PMID:18205967

Billstedt, E., Anckarsäter, H., Wallinius, M., & Hofvander, B. (2017). Neurodevelopmental disorders in young violent offenders: Overlap and background characteristics. *Psychiatry Research*, *252*, 234–241. doi:10.1016/j.psychres.2017.03.004 PMID:28285251

Bussing, R., Mason, D. M., Bell, L., Porter, P., & Garvan, C. (2010). Adolescent outcomes of childhood attention-deficit/hyperactivity disorder in a diverse community sample. *Journal of the American Academy of Child and Adolescent Psychiatry*, *49*(6), 595–605. doi:10.1016/j.jaac.2010.03.006 PMID:20494269

Carabellese, F., La Tegola, D., Margari, L., Craig, F., Ostuni, A., Scardaccione, E., Perrini, F., & Margari, F. (2016). ADHD and illegal conduct: A survey in Juvenile Justice Services in Puglia. *Rivista di Psichiatria*, *51*(4), 156–163. doi:10.1708/2342.25122 PMID:27727266

Carabellese, F., Tegola, D. L., Margari, L., Craig, F., & Ostuni, A. (2017). Scardaccione,E., Francesca Perrini,F., & Margari,F. (2017). Comorbidities and Correlates of Conduct Disorder Among Male Juvenile Detainees in South Korea. *Child and Adolescent Psychiatry and Mental Health*, *11*(1), 44. doi:10.118613034-017-0182-3 PMID:28924450

Charach, A., Yeung, E., Climans, T., & Lillie, E. (2011). Childhood attention-deficit/hyperactivity disorder and future substance use disorders: Comparative meta-analyses. *Journal of the American Academy of Child and Adolescent Psychiatry*, *50*(1), 9–21. doi:10.1016/j.jaac.2010.09.019 PMID:21156266

Choi, B., Kim, J. I., Kim, B., & Kim, B. (2017). Comorbidities and Correlates of Conduct Disorder Among Male Juvenile Detainees in South Korea. *Child and Adolescent Psychiatry and Mental Health*, *11*(1), 442017. doi:10.118613034-017-0182-3 PMID:28924450

Chou,W.J., Hsiao, R.C., Ni, H.C., Liang, S.H., Lin, C.F., Chan, H.L., Hsieh, Y.H., Wang, L.J., Lee, M.J., Hu, H.F., & Yen, C.F.(2019). Self-Reported and Parent-Reported School Bullying in Adolescents with High Functioning Autism Spectrum Disorder: The Roles of Autistic Social Impairment, Attention-Deficit/ Hyperactivity and Oppositional Defiant Disorder Symptoms. *International Journal of Environmental Research* and *Public Health, 16*(7). pii: E1117. doi: . doi:10.3390/ijerph16071117

Chou, W. J., Liu, T. L., Yang, P., Yen, C. F., & Hu, H. F. (2018). Bullying Victimization and Perpetration and Their Correlates in Adolescents Clinically Diagnosed With ADHD. *Journal of Attention Disorders*, *22*(1), 25–34. doi:10.1177/1087054714558874 PMID:25403369

Clark, D. B., & Cornelius, J. (2004). Childhood psychopathology and adolescent cigarette smoking: A prospective survival analysis in children at high risk for substance use disorders. *Addictive Behaviors*, *29*(4), 837–841. doi:10.1016/j.addbeh.2004.02.019 PMID:15135569

Copur, M., Turkcan, A., & Erdogmus, M. (2005). Substance Abuse, Conduct Disorder and Crime: Assessment in a Juvenile Detention House in Istanbul, Turkey. *Psychiatry and Clinical Neurosciences*, *59*(2), 151–154. doi:10.1111/j.1440-1819.2005.01350.x PMID:15823160

Davids, E., & Gastpar, M. (2003). Attention-deficit/hyperactivity disorder and substance abuse. *Psychiatrische Praxis*, *30*(4), 182–186. doi:10.1055-2003-39496 PMID:12768521

Dirks, H., Scherbaum, N., Kis, B., & Mette, C. (2017). ADHD in Adults and Comorbid Substance Use Disorder: Prevalence, Clinical Diagnostics and Integrated Therapy. *Fortschritte der Neurologie-Psychiatrie*, *85*(6), 336–344. doi:10.1055-0043-100763 PMID:28645126

Elkins, I. J., Saunders, G. R. B., Malone, S. M., Keyes, M. A., Samek, D. R., McGue, M., & Iacono, W. G. (2018). Increased Risk of Smoking in Female Adolescents Who Had Childhood ADHD. *The American Journal of Psychiatry*, *175*(1), 63–70. doi:10.1176/appi.ajp.2017.17010009 PMID:28838251

Epstein-Ngo, Q. M., McCabe, S. E., Veliz, P. T., Stoddard, S. A., Austic, E. A., & Boyd, C. J. (2016). Diversion of ADHD Stimulants and Victimization Among Adolescents. *Journal of Pediatric Psychology*, *41*(7), 786–798. doi:10.1093/jpepsy/jsv105 PMID:26590265

Estévez, N., Dey, M., Eich-Höchli, D., Foster, S., Gmel, G., & Mohler-Kuo, M. (2016). Adult attention-deficit/hyperactivity disorder and its association with substance use and substance use disorders in young men. *Epidemiology and Psychiatric Sciences*, *25*(3), 255–266. doi:10.1017/S2045796015000360 PMID:25989844

Fang, X., Massetti, G. M., Ouyang, L., Grosse, S. D., & Mercy, J. A. (2010). Attention-deficit/hyperactivity disorder, conduct disorder, and young adult intimate partner violence. *Archives of General Psychiatry*, *67*(11), 1179–1186. doi:10.1001/archgenpsychiatry.2010.137 PMID:21041619

Fletcher, J., & Wolfe, B. (2009). Long-term consequences of childhood ADHD on criminal activities. *The Journal of Mental Health Policy and Economics*, *12*(3), 119–138. PMID:19996475

Fogleman, N. D., Leaberry, K. D., Rosen, P. J., Walerius, D. M., & Slaughter, K. E. (2018). Relation between internalizing behaviors, externalizing behaviors, and peer victimization among children with and without ADHD. *Attention Deficit and Hyperactivity Disorders*, *10*(3), 209–222. doi:10.100712402-018-0248-y PMID:29330700

Fond, G., Loundou, A., Guillaume, S., Quantin, X., Macgregor, A., Lopez, R., Courtet, P., Bernard, P., Bailly, D., Abbar, M., Leboyer, M., & Boyer, L. (2014). Smoking behavior characteristics of non-selected smokers with childhood attention-deficit/hyperactivity disorder (AD/HD) history: A systematic review and meta-analysis. *European Archives of Psychiatry and Clinical Neuroscience*, *264*(5), 379–389. doi:10.100700406-014-0497-5 PMID:24619241

Freeman, R. B. (1996). Why do so many young American men commit crimes and what might we do about it? *The Journal of Economic Perspectives*, *10*(1), 25–42. doi:10.1257/jep.10.1.25

Galland, D., Tisserant, I., & Notardonato, L. (2017). Attention deficit hyperactivity disorder in forensic psychiatry: A review. *L'Encéphale*, *43*(3), 268–272. doi:10.1016/j.encep.2016.04.012 PMID:27637873

Giannotta, F., & Rydell, A. (2016). The Prospective Links Between Hyperactive/Impulsive, Inattentive, and Oppositional-Defiant Behaviors in Childhood and Antisocial Behavior in Adolescence: The Moderating Influence of Gender and the Parent-Child Relationship Quality. *Child Psychiatry and Human Development*, *47*(6), 857–870. doi:10.100710578-015-0617-0 PMID:26680210

Gokten, E. (2016). Effects of attention-deficit/hyperactivity disorder on child abuse and neglect. *Child Abuse & Neglect*, *62*, 1–9. doi:10.1016/j.chiabu.2016.10.007 PMID:27770673

Groenman, A. P., Janssen, T. W. P., & Oosterlaan, J. (2017). Childhood Psychiatric Disorders as Risk Factor for Subsequent Substance Abuse: A Meta-Analysis. *Journal of the American Academy of Child and Adolescent Psychiatry*, *56*(7), 556–569. doi:10.1016/j.jaac.2017.05.004 PMID:28647007

Groenman, A. P., Oosterlaan, J., Rommelse, N., Franke, B., Roeyers, H., Oades, R. D., Sergeant, J. A., Buitelaar, J. K., & Faraone, S. V. (2013). Substance use disorders in adolescents with attention deficit hyperactivity disorder: A 4-year follow-up study. *Addiction (Abingdon, England)*, *108*(8), 1503–1511. doi:10.1111/add.12188 PMID:23506232

Gunter, T. D., Arndt, S., Riggins-Caspers, K., Wenman, G., & Cadoret, R. J. (2006). Adult outcomes of attention deficit hyperactivity disorder and conduct disorder: Are the risks independent or additive? *Annals of Clinical Psychiatry*, *18*(4), 233–237. doi:10.1080/10401230600948415 PMID:17162622

Hechtman, L., Swanson, J. M., Sibley, M. H., Stehli, A., Owens, E. B., Mitchell, J. T., Arnold, L. E., Molina, B. S. G., Hinshaw, S. P., Jensen, P. S., Abikoff, H. B., Perez Algorta, G., Howard, A. L., Hoza, B., Etcovitch, J., Houssais, S., Lakes, K. D., Nichols, J. Q., Vitiello, B., ... Stern, K. (2016). Functional Adult Outcomes 16 Years After Childhood Diagnosis of Attention-Deficit/Hyperactivity Disorder: MTA Results. *Journal of the American Academy of Child and Adolescent Psychiatry*, *55*(11), 945–952.e2. doi:10.1016/j.jaac.2016.07.774 PMID:27806862

Hellström, L. (2019). A Systematic Review of Polyvictimization among Children with Attention Deficit Hyperactivity or Autism Spectrum Disorder. *International Journal of Environmental Research* and *Public Health, 16*(13). pii: E2280. doi:10.3390/ijerph16132280

Hofvander, B., Bering, S., Tärnhäll, A., Wallinius, M., & Billstedt, E. (2019). Few Differences in the Externalizing and Criminal History of Young Violent Offenders With and Without Autism Spectrum Disorders. *Front Psychiatry, 17*(10), 911. doi: . doi:10.3389/fpsyt.2019.00911

Huh, S. Y., Kim, S. G., Lee, J. S., Jung, W. Y., Choi, B. S., & Kim, J. H. (2019). A study on the school violence experience of children with attention-deficit hyperactivity disorder in the context of bullying. *Asia-Pacific Psychiatry*, *11*(3), e12353. doi:10.1111/appy.12353 PMID:30941893

Hunter, S. B., Miles, J. N., Pedersen, E. R., Ewing, B. A., & D'Amico, E. J. (2014). Temporal associations between substance use and delinquency among youth with a first time offense. *Addictive Behaviors*, *39*(6), 1081–1086. doi:10.1016/j.addbeh.2014.03.002 PMID:24656642

Jacob, L., Haro, J. M., & Koyanagi, A. (2018). Relationship between attention-deficit hyperactivity disorder symptoms and problem gambling: A mediation analysis of influential factors among 7,403 individuals from the UK. *Journal of Behavioral Addictions*, *7*(3), 781–791. doi:10.1556/2006.7.2018.72 PMID:30238788

Kolla, N. J., van der Maas, M., Erickson, P. G., Mann, R. E., Seeley, J., & Vingilis, E. (2018). Attention deficit hyperactivity disorder and arrest history: Differential association of clinical characteristics by sex. *International Journal of Law and Psychiatry*, *58*, 150–156. doi:10.1016/j.ijlp.2018.04.006 PMID:29853005

Koposov, R. A., Ruchkin, V. V., Eisemann, M., & Sidorov, P. I. (2005). Alcohol abuse in Russian delinquent adolescents. Associations with comorbid psychopathology, personality and parenting. *European Child & Adolescent Psychiatry*, *14*(5), 254–261. doi:10.100700787-005-0463-x PMID:15981137

Koumoula, A. (2012). The Course of Attention Deficit Hyperactivity Disorder (ADHD) Over the Life Span. *Psychiatriki*, *23*(S1), 49-59.

Kovács, I., Demeter, I., Janka, Z., Demetrovics, Z., Maraz, A., & Andó, B. (2020). Different aspects of impulsivity in chronic alcohol use disorder with and without comorbid problem gambling. *PLoS One*, *15*(1), e0227645. doi:10.1371/journal.pone.0227645 PMID:31999707

Kuppa, A., & Maysun, A. (2019). Risk of Alcohol Abuse in Humans with Attention-deficit/Hyperactivity Disorder Symptoms. *Cureus*, *11*(10), e5996. doi:10.7759/cureus.5996 PMID:31807384

Lambert, N. M., & Hartsough, C. S. (1998). Prospective study of tobacco smoking and substance dependencies among samples of ADHD and non-ADHD participants. *Journal of Learning Disabilities*, *31*(6), 533–544. doi:10.1177/002221949803100603 PMID:9813951

Lee, S. S., Humphreys, K. L., Flory, K., Liu, R., & Glass, K. (2011). Prospective association of childhood attention-deficit/hyperactivity disorder (ADHD) and substance use and abuse/dependence: A meta-analytic review. *Clinical Psychology Review*, *31*(3), 328–341. doi:10.1016/j.cpr.2011.01.006 PMID:21382538

Levin, F. R., & Kleber, H. D. (1995). Attention-deficit hyperactivity disorder and substance abuse: Relationships and implications for treatment. *Harvard Review of Psychiatry*, *2*(5), 246–258. doi:10.3109/10673229509017144 PMID:9384909

Lugoboni, F., Levin, F. R., Pieri, M. C., Manfredini, M., Zamboni, L., Somaini, L., Gerra, G., & Gics, G. S.Gruppo InterSert Collaborazione Scientifica (GICS). (2017). Co-occurring Attention Deficit Hyperactivity Disorder symptoms in adults affected by heroin dependence: Patients characteristics and treatment needs. *Psychiatry Research*, *250*, 210–216. doi:10.1016/j.psychres.2017.01.052 PMID:28473157

Mannuzza, S., & Klein, R. (2000). Long-term prognosis in attention-deficit/hyperactivity disorder. *Child and Adolescent Psychiatric Clinics of North America*, *9*(3), 711–726. doi:10.1016/S1056-4993(18)30114-7 PMID:10944664

Mason, W. A., & Windle, M. (2002). Reciprocal relations between adolescent substance use and delinquency: A longitudinal latent variable analysis. *Journal of Abnormal Psychology*, *111*(1), 63–76. doi:10.1037/0021-843X.111.1.63 PMID:11866180

Merrill, B. M., Molina, B. S. G., Coxe, S., Gnagy, E. M., Altszuler, A. R., Macphee, F. L., Morrow, A. S., Trucco, E. M., & Pelham, W. E. (2020). Functional Outcomes of Young Adults with Childhood ADHD: A Latent Profile Analysis. *Journal of Clinical Child and Adolescent Psychology*, *49*(2), 215–228. doi: 10.1080/15374416.2018.1547968 PMID:30689405

Mick, E., Biederman, J., Faraone, S. V., Sayer, J., & Kleinman, S. (2002). Case-control study of attention-deficit hyperactivity disorder and maternal smoking, alcohol use, and drug use during pregnancy. *Journal of the American Academy of Child and Adolescent Psychiatry*, *41*(4), 378–385. doi:10.1097/00004583-200204000-00009 PMID:11931593

Modesto-Lowe, V., Danforth, J. S., Neering, C., & Easton, C. (2010). Can We Prevent Smoking in Children With ADHD: A Review of the Literature. *Connecticut Medicine*, *74*(4), 229–236. PMID:20441004

Mohr-Jensen, C., Müller Bisgaard, C., Boldsen, S. K., & Steinhausen, H. C. (2019). Attention-Deficit/Hyperactivity Disorder in Childhood and Adolescence and the Risk of Crime in Young Adulthood in a Danish Nationwide Study. *Journal of the American Academy of Child and Adolescent Psychiatry*, *58*(4), 443–452. doi:10.1016/j.jaac.2018.11.016 PMID:30768385

Mohr-Jensen, C., & Steinhausen, H. C. (2016). A meta-analysis and systematic review of the risks associated with childhood attention-deficit hyperactivity disorder on long-term outcome of arrests, convictions, and incarcerations. *Clinical Psychology Review*, *48*, 32–42. doi:10.1016/j.cpr.2016.05.002 PMID:27390061

Molina, B. S. G., Howard, A. L., Swanson, J. M., Stehli, A., Mitchell, J. T., Kennedy, T. M., Epstein, J. N., Arnold, L. E., Hechtman, L., Vitiello, B., & Hoza, B. (2018). Substance use through adolescence into early adulthood after childhood-diagnosed ADHD: Findings from the MTA longitudinal study. *Journal of Child Psychology and Psychiatry, and Allied Disciplines*, *59*(6), 692–702. doi:10.1111/jcpp.12855 PMID:29315559

Mordre, M., Groholt, B., Kjelsberg, E., Sandstad, B., & Myhre, A. M. (2011). The impact of ADHD and conduct disorder in childhood on adult delinquency: A 30 years follow-up study using official crime records. *BMC Psychiatry*, *11*(1), 57. doi:10.1186/1471-244X-11-57 PMID:21481227

Ngo, Q. M., Veliz, P. T., Kusunoki, Y., Stein, S. F., & Boyd, C. J. (2018). Adolescent sexual violence: Prevalence, adolescent risks, and violence characteristics. *Preventive Medicine*, *116*, 68–74. doi:10.1016/j.ypmed.2018.08.032 PMID:30194960

Owens, E. B., & Hinshaw, S. P. (2016). Childhood conduct problems and young adult outcomes among women with childhood attention-deficit/hyperactivity disorder (ADHD). *Journal of Abnormal Psychology*, *125*(2), 220–232. doi:10.1037/abn0000084 PMID:26854507

Philipp-Wiegmann, F., Rösler, M., Clasen, O., Zinnow, T., Retz-Junginger, P., & Retz, W. (2018). ADHD modulates the course of delinquency: A 15-year follow-up study of young incarcerated man. *European Archives of Psychiatry and Clinical Neuroscience*, *268*(4), 391–399. doi:10.100700406-017-0816-8 PMID:28612143

Pingault, J. B., Côté, S. M., Lacourse, E., Galéra, C., Vitaro, F., & Tremblay, R. E. (2013). Childhood hyperactivity, physical aggression and criminality: A 19-year prospective population-based study. *PLoS One*, *8*(5), e62594. doi:10.1371/journal.pone.0062594 PMID:23658752

Román-Ithier, J. C., González, R. A., Vélez-Pastrana, M. C., González-Tejera, G. M., & Albizu-García, C. E. (2017). Attention deficit hyperactivity disorder symptoms, type of offending and recidivism in a prison population: The role of substance dependence. *Criminal Behaviour and Mental Health*, *27*(5), 443–456. doi:10.1002/cbm.2009 PMID:27455899

Romero-Martínez, Á., Lila, M., & Moya-Albiol, L. (2019). The importance of impulsivity and attention switching deficits in perpetrators convicted for intimate partner violence. *Aggressive Behavior*, *45*(2), 129–138. doi:10.1002/ab.21802 PMID:30474120

Sanctis, V. A. D., Trampush, J. W., Harty, S. C., Marks, D. J., Newcorn, J. H., Miller, C., & Halperin, J. M. (2008). Childhood Maltreatment and Conduct Disorder: Independent Predictors of Adolescent Substance Use Disorders in Youth With Attention Deficit/Hyperactivity Disorder. *Journal of Clinical Child and Adolescent Psychology*, *37*(4), 785–793. doi:10.1080/15374410802359650 PMID:18991129

Saules, K. K., Pomerleau, C. S., & Schubiner, H. (2003). Patterns of inattentive and hyperactive symptomatology in cocaine-addicted and non-cocaine-addicted smokers diagnosed with adult attention deficit hyperactivity disorder. *Journal of Addictive Diseases*, *22*(2), 71–78. doi:10.1300/J069v22n02_06 PMID:12703670

Sayal, K., Washbrook, E., & Propper, C. (2015). Childhood behavior problems and academic outcomes in adolescence: Longitudinal population-based study. *Journal of the American Academy of Child and Adolescent Psychiatry*, *54*(5), 360–8.e2. doi:10.1016/j.jaac.2015.02.007 PMID:25901772

Sibley, M. H., Pelham, W. E., Molina, B. S., Gnagy, E. M., Waschbusch, D. A., Biswas, A., MacLean, M. G., Babinski, D. E., & Karch, K. M. (2011). The delinquency outcomes of boys with ADHD with and without comorbidity. *Journal of Abnormal Child Psychology*, *39*(1), 21–32. doi:10.100710802-010-9443-9 PMID:20697799

Sitnick, S. L., Galán, C. A., & Shaw, D. S. (2019). Early childhood predictors of boys' antisocial and violent behavior in early adulthood. *Infant Mental Health Journal*, *40*(1), 67–83. doi:10.1002/imhj.21754 PMID:30576588

Ståhlberg, O., Boman, S., Robertsson, C., Kerekes, N., Anckarsäter, H., & Nilsson, T. (2017). A 3-year follow-up study of Swedish youths committed to juvenile institutions: Frequent occurrence of criminality and health care use regardless of drug abuse. *International Journal of Law and Psychiatry*, *50*, 52–60. doi:10.1016/j.ijlp.2016.09.004 PMID:27745884

Stickley, A., Koposov, R., Koyanagi, A., Inoue, Y., & Ruchkin, V. (2019). ADHD and depressive symptoms in adolescents: The role of community violence exposure. *Social Psychiatry and Psychiatric Epidemiology*, *54*(6), 683–691. doi:10.100700127-019-01662-5 PMID:30706080

Szobot, C. M., Rohde, L. A., Bukstein, O., Molina, B. S. G., Martins, C., Ruaro, P., & Pechansky, F. (2007). Is attention-deficit/hyperactivity disorder associated with illicit substance use disorders in male adolescents? A community-based case-control study. *Addiction (Abingdon, England)*, *102*(7), 1122–1130. doi:10.1111/j.1360-0443.2007.01850.x PMID:17567400

Taşkıran, S., Mutluer, T., Tufan, A. E., & Semerci, B. (2017). Understanding the associations between psychosocial factors and severity of crime in juvenile delinquency: A cross-sectional study. *Neuropsychiatric Disease and Treatment*, *18*(13), 1359–1366. doi:10.2147/NDT.S129517 PMID:28572731

Teixeira, M. C., Marino, R. L., & Carreiro, L. R. (2015). Associations between Inadequate Parenting Practices and Behavioral Problems in Children and Adolescents with Attention Deficit Hyperactivity Disorder. *The Scientific World Journal*, *683062*. Advance online publication. doi:10.1155/2015/683062 PMID:26844292

Tosto, M.G., Momi, S.K., Asherson, P., & Malki, K. (2015). A Systematic Review of Attention Deficit Hyperactivity Disorder (ADHD) and Mathematical Ability: Current Findings and Future Implications. *BMC Medicine, 27*(13), 204. doi: . doi:10.118612916-015-0414-4

Valero, S., Bosch, R., Corominas, M., Barrau, V., Ramos-Quiroga, J. A., & Casas, M. (2018). Remittance or persistence of attention deficit-hyperactivity disorder (ADHD) and its impact on recidivism in risky driving behaviors. *Traffic Injury Prevention, 19*(7), 701–707. doi:10.1080/15389588.2018.1505043 PMID:30485128

van de Glind, G., Konstenius, M., Koeter, M. W. J., van Emmerik-van Oortmerssen, K., Carpentier, P.-J., Kaye, S., Degenhardt, L., Skutle, A., Franck, J., Bu, E.-T., Moggi, F., Dom, G., Verspreet, S., Demetrovics, Z., Kapitány-Fövény, M., Fatséas, M., Auriacombe, M., Schillinger, A., Møller, M., ... van den Brink, W. (2014). Variability in the prevalence of adult ADHD in treatment seeking substance use disorder patients: Results from an international multi-center study exploring DSM-IV and DSM-5 criteria. *Drug and Alcohol Dependence, 134*, 158–166. doi:10.1016/j.drugalcdep.2013.09.026 PMID:24156882

van Emmerik-van Oortmerssen, K., van de Glind, G., Koeter, M. W., Allsop, S., Auriacombe, M., Barta, C., Bu, E. T. H., Burren, Y., Carpentier, P.-J., Carruthers, S., Casas, M., Demetrovics, Z., Dom, G., Faraone, S. V., Fatseas, M., Franck, J., Johnson, B., Kapitány-Fövény, M., Kaye, S., ... Schoevers, R. A. (2014). Psychiatric comorbidity in treatment-seeking substance use disorder patients with and without attention deficit hyperactivity disorder: Results of the IASP study. *Addiction (Abingdon, England), 109*(2), 262–272. doi:10.1111/add.12370 PMID:24118292

Watts, S. J. (2018). ADHD Symptomatology and Criminal Behavior During Adolescence: Exploring the Mediating Role of School Factors. *International Journal of Offender Therapy and Comparative Criminology, 62*(1), 3–23. doi:10.1177/0306624X16639970 PMID:27056790

Wilens, T. E., & Biederman, J. (2006). Alcohol, drugs, and attention-deficit/ hyperactivity disorder: A model for the study of addictions in youth. *Journal of Psychopharmacology (Oxford, England), 20*(4), 580–588. doi:10.1177/0269881105058776 PMID:16174669

Wymbs, B. T., Dawson, A. E., Suhr, J. A., Bunford, N., & Gidycz, C. A. (2017). ADHD Symptoms as Risk Factors for Intimate Partner Violence Perpetration and Victimization. *Journal of Interpersonal Violence, 32*(5), 659–681. doi:10.1177/0886260515586371 PMID:26025345

Yoshimasu, K. (2016). Substance-Related and Addictive Disorders as a Risk Factor of Suicide and Homicide among Patients with ADHD: A Mini Review. *Current Drug Abuse Reviews, 9*(2), 80–86. doi:10.2174/1874473709666160802112215 PMID:27492359

Young, S., González, R. A., Mullens, H., Mutch, L., Malet-Lambert, I., & Gudjonsson, G. H. (2018). Neurodevelopmental disorders in prison inmates: Comorbidity and combined associations with psychiatric symptoms and behavioural disturbance. *Psychiatry Research, 261*, 109–115. doi:10.1016/j.psychres.2017.12.036 PMID:29291476

Young, S., Wells, J., & Gudjonsson, G. H. (2011). Predictors of offending among prisoners: The role of attention-deficit hyperactivity disorder and substance use. *Journal of Psychopharmacology (Oxford, England), 25*(11), 1524–1532. doi:10.1177/0269881110370502 PMID:20558498

Zulauf, C. A., Sprich, S. E., Safren, S. A., & Wilens, T. E. (2014). The complicated relationship between attention deficit/hyperactivity disorder and substance use disorders. *Current Psychiatry Reports, 16*(3), 436. doi:10.100711920-013-0436-6 PMID:24526271

Chapter 18
ADHD, Parental Stress, Stigma, and Mindfulness Training

Rejani Thudalikunnil Gopalan
https://orcid.org/0000-0002-5957-8144
Mahatma Gandhi Medical College and Hospital, India

ABSTRACT

Many studies have proven that parental stress was associated with childhood mental disorders and disabilities, and in recent years, studies have shown that parents of children with neurodevelopmental disorders (NDDs) experience more parenting stress than parents of typically developing children. Parents living with a child with ADHD experienced stress as they struggled to cope with the child's symptoms amidst the stigmatizing attitudes from family and community members. The chapter tried to explore various factors related with parental stress and ADHD such as quality of life, parental rating of ADHD symptoms and related issues, treatment outcome, marital life, and mental health. One of the important factors contributing to stress is stigma, and the chapter also attempted to explore the link between parental stress and stigma, especially related to ADHD and its interventions. The chapter emphasized the role of mindfulness training for treating ADHD and parental stress while pointing out the methodological limitations.

INTRODUCTION

Attention Deficit Hyperactivity Disorder (ADHD) is the most commonly diagnosed behavioural disorder of childhood. Its core symptoms include developmentally inappropriate levels of attention, concentration, activity, distractibility and impulsivity. Children with ADHD usually have functional impairment across multiple settings including home, school and peer relationship. It has also been shown to have long-term adverse effects on academic performance, vocational success and socio-emotional development (NIH Consensus Development Conference Statement, 2000).

Attention Deficit Hyperactivity Disorder has a long history that spans over a century. The understanding of its nature, conceptualization and treatment has undergone a lot of changes and the current understanding of this disorder represents a varying developmental history. The first reference of hyper-

DOI: 10.4018/978-1-7998-5495-1.ch018

activity could be traced back to a poem written by a German physician Heinrich Hoffman in 1865, which described the activities of a hyperactive or ADHD child named Fidgety Phil. George Still and Alfred Tredgold carried out the first scientific work on ADHD. Still, in 1902, described the clinical condition of 43 children who were similar to what is today known as ADHD and he attributed all these symptoms to 'defect in moral control', which could arise from defect of cognitive relation to the environment, defect of moral consciousness or defect in inhibitory volition. But later he proposed that early, mild and undetected brain damage could lead to such a condition. Tredgold (1908) and Pasamanick, Rogers and Lilienfeld (1956) supported the same conceptualization.

Studies focused on the relation between behavioural problems and brain lesions found an association between defects in forebrain structures and severe restlessness. Milder forms of hyperactivity were attributed to psychological causes such as 'spoiled' child-rearing practices or delinquent family environments. This gave way for the concept of 'brain injured child' (Strauss and Lehtinen, 1947) and it was modified as the concept of Minimal Brain Damage and Minimal Brain Dysfunction (MBD) by the 1950s and 1960s. Laufer, Denhoff and Solomons (1957a) coined the term 'Hyperkinetic impulse disorder' to refer to this disorder and they conceptualized that it could be caused by a central nervous system deficit occurring in the thalamic area due to the poor filtering of the stimulation. Laufer and Denhoff (1957) and Chess (1960) developed the concept of 'Hyperactive child syndrome', which emphasized hyperactivity as the major feature and thus the concept of a syndrome of hyperactivity was separated from the concept of a brain-damage syndrome. The disorder was included in the second edition of the Diagnostic and Statistical Manual of Mental Disorders (DSM-II) (American Psychiatric Association (APA), 1968) and it described the hyperkinetic reaction of childhood disorder as characterized by overactivity, restlessness, distractibility and short attention span, especially in younger children, which usually diminishes by adolescence. The difference in the conceptualization of ADHD between Europe and North America started during the 1960's and it was reflected in the classification of the disorder in DSM and ICD (International Classification of Diseases, World Health Organization). Clinicians in Europe considered this disorder as a rare syndrome with excessive motor activity and a sign of brain damage but in North America, this disorder was considered relatively common and not necessarily associated with brain damage.

During the 1970's, two different models to explain the nature of ADHD had developed-Wender's theory of MBD and Douglas' model of attention impulse control. Thus the emphasis was shifted from overactivity to the attention aspect of the disorder especially focusing on deficits in sustained attention as the core feature and the disorder was renamed Attention Deficit Disorder (ADD) with the publication of DSM-III (APA, 1980). The use of stimulant medication, special education programs, classroom behaviour `modification, dietary management and parent training were the treatment modalities employed during that period. Unhealthy environment was considered as the etiology of hyperactivity such as poor child rearing practices and child behaviour management. Studies also focused on the psychophysiology of hyperactivity in children and adult hyperactivity.

During the 1980's and 1990's researchers questioned the concept of inattention as the core feature. During the 1980's research was focused on criteria, assessment and treatment of this disorder. Research focused on the genetic and neurobiological basis of the disorder and the relative efficacy of different treatment modalities during the 1990's. The comparison of single versus combined modalities, multimodal treatments, parent training, classroom management, social skill training and the development of management guidelines were emphasized. Recent studies focused more on the neurological aspects like frontal lobe functions, metabolic activities, structure of the brain and the genetic aspects of ADHD (hereditary transmission, gene related to this disorder). It is recognized that ADHD is more influenced by neurological and genetic factors than social and environmental factors (Barkley, 1998).

ADHD is a highly comorbid condition and it is associated with externalizing disorders (oppositional defiant disorder and conduct disorder), internalizing disorders (anxiety and depression), mood disorders (major depression, bipolar disorder) and somatization disorder (Barkley, 1998). When ADHD occurs with another disorder, its presentation and management become more complex and it is often necessary to treat the comorbid disorder in addition to the ADHD. Comorbidity with CD influences the impairments associated with ADHD like greater symptom severity, parental psychopathology, social adversity, peer rejection, impulsivity (Abikoff and Klein, 1992), poor school performance and antisocial behaviour (Fergusson, Horwood and Lynskey, 1993). Children displayed more negative and fewer positive interactions with their mothers, decreased language-based skills and transgenerational transmission, showed greater maternal depression, psychological distress and marital discord when comorbid with ODD (Barkley, Fischer, Edelbrock and Smallish, 1991; Vance and Luk, 2000). The co morbidity of anxiety or mood disorder was often associated with a history of greater family and personal stress, greater parental symptoms of anxiety and mood disturbances and reduced responsiveness to stimulant medication (Jensen et al., 1997).

By considering the complexity of ADHD and its impact on parents and other family members, this chapter mainly focused on discussing the parental stress, coping, stigma and intervention to reduce stigma, and mindfulness training to reduce the parental stress.

Parental Stress and Disabilities

Parenting itself can be a generally stressful life event and the manifestation of major and persistent child problems may be the most significant dimension of stress across a range of unpleasant parental effects (Weinberg and Richardson, 1981).

The challenges that family caregivers face in meeting the needs of their children increase dramatically when the child has a severe emotional or behavioural disorder (Friesen, 1989). Many studies have focused on the impact of children with internalizing or externalizing disorders on the parental stress and coping patterns. Most of the studies have focused on the developmental delay, disability or chronic /serious medical illness.

Krauss (1993) investigated the differences in child-related and parenting stress between mothers and fathers of 121 toddlers with disabilities. He found that mothers and fathers reported similar levels of parenting–related stress, mothers had more difficulty in adjusting to the personal aspects of parenting and parenthood (parental health, restrictions in role and relation with spouse while fathers reported more stress related to their child's temperament (like child's mood and adaptability) and their relationship to the child. Prematurity status of the child was the major source of the mothers stress where as fathers stress was more sensitive to the effects of the family environment.

Dyson (1993) studied 74 families with a child with disabilities and found high level of parental stress. He reported that the presence or absence of disabilities and the quality of family relationship were the best predictors of parental stress. Seltzer, Greenberg, Floyd, Pettee and Hong, (2001) found that parents of a child with a developmental disability had lower rates of employment, larger families and lower rates of social participation but were similar to parents without a child with a disability in educational and marital status, physical health and psychological well being. Parents whose child had a serious mental health problem had normative patterns of educational and occupational attainment and marriage, but elevated levels of physical symptoms, depression and alcohol symptoms at mid-life.

Patterson (1980) reported that mothers of aggressive boys have a negative self-image, low self-esteem, and experience feelings of depression, anxiety, fatigue, anger and isolation. Wahler and Afton (1980) suggested that mothers of problem children may be isolated from social support, such as contacts with friends, and that this insularity may be predictive of higher levels of maternal negativism and poorer treatment outcomes. Other studies have suggested that social support may be a particularly critical factor when a family is under particular stress, such as associated with an irritable child. Parents were worried about their child's problem and expressed difficulties in managing the child. Most of them felt disappointed, guilty and upset about their child's condition and thought that it was due to the 'bad karma' in their past life and god has punished them through the child's problem and some parents accepted it as a method of coping. Some parents were worried about the child's excessive talk and physical aggression (Gopalan,Oommen, Srinath & Kapur, 2006).

In a systematic review of parenting stress and child behavior problems among different clinical groups (i.e., Autism Spectrum Disorders (ASD)/Developmental Delays(DD), chronic illness, with or at-risk for behavioral and/or mood disorders), Barroso, Mendez, Graziano, & Bagner (2018) reported that parenting stress was more strongly related to child externalizing than internalizing problems and the association between parenting stress and behavior problems was stronger among studies which had mostly male and clinic-recruited samples. Overall, parenting stress levels were higher for parents of children with ASD/DD compared to parents of children from other clinical groups.

Many studies have proven that parental stress was associated with childhood mental disorders and disabilities and the stress level varies with severity of disabilities and clinical conditions and many psychosocial factors were also contributed to it.

Parental Stress and Childhood ADHD

In recent years, studies have shown that parents of children with Neurodevelopmental Disorders (NDDs) experience more parenting stress than parents of typically developing children, especially parents of children with Autism Spectrum Disorders or ADHD report the highest scores of parenting stress (Craig, Operto, Giacomo, Margari, Frolli, Conson, Ivagnes, Monaco, & Margari,2016). High level of parental stress and poor quality of life were observed among parents with children a diagnosis of ADHD than children with anxiety disorders, autism spectrum disorder and typically developing children (Telman,van Steensel, Maric, & Bögels,2017) and the risk of stress increased when these parents reported having their own disorder/disease (Almogbel, Goyal, & Sansgiry, 2017). Parents living with a child with ADHD experienced stress as they struggle to cope with the child's symptoms amidst the stigmatizing attitudes from family and community members. Parents experienced burdensome emotions, unable to meet their own needs, interfered family activities and family cohesion, highest levels of depression, stress and impaired social and occupational functioning(Mofokeng, & van der Wath,2017;Klassen,Miller,& Fine,2004;Rockhill, Violette, Stoep, Grover, & Myers, 2013).

Anastopoulos, Guevremont, Shelton and Dupaul (1992) found that parental stress was associated with frequent aggressive behaviour, severe ADHD symptoms and higher incidents of child health problems. Mother's psychopathology and who were not working outside of home were associated with mothers stress under parental characteristics and it was more in single vs. two-parent families. Parental stress was more in children with ADHD with ODD than ADHD alone. Parents of children with ADHD very often experience considerable stress in their parenting roles. This increased stress would emerge from the increased care taking demands due to defiant behaviour (Cunningham and Barley, 1979; Tallmadge, Paternite and Gordon, 1989), younger age (Mash and Johnston, 1983) and first-born birth order of the children with ADHD (Mash and Johnston, 1990).

In a qualitative research aimed at understanding the stress of parents of children with ADHD, Leitch, Sciberras, Post, Gerner, Rinehart, Nicholson, & Evans (2019) have identified four primary themes such as The child's behaviour feels like a "wrecking ball"; Coping with the "war at home"; A divided family: "relationships don't survive"; and Craving support: and "it's goddamn hard work". Parents attribute their high stress to their children's behaviour, unmet needs for support, and social stigma. In another review of qualitative studies on experiences of parents of children with attention deficit hyperactivity disorder, Laugesen and Groenkjaer (2015) reported categories which generated six synthesized findings: 1) An emotional roller coaster between hope and hopelessness, 2) Mothers as advocates in a battlefield within the system and family, 3) Parental experiences in a crossfire of blame, self-blame and stigmatization, 4) Shuttling between supportive and non-supportive services and professionals, 5) Routines, structures and strategies within everyday life, and 6) Despite multiple challenges, it is not all bad. The findings illustrated the complexity of parental experiences that are influenced by guilt, hope, blame, stigmatization, exhaustion, reconciliation and professional collaboration and it addressed the impact attention deficit hyperactivity disorder has on the everyday family, and how parents seem to adapt to their life situation in the process of accepting their child's disorder.

Parental Stress and Adolescents with ADHD

Increased level of parenting stress was found be associated with adolescents with ADHD. Muñoz-Silva, Lago-Urbano, Sanchez-Garcia, & Carmona-Márquez,(2017) have studied 126 mothers of girls and boys aged 6-17 years old and reported that ADHD symptoms and conduct disorder negatively affected the family's social life which in turn affected the mother's parenting stress. In another study comprised 84 adolescents with ADHD, aged 13 to 18 and their parents, Wiener, Biondic, Grimbos, & Herbert (2017) reported that mothers and fathers of adolescents with ADHD reported more stress, and mothers experienced elevated levels of stress in terms of role restrictions, feelings of social alienation, conflict with their partner, feelings of guilt and incompetence and relationship with their children.

The lifetime maternal caregiver strain (CS) associated with raising a child with attention-deficit/hyperactivity disorder (ADHD) into adolescence and young adulthood was examined in the Pittsburgh ADHD Longitudinal Study (PALS), a longitudinal study of individuals diagnosed with ADHD in childhood and recontacted in adolescence and young adulthood for yearly follow-up. Babinski, Mazzant, Merrill, Waschbusch, Sibley, Gnagy, Molina, & Pelham (2020) reported that adolescent/young adult ODD, delinquency, and school discipline mediated the association between childhood ADHD and lifetime maternal caregiver strain. In another study it was noticed that the association between child and adolescent's ADHD and parenting stress was mediated by children's conduct problems and by negative impact on family's social life and a pathway from child/adolescent's ADHD through children's conduct problems and then through their negative impact on family's social life to mother's parenting stress (Muñoz-Silva, Lago-Urbano, Sanchez-Garcia, & Carmona-Márquez, 2017).

Bussing, Meyer, Zima, Mason, Gary, Garvan (2015) examined the associations of childhood attention-deficit/hyperactivity disorder (ADHD) risk status with subsequent parental social network characteristics and caregiver strain in adolescence; and examined predictors of adolescent mental health service use at eight-year follow-up. They found that parents of youth with childhood ADHD reported support networks consisting of fewer spouses but more healthcare professionals, and lower levels of support and caregiver strain increased with adolescent age and psychopathology. Increased parental network support, youth ADHD symptoms, and caregiver strain, but lower youth stigma perceptions were independently associated with increased service use. Raising children with ADHD appears to significantly impact parental social network experiences and reduced spousal support and overall lower network support levels may contribute to high caregiver strain commonly reported among parents of ADHD youth. It was also noticed that parental social network experiences influence adolescent ADHD service use.

Studies have shown that adolescents with ADHD may show high levels of defiance, posing significant challenges for parents, increased parental stress and reactivity and some of these parents have ADHD or other psychopathology that may contribute to maladaptive parenting. The kind of stress associated with childhood ADHD and adolescence ADHD were found to be different in terms of symptoms, co-morbidity and psychosocial factors. Some parents adjust and demonstrate optimism and resilience in the face of their teens' ADHD and parental factors (eg, emotional intelligence) and interventions (eg, mindfulness training) that may improve parenting/teen relationships and the developmental outcomes of teens. Researchers suggest that both child/adolescent's and family factors should be considered in the designing of interventions for reducing parenting stress in families of children and adolescents with ADHD (Modesto-Lowe, Chaplin, Godsay, & Soovajian, 2014;Muñoz-Silva, Lago-Urbano, Sanchez-Garcia,& Carmona-Márquez, 2017).

Maternal Stress and ADHD

Attention deficit/hyperactivity disorder can result in stress for the mother, resulting in poor health and this issue has important clinical and treatment implications(Babakhanian, Sayar, Babakhanian, &Mohammadi, 2016;Samiei, Daneshmand, Keramatfar, Khooshabi, Amiri, Farhadi, Farzadfard, Kachooi, Samadi, 2015). Mash and Johnston (1983) reported that maternal stress is associated with child distractibility and degree of bother and it was more for mothers of younger children who also showed more self-blaming and depression. Mothers of hyperactives reported more stress related to the parent child interaction, as well as feelings of depression, social isolation, self-blame, role restriction and lack of attachment to the child.

Clinical features and symptom severity influence the maternal stress as noticed by Weinberger, Gardner, & Gerdes (2018) that mothers of children with ADHD, Predominantly Hyperactive-Impulsive or Combined Type (ADHD-HI/C)reported significantly greater parenting stress and engaged in more negative parenting behaviors than mothers of children with ADHD, Predominantly Inattentive Type (ADHD-I). In a longitudinal five years study, Gordon and Hinshaw (2017) noted that parenting stress-parental distress by mothers of girls with attention-deficit/hyperactivity disorder (ADHD)during the participants' childhood was positively associated with adolescent externalizing and internalizing behaviors, and parental stress due to dysfunctional interactions during adolescence was associated with contemporaneous adolescent depressive symptoms and externalizing behaviors.

Many potential protective factors along with risk factors in maternal functioning and the impact on child treatment outcome and maternal ADHD-symptoms and degree of resilience were significantly correlated to symptom reduction in offspring diagnosed with ADHD (Rasmussen, Storebø, Shmueli-Goetz,

Bojesen, Simonsen, & Bilenberg, 2018).Personality traits or ADHD characteristics do not appear operative for the high parenting stress of mothers of a child with ADHD. However, high maternal ADHD or low conscientiousness were associated with stress levels similar to raising a child with ADHD(Algorta, Kragh, Arnold, Molina, Hinshaw, Swanson, Hechtman, Copley, Lowe, & Jensen, 2018).

Parental Stress, Related Factors and Impact

Many factors were related with parental stress and ADHD such as type of ADHD, symptom severity, child-parent characteristics, and self-efficacy beliefs on parenting. Parental stress affects the quality of life, parental rating of ADHD symptoms and related issues, treatment outcome, marital life and mental health. This section tried to explore all these aspects.

Parents of children of the combined subtype experienced higher parenting stress and felt their children displayed qualities that made it difficult for them to fulfill their parenting roles Higher ADHD symptom severity was associated to poor quality of life, and combined and inattentive subtypes are associated with greater disorder severity, more comorbid psychiatric disorders, and worse quality of life than the subtype with hyperactivity/impulsivity predominance(Yang, Jong, Hsiu-Yi Hsu, & Tsai, 2007;Escobar, Hervas, Soutullo, Mardomingo, Uruñuela, & Gilaberte, 2008).

Child and parent characteristics influenced parenting stress and child's oppositional-defiant behavior and maternal psychopathology were especially potent predictors. The severity of the child's ADHD, the child's health status, and maternal health status, IQ level or emotional and behavioral problems were associated with the higher levels of parenting stress (Anastopoulos, Guevremont, Shelton, & DuPaul, 1992; Craig et al., 2016). Mash and Johnston (1990) proposed that child characteristics such as temperament have an influence on parent-child interactive stress. In support of this notion, research indicated that mothers of temperamentally difficult children reported higher levels of parenting stress, depression and psychosocial problems such as doubts about their parenting competence.

McBride, Shoppe and Rane (2002) examined variations in the relationships among child characteristics, parenting stress and parental involvement. Participants were 100 two-parent families with preschool-aged children. Parental involvement, perceptions of child temperament and parental stress were collected by interview and self-report. Result showed association between child temperament and parental stress. There was significant association between temperament and parental involvement for fathers than for mothers. For both fathers and mothers, children perceived as less emotionally intense were less stressful. However, the difference in stress associated with low versus high levels of emotional intensity appeared to exist mainly for mothers of boys and fathers of girls. This may be because opposite –sex parent –child relationship is more challenging and less scripted.

Parenting stress was also predicted by lower socioeconomic status (SES) and number of family members and higher ADHD symptoms, and child sleep problems (Bonifacci, Massi, Pignataro, Zocco, & Chiodo, 2019; Martin, Papadopoulos, Chellew, Rinehart, & Sciberras,2019).Cultural factors affect the parenting stress as noticed in a study that Korean mothers reported significantly higher parenting stress yet significantly lower childhood problem behaviors compared to US mothers (Chung,Ebesutani, Bang, Kim, Chorpita, Weisz, Suh, & Byun, 2013).

Parenting ability and confidence were influenced by the diagnosis of ADHD, and parenting self-efficacy beliefs found to be a robust predictor of parenting stress (Williamson & Johnston, 2019).Compared to parents of children without ADHD, parents of children with ADHD reported lower self-efficacy in their ability to help their children, felt less welcome and supported by their children's schools and teachers, and perceived less time and energy for involvement in their children's academic lives. Mothers of children with and without ADHD reported similar types and levels of involvement behaviors in the home. Fathers of children with ADHD reported being more disengaged from their children's learning and using more coercive and punitive interactions regarding their children's achievement compared to fathers of children without ADHD (Rogers, Wiener, Marton, & Tannock, 2009). Increment in age and education level of children with ADHD may be associated with lower level of parenting self efficacy (Gohari, Dehghani, Gilda Rajabi, & Mahmoudi-Gharaei, 2012).

Parenting variables such as parenting attitude and sense of competence have been suggested as significant determinants of socio-emotional development of children with attention deficit hyperactivity disorder. Higher levels of affectionate parenting attitude of mothers and non-co-morbid status of children were associated with higher self-esteem of children, and higher levels of rejecting parenting attitude of mothers contributed to the lower social competence in children with attention deficit hyperactivity disorder (Oh,Park, Suk,Song, & Im,2012).

Inconsistent parental discipline is a robust correlate of child attention-deficit/hyperactivity disorder (ADHD) symptoms and it was found that child ADHD symptoms were associated with variability in warm parenting behaviors, and higher levels of parenting-related stress were related to greater variability in harsh parenting behaviors. James and Lansford (2018) suggested that Parent-based treatment programs for children with ADHD should include a stronger focus on reducing stress from parenting (e.g., teaching coping skills for parents), as this may lead to greater consistency in parental behavior more generally, and presumably better child outcomes.

Parent characteristics and family-environment circumstances are reciprocally interacting with child characteristics, which would result in elevated parenting stress (Mash and Johnston, 1990). The other factors, which increase the parental stress, are parental mood, independent of whether or not psychopathology is involved (Jouriles, Murphy and O'Leary, 1989). Depression and other types of parental psychopathology (Lahey et al., 1988), marital dysfunction (Barkley et al., 1990), problematic interaction between ADHD children and their siblings and negative life events (Campbell, Breaux, Ewing and Szumowski, 1986) also increase parental stress. However studies have shown that child's ADHD and other clinically relevant child characteristics were primary determinants of parental stress (Barkley, 1990) and the improvement in child's ADHD would make changes in parent behaviour like issue of fewer commands, less criticism and more warmth (Barkley, 1989: Schachar, Taylor, Wieselberg, Thorley and Rutter, 1987).

Parents of children with attention-deficit hyperactivity disorder (ADHD) and oppositional defiant disorder (ODD) often have elevated ADHD and depressive symptoms, both of which increase the risk of ineffective parenting and interparental discord. Wymbs, Dawson, Egan, Sacchetti, Tams, & Wymbs (2017) reported that child ADHD/ODD behavior predicted less positive and more negative parenting and communication, and parent couples including two parents with elevated ADHD communicated more positively while managing children exhibiting ADHD/ODD behavior. The study emphasized that depending on the similarity of ADHD and depressive symptom levels in parent couples, adults managing children exhibiting ADHD/ODD behavior may parent or communicate positively or negatively and it highlighted the need to consider the psychopathology of both parents when treating children with ADHD in two-parent homes.

Similarity in parent and child characteristics influence the quality of parenting and Psychogiou, Daley, Thompson, & Sonuga-Barke (2008) have examined the interaction between mother and child attention-deficit/hyperactivity disorder (ADHD) symptoms on parenting and found that parental response to children with high ADHD symptoms was more positive and affectionate when the mother also had high ADHD symptoms which highlights the importance of considering both child and maternal ADHD symptoms in studies of parenting.

The level of family impact was dependent on a number of factors, including the severity of child's emotional and behavioural problems, family strengths, cultural acceptance of the child's difficulties and the parent's social support systems. High family stress was associated with the families using inpatient hospitalization and intermediate non-residential services for their children and lower family stress has been associated with the families using traditional outpatient services alone (Bickman, Foster and Lambert, 1996: Foster, Saunders and Summerfelt, 1996). Gottlieb (1981) reported that friends or family might cause stress due to their own attitudes and beliefs about mental illness. They may blame parent/s for causing the mental illness. Feeling of stigma and withdrawal of family support may also be a good reason for stress in the care giving family.

Parent training programmes are psychosocial interventions aimed at training parents in techniques to enable them to manage their children's challenging behavior and it was found to be effective in managing behavioural problems and reducing parental stress and enhancing parental confidence, and improving the quality of their ADHD children (Zwi, Jones, Thorgaard, York, & Dennis, 2011; Kousha, & Kakrodi, 2019). Parent training and medical management were found to decrease the stress. In a child management and parent training study, Kazdin and Wassell (2000) found that after intervention, improvements in parents were also noticed such as decreased depression, overall symptoms and stress. In an outcome study of success-based, non coercive treatment of oppositional behaviour in children from violent homes, Ducharme et al. (2000) found that training improved maternal perception of the child and reduced maternal stress. Family support services produced effective and lasting change in family's ability to cope with the child's problem. It has been found effective in strengthening intrafamily support, informal social ties outside the family and formal ties between parents and professionals (Hawkins and Singer, 1989; Singh, 1995). ADHD children's behavioral problems and parental self-awareness of psychological and emotional problems were reported as the most influential on parenting stress, and recognition of the pathological cause was the most influential factor in willingness to accept treatment (Lin & Chung, 2002).

The severity of parental stress affects the perception of their child's problem. Schaughency and Lahey (1985) found that maternal rating of child behaviour is influenced by maternal stress and depression. They may tend to exaggerate the child behaviour problems and label them as deviant. Parent and teacher ratings of child behaviors are often discrepant, and these discrepancies may be correlated with parenting stress (Chen, Hwang-Gu, Ni, Liang, Lin, Lin, Tseng, &Gau, 2017). Adolescent ADHD classification, mothers' self-reported ADHD symptoms were associated with higher parenting stress and the extent to which clinical levels of adolescent Oppositional Defiant Disorder (ODD) symptoms or externalizing behavior in general were associated with parenting stress depended on the rater of these behaviors. Parenting stress was associated with higher levels of ODD and other externalizing behaviors when these behaviors were rated by parents but not when they were rated by teachers (Wiener, Biondic, Grimbos, & Herbert, 2016).

Parental stress also affects the adherence to treatment. Maternal expressed emotion (EE), attributions, depression and parenting stress in mothers of children with behaviour problems referred for therapy, were tested for associations with entry to therapy. Calam, Bolton and Roberts (2002) found that mothers who did not attend the therapy scored higher on EE dimensions of critical comments, hostility or emotional over-involvement, maternal depression and parental stress. Parental distress not only affects the rating of symptoms but also the outcome in adolescent and adulthood. Gordon and Hinshaw (2017) reported that parenting stress, particularly related to maternal perceptions of dysfunctional interactions with adolescent daughters, serves as a key mediator in the association between childhood ADHD status and important domains of young adult functioning and they suggested that minimizing parenting stress and dysfunctional mother-daughter interactions during adolescence might reduce the risk of adverse adult outcomes for girls with ADHD.

Marital Discord

Parents of children and adolescents with psychiatric disorders may experience perceived family burden. Although previous research has extensively addressed the contribution of clinical factors to perceived family burden, the contribution of marital and parental factors to family burden has rarely been studied in the context of parents whose children have a psychiatric disorder and reported that parental satisfaction marital satisfaction and perceived family burden (Hasson-Ohayon, Ben-Pazi, Silberg, Pijnenborg, & Goldzweig, 2019). Mothers of children with developmental delay suffer more from depression and have less marital satisfaction compared to mothers of healthy children (Doulabi, Sajedi, Vameghi,Mazaheri, Baghban, & Afraz, 2019).

Parents of children with ADHD often experience low marital satisfaction than parents with normal children, since the child's increased susceptibility to maladjustment can affect family dynamics as a whole. Higher parental stress and lower self-efficacy were found to affect marital satisfaction suggesting that personal characteristics and situation appraisal are tapped when facing strain and hardship (Ben-Naim, Gill, Laslo-Roth, &Einav,2019; Mohammadi, Farokhzadi, Alipour, Rostami, Dehestani, & Salmanian,2012).

It was noticed that employment and reasonable income may contribute to a lower level of stress and improved relationship among mothers with ADHD children(Kachooei, Daneshmand, Dolatshahi, Samadi, & Samiei, 2016).

Impact on Mental Health

The mothers of children with attention-deficit hyperactivity disorder tend to experience depression at higher levels because of the poor social interaction and deviant behaviors of their children. These depressed mothers often harm themselves and negatively impact their family and community. Among the sample of 100 mothers of school-age children with attention-deficit hyperactivity disorder, almost half of the mothers suffered higher parenting stress and that 34% required professional psychiatry referral and 40% of the participants suffered from depression. Higher levels of parenting stress and low socioeconomic status were associated with a higher incidence of depression, and better social support had lower depression levels (Chen, Tsai, Chou, & Hu,2015). Studies have noted that high prevalence rate of disorders and background of ADHD in families of individuals with ADHD shows the probability of effect of inheritance in the disorder and it also shows that parents of children with ADHD have more substance abuse and history of ADHD in their background (Farokhzadi, Mohammadi, Alipour, Rostami, & Dehestani, 2012).

Several factors, which limit our current understanding of parent stress in children with ADHD, are differences in defining parent stress, the different tools used for assessing stress and the methodologies to evaluate its influence on treatment effectiveness. The association between parent and child characteristics with parent stress and coping is not fully known.

STRESS, STIGMA AND INTERVENTIONS

While discussing about parental stress related to ADHD, it is important to consider the source of parenting stress such as symptom severity, comordities, parent-child characteristics, parenting style and one of the important factors contributing o stress is stigma. This section attempted to explore the link between parental stress and stigma, especially related to ADHD and its interventions.

Patients suffering from ADHD are at high risk to be confronted with stigma, prejudices, and discrimination. Stigma refers to the undesirable characteristics linked to mental illness and the adverse cognitive and behavioral consequences. Stigma causes a spiral of alienation and discrimination, leading to social isolation that diminishes chances for recovery. The contribution of stigma associated with ADHD can be conceptualized as an underestimated risk factor, affecting treatment adherence, treatment efficacy, symptom aggravation, life satisfaction, and mentally well-being of individuals affected by ADHD. Public as well as health professionals' concepts about ADHD were found to be highly diverse, setting individuals with an ADHD diagnosis at greater risk to get stigmatized (Mueller, Fuermaier, Koerts, & Tucha, 2012).

Parental affiliate stigma about their children's inattentive and hyperactive/impulsive symptoms may have negative ramifications for parent-child interactions and children's social functioning. Mikami, Chong, Saporito, & Na (2015) examined parents' perceptions/awareness and internalization of public courtesy stigma (affiliate stigma) about their children's inattentive and hyperactive/impulsive symptoms, and associations between parental affiliate stigma, parental negativity expressed toward the child, and child social functioning and reported that parents' self-reports of greater affiliate stigma were associated with more observed negative parenting. The associations between high parental affiliate stigma and children's poorer adult informant-rated social skills and greater observed aggression were partially mediated by increased parental negativity. The positive association between children's adult informant-rated aggressive behavior and parental negativity was partially mediated by parents' increased affiliate stigma.

Multiple factors of caregivers and children were related to affiliate stigma in caregivers of children with ADHD. In a sample of 400 caregivers of children with ADHD showed that female caregivers and those caring for girls with ADHD had higher levels of affiliate stigma than did male caregivers and those caring for boys. Higher education levels in caregivers and more severe inattention symptoms in children were associated with higher levels of affiliate stigma. A higher level of affiliate stigma was also significantly associated with unfavorable attitudes toward children's diagnoses, pharmacotherapy and behavioral therapy, and etiological explanations for ADHD (Chang, Chen, Liu, Hsiao, Chou,& Yen, 2020).

Masuch, Bea, Alm, Deibler, & Sobanski (2019) have assessed internalized stigma, perceived public stigma, anticipated discrimination and their associations with demographic, psychiatric and psychosocial characteristics in a sample of 104 adults with ADHD and they reported high internalized stigma, anticipated discrimination in daily life and perceived public stigma among the sample. Internalized stigma and/or anticipated discrimination correlated with ADHD symptoms, psychological distress, self-esteem, functional impairment and quality of life were associated with ADHD family history and employment status and most frequently perceived stereotypes were doubts about the validity of ADHD as a mental disorder. This study emphasis that ADHD is associated with characteristic public stereotypes, which are distinct from stereotypes related to other mental disorders and stigmatization.

There is a great need for antistigma programs in order to decrease stigma related to persons with mental health problems. The antistigma program on Sixty-three students from high schools showed that social discrimination and the tendency towards social restriction were reduced, while, at the same time, social awareness of mental health-related problems was increased among young people six months after program implementation (Pejović-Milovancević, Lecić-Tosevski, Tenjović, Popović-Deusić, & Draganić-Gajić, 2009).

Children and adolescents demonstrate stigmatizing responses to peers with common mental health problems and the nature and extent of these responses depends on the type of problem and the type of measurement (O'Driscoll, Heary, Hennessy,& McKeague, 2012). Giannakopoulos, Assimopoulos, Petanidou, Tzavara, Kolaitis, & Tsiantis (2012) evaluated the effectiveness of a school-based educational intervention for improving adolescents' attitudes and reducing the desire for social distance from people with mental illness living in their community and found that all attitude dimensions and half of the measured social distance statements were significantly improved in the intervention group at follow up assessment compared to controls. However, the statements measuring more intimate types of social relationships did not change significantly post intervention. It shows that short educational interventions can be effective to some extent in reducing discriminatory attitudes towards people with mental illness.

Intervention for reducing social stigma towards mental illness in adolescents within the school environment consisted of providing information via a documentary film and of contact with healthcare staff and found to be effective in authoritarianism and social restrictiveness especially with those who knew someone with mental illness(Vila-Badia, Martínez-Zambrano, Arenas, Casas-Anguera, García-Morales, Villellas et al.,2016).Educational mental health intervention can have a positive impact on adolescents' perceptions towards people with mental illness and improvements in the knowledge of mental health and illness among adolescents(Sakellari, Lehtonen, Sourander, Kalokerinou-Anagnostopoulou, &Leino-Kilpi, 2014; Sakellari, Leino-Kilpi, & Kalokerinou-Anagnostopoulou,2011). In an intervention program consisted in providing information and contact with users of mental health in order to reduce social stigma in the school environment, improvement was noticed in the students' perception of mental disorders and reduction in their levels of stigma, especially in the area of authoritarianism(Martínez-Zambrano, García-Morales, García-Franco, Miguel, Villellas, Pascual, Arenas, Ochoa, 2013). Yamaguchi, Mino, & Uddin (2011) reviewed forty studies on effects of educational interventions (educational condition, video-based contact condition and contact condition) to reduce stigmatization and improve awareness of mental health problems among young people and noticed significant improvements in knowledge, changes in attitudes towards people with mental illness, significant effects in social distance and improved young people's awareness of mental illness. From the comparison of the three types of educational interventions, direct contact with people with mental illness (Contact condition) seems to be key factor in reducing stigmatization, while the components of Education and Video-based contact conditions are still arguable.

Interventions to reduce stigma among primary healthcare providers towards persons with mental illness showed changes in perceptions of violence (survival threats) and the ability to treat mental illness effectively (professional threats), and increased willingness to interact with a person with mental illness and observed clinical competency (Kohrt, Turner, Rai, Bhardwaj, Kathleen Sikkema, Adelekun, Dhakal, Luitel, Lund, Patel, & Jordans,2020). In another study on the effectiveness of interventions designed to reduce mental illness stigma among healthcare students and professionals, interventions involving direct contact, indirect filmed contact or an educational email was effectively reduced stigma in the short term. There was not enough evidence to suggest that any intervention can maintain stigma reduction over time. Stigma reduction in healthcare students and professionals needs to be sustained over time if it is to result in positive changes for people living with mental illness. Further research is needed to determine which interventions, if any, can achieve this. Only then will large-scale implementation of a stigma reduction intervention be feasible and beneficial to people living with mental illness (Stubbs, 2014).

Multiple psychosocial factors influence the stigma and stigma reduction programs. Individuals with mental illness living in countries with less stigmatizing attitudes, higher rates of help-seeking and treatment utilization and better perceived access to information had lower rates of self-stigma and perceived discrimination and those living in countries where the public felt more comfortable talking to people with mental illness had less self-stigma and felt more empowered. Targeting the general public through mass anti-stigma interventions may lead to a virtuous cycle by disrupting the negative feedback engendered by public stigma, thereby reducing self-stigma among people with mental health problems. A combined approach involving knowledge, attitudes and behaviour is needed and mass interventions that facilitate disclosure and positive social contact may be the most effective. Improving availability of information about mental health issues and facilitating access to care and help-seeking also show promise with regard to stigma (Evans-Lacko, Brohan, Mojtabai, & Thornicroft, 2012).

ADHD AND COPING

Hans Selye (1956, 1976) often referred to as the 'father of stress research' first studied the phenomenon of stress. According to him stress is a 'non-specific response of the body to any demand and he explained about General Adaptational Syndrome (GAS). The current conceptualization of stress as interactional in nature (Lazarus and Launier, 1978), involves some sort of transaction between the individual and the environment. According to Lazarus (1993) stress is dependent upon cognitive processes related to the perception of events and their meaning to the individual. Coping traditionally has been defined as a series of responses that are designed to help the organism adjust to an ongoing stress. Folkman and Lazarus (1985) state that coping refers to cognitive and behavioural efforts to manage (master, reduce or tolerate) a troubled person environment relationship. Thus, coping responses are distinguished from other adaptation responses only in that they are inextricably linked to stress. Current theory and research rests on the notion that coping primarily involves conscious styles or strategies of responding to stressful or negative events. (Folkman and Lazarus, 1988). The individual chooses the coping strategies to utilize in a particular situation, based on his /her coping resources, that is the relatively stable characteristics of the person's disposition and social environment and the appraisal of the event.

Care for a child with a disability is a stressful experience for parents which triggers a range of emotions and feelings that require a set of behaviors and attitudes to manage daily life. To face this situation, parents use coping strategies. The range of coping strategies used includes religion active coping, planning, acceptance, focus and venting of feelings, and seeking emotional social support . Parents mainly used emotion-focused and problem-centered coping and the coping strategy choice was significantly correlated with gender. Mothers preferentially used emotion-focused coping and it was also correlated with low levels of education and socioeconomic status. Depressed or anxious parents more frequently used emotion-focused strategies. Religious faith was correlated with a strategy centered on religious coping (Ben Thabet, Sallemi, Hasïri et al., 2013). Sadati,Salehzade, Hemmati, Darvish, Heydari, & Tabrizi (2015) have noticed a was a significant relationship between mothers' loving care towards disabled children and purpose in life religious attitude and life satisfaction. Gopalan, Oommen, Srinath and Kapur (2006) observed in their study on ADHD that most of the parents felt disappointed, guilty and upset about their child's condition and thought that it was due to the 'bad karma' in their past life and god has punished them through the child's problem and some parents accepted it as a method of coping. McKee, Harvey, Danforth, Ulaszek, Friedman (2004) reported that parents use different styles of coping styles which reflected in their parenting style. For mothers, use of more maladaptive and less adaptive coping styles was related to more self-reported lax and overreactive discipline, more observed coercive parenting, and more observed child misbehavior. For fathers, use of more maladaptive and less adaptive coping styles was related to self-reported lax discipline. It is also reported that parent coping by more use of positive reframing (thinking about problems as challenges that might be overcome) was associated with higher role satisfaction for both mothers and fathers (Podolski & Nigg, 2001). Cappe, Bolduc, Rougé, Saiag, & Delorme (2017) have studied quality of life and adjustment mechanisms in ninety parents of children with Attention-Deficit/Hyperactivity Disorder (ADHD) and found that the severity of the disorder, perceiving the situation as a threat or a loss, feeling guilty and holding on to irrational beliefs were related to emotion-focused coping strategies and to a poorer quality of life. In contrast, perceiving the situation as challenging was related to a greater sense of control and personal fulfillment. Moreover, perceiving the situation as challenging and adopting problem-focused coping strategies predicted better quality of life.

In a systematic review on coping strategies used by parents of children with ADHD, Craig, Savino, Fanizza, Lucarelli, Russo, & Trabacca (2020) found that parents of ADHD children used more avoidant-focused coping strategies than parents of typical children. Mothers of ADHD children sought significantly more support and used more indirect means than mothers of typically developing (TD) children. More or less similar finding was noticed in parents of a child with Autism Spectrum Disorders that parents used more avoidance strategies and less social support-seeking strategies than those of typical children. Furthermore, problem-focused coping protects parental stress and quality of life, that on the contrary, emotion-focused coping is a risk factor for alteration. The studies illustrates the need to adapt psychoeducational interventions for parents of children with disabilities (Vernhet, Dellapiazza, Blanc et al., 2019).

MINDFULNESS TRAINING, ADHD AND PARENTAL STRESS

While hyperactivity declines over time, inattention and executive function difficulties persist, leading to functional deficits. Adolescents and adults with ADHD have pervasive impairment in interpersonal and family relationships and they may develop addiction, delinquent behavior and comorbid psychiatric disorders. Both pharmacological and non-pharmacological interventions were proved to be effective in dealing with ADHD but with limitations. Despite advances in diagnosis and treatment, persistent residual symptoms are common, highlighting the need for novel treatment strategies. Mindfulness training, derived from Eastern meditation practices, may improve self-regulation of attention and may also be a useful strategy to augment standard ADHD treatments (Modesto-Lowe, Farahmand, Chaplin, & Lauren Sarro, 2015).

Mindfulness means paying attention and being aware of the experiences occurring in the present moment, and it is usually developed by the practice of meditation. Mindfulness training may be one self-regulatory method for strengthening attentional processes (orienting, alerting, and executive attention) and Preliminary findings from the review articles suggested significant improvements in attentional processes. It may be used as a potential tool to reduce impairments in patients with residual symptoms of ADHD. Clinically, this would manifest by an increased ability to suppress task-unrelated thoughts and distractions resulting in improved attention, completion of tasks and potential improvement in occupational and social function (Cassone, 2015;Modesto-Lowe, Farahmand, Chaplin, & Lauren Sarro, 2015; Schmiedeler, 2015).

Mindfulness training is a feasible intervention in a subset of ADHD adults and adolescents and may improve behavioral and neurocognitive impairments. Twenty-four adults and eight adolescents with ADHD enrolled in a feasibility study of an 8-week mindfulness training program and majority of participants completed the training and reported high satisfaction with the training. Pre-post improvements in self-reported ADHD symptoms and test performance on tasks measuring attention and cognitive inhibition were noted and improvements in anxiety and depressive symptoms were also observed (Zylowska, Ackerman, Yang, Futrell, Horton, Hale, Pataki, & Smalley, 2008). Aadil, Cosme, & Chernaik(2017) have reviewed 17 articles to look for the beneficial effects of mindfulness-based cognitive behavioral therapy for treatment of attention deficit hyperactivity disorder in adults and reported that there was a clear beneficial effect of such therapies, especially when used in adjunct with stimulant medication and may increase overall compliance. In a randomized clinical trial, Behbahani, Zargar, Assarian, & Akbari (2018) found reduction in children's problematic characteristics and improvement in ADHD symptoms in the mindful parenting training group. Lee, Ma, Ho, Tsang, Zheng, & Wu (2017) reviewed studies related to effectiveness for individuals (children, adolescents and adults) with ADHD to improve attention and it was found that mindfulness-based intervention was comparatively more popularly used in adults with ADHD to improve attention, and the improvement was significant.

Mindfulness-based intervention has received more clinical interest and empirical support for individuals with ADHD especially to improve attention. It is still unclear whether mindfulness-based intervention is effective for children and adolescence with ADHD due to limited studies available and the limitations of the study design in the reviewed studies. For better understanding, large, well-designed studies should be conducted with robust strategies, allowing more comparison studies with the better analytical outcome (Lee et al., 2017; Schmiedeler, 2015; Aadil, Cosme, & Chernaik,2017).

Mindfulness training has been used for reducing parental stress and found to be effective. Rayan & Ahmad (2018) reviewed effectiveness of mindfulness-based interventions (MBIs) for management of parenting distress in parents of children with disabilities and found to be effective and the interventions used a variety of approaches to implement mindfulness training, including MBIs and combined mindfulness and other interventions. Lunsky, Hastings, Weiss, Palucka, Hutton, & White (2017) evaluated two community based interventions for parents of adults with autism spectrum disorder and other developmental disabilities. Parents in the mindfulness group reported significant reductions in psychological distress, while parents in the support and information group did not and reduced levels of distress in the mindfulness group were maintained at 20 weeks follow-up. Results suggested the psychological components of the mindfulness based group intervention were effective over and above the non-specific effects of group processes and informal support.

The central tenants of mindful parenting appear to be emotional awareness, emotional regulation, attention regulation, intentionality and non-judgmental acceptance. In a review included randomized controlled trials on parenting programs that drew upon mindfulness-based stress reduction, mindfulness-based cognitive therapy, mindfulness-based cognitive behavior therapy, dialectical behavior therapy or acceptance commitment therapy, Townshend, Jordan, Stephenson, & Tsey (2016) indicated that mindful parenting programs may reduce parental stress, increase parents' emotional awareness of their 10-14-year-old children and reduce preschool children's symptoms associated with externalizing disorders and a recurring finding was that the mindful parenting programs reduced parents' emotional dismissal of their adolescents and preschoolers. In another systematic review and meta-analysis, Burgdorf, Szabó, & Abbott (2019) evaluated the effectiveness of mindfulness interventions for parents, in reducing parenting stress and improving youth psychological outcomes and found reduction in parenting stress, growing to a moderate reduction at 2 month follow-up. Change in parenting stress predicted change in youth externalizing and cognitive effects, and improved youth psychological functioning. Behbahani, Zargar, Assarian, & Akbari (2018) reported reduction in parenting stress, negative parent-child interactions, and children's problematic characteristics in the mindful parenting training group compared with the control group in the posttest and follow-up.

Analysis of the randomized controlled trials showed that mindfulness-based parenting interventions had significant positive treatment effects on symptoms of depression in parents. Samples of parents with culturally, economically, or racially diverse backgrounds have not been well-studied in relation to mindfulness-based parenting. Consistent use of frameworks, intervention types, and measurement tools across studies will strengthen the body of evidence (Alexander, 2018).

CONCLUSION

Attention-deficit hyperactivity disorder (ADHD) is a complex disorder that can affect individuals across the lifespan. It is associated with substantial heterogeneity in terms of aetiology, clinical presentation and treatment outcome and is the subject of extensive research. Because of this, it can be difficult for clinicians to stay up to date with the most relevant findings and know how best to respond to parents' questions and concerns about the disorder and interventions. Despite extensive advances in understanding this complex disorder, it is clear that there is still a long way to go. There is need for future non-pharmacological interventions to be more specifically targeted for ADHD symptoms and its commonly associated functioning deficits in order to ensure the best long-term outcomes for children with ADHD (Tarver, Daley, &Sayal, 2014).

Findings from the multiple studies highlighted the negative effects of ADHD on parent psychological adjustment and underline the need to recommend training programs that improve parenting skills, parents' perceptions concerning their child's behavior disorder and parental functioning. Also to explore the coping mechanisms of parents of children with ADHD in order to promote positive coping strategies for parents of children with ADHD, and to help such parents to identify people who can support them. (Craig, Savino, Fanizza, Lucarelli, Russo, & Trabacca,2020). Health care providers need to develop and apply a parenting skills improvement program to improve positive parenting attitudes, which will benefit self-esteem and social competence in children with attention deficit hyperactivity disorder (Oh, Park, Suk, Song, & Im, 2012).Both child/adolescent's and family factors should be considered in the designing of interventions for reducing parenting stress in families of children and adolescents with ADHD (Muñoz-Silva, Lago-Urbano, Sanchez-Garcia, & Carmona-Márquez,2017).

Reduction of stigma and associated issues are also need to be addressed while trying reduce the parenting stress and multi-disciplinary interventions are to be considered. Though mindful training is found to be effective in reducing parental stress, the studies suffer methodological limitations such as small sample size, information bias and future studies need to confirm its effectiveness on different co morbidities, symptom severities and cultural suitability.

REFERENCES

Aadil, M., Cosme, R. M., & Chernaik, J. (2017). Mindfulness-Based Cognitive Behavioral Therapy as an Adjunct Treatment of Attention Deficit Hyperactivity Disorder in Young Adults: A Literature Review. *Cureus*, *9*(5), e1269. doi:10.7759/cureus.1269 PMID:28775916

Abikoff, H., & Klein, R. (1992). Attention Deficit Hyperactivity and Conduct Disorders: Comorbidity and implications for treatment. *Journal of Consulting and Clinical Psychology*, *60*(6), 881–892. doi:10.1037/0022-006X.60.6.881 PMID:1360990

Alexander, K. (2018). Integrative Review of the Relationship Between Mindfulness-Based Parenting Interventions and Depression Symptoms in Parents. *Journal of Obstetric, Gynecologic, and Neonatal Nursing*, *47*(2), 184–190. doi:10.1016/j.jogn.2017.11.013 PMID:29294315

Algorta, P. G., Kragh, C. A., Arnold, L. E., Molina, B. S. G., Hinshaw, S. P., Swanson, J. M., Hechtman, L., Copley, L. M., Lowe, M., & Jensen, P. S. (2018). Maternal ADHD Symptoms, Personality, and Parenting Stress: Differences Between Mothers of Children With ADHD and Mothers of Comparison Children. *Journal of Attention Disorders*, *22*(13), 1266–1277. doi:10.1177/1087054714561290 PMID:25525155

Almogbel, Y. S., Goyal, R., & Sansgiry, S. S. (2017). Association Between Parenting Stress and Functional Impairment Among Children Diagnosed with Neurodevelopmental Disorders. *Community Mental Health Journal*, *53*(4), 405–414. doi:10.100710597-017-0096-9 PMID:28176211

American Psychiatric Association. (1968). *Diagnostic and Statistical Manual of Mental Disorders* (2nd ed.). Author.

American Psychiatric Association. (1980). *Diagnostic and Statistical Manual of Mental Disorders* (3rd ed.). Author.

Anastopoulos, A. D., Guevremont, D. C., Shelton, T. L., & Dupaul, G. J. (1992). Parenting stress among families of children with Attention Deficit Hyperactivity Disorder. *Journal of Abnormal Child Psychology*, *20*(5), 503–520. doi:10.1007/BF00916812 PMID:1487593

Babakhanian, M., Sayar, S., Babakhanian, M., & Mohammadi, G. (2016). Iranian Children With ADHD and Mental Health of Their Mothers: The Role of Stress. *Iranian Journal of Psychiatry and Behavioral Sciences*, *10*(1), e2026. doi:10.17795/ijpbs-2026 PMID:27284276

Babinski, D. E., Mazzant, J. R., Merrill, B. M., Waschbusch, D. A., Sibley, M. H., Gnagy, E. M., Molina, B. S. G., & Pelham, W. E. (2020). Lifetime caregiver strain among mothers of adolescents and young adults with attention-deficit/hyperactivity disorder. *Journal of Family Psychology*, *34*(3), 342–352. doi:10.1037/fam0000609 PMID:31750692

Barkley, R. A. (1989). Hyperactive girls and boys: Stimulant drug effects on mother-child interactions. *Journal of Child Psychology and Psychiatry, and Allied Disciplines*, *30*(3), 379–390. doi:10.1111/j.1469-7610.1989.tb00253.x PMID:2663900

Barkley, R. A. (1990). *Attention Deficit Hyperactivity Disorder: A handbook for diagnosis and treatment*. Guilford Press.

Barkley, R. A. (1998). *Attention Deficit Hyperactivity Disorder: A handbook for diagnosis and treatment* (2nd ed.). Guilford press.

Barkley, R. A., Fischer, M., Edelbrock, C., & Smallish, L. (1991). The adolescent outcome of hyperactive children diagnosed by research criteria, III: Mother child interactions, family conflicts and maternal psychopathology. *Journal of Child Psychology and Psychiatry, and Allied Disciplines*, *32*(2), 233–255. doi:10.1111/j.1469-7610.1991.tb00304.x PMID:2033106

Barroso, N. E., Mendez, L., Graziano, P. A., & Bagner, D. M. (2018). Parenting Stress through the Lens of Different Clinical Groups: A Systematic Review & Meta-Analysis. *Journal of Abnormal Child Psychology*, *46*(3), 449–461. doi:10.100710802-017-0313-6 PMID:28555335

Behbahani, M., Zargar, F., Assarian, F., & Akbari, H. (2018). Effects of Mindful Parenting Training on Clinical Symptoms in Children with Attention Deficit Hyperactivity Disorder and Parenting Stress: Randomized Controlled Trial. *Iranian Journal of Medical Sciences*, *43*(6), 596–604. PMID:30510336

Ben-Naim, S., Gill, N., Laslo-Roth, R., & Einav, M. (2019). Parental Stress and Parental Self-Efficacy as Mediators of the Association Between Children's ADHD and Marital Satisfaction. *Journal of Attention Disorders*, *23*(5), 506–516. doi:10.1177/1087054718784659 PMID:29985090

Ben Thabet, J., Sallemi, R., Hasïri, I., Zouari, L., Kamoun, F., Zouari, N., Triki, C., & Maâlej, M. (2013). Psycho-emotional impact of a child's disability on parents. *Archives of Pediatrics*, *20*(1), 9–16. doi:10.1016/j.arcped.2012.10.024 PMID:23266169

Bickman, L., Foster, E. M., & Lambert, E. W. (1996). Who gets hospitalized in a continuum of care? *Journal of the American Academy of Child and Adolescent Psychiatry*, *35*(1), 74–80. doi:10.1097/00004583-199601000-00015 PMID:8567616

Bonifacci, P., Massi, L., Pignataro, V., Zocco, S., & Chiodo, S. (2019). Parenting Stress and Broader Phenotype in Parents of Children with Attention Deficit Hyperactivity Disorder, Dyslexia or Typical Development. *International Journal of Environmental Research and Public Health*, *16*(11), 1878. doi:10.3390/ijerph16111878 PMID:31141931

Burgdorf, V., Szabó, M., & Abbott, M. J. (2019). The Effect of Mindfulness Interventions for Parents on Parenting Stress and Youth Psychological Outcomes: A Systematic Review and Meta-Analysis. *Frontiers in Psychology*, *10*, 1336. doi:10.3389/fpsyg.2019.01336 PMID:31244732

Bussing, R., Meyer, J., Zima, B. T., Mason, D. M., Gary, F. A., & Garvan, C. W. (2015). Childhood ADHD Symptoms: Association with Parental Social Networks and Mental Health Service Use during Adolescence. *International Journal of Environmental Research and Public Health*, *12*(9), 11893–11909. doi:10.3390/ijerph120911893 PMID:26402692

Calam, R., Bolten, C., & Roberts, J. (2002). Maternal expressed emotion, attributions and depression and entry into therapy for children with behaviour problems. *British Journal of Clinical Psychology*, *41*(2), 213–216. doi:10.1348/014466502163985 PMID:12034007

Campbell, S. B., Breaux, A. M., Ewing, L. J., & Szumowski, E. K. (1986). Correlates and predictors of hyperactivity and aggression: A longitudinal study of parent – referred problem preschoolers. *Journal of Abnormal Child Psychology*, *14*(2), 217–234. doi:10.1007/BF00915442 PMID:3722619

Cappe, E., Bolduc, M., Rougé, M. C., Saiag, M. C., & Delorme, R. (2017). Quality of life, psychological characteristics, and adjustment in parents of children with Attention-Deficit/Hyperactivity Disorder. *Quality of Life Research: An International Journal of Quality of Life Aspects of Treatment, Care and Rehabilitation, 26*(5), 1283–1294. doi:10.100711136-016-1446-8 PMID:27798755

Cassone, A. R. (2015). Mindfulness training as an adjunct to evidence-based treatment for ADHD within families. *Journal of Attention Disorders, 19*(2), 147–157. doi:10.1177/1087054713488438 PMID:23704114

Chang, C. C., Chen, Y. M., Liu, T. L., Hsiao, R. C., Chou, W. J., & Yen, C. F. (2020). Affiliate Stigma and Related Factors in Family Caregivers of Children with Attention-Deficit/Hyperactivity Disorder. *International Journal of Environmental Research and Public Health, 17*(2), 576. doi:10.3390/ijerph17020576 PMID:31963190

Chen, W. L., Tsai, S. T., & Chou, F. H. (2015). Depression and Related Factors in Mothers of School-Aged Children With Attention-Deficit Hyperactivity Disorder. *Hu Li Za Zhi, 62*(1), 39–49. doi:10.6224/JN.62.1.39 PMID:25631183

Chen, Y. C., Hwang-Gu, S. L., Ni, H. C., Liang, S. H., Lin, H. Y., Lin, C. F., Tseng, Y. H., & Gau, S. S. F. (2017). Relationship between parenting stress and informant discrepancies on symptoms of ADHD/ODD and internalizing behaviors in preschool children. *PLoS One, 12*(10), e0183467. doi:10.1371/journal.pone.0183467 PMID:29016602

Chess, S. (1960). Diagnosis and treatment of the hyperactive child. *New York State Journal of Medicine, 60*, 2379–2385. PMID:13809736

Chung, K. M., Ebesutani, C., Bang, H. M., Kim, J., Chorpita, B. F., Weisz, J. R., Suh, D., & Byun, H. (2013). Parenting stress and child behavior problems among clinic-referred youth: Cross-cultural differences across the US and Korea. *Child Psychiatry and Human Development, 44*(3), 460–468. doi:10.100710578-012-0340-z PMID:23073610

Craig, F., Operto, F. F., De Giacomo, A., Margari, L., Frolli, A., Conson, M., Ivagnes, S., Monaco, M., & Margari, F. (2016). Parenting stress among parents of children with Neurodevelopmental Disorders. *Journal of Psychiatric Research, 242*, 121–129. doi:10.1016/j.psychres.2016.05.016 PMID:27280521

Craig, F., Savino, R., Fanizza, I., Lucarelli, E., Russo, L., & Trabacca, A. (2020). A systematic review of coping strategies in parents of children with attention deficit hyperactivity disorder (ADHD). *Research in Developmental Disabilities, 98*, 103571. doi:10.1016/j.ridd.2020.103571 PMID:31931455

Cunningham, C. E., & Barley, R. A. (1979). The interactions of normal and hyperactive children with their mothers during free play and structured tasks. *Child Development, 50*(1), 217–224. doi:10.2307/1129059 PMID:446207

Doulabi, M. A., Sajedi, F., Vameghi, R., Mazaheri, M. A., Baghban, A. A., & Afraz, F. (2019). Marital Satisfaction and Depression in Mothers of 3-4 Year Old Children with Developmental Delay in Comparison with Mothers of Normal Children. *Iranian Journal of Child Neurology, 13*(4), 91–108. PMID:31645870

Ducharme, J. M., Atkinson, L., & Poulton, L. (2000). Success-based, Non-coercive treatment of oppositional behaviour in children from violent homes. *Journal of the American Academy of Child and Adolescent Psychiatry*, *39*(8), 995–1004. doi:10.1097/00004583-200008000-00014 PMID:10939227

Dyson, L. L. (1993). Response to the presence of a child with disabilities: Parental stress and Family functioning over time. *American Journal of Mental Retardation*, *98*, 207–218. PMID:7691096

Escobar, R., Hervas, A., Soutullo, C., Mardomingo, M. J., Uruñuela, A., & Gilaberte, I. (2008). Attention deficit/hyperactivity disorder: Burden of the disease according to subtypes in recently diagnosed children. *Actas Españolas de Psiquiatría*, *36*(5), 285–294. PMID:18830848

Evans-Lacko, S., Brohan, E., Mojtabai, R., & Thornicroft, G. (2012). Association between public views of mental illness and self-stigma among individuals with mental illness in 14 European countries. *Psychological Medicine*, *42*(8), 1741–1752. doi:10.1017/S0033291711002558 PMID:22085422

Farokhzadi, F., Mohammadi, M. R., Alipour, A., Rostami, R., & Dehestani, M. (2012). Substance abuse disorders in the parents of ADHD children, and parents of normal children. *Acta Medica Iranica*, *50*(5), 319–327. PMID:22837085

Ferguson, J. H. (2000). National Institutes of Health Consensus Development Conference Statement: Diagnosis and Treatment of Attention-Deficit/Hyperactivity Disorder (ADHD) (2000). *Journal of the American Academy of Child and Adolescent Psychiatry*, *39*(2), 182–193. doi:10.1097/00004583-200002000-00018 PMID:10673829

Fergusson, D. M., Horwood, L. J., & Lynskey, M. T. (1993). The effects of conduct disorder and Attention Deficit in middle childhood on offending and scholastic ability at age 13. *Journal of Child Psychology and Psychiatry, and Allied Disciplines*, *34*(6), 899–916. doi:10.1111/j.1469-7610.1993.tb01097.x PMID:8408374

Folkman, S., & Lazarus, R. S. (1985). If it changes it must be a process: Study of emotion and coping during three stages of a college examination. *Journal of Personality and Social Psychology*, *48*(1), 150–170. doi:10.1037/0022-3514.48.1.150 PMID:2980281

Folkman, S., & Lazarus, R. S. (1988). Coping as a mediator of emotion. *Journal of Personality and Social Psychology*, *54*(3), 466–475. doi:10.1037/0022-3514.54.3.466 PMID:3361419

Foster, E. M., Saunders, R. C., & Summerfelt, W. T. (1996). A comparison of multiple methods of predicting level of care in mental health services. *Evaluation and Program Planning*, *19*, 143–153. doi:10.1016/0149-7189(96)00005-5

Friesen, B. J. (1989). National study of parents whose children have serious emotional disorders. In A. Algarin, R. Friedman, A. Duchnowski, K. Kutash, S. Silver, & M. Johnson (Eds.), *Children's mental health service and policy. Building a research base*. University of South Florida Research and Training Centre for Children's Mental Health.

Giannakopoulos, G., Assimopoulos, H., Petanidou, D., Tzavara, C., Kolaitis, G., & Tsiantis, J. (2012). Effectiveness of a school-based intervention for enhancing adolescents' positive attitudes towards people with mental illness. *Mental Illness*, *4*(2), e16. doi:10.4081/mi.2012.e16 PMID:25478117

Gohari, Z., Dehghani, F., Rajabi, G., & Mahmoudi-Gharaei, J. (2012). Parenting Self Efficacy in Mothers of Children with Attention Deficit Hyperactivity Disorder vs. Normal Children. *Iranian Journal of Psychiatry, 7*(2), 57–60. PMID:22952546

Gopalan, R. T., Oomme, A., Srinath, S., & Kapur, M. (2006). *Clinic based multimodal intervention for children with Attention Deficit Hyperactivity Disorder* (PhD Thesis). National Institute of Mental Health and Neuro Sciences, Bengaluru, India.

Gordon, C. T., & Hinshaw, S. P. (2017). Parenting Stress as a Mediator Between Childhood ADHD and Early Adult Female Outcomes. *Journal of Clinical Child and Adolescent Psychology, 46*(4), 588–599. doi:10.1080/15374416.2015.1041595 PMID:26042524

Gordon, C. T., & Hinshaw, S. P. (2017). Parenting Stress and Youth Symptoms among Girls with and without ADHD. *Parenting, Science and Practice, 17*(1), 11–29. doi:10.1080/15295192.2016.1262178 PMID:29308056

Gottlieb, B. H. (1981). *Social networks and social support.* Sage Publications.

Hasson-Ohayon, I., Ben-Pazi, A., Silberg, T., Pijnenborg, G. H. M., & Goldzweig, G. (2019). The mediating role of parental satisfaction between marital satisfaction and perceived family burden among parents of children with psychiatric disorders. *Journal of Psychiatric Research, 271*, 105–110. doi:10.1016/j.psychres.2018.11.037 PMID:30472503

Hawkins, N. E., & Singer, G. H. S. (1989). A skills training approach from assisting parents to cope with stress. In G.H.S. Singer & L.K Irwin (Eds.), Support for caregiving families: Enabling positive adaptation to disability. Baltimore, MD: Paul Brookes.

Jensen, P. S., Martin, D., & Cantwell, D. P. (1997). Comorbidity in ADHD: Implications for future research, practice and DSM-IV. *Journal of the American Academy of Child and Adolescent Psychiatry, 36*(8), 1065–1079. doi:10.1097/00004583-199708000-00014 PMID:9256586

Jouriles, E. N., Murphy, C. M., & O'Leary, K. D. (1989). Effects of maternal mood on Mother-son interaction patterns. *Journal of Abnormal Child Psychology, 17*(5), 513–525. doi:10.1007/BF00916510 PMID:2808944

Kachooei, H., Daneshmand, R., Dolatshahi, B., Samadi, R., & Samiei, M. (2016). Attention-Deficit/Hyperactivity Disorder and Martial Satisfaction: The Preliminary Roles of Employment and Income. *Iranian Journal of Psychiatry and Behavioral Sciences, 10*(2), e4012. doi:10.17795/ijpbs-4012 PMID:27803722

Kazdin, A. E., & Wassell, G. (2000). Therapeutic changes in children, parents and families resulting from treatment of children with conduct problems. *Journal of the American Academy of Child and Adolescent Psychiatry, 39*(4), 414–420. doi:10.1097/00004583-200004000-00009 PMID:10761342

Klassen, A. F., Miller, A., & Fine, S. (2004). Health-related quality of life in children and adolescents who have a diagnosis of attention-deficit/hyperactivity disorder. *Pediatrics, 114*(5), e541–e547. doi:10.1542/peds.2004-0844 PMID:15520087

Kohrt, B.A., Turner, E.L., Rai, S., Bhardwaj,A., Sikkema,K.J., Adelekun,A., Dhakal,M., Luitel,N.P, Lund,C., Patel,V., & Jordans, M. (in press). Reducing mental illness stigma in healthcare settings: Proof of concept for a social contact intervention to address what matters most for primary care providers. *Social Science & Medicine*, *250*, 112852. doi:10.1016/j.socscimed.2020.112852

Kousha, M., & Abbasi Kakrodi, M. (2019). Can Parents Improve the Quality of Life of Their Children with Attention Deficit Hyperactivity Disorder? *Iranian Journal of Psychiatry*, *14*(2), 154–159. doi:10.18502/ijps.v14i2.995 PMID:31440297

Krauss, M. W. (1993). Child-related and parenting stress: Similarities and differences between mothers and fathers of children with disabilities. *American Journal of Mental Retardation*, *97*, 393–404. PMID:8427694

Lahey, B. B., Pelham, W. E., Schaughency, E. A., Atkins, M. S., Murphy, H. A., Hynd, G. W., Russo, M., Hartdagen, S., & Lorys-Vernon, A. (1988). Dimensions and types of Attention Deficit Disorder with Hyperactivity children. A factor analytic and cluster analytic approach. *Journal of the American Academy of Child and Adolescent Psychiatry*, *27*(3), 330–335. doi:10.1097/00004583-198805000-00011 PMID:3379015

Laufer, M., & Denhoff, E. (1957). Hyperkinetic behaviour syndrome in children. *The Journal of Pediatrics*, *50*(4), 463–473. doi:10.1016/S0022-3476(57)80257-1 PMID:13406705

Laufer, M. W., Denhoff, E., & Solomons, G. (1957). Hyperkinetic Impulse Disorder in children's behaviour problems. *Psychosomatic Medicine*, *19*(1), 38–49. doi:10.1097/00006842-195701000-00005 PMID:13400991

Laugesen, B., & Groenkjaer, M. (2015). Parenting experiences of living with a child with attention deficit hyperactivity disorder: A systematic review of qualitative evidence. *JBI Database of Systematic Reviews and Implementation Reports*, *13*(11), 169–234. doi:10.11124/jbisrir-2015-2449 PMID:26657468

Lazarus, R. S. (1993). Coping theory and research: Past, present and future. *Psychosomatic Medicine*, *55*(3), 234–247. doi:10.1097/00006842-199305000-00002 PMID:8346332

Lazarus, R. S., & Launier, R. (1978). Stress-Related Transactions between Person and Environment. In L. A. Pervin & M. Lewis (Eds.), *Perspectives in Interactional Psychology* (pp. 287–327). Plenum. doi:10.1007/978-1-4613-3997-7_12

Lee, C. S. C., Ma, M. T., Ho, H. Y., Tsang, K. K., Zheng, Y. Y., & Wu, Z. Y. (2017). The Effectiveness of Mindfulness-Based Intervention in Attention on Individuals with ADHD: A Systematic Review. *Hong Kong Journal of Occupational Therapy*, *30*(1), 33–41. doi:10.1016/j.hkjot.2017.05.001 PMID:30186078

Leitch, S., Sciberras, E., Post, B., Gerner, B., Rinehart, N., Nicholson, J. M., & Evans, S. (2019). Experience of stress in parents of children with ADHD: A qualitative study. *International Journal of Qualitative Studies on Health and Well-being*, *14*(1), 1690091. doi:10.1080/17482631.2019.1690091 PMID:31713473

Lin, Y. F., & Chung, H. H. (2002). Parenting stress and parents' willingness to accept treatment in relation to behavioral problems of children with attention-deficit hyperactive disorder. *The Journal of Nursing Research*, *10*(1), 43–56. doi:10.1097/01.JNR.0000347582.54962.04 PMID:11923900

Lunsky, Y. P., Hastings, R., Weiss, J. A. M., Palucka, A., Hutton, S., & White, K. (2017). Comparative Effects of Mindfulness and Support and Information Group Interventions for Parents of Adults with Autism Spectrum Disorder and Other Developmental Disabilities. *Journal of Autism and Developmental Disorders*, *47*(6), 1769–1779. doi:10.100710803-017-3099-z PMID:28374207

Martin, C. A., Papadopoulos, N., Chellew, T., Rinehart, N. J., & Sciberras, E. (2019). Associations between parenting stress, parent mental health and child sleep problems for children with ADHD and ASD: Systematic review. *Research in Developmental Disabilities*, *93*, 103463. doi:10.1016/j.ridd.2019.103463 PMID:31446370

Martínez-Zambrano, F., García-Morales, E., García-Franco, M., Miguel, J., Villellas, R., Pascual, G., Arenas, O., & Ochoa, S. (2013). Intervention for reducing stigma: Assessing the influence of gender and knowledge. *World Journal of Psychiatry*, *3*(2), 18–24. doi:10.5498/wjp.v3.i2.18 PMID:24175182

Mash, E. J., & Johnston, C. (1983). Parental perceptions of child behaviour problems, parenting self-esteem. And mothers' reported stress in younger and older Hyperactive and normal children. *Journal of Consulting and Clinical Psychology*, *51*(1), 86–99. doi:10.1037/0022-006X.51.1.86 PMID:6826870

Mash, E. J., & Johnston, C. (1990). Determinants of parenting stress: Illustrations from families of hyperactive children and families of physically abused children. *Journal of Clinical Child Psychology*, *19*(4), 313–328. doi:10.120715374424jccp1904_3

Masuch, T. V., Bea, M., Alm, B., Deibler, P., & Sobanski, E. (2019). Internalized stigma, anticipated discrimination and perceived public stigma in adults with ADHD. *ADHD Attention Deficit and Hyperactivity Disorders*, *11*(2), 211–220. doi:10.100712402-018-0274-9 PMID:30341693

McBride, B. A., Shoppe, S. J., & Rane, T. R. (2002). Child characteristics, parenting stress and parental involvement: Fathers Vs mothers. *Journal of Marriage and the Family*, *64*(4), 998–1011. doi:10.1111/j.1741-3737.2002.00998.x

McKee, T. E., Harvey, E., Danforth, J. S., Ulaszek, W. R., & Friedman, J. L. (2004). The relation between parental coping styles and parent-child interactions before and after treatment for children with ADHD and oppositional behavior. *Journal of Clinical Child and Adolescent Psychology*, *33*(1), 158–168. doi:10.1207/S15374424JCCP3301_15 PMID:15028550

Mikami, A. Y., Chong, G. K., Saporito, J. M., & Na, J. J. (2015). Implications of parental affiliate stigma in families of children with ADHD. *Journal of Clinical Child and Adolescent Psychology*, *44*(4), 595–603. doi:10.1080/15374416.2014.888665 PMID:24697640

Modesto-Lowe, V., Chaplin, M., Godsay, V., & Soovajian, V. (2014). Parenting teens with attention-deficit/hyperactivity disorder: Challenges and opportunities. *Clinical Pediatrics*, *53*(10), 943–948. doi:10.1177/0009922814540984 PMID:24982442

Modesto-Lowe, V., Farahmand, P., Chaplin, M., & Sarro, L. (2015). Does mindfulness meditation improve attention in attention deficit hyperactivity disorder? *World Journal of Psychiatry*, *5*(4), 397–403. doi:10.5498/wjp.v5.i4.397 PMID:26740931

Mofokeng, M., & van der Wath, A. E. (2017). Challenges experienced by parents living with a child with attention deficit hyperactivity disorder. *Journal of Child and Adolescent Mental Health, 29*(2), 137–145. doi:10.2989/17280583.2017.1364253 PMID:28974169

Mohammadi, M. R., Farokhzadi, F., Alipour, A., Rostami, R., Dehestani, M., & Salmanian, M. (2012). Marital Satisfaction amongst Parents of Children with Attention Deficit Hyperactivity Disorder and Normal Children. *Iranian Journal of Psychiatry, 7*(3), 120–125. PMID:23139693

Mueller, A. K., Fuermaier, A. B., Koerts, J., & Tucha, L. (2012). Stigma in attention deficit hyperactivity disorder. *Attention Deficit and Hyperactivity Disorders, 4*(3), 101–114. doi:10.100712402-012-0085-3 PMID:22773377

Muñoz-Silva, A., Lago-Urbano, R., Sanchez-Garcia, M., & Carmona-Márquez, J. (2017). Child/Adolescent's ADHD and Parenting Stress: The Mediating Role of Family Impact and Conduct Problems. *Frontiers in Psychology, 8*, 2252. doi:10.3389/fpsyg.2017.02252 PMID:29312090

O'Driscoll, C., Heary, C., Hennessy, E., & McKeague, L. (2012). Explicit and implicit stigma towards peers with mental health problems in childhood and adolescence. *Journal of Child Psychology and Psychiatry, and Allied Disciplines, 53*(10), 1054–1062. doi:10.1111/j.1469-7610.2012.02580.x PMID:22823158

Oh, W. O., Park, E. S., Suk, M. H., Song, D. H., & Im, Y. (2012). Parenting of children with ADHD in South Korea: The role of socio-emotional development of children with ADHD. *Journal of Clinical Nursing, 21*(13-14), 1932–1942. doi:10.1111/j.1365-2702.2011.03968.x PMID:22340017

Pasamanick, B., Rogers, M. E., & Lilienfeld, A. M. (1956). Pregnancy experience and the development of behaviour disorder in children. *The American Journal of Psychiatry, 112*(8), 613–618. doi:10.1176/ajp.112.8.613 PMID:13292548

Patterson, G.R. (1980). Mothers: The unacknowledged victims. *Monographs of the Society for Research in Child Development, 45*(5).

Pejović-Milovancević, M., Lecić-Tosevski, D., Tenjović, L., Popović-Deusić, S., & Draganić-Gajić, S. (2009). Changing attitudes of high school students towards peers with mental health problems. *Psychiatria Danubina, 21*(2), 213–219. PMID:19556951

Podolski, C. L., & Nigg, J. T. (2001). Parent stress and coping in relation to child ADHD severity and associated child disruptive behavior problems. *Journal of Clinical Child Psychology, 30*(4), 503–513. doi:10.1207/S15374424JCCP3004_07 PMID:11708238

Psychogiou, L., Daley, D. M., Thompson, M. J., & Sonuga-Barke, E. J. (2008). Do maternal attention-deficit/hyperactivity disorder symptoms exacerbate or ameliorate the negative effect of child attention-deficit/hyperactivity disorder symptoms on parenting? *Development and Psychopathology, 20*(1), 121–137. doi:10.1017/S0954579408000060 PMID:18211731

Rasmussen, P. D., Storebø, O. J., Shmueli-Goetz, Y., Bojesen, A. B., Simonsen, E., & Bilenberg, N. (2018). Childhood ADHD and treatment outcome: The role of maternal functioning. *Child and Adolescent Psychiatry and Mental Health, 12*(1), 31. doi:10.118613034-018-0234-3 PMID:29983736

Rayan, A., & Ahmad, M. (2018). Mindfulness and parenting distress among parents of children with disabilities: A literature review. *Perspectives in Psychiatric Care*, *54*(2), 324–330. doi:10.1111/ppc.12217 PMID:28247409

Rockhill, C., Violette, H., Vander Stoep, A., Grover, S., & Myers, K. (2013). Caregivers' distress: Youth with attention-deficit/hyperactivity disorder and comorbid disorders assessed via telemental health. *Journal of Child and Adolescent Psychopharmacology*, *23*(6), 379–385. doi:10.1089/cap.2013.0019 PMID:23952184

Rogers, M. A., Wiener, J., Marton, I., & Tannock, R. (2009). Parental involvement in children's learning: Comparing parents of children with and without Attention-Deficit/Hyperactivity Disorder (ADHD). *Journal of School Psychology*, *47*(3), 167–185. doi:10.1016/j.jsp.2009.02.001 PMID:19328285

Sadati, A. K., Salehzade, H., Hemmati, S., Darvish, M., Heydari, S. T., & Tabrizi, R. (2015). The Causal Factors Associated with the Loving Care of the Mothers of Children with Multiple Disabilities. *International Journal of Community Based Nursing and Midwifery*, *3*(4), 309–317. PMID:26448958

Sakellari, E., Lehtonen, K., Sourander, A., Kalokerinou-Anagnostopoulou, A., & Leino-Kilpi, H. (2014). Greek adolescents' views of people with mental illness through drawings: Mental health education's impact. *Nursing & Health Sciences*, *16*(3), 358–364. doi:10.1111/nhs.12113 PMID:24382318

Sakellari, E., Leino-Kilpi, H., & Kalokerinou-Anagnostopoulou, A. (2011). Educational interventions in secondary education aiming to affect pupils' attitudes towards mental illness: A review of the literature. *Journal of Psychiatric and Mental Health Nursing*, *18*(2), 166–176. doi:10.1111/j.1365-2850.2010.01644.x PMID:21299729

Samiei, M., Daneshmand, R., Keramatfar, R., Khooshabi, K., Amiri, N., Farhadi, Y., Farzadfard, S. Z., Kachooi, H., & Samadi, R. (2015). Attention Deficit Hyper Activity Disorder (ADHD) and Stress: A Mutual Relationship between Children and Mothers. *Basic and Clinical Neuroscience*, *6*(2), 113–121. PMID:27307956

Schachar, R., Taylor, E., Wieselberg, M., Thorley, G., & Rutter, M. (1987). Changes in family function and relationships in children who respond to Methylphenidate. *Journal of the American Academy of Child and Adolescent Psychiatry*, *26*(5), 728–732. doi:10.1097/00004583-198709000-00019 PMID:3667503

Schaughency, E. A., & Lahey, B. B. (1985). Mothers' and Fathers' perceptions of child deviance: Roles of child behaviour, parental depression and marital satisfaction. *Journal of Consulting and Clinical Psychology*, *53*(5), 718–723. doi:10.1037/0022-006X.53.5.718 PMID:4056189

Schmiedeler, S. (2015). Mindfulness-based intervention in attention-deficit-/hyperactivity disorder (ADHD. *Zeitschrift fur Kinder- und Jugendpsychiatrie und Psychotherapie*, *43*(2), 123–131. doi:10.1024/1422-4917/a000341 PMID:25769764

Seltzer, M. M., Greenberg, J. S., Floyd, F. J., Pettee, Y., & Hong, J. (2001). Life course impacts of parenting a child with a disability. *American Journal of Mental Retardation*, *106*(3), 265–286. doi:10.1352/0895-8017(2001)106<0265:LCIOPA>2.0.CO;2 PMID:11389667

Selye, H. (1956). *The stress of life*. McGraw-Hill.

Selye, H. (1976). *The stress of life* (rev. ed). McGraw-Hill.

Singh, N. N. (1995). In search of unity: Some thoughts on the family- professional relationships in service delivery systems. *Journal of Child and Family Studies*, *4*(1), 3–18. doi:10.1007/BF02233951

Strauss, A. A., & Lehtinen, L. E. (1947). *Psychopathology and Education of the Brain-Injured Child*. Grune and Stratton.

Stubbs, A. (2014). Reducing mental illness stigma in health care students and professionals: A review of the literature. *Australasian Psychiatry*, *22*(6), 579–584. doi:10.1177/1039856214556324 PMID:25371444

Tallmadge, J. M., Paternite, C. E., & Gordon, M. (1989). *Hyperactivity and aggression in parent-child interaction: Test of a two-factor theory*. Paper presented at the meeting of the Society for Research in Child Development, Kanas City, MO.

Tarver, J., Daley, D., & Sayal, K. (2014). Attention-deficit hyperactivity disorder (ADHD): An updated review of the essential facts. *Child: Care, Health and Development*, *40*(6), 762–774. doi:10.1111/cch.12139 PMID:24725022

Telman, L. G. E., van Steensel, F. J. A., Maric, M., & Bögels, S. M. (2017). Are Anxiety Disorders in Children and Adolescents Less Impairing Than ADHD and Autism Spectrum Disorders? Associations with Child Quality of Life and Parental Stress and Psychopathology. *Child Psychiatry and Human Development*, *48*(6), 891–902. doi:10.100710578-017-0712-5 PMID:28176178

Townshend, K., Jordan, Z., Stephenson, M., & Tsey, K. (2016). The effectiveness of mindful parenting programs in promoting parents' and children's wellbeing: A systematic review. *JBI Database of Systematic Reviews and Implementation Reports*, *14*(3), 139–180. doi:10.11124/JBISRIR-2016-2314 PMID:27532143

Tredgold, A. F. (1908). *Mental Deficiency (Amentia)*. Wood.

Vance, A. L. A., & Luk, E. S. L. (2000). Attention Deficit Hyperactivity Disorder: Current progress and controversies. *The Australian and New Zealand Journal of Psychiatry*, *34*(5), 719–730. doi:10.1080/j.1440-1614.2000.00809.x PMID:11037357

Vernhet, C., Dellapiazza, F., Blanc, N., Cousson-Gélie, F., Miot, S., Roeyers, H., & Baghdadli, A. (2019). Coping strategies of parents of children with autism spectrum disorder: A systematic review. *European Child & Adolescent Psychiatry*, *28*(6), 747–758. doi:10.100700787-018-1183-3 PMID:29915911

Vila-Badia, R., Martínez-Zambrano, F., Arenas, O., Casas-Anguera, E., García-Morales, E., Villellas, R., Martín, J. R., Pérez-Franco, M. B., Valduciel, T., Casellas, D., García Franco, M., Miguel, J., Balsera, J., Pascual, G., Julia, E., & Ochoa, S. (2016). Effectiveness of an intervention for reducing social stigma towards mental illness in adolescents. *World Journal of Psychiatry*, *6*(2), 239–247. doi:10.5498/wjp.v6.i2.239 PMID:27354967

Wahler, R. G., & Afton, A. D. (1980). Attentional processes in insular and non-insular mothers. Some differences in their summary reports about child problem behaviours. *Child Behaviour Therapy*, *2*, 25–41. doi:10.1300/J473V02N02_02

Weinberg, S. L., & Richardon, M. S. (1981). Dimensions of Stress in early parenting. *Journal of Consulting and Clinical Psychology*, *49*(5), 686–693. doi:10.1037/0022-006X.49.5.686 PMID:7287978

Weinberger, K. A., Gardner, D. M., & Gerdes, A. C. (2018). Maternal Functioning Differences Based on ADHD Subtype. *Journal of Attention Disorders*, *22*(13), 218–1223. doi:10.1177/1087054714567132 PMID:25589371

Wiener, J., Biondic, D., Grimbos, T., & Herbert, M. (2016). Parenting Stress of Parents of Adolescents with Attention-Deficit Hyperactivity Disorder. *Journal of Abnormal Child Psychology*, *44*(3), 561–574. doi:10.100710802-015-0050-7 PMID:26183609

Williamson, D., & Johnston, C. (2019). Maternal ADHD Symptoms and Parenting Stress: The Roles of Parenting Self-Efficacy Beliefs and Neuroticism. *Journal of Attention Disorders*, *23*(5), 493–505. doi:10.1177/1087054717693373 PMID:28201945

Wymbs, B. T., Dawson, A. E., Egan, T. E., Sacchetti, G. M., Tams, S. T., & Wymbs, F. A. (2017). ADHD and Depression Symptoms in Parent Couples Predict Response to Child ADHD and ODD Behavior. *Journal of Abnormal Child Psychology*, *45*(3), 471–484. doi:10.100710802-016-0220-2 PMID:27796690

Yamaguchi, S., Mino, Y., & Uddin, S. (2011). Strategies and future attempts to reduce stigmatization and increase awareness of mental health problems among young people: A narrative review of educational interventions. *Psychiatry Journal of Clinical Neuroscience*, *65*(5), 405–415. doi:10.1111/j.1440-1819.2011.02239.x PMID:21851449

Yang, P., Jong, Y. J., Hsu, H. Y., & Tsai, J. H. (2007). Psychiatric features and parenting stress profiles of subtypes of attention-deficit/hyperactivity disorder: Results from a clinically referred Taiwanese sample. *Journal of Developmental and Behavioral Pediatrics*, *28*(5), 369–375. doi:10.1097/DBP.0b013e3181131f8e PMID:18049319

Zwi, M., Jones, H., Thorgaard, C., York, A., & Dennis, J. A. (2011). Parent training interventions for Attention Deficit Hyperactivity Disorder (ADHD) in children aged 5 to 18 years. *Cochrane Database of Systematic Reviews*, *12*, CD003018. doi:10.1002/14651858.CD003018.pub3 PMID:22161373

Zylowska, L., Ackerman, D. L., Yang, M. H., Futrell, L., Horton, N. L., Hale, T. S., Pataki, C., & Smalley, S. L. (2008). Mindfulness meditation training in adults and adolescents with ADHD: A feasibility study. *Journal of Attention Disorders*, *11*(6), 737–746. doi:10.1177/1087054707308502 PMID:18025249

Chapter 19
Yoga as a Complementary Therapy for ADHD

Nikita Naresh Ahuja
Hospital for Mental Health, Vadodara, India

ABSTRACT

Attention deficit hyperactivity disorder (ADHD) is a neurodevelopmental disorder that commonly occurs among children between the age ranges of 3-10 years. Though pharmacotherapy in combination of play therapy and behavior therapy has been proved to be effective for the treatment of ADHD, but the results derived from them does not seem to sustain for a longer period of time. There are other alternative therapies too, which can help in management of the symptoms of ADHD. This chapter talks about the different aspects of yoga and effect of different asanas, pranayama, and meditation on ADHD. As medication has its own negative side effects, practitioners have started to research other techniques to be helpful for managing ADHD, and Yoga is proved to be one of the effective ways to reduce the symptoms of ADHD. Yoga is not only limited to the physical exercise; it also includes breathing exercises, meditation, and relaxation exercises, which help to have a balance between mind and body. Through regular practice of yoga, one can attain peace of mind and can lead a happy and healthy life.

INTRODUCTION

Attention deficit hyperactivity disorder (ADHD) is a neurodevelopmental disorder that commonly occurs among children between the age range of 3- 10 years. It is characterized by low attention span, excessive activity and impulsivity. Most of the children with ADHD also find it difficult to regulate their emotions. Moreover, the symptoms of the disorder persist into adulthood in up to 60% of childhood cases, meaning that roughly 4% of adults suffer from ADHD. ADHD has been identified as a *complex trait* disorder that it is affected by many susceptibility genes(Gizer et al., 2009).The exact cause of ADHD has not been known till date. There are various different etiological reasons.Though medications can subside the ADHD symptoms but it also has a negative side effect like sleep disturbance, mood disorder or reduced appetite. Other form of psychotherapies and cognitive behaviour therapy also prove to be affective for management of ADHD but no sustainable positive effects have been found yet. From a holistic

DOI: 10.4018/978-1-7998-5495-1.ch019

point of view, chemical overstimulation of the nervous system is not healthy. A study by Esparham et al.(2014)stated, there are many alternative therapies that are effective both alone and in collaboration with pharmacotherapy

Yoga is a group of physical, mental and spiritual practices. According to Yoga sutra of Patanjali YogasChittavrittinirodhah(1.2)

Yoga is calming down the fluctuations/patterns of consciousness

Yoga as exercise is a physical activity consisting of different form ofasana (physical postures), pranayamas (breathing exercises), and dharana/dhyana (meditation). These components help to connect the breathing, thoughts, emotions, and body into awareness of the present moment.Physical exercise is proven to have positive effects on general health and well-being and also improves mood and quality of life.Swami SivanandaSaraswati explained yoga as an "integration and harmony between thought, feeling and deed, or integration between head, heart and hand".Swami Satyananda Saraswati stated "Yoga is an aid which helps in forming a new perspective of what is real and what is necessary in life, and how to become established in a way of life which embraces both inner and outer realities."

By regular yoga practices, an individual can enhance and develop his emotional intelligence. Yoga is an effective instrument of modification of human emotions. The practice of yoga, with its philosophical core strives to improve emotional intelligence by building a sense of empowerment while strengthening body, mind and spirit. Yogic philosophy recognizes the human being dilemmas when it comes to the emotions. Yoga in its original recognition is the applied science of modifying and enriching human emotions.

Patanjali known as the "father of yoga," has codified his thoughts and knowledge of yoga in *The Yoga Sutra of Patanjali.The Yoga Sutra* is considered text on the system of yoga. This is a guide for living the right life. Essentially, Patanjali says, "you can't practice asanas in yoga class, feel the stretch, and then go home to play with your kids, cook a meal, yell at your employees, and cheat on your taxes. There is more to yoga than that — yoga can help you cultivate body, mind, and spiritual awareness." (Roberts,n.d.)

Patanjali explained Yoga teachings by dividing it into eightfold path of yoga, which are also called the eight limbs of Patanjali. The eight limbs of Patanjali are as follows:

Yama

Yama is social behavior, how onetreat others and the world around them. These are moral principles. There are five yamas:

- **Nonviolence** (*ahimsa*): No harm to others in thought or deed.
- **Truth and honesty** (*satya*): Tell no lies.
- **Nonstealing** (*asteya*): Do not steal anything either be it materialistic or intangible things.
- **Nonlust** (*brahmacharya*): Avoid meaningless sexual encounters.
- **Nonpossessiveness** (*aparigraha*):Living a simple life without greed and attachment and not persevering the things.

Niyama

Niyama is inner discipline and responsibility, how one treats themselves. They are also called observances. There are five niyamas:

- **Purity** (*shauca*):This refers to internal and external cleanliness. Regular practice of yamas provides internal cleanliness.
- **Contentment** (*santosha*):Being happy and satisfied with what one has, accepting oneself and others and living in the moment.
- **Austerity** (*tapas*): Discipline in body, speech, and mind.
- **Study of the sacred text** (*svadhyaya*):Read Inspirational books which changes the individual's perspective towards life.
- **Living with an awareness of the Divine** (*ishvara-pranidhana*):Total devotion to GOD.

Asana

Asana is a steady posture. It is a form of a exercise that includes different physical postures which affect the physical, mental and spiritual health of the individual.Having mastered the physical body is the first step towards letting go of attachment. (Feuerstein, 2003)

Pranayama

Prana is the life force.*Pranayama* is the control of breath. "The real meaning of Pranayama, according to Patanjali, the founder of Yoga philosophy, is the gradual cessation of breathing, the discontinuance of inhalation and exhalation". (Paramhansa Yogananda, 2005)

Pratyahara

Pratyahara is withdrawal of the senses. Pratyahara is going into one's awareness by detaching onself from the outer objects. Pratyahara empowers one to stop being controlled by the external world, fetch one's attention to seek self-knowledge and experience the freedom innate in one's inner world. (Bell, 2007)

Dharana

Dharana means concentration. Focusing on one point is called concentration. Concentration calms the mind and makes it stable.

Dhyana

Uninterrupted meditation without an object is called *dhyana*. Concentration (dharana) leads to the state of meditation. The goal of meditation is not unconsciousness or nothingness. It is heightened awareness and oneness with the universe. (Campbell, 2015)

Samadhi

The ultimate goal of the eightfold path to yoga is *samadhi* or absolute bliss. ParamahansaYogananda (2014) called it a blissful super consciousness state in which a yogi perceives the identity of the individualized soul and Cosmic Spirit.

Benefits of Yoga

Many studies state on how yoga affects the human body and mind on a very basic level. In article by Dennis Thompson Jr (2013) he talked about how yoga helps to regulate the level of chemicals and hormones which include cortisol, stress hormone, GABA (gamma amino butyric acid), and Serotonin, all of which play a major role in person's mental health

McClafferty (2011) studied yoga as therapy for the treatment of stress, chronic pain, asthma, irritable bowel syndrome, and ADHD and found that yoga improves concentration and attention span and teaches focus. When kids concentrate on their breath or feel a stretch in their arms, they learn body awareness. This teaches them to keep their minds in one place, instead of all over the place. With the regular practice of yoga, kids eventually learn to apply self control in their other activities of the day to day life. The practice of yoga can calm the kids as it boosts up their confidence by practising the same posture regularly. Holding a pose is meant to be hard work both physically and mentally. People with ADHD spend way too much time inside their heads. They tend to more aware about their surroundings rather than their own self. Yoga helps to balance between the mind and the body. Harrison et al.(2004) reported that yoga has beneficial effects such as reduced hyperactivity, inattention, and anxiety and sleep patterns in children with ADHD.

Physiological Effects of Yoga

Where a specific muscle is weak, one can do exercise to make it stronger. The same happens with our brain. Regular practice of Yoga releases several important chemicals A hormone Endorphins,that regulates mood, pleasure, and pain. The physical activity also elevates the brain's dopamine, norepinephrine, and serotonin levels. These brain chemicals turns on the attention system, the executive functions like sequencing, working memory, inhibiting and sustaining attention, which is most affected in ADHD. A study by pal et al.(2014) and Del Campo (2011) reported that the increase in dopamine levels result to increase in the attention system's ability to be more consistent and alert and less impulsive.

Benefits of Asanas (Physical Exercise)

An **asana** is a sanskrit term which means "posture" or "pose". Asana is a general term used for sitting in a meditative pose. The Yoga Sutras of Patanjali define "asana" as a position that is steady and comfortable. In hatha yoga, the word asanas is also referred to physical exercise that comprises of different physical poses like standing, twisting, reclining and balancing poses. In hatha yoga, Asanas are meant to provide both spiritual and physical benefits. Many studies (Ross,2010; Alexander,2008; Hayes, 2010) have reported that they improve flexibility, strength, and balance; and it also reduces stress and helps in coping with different physical and mental ailments like asthma, diabetes.

By placing the body in specific positions, it increases awareness, concentration and relaxes the body and mind. It is a step by step methodical way of freeing up spine, limbs and other parts of the body. By regular practice of yoga, one gains steadiness, health and lightness of limbs. In a book by Iyengar (1979), 'Light on Yoga', he mentioned that a steady and pleasant posture produces mental equilibrium and prevents fickleness of mind.

Effects of Yoga on Cardiovascular Diseases

Cardiovascular diseases (CVDs) are a group of disorders of the heart and blood vessels and it is found to be the number one cause of death globally. According to WHO, An estimated 17.9 million people died from CVDs in 2016, representing 31% of all global deaths. Of these deaths, 85% are due to heart attack and stroke (WHO Factsheet 2017).

Heart attacks and strokes are caused due to the blockage in veins and arteries that prevents blood to flow in other parts of the body. The causes and effects of heart failure involves both the nervous system, through which mental and emotional processes influence the cardiac functions and the metabolic, digestive and other systems which depends on heart(Swami Karmananda,1983).

Many different treatments are available for the cure of the cardiovascular diseases but yoga is also found to be useful in managing the symptoms of cardiovascular diseases (La Forge,1997). Yoga effects on three mechanisms: vagal nerve stimulation, reduction in perceived stress, and musculoskeletal stimulation. By performing certain types of asanas that impact the vagal nerve directly, it may help to activate parasympathetic system which results in decreased heart rate and blood pressure.

The patients with cardiovascular diseases are always advised to exercise as it helps in improving the vascular reactivity and inflammatory markers, but the people suffering from cardiovascular disease have many do's and don'ts due to which they are not able to perform a lot of physical activities but yoga is very flexible as it has variety of different postures and relaxation exercises which helps the person to do the physical activity and feel relaxed at the same time. In studies done by Stamler(1989) and Appel (2003) reported that by regular practice of yoga and meditation there was a reduction in BP and it has been estimated that reducing systolic BP by 3 mm Hg in general population has potential to reduce stroke mortality by 8% and coronary heart disease (CHD) by 5%.

In a recently published scientific statement by Brook et al., (2013) on alternative methods to lower blood pressure (BP) and reduce CVD risk, the American Heart Association (AHA) reported that Transcendental Meditation techniques may be considered in clinical practices to lower BP. The AHA also reported research that TM may reduce heart attacks, stroke and deaths in CVD patients

Yoga for Cardiovascular diseases:

- Pawanmuktasasna part 1 and 2
- Vajrasana
- Shashankasana
- Sarpasana
- Nadi shodhan pranayama
- Ujjayi pranayama
- Yoga Nidra

(Swami Karmananda, 'Yogic Management of Common Diseases', 1983)

Effects of Yoga on Thyroid Diseases

Thyroid is a small gland which plays a huge role in our body. It is one of the endocrine gland which creates hormones that regulate our body's metabolism. Women are likely to suffer more than men. The most common thyroid problems involve abnormal production of thyroid hormones. When the gland produces high amount of thyroid hormone it's called as hyperthyroidism. The symptoms include restlessness, anxiety, nervousness, increased sweating, weight loss, muscle weakness and sleep problems. When the gland produces insufficient thyroid hormone it's called hypothyroidism. The symptoms include fatigue, weight gain, mood swings, and depression and memory problems (Murrell, 2017).

Though thyroid can be managed with pharmacological treatment, but there are ample of studies supporting the use of alternative therapy for the regulation of hormone levels (Chatterjee &Mondal, 2017).Yoga helps to create balance among all the glands and hormones leading to healthy functioning of every organ of the body. Yoga is one of the alternative approaches that have been observed to have some long term benefits in thyroid diseases and regular yoga practices are capable of making changes in the secretions of bodily hormones (Maske & Barnwal, 2016).

Werner et al. (1986) &Gorden et al.(2008), reported that yoga along with transcendental meditation affected the TSH levels. Yoga seems to improve psychological conditions to manage stress, reduce negative emotions and anxiety while simultaneously raising positive emotions and the ultimate improvement of emotional balance (Mondal, Kuhu, & Saha, 2018).

Yogic practices for thyroid diseases:

- Ustrasana
- Sarvangasana
- Matsyasana
- Simhasana
- Suryanamaskar
- Shhetali Pranayama
- Ujjayayi Pranayama

(Swami Karmananda, 1983)

Benefits of Yoga and ADHD

In regards to ADHD symptoms, asanas can help in minimizing the symptoms, as the regular practice of asanas increases oxygen and blood flow to the brain which has a balancing effect on the nervous system. Yoga helps the children with ADHD to establish connection between body and mind and increase concentration and attention. Chou and Huang (2017) found that an eight-week yoga program significantly improved sustained attention and discrimination function in children with ADHD. Findings revealed that the group who underwent yoga intervention had significantly better reaction time and response accuracy than the other group.

In an article ADHD weekly (2018) by CHADD organization it stated that for practising yoga one does not need any kind of equipment or materials. One just needs a calm and serene environment with open space where a child can practice different forms of asanas, pranayama and meditative exercises.

YOGIC POSES (ASANAS) FOR ADHD

According to Swami Satyananda Saraswati, some of the yogic physical postures that can help the child to increase attention and concentration and calm the mind are listed below:

Tadasana (Palm Tree Pose)

It requires the child to balance on one foot, with his palms together over his head and his other foot placed against the inner thigh of the leg holding the weight. This exercise is to be done in coordination with the breath. The child has to fix the eyes at a point on the wall and the eyes should remain fixed throughout the practice.

Shashankasana (Pose of the Moon or Hare Pose)

In this the child is asked to sit in vajrasana, placing the palms on the thighs just above the knees. Then after While inhaling, raise the arms above the head, keeping them straight and shoulder width apart. Exhale while bending forward from the hips, keeping the arms and head straight. The hands and forehead should rest on the floor in front of the knees and touch the floor. Retain the breath for up to 5 seconds in the final position. Then simultaneously inhale and slowly raise the arms and trunk to the vertical position. Keep the arms and head in line. Exhale while lowering the hands to the knees.

Simhagarjanasana (Roaring Lion Pose)

Sit in simhasana. Open the eyes and gaze at the eyebrow centre, which is also called as shambhavimudra. Relax the whole body. Inhale slowly through the nose. After inhalation, open the mouth and extend the tongue out as far as possible towards the chin. While slowly exhaling, produce a clear, steady 'aaa' sound from the throat, keeping the mouth wide open. Do not strain or force the sound in any way. At the end of exhalation, close the mouth and breathe in.

Shalabhasana (Locust Pose)

Lie flat on the stomach with the legs and feet together and the soles of the feet uppermost. The arms may be placed either under the body or by the sides, with the palms Stretch the chin slightly forward and rest it on the floor throughout the practice. Close the eyes and relax the body. Slowly raise the legs as high as possible without straining, keeping them straight and together. The legs are elevated by applying pressure with the arms against the floor and contracting the lower back muscles. Hold the final position for as long as is comfortable without strain. Slowly lower the legs to the floor.

Padahastasana (hand to Foot Pose)

Stand with the spine straight, feet together and hands beside the body. Relax the body. Divide the weight of the body evenly on both feet. Slowly bend forward, While bending forward, imagine that the body has no bones or muscles. Do not strain or force the body. Place the fingers underneath the toes or bring the palms to the floor beside the feet. If this is not possible, bring the fingertips as near to the floor as possible. Relax the back of the neck. Hold the position, relaxing the whole back. Slowly return to the starting position in the reverse order.

Benefits

All this asana helps to develop physical and mental balance. The entire spine is stretched and loosened, helping to clear up congestion of the spinal nerves at the points where they emerge from the spinal column. It relieves frustration and releases emotional tension. Tension is removed from the chest and diaphragm. Simhagarjanasana is useful for people who stutter or who are nervous and introverted. Spinal nerves are stimulated and toned. Inverting the trunk can increase vitality, improve metabolism and concentration and help with nasal and throat diseases. (Swami Satyananda Saraswati pg 235)

Pranayama (Breathing Exercises)

The breath is the most essential process of the body. It influences the activities of each and every cell and, most importantly, it plays a very eminent role in performance of the brain. Pranayama is the practice of breath control in yoga. *Pranayama* (*prāna*, energy + *ayām*, expansion) is expansion of individual energy into cosmic energy. It is the first and the last thing in our lives. Without breath there is no life Human beings breathe about 15 times per minute and 21,600 times per day. Respiratory system places a important role in producing energy in the body and providing power to every muscular contraction mental process and glandular secretion.Breath is the essential and the easiest doorstep to the human nervous system as it touches every aspect of our life: physical, psychological, emotional and spiritual. Daily stressors and our life style can affect our breathing which in turn gives birth to various physical and mental diseases. By practising pranayama we allow the life energy flow into the whole body which energizes and heals the body by providing life force to the system. Swami Muktibodhanandha (1998), states that although breathing is an unconscious process, conscious control of it may be taken at any time,by controlling prana, mind is automatically controlled. Prana and mind influence each other.

With regular practice of pranayama, it strengthens our whole body organs. It stimulates the parasympathetic system. Pranayama practices, stretches the lung tissue producing inhibitory signals from action of slowly adapting receptors and hyperpolarising currents. These inhibitory signals coming from cardiorespiratory region involving vagi are believed to synchronize neural elements in the brain leading to changes in the autonomic nervous system; and a resultant condition characterized by reduced metabolism and parasympathetic dominance. The breathing patterns are closely associated with our emotional states. And by consciously changing our breathing pattern one can change their emotional state of mind. In children with ADHD, regular practice of pranayama helps them to ease their mind and become aware about their surroundings.

Types of Pranayama (Breathing Exercise)(Swami Satyanand Saraswati)

Abdominal (or diaphragmatic) Breathing:

Instructions:

Sit in any meditative posture. Place the right hand on the abdomen just above the navel and the left hand over the centre of the chest. Observe the breath without controlling it. Let it be absolutely natural.

Figure 1.

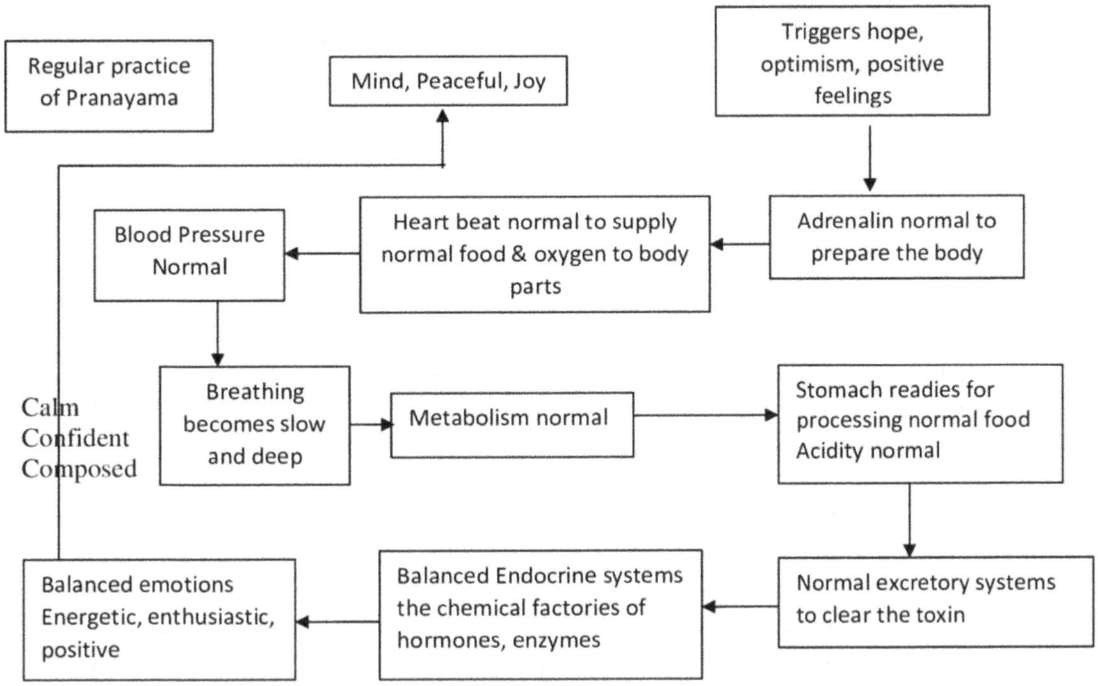

To practise abdominal breathing, feel as though you are drawing the energy and breathe in and out directly through the navel. Inhale while expanding the abdomen as much as is comfortable. At the end of the inhalation, the diaphragm will be compressing the abdomen and the navel will be at its highest point. On exhalation, the diaphragm moves upward and the abdomen moves downward. At the end of the exhalation, the abdomen will be contracted and the navel compressed towards the spine.

AnulomVilom Pranayama:

Instructions:

Sit in a meditative posture. Block the right nostril though the right thumb for 2 seconds. Inhale through left nostril. Block both the nostrils and hold the breath for 4 seconds. After that keep the left nostril blocked and release the right nostril. Exhale through the right nostril for 2 seconds. Now inhale through the right nostril for 2 seconds, block both nostrils, and hold the breath for 4 seconds. Keep the right nostril blocked and release the left nostril.

Bhramari Pranayama (Humming bee Breath)

Instructions

Sit in a comfortable meditation asana, Close the eyes and relax the whole body. The lips should remain gently closed with the teeth slightly separated throughout the practice. Raise the arms sideways and bend the elbows, bringing the hands to the ears. Use the index or middle finger to plug the ears or the flaps of the ears may be pressed without inserting the fingers. Inhale through the nose. Exhale slowly while making a deep, steady humming sound like that of the black bee.

Benefits: Pranayama relieves stress and cerebral tension, and so helps in alleviating anger, anxiety and insomnia, increasing the healing capacity of the body.Bhramarihelps in calming the mind and directing the awareness inward. The vibration of the humming sound creates a soothing effect on the mind and nervous system. (Swami Satyanand Saraswati pg. 241)

Meditation

Meditation is a practice where an individual focuses his mind on a particular object, thought or activity which helps to increase attention and awareness. And become mentally and emotionally calm and stable. Swami Satchitananda (2011) stated that the aim of meditation is to keep the mind fully occupied on one thing. When the mind is fully occupied on one thing, it is kept away from many things, and it becomes quiet. Meditation is found to be effective in reducing stress, anxiety and increasing peace, self-concept and wellbeing.

Meditation and yogic therapy are good ways to manage ADHD symptoms. Many researches shows that mindfulness meditation – where one actively observes his moment to moment Swami Satchitananda (2011) foused thoughts and feelings. It may also be a good way to calm the mind and improve the focus. Mindfulness meditation strengthens the ability to control the attention. It teaches us how to observe and focus on oneself. It also helps to be aware about one's emotions, which decreases the risk of acting impulsively.

Meditation is helpful in children with ADHD as it thickens the prefrontal cortex that is involved in focus, planning and impulse control. Gersten (2011) states that the purpose of meditation is to center and balance the mind. As children with ADHD have trouble getting their work done on time and can become forgetful about things, but mindfulness meditation can actually help the child to tune out the judgemental voice in the head.

A review done by Kaunhoven et al. (2007) reported that "The practice of mindfulness meditation is a conscious exercise that builds attention and inhibitory skills." It teaches the child to pay attention to paying attention. Meditation also relaxes the human mind and helps the child to experience inner peace.

Relaxation Exercise

Relaxation exercise is proved to be one of the most effective exercises for the children with ADHD as it helps the child to relax his body and mind. The mind of an ADHD child is always into something that creates chaos in the mind due to which sometimes the child feels frustrated and irritated. The relaxation exercise helps the child to calm his inner chaos and experience peace. It relaxes the whole psycho-physiological system and develops body awareness.

Shavasana is meant to be the most effective and easiest way of relaxing oneself. In this the child is asked to lie down on bed in a comfortable manner. He is asked to relax his whole body and stop all the body movements and gradually becoming aware of his own breath and allow the breath to be relaxed. Slowly the child is asked to become aware about his body parts and feel that his body parts are getting relaxed and feel that he is completely getting relaxed.

CONCLUSION

Regular practice of yoga can not only be affective to the children of ADHD but it can also be helpful for the parents of the children with ADHD. Many studies have shown that the parents of children with ADHD undergo a lot of stress and relationship problems and many a times they find it difficult to manage their child, so through practice of yoga or meditation the adults can calm themselves and gain inner peace which increases their self esteem and gives them motivation and creative ideas to understand their children in a more deeper sense.

Regular practice of yoga can lead to self-awareness. Yoga cannot provide a cure for life, but it does present a proven method for coping with it. In recent years, yoga has been exposed in ADHD populations to address ongoing distractibility, emotional dysregulation and impulsivity. Evidence suggests that certain yogic postures and meditative practices improve attention and help to manage the symptoms of ADHD by activating hormones and chemicals implicated in both sustaining and directing attention. Yoga may also help increase time on task for students with ADHD in the educational setting. A study done by Peck et al.(2005) investigated the effect of a yoga practice intervention on children's time on task in school and stated that Yoga may have the potential to increase time on task in class and be an enjoyable and cost-effective treatment for children with attention problems. In ADHD, it will help children to increase their focus pertaining to increased attention and concentration which results in good performance in every aspect of the life. In Nutshell, we can say that Yoga is not only limited to physical form of exercises but it compromises of asanas, pranayamas and dhyana. Though lot of researches have been carried out on the yogic management of ADHD but still an ample of researches are yet to be done to prove the longer and sustaining effects of yoga in management of ADHD.

REFERENCES

Alexander, G. K., Taylor, A. G., Innes, K. E., Kulbok, P., & Selfe, T. K. (2008). Contextualizing the effects of yoga therapy on diabetes management: A review of the social determinants of physical activity. *Family & Community Health*, *31*(3), 228–239. doi:10.1097/01.FCH.0000324480.40459.20

Appel, L. (2003). Lifestyle modification as a means to prevent and treat high blood pressure. *Journal of the American Society of Nephrology*, *14*(90002), S99–S102. doi:10.1097/01.ASN.0000070141.69483.5A

Bell. (2007). *Mindful Yoga, Mindful Life: A Guide for Everyday Practice*. Rodmell Press.

Brook, R. D., Appel, L. J., Rubenfire, M., Ogedegbe, G., Bisognano, J. D., Elliott, W. J., Fuchs, F. D., Hughes, J. W., Lackland, D. T., Staffileno, B. A., Townsend, R. R., & Rajagopalan, S. (2013). Beyond medications and diet. Alternative approaches to lowering blood pressure. A Scientific Statement from American Heart Association. *Hypertension*, *61*(6), 1360–1363. doi:10.1161/HYP.0b013e318293645f

Campbell, W. (2015). *Eight limbs of yoga*. Retrieved from https://www.wendycampbellyoga.com/newsposts/2015/9/13/7-practical-tips-for-yoga-beginners

Cardiovascular Diseases (CVDs). (2017). Retrieved from https://www.who.int/news-room/fact-sheets/detail/cardiovascular-diseases-(cvds)

CHADD ADHD Weekly. (2018). Retrieved from https://chadd.org/adhd-weekly/yoga-could-benefit-children-with-adhd/

Chatterjee, S., & Mondal, S. (2017). Effect of combined yoga programme on blood levels of thyroid hormones: a quasi-experimental study. *Indian Journal of Traditional Knowledge*, *16*, S9-S16.

Chou, C.C., & Huang, C.J. (2017). Effects of an 8-week yoga program on sustained attention and discrimination function in children with attention deficit hyperactivity disorder. *PeerJ.com*, *5*, e2883. doi:10.7717/peerj.2883

Del Campo, N., Chamberlain, S. R., Sahakian, B. J., & Robbins, T. W. (2011). The roles of dopamine and noradrenaline in the pathophysiology and treatment of attention-deficit/hyperactivity disorder. *Biological Psychiatry*, *69*(12), e145–e157. doi:10.1016/j.biopsych.2011.02.036

Esparham. A., Evans, R.G., Wagner, L.E., & Drisko, J.A. (2014). Pediatric integrative medicine approaches to attention deficit hyperactivity disorder (ADHD) Children. *mdpi.com*, *1*, 186–207. doi:10.3390/children1020186

Everyday Health. (2011). *7 ADHD stress reduction techniques*. Retrieved from https://www.everydayhealth.com/adhd-pictures/adhd-stress-reduction-techniques.aspx

Everyday Times. (2013). *ADHD kids:Benefit from Yoga*. Retrieved from https://www.everydayhealth.com/adhd/bending-energy-adhd-kids-benefit-from-yoga.aspx

Feuerstein, G. (2003). *The Deeper Dimensions of Yoga: Theory and Practice*. Shambhala Publications.

Gizer, I., Ficks, C., & Waldman, I. (2009). Candidate gene studies of ADHD: A meta-analytic review. *Human Genetics*, *126*(1), 51–90. doi:10.100700439-009-0694-x

Gordon, L., Morrison, E. Y., McGrowder, D., Penas, Y. E., Zamoraz, E. M., Garwood, D., Alexander-Lindo, R., & Irving, R. (2008). Effect of yoga and traditional physical exercise on hormones and percentage insulin binding receptor in patients with type 2 diabetes. *American Journal of Biotechnology & Biochemistry*, *4*(1), 35–42. doi:10.3844/ajbbsp.2008.35.42

Harrison, L., Manocha, R., & Rubia, K. (2004). Sahaja yoga meditation as a family treatment programme for children with attention deficits-hyperactivity disorder. *Clinical Child Psychology and Psychiatry*, *9*(4), 479–497. doi:10.1177/1359104504046155

Hayes, M., & Chase, S. (2010). Prescribing Yoga. *Primary Care*, *37*(1), 31–47.

Healthline. (2017). *A review by Daniel Murrell, '6 common thyroid disorders and problems'*. Retrieved from https://www.healthline.com/health/common-thyroid-disorders

Hegde, V. (2007). *The science of stress and The Art of managing it*. Mind Tree Consulting.

Iyengar, B. K. S. (1979). *Light on Yoga: Yoga Dipika*. Thorsons.

Karmananda S. (1983). *Yogic management of common diseases*. Yoga Publication Trust.

Kaunhoven, R. J., & Dorjee, D. (2017). How does mindfulness modulate self-regulation in pre-adolescent children? An integrative neurocognitive review. *Neuroscience and Biobehavioral Reviews*, *74*, 163–184. doi:10.1016/j.neubiorev.2017.01.007

La Forge, R. (1997). Mind–body fitness: Encouraging prospects for primary and secondary prevention. *The Journal of Cardiovascular Nursing*, *11*(3), 53–65. doi:10.1097/00005082-199704000-00006

Maske, U., & Barnwal, S. (2016). Effect of hatha yogic practices on the level of triiodothyronine (T3) in patients of hyperthyroidism. *International Journal of Applied Research*, *2*(7), 754–757.

McClafferty, H. (2011). (in Review). Complementary, holistic and integrative medicine. *Pediatrics*, *32*, 201–203. doi:10.1542/pir.32-5-201

Mondal, S., Kundu, B., & Saha, S. (2018). Yoga as therapeutic intervention for the management of type 2 diabetes mellitus. *International Journal of Yoga*, *11*(2), 129–138. doi:10.4103/ijoy.IJOY_74_16

Muktibodhananda, S. (1998). *Hatha Yoga Pradipika*. Yoga Publication Trust.

Pal, R., Singh, S. N., Chatterjee, A., & Saha, M. (2014). Age-related changes in cardiovascular system, autonomic functions, and levels of BDNF of healthy active males: Role of yogic practice. *Age (Dordrecht, Netherlands)*, *36*(4), 9683. doi:10.100711357-014-9683-7

Peck, H., Kehle, T., Bray, M., & Theodore, L. (2005). Yoga as an intervention for children with attention problems. *School Psychology Review*, *34*, 415–424.

Roberts, S. (n.d.). *Patanjali's Eightfold path of yoga*. Retrieved from https://yoga.sherry-roberts.com/patanjali-and-his-eightfold-path-of-yoga/

Ross, A., & Thomas, S. (2010). The health benefits of yoga and exercise: A review of comparison studies. *Journal of Alternative and Complementary Medicine (New York, N.Y.)*, *16*(1), 3–12. doi:10.1089/acm.2009.0044

Saraswati, S. S. (1969). *Asana Pranayama Mudra Bandha. Yoga Publication Trust.*

Satchitananda, S. (2011). Meditation. Internal Yoga Publication.

Stamler, J., Rose, G., Stamler, R., Elliott, P., Dyer, A., & Marmot, M. (1989). INTERSALT study findings. Public health and medical care implications. *Hypertension*, *14*(5), 570–577. doi:10.1161/01.HYP.14.5.570

Werner, O., Wallace, R. K., Charles, B., Janssen, G., Stryker, T., & Chalmers, R. A. (1986). Long-term endocrinologic changes in subjects practicing the transcendental meditation and TM sidhi program. *Psychosomatic Medicine*, *48*(1-2), 59–65. doi:10.1097/00006842-198601000-00004

Yogananda, P. (2005). *The Essence of Kriya Yoga* (1st ed.). Alight Publications.

Yogananda, P. (2014). Autobiography of a yogi (13th ed.). Self Realization Fellowship.

Chapter 20
Rehabilitation Strategies for Persons With ADHD

Yesha A. Vyas
https://orcid.org/0000-0002-6537-9424
Samanjasya, India

ABSTRACT

ADHD is a neurodevelopmental disorder affecting a significant number of people. It is characterized by inattention and/or hyperactivity and/or impulsivity. It impacts various aspects of an individual's life. Rehabilitation is a holistic process, aiming at restoring and training an individual to improve their quality of life, increase independence, increase social participation and social inclusion. A combination of various rehabilitation strategies are used depending on the individual's needs, severity of the disorder, and developmental phase. Apart from the client, involving parents, caregivers, teachers, schools, and employers and co-workers ensure a consistent and effective rehabilitation process. This chapter focuses on the rehabilitation strategies like medication, behavioral training, psychoeducation, psychotherapy, social skills training, remediation methods, classroom management, parent training, coaching, support groups, lifestyle changes, and career and vocational guidance. Using timely intervention strategies and training enhances the rehabilitation process.

ATTENTION DEFICIT / HYPERACTIVITY DISORDER

Attention deficit / hyperactivity disorder (ADHD) is a neurodevelopmental disorder that affects many children and adults. This is characterized by a persistent pattern of inattention and/or hyperactivity and/or impulsivity or the combined type. The symptoms can be presented in a combined or predominant style.

Farone (2001), describes ADHD as a "chronic, debilitating disorder" that could have impacts on many aspects of an individual's life. The various areas of an individual's life that are impacted are academic, social and interpersonal relationships. Weiss & Hechtman(1993) in a study stated that about 30-60% people who are diagnosed with ADHD continue to show significant symptoms of the disorder in their adulthood too. Mannuzza & Klien (1993), state that children with the disorder are at greater risks for negative outcomes like lower educational rates and employment opportunities.

DOI: 10.4018/978-1-7998-5495-1.ch020

Rehabilitation

Riggar & Maki (2003) in their Handbook of Rehabilitation Counseling have described the concept of rehabilitation as "a holistic and integrated program of medical, physical, psychosocial, and vocational interventions that empower a person with disability to achieve a personally fulfilling, socially meaningful, and functionally effective interaction with the world" (Banja, 1990). Sherwin Elisabeth, in the Oxford Handbook of Rehabilitation Psychology has described rehabilitation, "as a profession that assists persons with disabilities in adapting to the environment, assists environments in accommodating the 'needs of the individual, and works toward full participation of persons with disabilities in all aspects of society, especially work"(Szymanski, 1985).

Rehabilitation counselling can also be described as a process which facilitates people with physical, psychological, developmental, cognitive and emotional disabilities to achieve their goals (personal, professional and living independently) in a holistic way. "The counseling process involves communication, goal setting, and beneficial growth or change through self-advocacy, psychological, vocational, social, and behavioral interventions" (Commission on Rehabilitation Counselor Certification - CRCC).

Maki (2012) has described some of the techniques and modalities used in the rehabilitation counseling process. They are: -

- Assessment and appraisal
- Diagnosis and treatment planning
- Career (vocational) planning
- Individual and group counselling treatment interventions
- Case management, referral, and service coordination
- Program evaluation and research
- Interventions to remove environmental, employment, and attitudinal barriers
- Consultation services
- Assistance in job analysis, job development and placement services
- Provision of consultation about and access to rehabilitation technology (Commission on Rehabilitation Counselor Certification, 1994)

Rehabilitation Strategies

The rehabilitation of persons with ADHD requires a "multimodal" approach. It consists of the client, parents, teachers, school, peer and environment to some extent. The rehabilitation process of a person with ADHD is a continuous and lifelong process, as each developmental stage of a person's life could bring a different level of challenge and issues. The process of rehabilitation covers the medical, psychological, cognitive, social, physical, emotional and vocational aspects. Rehabilitation of persons with ADHD is essential to reduce the impact of the disorder, to improve quality of life and enhance personal and emotional wellbeing.

The rehabilitation strategies are used singularly or in combination depending on the diagnosis and the presenting complaints of the person with ADHD. Further, rehabilitation strategies, along with their applications and impact specifically for ADHD have been discussed.

Medication

Medication is the first line of treatment for a majority of the people diagnosed with ADHD. The medication administered would vary with age, severity, and combination type presented by the client. There are a few interventions in all of medicine that are as quickly and dramatically effective as stimulant medication when used to treat ADHD. The stimulant medications that are so important in treating ADHD fall into two groups. They are the amphetamines and methylphenidate compounds. Amphetamine was introduced in the late 1930s. Methylphenidate was first synthesized in 1955 and began to be used in the early 1970s. Between 70-80 percent of children with ADHD respond well to medication. For some the benefits are extraordinary, for others, medication is quite helpful and for others the benefits are modest. (Wender et al.,2017)

Dupar (2017), suggests a few ways in which medication could work on individuals -

1. Sustained focus
2. Less impulsivity
3. Improved mood
4. Greater attention to detail
5. Better Memory
6. Better sleep
7. Demonstrate an improvement in school performance (listening, following instructions, completing tasks, getting better grades) (Powers et al., 2008)

It is important to note here that the effects of medication are not long lasting. Their effects last only for a short period of time. Hence they need to be continued as per the dosage and length as prescribed by the doctor. The medication only covers up for the chemical differences that affect behavior in many diverse areas. The medication primarily works on improving the self-control of the person with ADHD. The result is seen in behavior and improved adjustment at home, school and with peers (Paul & David, 2016).

Along with medication being an important aspect of the rehabilitation process, other aspects such as cognitive, psychological, emotional, physical and social also need to be addressed simultaneously.

Behavior Therapy

Behavior therapy derives its fundamentals from the theories of classical and operant conditioning. Children and adults diagnosed with ADHD often show behavior that can be disruptive, unhealthy or at times harmful to self or others. Once diagnosed with ADHD, behavior therapy can be initiated. Behavior therapy works and aims towards reducing the presented disruptive, unhealthy or harmful behaviors. The goals of behavior therapy are to encourage and increase the frequency of desired and healthy behaviors and reduce the intensity and frequency of undesired behaviors. (Evans et.al, 2013)

Miltenberger R. G (2008), in his book has described some key principles and techniques of behavior therapy. Behavior therapy is customized for the person with ADHD after detailed assessment of their functional behaviors. The first step to behavior therapy and modification involves identifying the target behavior to increase (positive behavior) and decrease(negative behavior). The antecedent and the consequence of the behavior are analysed along with the modified behavior that needs to be developed.

"This will also help in identifying the "functions" of the behavior". The functions of behavior can be identified as the reasons for the occurence of a particular behavior. They are: -

- *Skill deficit*

The lack of skills required to complete a task is referred to as "skill deficit". The client may not be able to concentrate due to lack of skills. Meaninglessness of the stimulus for the child leads to the brain being passive and so, the expected response may not be elicited.

- *Attention-seeking behavior*

The undesirable behavior may be noticed or desirable behavior could be absent due to the need of attention. Attention seeking in general behavior takes place to gain attention from others at home or public places. Emotional disturbances and genetics may be crucial factors.

- *Escape*

The client wishes to escape the situation by not participating or completing the task on hand. This function can be presented in a cognitive way (daydreaming) or behavioral (moving away from the task)

- *Tangible rewards*

Reinforcing incorrect behavior results in tangible function of behavior being encouraged. When a client is given a toy, food item or a gadget to stop him from crying, this reinforces the behavior of crying to achieve materialistic rewards.

- *Self-stimulatory behavior*

The client has no or very little control over impulsiveness, anxiety, irritation, sensory issues, restlessness due to temperamental, genetic, physiological or environmental factors.

Consistency is the key in making behavior modification effective. Behavior therapy and modification work best when the client, families, caregivers and teachers work as a team.

Some of the techniques used in behavior therapy for treating persons with ADHD are: -

- *Restructuring of the environment*

In this technique the necessary environmental changes are made that support the desired behavioral goal. Distraction is taken away and a conducive environment is created to encourage desired behavior. For e.g. For a child who constantly moves out of the class due to hyperactivity, his sitting position can be changed to a place where it would be difficult for him to move out of the class; distraction can be minimized by removing extra objects from the desk and room.

- *Restructuring of activities*

In this technique the activities are customized according to the person with ADHD. For e.g. Introducing time bound tasks, larger tasks broken down into smaller activities.

- *Token economy*

This technique is more of a reinforcement technique to increase desired behavior. The client is given a token after each favourable response and in the absence of the favourable response a certain predetermined amount of tokens are withdrawn. After collecting a number of predetermined tokens, a favourable reinforcement is given to the client. For e.g. collecting a certain number of starts or points against a gift or reward.

- *Positive reinforcement*

This technique uses complimenting and providing rewards and in response to desired behavior. For e.g. When the client completes his/her task, he/she is allowed to watch a show.

- *Time out*

This technique involves separating the client from others or the activity in which he/she is involved. This is done in response to an undesirable behavior. The client is given isolation and no one talks to him/her. Also the access to any desired activity is taken away due to the undesired behavior. For e.g. Hitting siblings, other kids during play leads to him being removed from the play time.

- *Teaching new behavior*
    - Modelling - It is also called observational learning or imitation.
    - Prompting - A cue or hint meant to help the client to perform a desired skill, behavior or a part of a skill. Prompting can be physical or verbal.
    - Shaping - It is a way of adding behaviors to a person's repertoire. It is used when the client does not display the desired behavior (ref. Rhonda Black). In shaping, any behavior that resembles the desired behavior is reinforced.
    - Chaining - It is a series of behaviors that are related to each other and usually one behavior works as the cue for the next behavior
    - Fading - Fading is simply gradually reducing the strength of prompt. The overall goal of the client is to ultimately need no prompts.

Behavior therapy can be used for improving the sitting tolerance, increasing the attention span and encouraging the completion of the task with fewer challenges. It can also be used to shape and determine social behavior in groups, with peers, in school and at home. Behavior therapy is usually used and works best with children and teenagers.

Psychoeducation

Psychoeducation refers to the process of providing the client and their families with sufficient education and information about the mental illness, disorder or disability the client is diagnosed with. It is generally known that those who have a thorough understanding of their challenges they are facing along with the knowledge of their coping ability, resources available and their strength and limitations are better able to handle their challenges and presenting problems. Knowledge and information about their condition helps their families, caregivers and peers to support them better.

Bauml et al. (2006) have stated that psychoeducation when administered in groups, schools, hospitals, clinical settings or otherwise often leads to better and improved treatment compliances. It is proposed that psychoeducation works towards reducing the stigma associated with illness or disability. Reyes, states that family psychoeducation increases compliance with the treatment plan and also ensures that the client receives adequate support in terms of emotional, resources and others while under treatment.

Psychoeducation is one of the important pillars to rehabilitation. In the childhood stage - parents, family, peers, teachers, school and caregivers are given psychoeducation to increase understanding about the child's diagnosis. This also increases the support and ensures the application of the treatment plan in various areas of the child's life. Psychoeducation at this stage also involves advocacy in terms of accomodation and relaxation in learning and education to ensure social participation and provide an opportunity to have an inclusive education. In the adulthood stage - self, parents, family, partners, peers, college, workplace can be provided with psychoeducation.

Another extremely important aspect covered by psychoeducation is reducing the stigma, discrimination, prejudice and marginalization related to the disorder, creating a socially inclusive environment, encouraging social participation and changing the attitude of people.

Psychotherapy

Psychotherapy is an effective psychological intervention for a multitude of psychological, behavioral, and somatic problems, symptoms, and disorders and thus rightfully considered as a main approach in mental and somatic health care management (Prince et al., 2007; Goldfried, 2013).

Psychotherapy is not a standalone effective treatment for the symptoms of ADHD. Along with the ADHD symptoms the clients, most times also present secondary symptoms that are a result of their present challenges. However it is useful in teenagers and adults where there are associated symptoms of low self-image, low self-esteem, low self-worth, identity issues, anger, emotional disturbances, anxiety, stress and difficult interpersonal relationships.

These emotional difficulties along with their accompanying thought and inability to finish their tasks and achieve their goals also add up and lead to the client's present challenges. For teenagers and adults, especially, psychotherapy helps to relieve these emotional and thought challenges. Psychotherapy also helps in working directly with symptoms and behaviors as a result of ADHD like procrastination, anger and self-worth and self-image. There are multiple exercises and techniques that are used in therapy that the client learns to practice and apply in their life. Psychotherapy also helps the client focus on their strengths and think beyond their disorder (Honos-Webb,2010).

Younger children may not always be able to comprehend their situation and fathom the reasons for their behavior. Comparison with their peers, inability to function similarly as them and inability to function age appropriately at times also leaves them feeling anxious, angry, stressed and with a low self-image and experiencing disturbing emotions. Younger children may not be able to fully express their emotions and thoughts. This at times comes out as difficult behavior. Play therapy is often used as a therapeutic tool to encourage children to share their thoughts and emotions.

In the past decade many multi modal interventions have included Cognitive Behavior Therapy (CBT) for ADHD (McDermott, 2000, 2009; Ramsay & Rostain, 2003, 2008; Rostain & Ramsay, 2006; Safren et.al, 2005). CBT is adapted from Beck's traditional cognitive model that focuses on the interplay of thoughts, emotions and behaviors through understanding individual's beliefs about and interpretation of their experiences. CBT also works to explore the individual's thoughts regarding the self, others and the world.

Ramsay (2010) says "Understanding how you think is an effective start to making changes in your life". Although ADHD is not the result of negative thoughts, cognitive and behavioral modification often open the way for patients to implement new coping skills and gain new experiences that promote new outlooks on themselves and new coping options (Ramsay, 2007; Safren, 2006).

Demoralizing thoughts and beliefs often keep many adults with ADHD from achieving their goals and realising them. CBT helps the individual's with ADHD understand and deal with their distorting thinking process and targets their ongoing struggles primarily with disorganization and procrastination. The combination of medication and CBT is often the treatment of choice for dealing with the wide-range effects of ADHD (ADDitude, ADHD Medication and Treatment).

Psychotherapy alleviates the symptoms, makes the client more functional and improves their quality of life. This is vital as the ultimate goal of rehabilitation is to "restore client's health and normal life by training and therapy".

Social Skills Training

Social skills include our verbal and non-verbal interactions with others. This also includes how one conducts themselves with others. Social skills are important because they help connect with other people, allow expression of thoughts, emotions and opinions and develop healthy interpersonal relationships which are important.

The impulsiveness, hyperactivity, and inattention associated with ADHD can wreak havoc on a child's attempts to connect with others in positive ways (Bunford et al,2018). Research finds that children with ADHD tend to be extremely poor monitors of their own social behavior (Hoza,2007). Children with ADHD have difficulty learning by experiences and situations that they are a part of. They often react without thinking through consequences (Gardner & Gerdes, 2015).

To make social skills training further effective it can be done with all the significant people involved in caregiving and training in the person with ADHD's life. One of the key organizations "Children and Adults with Attention-Deficit/Hyperactivity Disorder (CHADD)" working in the field of ADHD since, 1987, has mentioned various ways of identifying lack of social skills and their development in persons with ADHD.

Some of the key areas that can be worked upon in social skills training are: -

1. Understanding social situation

This involves understanding social cues and social participation. Further, understanding other people's body language, meaning of words and tone and non-verbal gestures. On a larger scale this also involves understanding group dynamics and behavior. Developing an understanding for social cues also involves setting up boundaries for the self and others.

2. Communication and language

For clients with ADHD increasing vocabulary and developing spoken language is an important aspect of social skill training. Having a sufficient vocabulary and practicing it, assists in expressing their emotions and thoughts to others.

Communication involves interacting with others, the mode of expression, use of words, tone and pitch, timing of communication and more. Communication largely depends on language and understanding social cues.

3. Group play/activities

Group play/activities are a ground for clients to practice their learnt and known social skills. Encouraging the client to participate in group work according to their likes and comforts encourages social participation, self-expression and understanding others. For younger children, meeting and playing with children of their age, provides an opportunity for the caregivers and parents to introduce and shape positive social skills.

4. Social problem solving skills

These involve resolving and using problem solving skills to deal with the social situations and challenges. This requires adaptability and coping skills along with thinking and expression. In social situations there are chances that a problem situation may arise. The ability to deal with them at a cognitive and emotional level is a part of the social skills training.

5. Assertiveness training

Being assertive means being able to communicate your thoughts, opinions and emotions to others in a healthy and balanced way. People with ADHD do often experience anxiety, anger, stress and difficult emotions among many others things. Developing the skill for being assertive allows people with ADHD a scope to express themselves confidently. Assertiveness training often involves psychotherapy (mostly CBT) to primarily increase self-acceptance, self-worth and increase self-awareness. If the client is aware of the thoughts, feelings and emotions and has an increased understanding of the self, his chances of expression and communication become better.

The development of social skills can be initiated and customized according to the client's needs, diagnosis and current level of skills. These skills can be developed as close to as their age appropriate social skills. Practicing these skills at a holistic level(including therapist, parents, teachers, school and peers) increases the chances of its application and learning. It also increases the scope of practice and adapting the social skills. Shape positive behaviors with immediate rewards (Mikami et al, 2017)

Parent Training

Parents of the person with ADHD often experience difficult emotions. These emotions are often to do primarily with acceptance of the client and the disorder, fear and uncertainty around social acceptance, stigma and prejudice against the disorder, feelings of denial or grief and anger and many times difficulty coping with the client and balancing their needs and other disturbing emotions.

Parent training is a vital part of the rehabilitation process. The primary step is providing psychoeducation and psychotherapy or counselling of the parents and caregivers. This helps parents to deal with the emotional disturbances, parental expectations and encourages acceptance of their child with ADHD.

Parents are also involved in the Behavior Parent Training(BPT). Behavioral Parent Training (BPT) is the predominant mode of behavior management treatment targeting home-based problems for school-age youth with ADHD (Pfiffner & Kaiser; 2010; Anastopoulos & Farley, 2003).

Parent training involves working with acceptance, psychoeducation of the disorder, discipline strategies and instructions, communication strategies, working with self, creating a balance between self, the child and their professional life, adjusting and adapting, dealing with self ADHD(some parents of children with ADHD, also have ADHD), seeking help, working on relationship with spouse and other challenges (Tuckman, 2009).

Parents are taught techniques that they implement with the client and discuss progress, problem-solve, and learn new techniques. Interventions need to be feasible and palatable for families so they can be maintained in the long run. Parent training equips the parents with skills for giving instructions and training them in dealing with the client. Improvement is often gradual. Contingency should be kept for major developmental changes and transitions that could affect the client.

Parent training also ensures that the parents are equally involved which in turn increases the support system for the person with ADHD, increases independence of the parents in dealing with the challenges and higher chance in the process of rehabilitation. This increases the support system for the client and makes the process more holistic.

Support Groups

Support groups offer education, emotional support and encouragement to parents and families of people with ADHD and also to individuals with ADHD. Being with people who understand the struggles and challenges without having to explain to them offers a sense of comfort and a sense of belonging. People in support groups often express their concerns and share their emotions without having to worry about bias and stigma.

People in support groups share their struggles, challenges, coping strategies and their journey. This offers a chance to others in the group to learn from others sharings. People with different age groups who are diagnosed with ADHD and their families are a part of the group. The sharings of the group gives a chance to the younger children to learn and adapt from others and be better prepared for other developmental, emotional and practical challenges in the future.

Support groups offer information about the resources and specialists of the field. There are various groups that work to advocate for the rights of the people with ADHD. These support groups provide information to new parents of children diagnosed with ADHD about the various facilities, provisions, accommodations and relaxations provided to the people with ADHD and their families by the law.

Larger groups often have specialists and concerned practitioners on their panel and often invite them to talk about their concerned issues. In the rehabilitation process, support groups offer a scope for social inclusion and social participation.

Coaching

"The notion of "coaching" for adult ADHD was originally used as a metaphor for the need to adopt a more interactive, directive therapeutic alliance than is seen in traditional therapy (Hallowell & Ratey, 1994). The field of ADHD coaching arose as a profession designed to help adults with ADHD develop the necessary organization, time management, and other skills to handle the challenges of daily life (National Resource Center on AD/HD [NRC], 2003). ADHD coaching is not a psychosocial treatment per se, to the extent that it is not a traditional psychological treatment; does not require a degree or credentialing in a mental health profession; and does not involve the comprehensive assessment and treatment of various cognitive, emotional, behavioral, developmental, and personality factors. Instead, it is a targeted support service that uses various cognitive and behavior modification principles to promote the use of adaptive coping skills.

ADHD coaching is a specialty that is an outgrowth of life and executive coaching movements (Berman & Bradt, 2006; Neenan & Dryden, 2002). ADHD coaching builds on the foundation of positive psychology (Seligman & Csikszentmihalyi,2000), a wellness model that emphasizes factors involved in healthy development, the acquisition of adaptive living skills, and the notion that individuals can be encouraged to discover solutions to their problems.

ADHD coaching is a personal education approach, focusing on recognizing and using psychological strengths, and making use of existing aptitudes and talents, rather than directly focusing on problem reduction (Ratey, 2008).

ADHD coaching strives to bridge the gap between ability and performance (Young & Giwerc, 2003). Ratey (2002) proposed that five main ways ADHD coaching is helpful are by maintaining arousal, modulating emotions, maintaining motivation and providing immediate reward, supporting the client's ability to carry out self-directed actions and change behavior patterns.

ADHD coaching helps the client in setting up a structure, setting goals, task management, time management, developing new skills, learning household tasks, routine activities, dealing with challenges, developing new habits and integrating them in the client's life. The ADHD coach works as a personal mentor who is present while the client performs and learns tasks. This allows the person with ADHD to increase their focus on tasks and physical activities and reduces their anxiety to some extent. Coaching gives the person with ADHD someone to rely on and learn and practice hands on skills and tasks.

Remedial Teaching

In remediation, the deficit in learning is identified and strategies are used to equip the person with ADHD to improve and reduce the deficit. Through remedial teaching, the various educational skills of the student are worked upon and improved. The process of remediation is different for different needs because there is a lot of variation in strengths and deficits for each individual with special needs. Some common basic principles and strategies that remain common for all are: -

1. Acquisition - learning new task or skill

2. Fluency - working on acquired skill independently with more accuracy
3. Maintenance - maintaining the same fluency and accuracy level while learning another task
4. Generalization - ability to identify and use the learnt skill in different situations

Remedial instruction is focused on the specific concepts with which the student struggles. Remediation strategies include differential and alternate instruction strategies, determining the individual needs, reteaching, task analysis, additional practice and one-on-one tutoring.

Various strategies are used with students, when they face difficulty in the academic area. Remediation strategies are one type of intervention. Some of the steps involve designing Individual education plan (IEP), frequent evaluation - specially after a short term objective or learning a new skill, Test-Teach-Test(TTT) to redefine the present level of the student and regular upgradation of the IEP of the student.

Effective remediation involves assessing the student's needs, providing intervention and evaluating student outcomes. Effective rehabilitation of the child with ADHD also involves accommodation and modification of the content being taught and instructional modification. Modifications in techniques of evaluation and relaxation in evaluations also provide encouragement and support to continue with the educational facilities available. For inclusive education it is necessary that the person with ADHD learn and are assessed keeping in mind their needs and the age appropriate level.

Effective remediation usually involves customizing the remedial teaching in accordance to the ways in which the person with ADHD can learn. Remedial strategies are an important aspect of rehabilitation as they provide the scope of education at par with their current age appropriate level and promote inclusive education at the same time.

Classroom Management

Persons with ADHD who are in school benefit from the Daily Report Card system. This approach sets specific goals for the students, gives feedback on their performance towards achieving their goals and rewards them for achieving their goals. Daily report cards are designed especially for each student keeping in mind their individual academic and social goals.

In classroom management, teachers are trained with strategies that help in dealing with the behavioral problems of children with ADHD. Strategies like building a structure, restructuring of environment, rescheduling of activities, being aware of the disorder and its impact on behavior and cognition, incorporating firm instructional styles, bringing in humor, being empathetic to the needs of the child with ADHD and establishing a connect are some of the strategies that the teacher can use at a classroom level.

Classroom management is a vital part of the rehabilitation process of the individual with ADHD. The person with ADHD spends half of his waking hours at school or with peers. So if rehabilitation strategies are followed at any singular level, it will not reflect in all areas and it will be incomplete. Hence, just as the parents, caregivers and family are provided psychoeducation, psychotherapy and parental training to equip them to deal with the client, similarly teachers and school staff can be equipped with strategies to deal with the behavioral, emotional and academic challenges that the client may present at the school.

Classroom management as a part of the rehabilitation process also reinforces the application of strategies and techniques at a holistic level.

Lifestyle Changes

Dietary treatments have been highly publicized in the past, but numerous and recent studies have found them to be of little or no value (Paul et al., 2017). It is recommended to eat a healthy and balanced diet. However, it is vital to be aware of allergies and the effects various foods have on the behavior and mood (Tuckman, 2009).

Along with the diet, exercising regularly and sleeping well are also essential. Maintaining a daily routine and structuring the day in a way to incorporate activities that are productive and enjoyable also help in achieving goals and staying healthy emotionally and physically. For younger children with ADHD routines can be set with the assistance of their parents, caregivers or teachers. For adults with ADHD a coach can assist and follow up (ADDitude, 2017).

These lifestyle changes work as a part of the rehabilitation process as they facilitate the person with ADHD to stay healthy; emotionally and behaviorally, and also work towards their goals.

Career Counselling and Workplace Support

Regardless of one's particular occupational path, the ability to function in a work setting, including self-employment and stay-at-home parenting, is an inescapable feature of adult life that requires individuals to function relatively independently in terms of organization; time management; planning, prioritizing, and following through on tasks; and other skills related to self-management (Evans et al., 2018).

Individuals with ADHD, seek jobs that allow them to use their skills and aptitudes and that do not emphasize on their various academic skills that may represent areas of relative weakness for them. Career counselling identifies the areas and aptitudes that the individual can perform well in and based on that a career choice can be made. Career counselling also encompasses identification of interests and personality of the individual. Hence the career choice made thereafter is more scientific as it employs their strengths, personality, aptitude and interests. To broaden the scope and make it further relevant, vocational assessment can be done. Vocational assessment must take into account the relationship of work related abilities and skills being measured in the context of a variety of other related factors.

However, this may be subjective as each individual with ADHD has a varied set of emotional, behavioral and cognitive challenges that they are coping with.

Through ADHD coaching strategies, individuals with ADHD can be coached to learn skills, behavior patterns and coping skills that are required at the workplace. However, for this the workplace and the co-workers need to be sensitized and given psychoeducation about the needs of the individual with ADHD. After being placed in the job, during the job training, induction and skill training, counseling process is introduced to make the transition and adaptation effective. Even after the individual is placed into a workplace, regular follow ups with the employer, co-workers and the individual with ADHD is required to ensure healthy adjustment to the workplace.

Integration of the workplace, therapist, ADHD coach and the individual with ADHD is vital for a successful vocational rehabilitation to take place.

CONCLUSION

For rehabilitation of people with ADHD it is required that a holistic approach is used. As the disorder is a continuous and rather permanent one, it is required that rehabilitation strategies are applied at all strategies. Each developmental stage and age, right from the diagnosis, provides a different set of challenges which are in varied domains. To reduce the gap between the ability and the age appropriate behavior for the individual with ADHD, timely interventions along with appropriate rehabilitation strategies are recommended.

REFERENCES

Anastopoulos, A. D., & Farley, S. E. (2003). A cognitive-behavioral training program for parents of children with attention-deficit/hyperactivity disorder. In A. E. Kazdin & J. R. Weisz (Eds.), *Evidence-based psychotherapies for children and adolescents*. Guilford Press.

Bagwell, C.L., & Molina, B.S., Pelham, & W.E. (. (2001). ADHD and problems in peer relations: Predictions from childhood to adolescence. *Journal of the American Academy of Child and Adolescent Psychiatry*, *40*, 1285–1292. doi:10.1097/00004583-200111000-00008 PMID:11699802

Bauml, J., Froböse, T., Kraemer, S., Rentrop, M., & Pitschel-Walz, G. (2006). Psychoeducation: A basic psychotherapeutic intervention for patients with schizophrenia and their families. *Schizophrenia Bulletin*, *32*(1), S1–S9. https://www.ncbi.nlm.nih.gov/pmc/articles/PMC2683741. doi:10.1093chbulbl017 PMID:16920788

Black Rhonda. (n.d.). *Special Education: Behavioral Terms*. Retrieved from https://www.studyblue.com/notes/note/n/behavioral-terms/deck/17764131

Bunford, N., Evans, S. W., & Langberg, J. M. (2018). Emotion Dysregulation Is Associated With Social Impairment Among Young Adolescents With ADHD. *Journal of Attention Disorders*, *22*(1), 66–82. doi:10.1177/1087054714527793 PMID:24681899

Children and Adults with Attention-Deficit/Hyperactivity Disorder (CHADD). (n.d.). *Relationships and Social Skills*. Retrieved from https://chadd.org/for-adults/relationships-social-skills/

Dupar, L. (2017). *ADDitude, Expert eBook*. ADHD Medication & Treatment.

Evans, S., Owens, J. S., & Bunford, N. (2013). Evidence-Based Psychosocial Treatments for Children and Adolescents with Attention-Deficit/Hyperactivity Disorder. *Journal of Clinical Child & Adolescent Psychology*, *43*(4), 527-551. doi:10.1080/15374416.2013.850700

Faraone, S. V., Biederman, J., & Monuteaux, M. C. (2001). A psychometric measure of learning disability predicts educational failure four years later in boys with ADHD. *Journal of Attention Disorders*, 220–230. doi:10.1177/108705470100400404

Gardner, D. M., & Gerdes, A. C. (2015). A Review of Peer Relationships and Friendships in Youth With ADHD. *Journal of Attention Disorders*, *19*(10), 844–855. doi:10.1177/1087054713501552 PMID:24062277

Honos-Webb, L. (2010). The Gift of ADHD. *New Harbinger Publications., ISBN-13*, 978–1572248502.

Hoza, B. (2007). Peer functioning in children with ADHD. *Ambulatory Pediatrics*, *7*(1), 101–106. doi:10.1016/j.ambp.2006.04.011 PMID:17261489

Johnston, C., & Mash, E. J. (2001). Families of children with ADHD: Review and recommendations for future research. *Clinical Child and Family Psychology Review*, *4*(3), 183–207. doi:10.1023/A:1017592030434 PMID:11783738

Maki, D. R., & Tarvydas, V. M. (2012). The Professional Practice of Rehabilitation Counseling: Concepts and Paradigms in Rehabilitation Counseling. Academic Press.

Mannuzza, S., Klein, R. G., & Bessler, A. (1993). Adult outcome of hyperactive boys: Educational achievement, occupational rank and psychiatric status. *Archives of General Psychiatry*, *50*(7), 565–576. doi:10.1001/archpsyc.1993.01820190067007 PMID:8317950

Mikami, A. Y., Smit, S., & Khalis, A. (2017). Social Skills Training and ADHD-What Works? *Current Psychiatry Reports*, *19*(12), 93. doi:10.100711920-017-0850-2 PMID:29082428

Miltenberger, R. G. (2008). *Behavior Modification: Principles and Procedures* (4th ed.). Thomas Learning Inc.

Pfiffner, L., & Kaiser, N. (2010). Behavioral parent training, Dulcan's textbook of child and adolescent psychiatry. American Psychiatric Association.

Psychoeducation: Definition, goals and methods. (2014). Retrieved from http://www.aipc.net.au/articles/psychoeducation-definition-goals-and-methods

Ramsay, R. J. (2010). *Nonmedication Treatments for Adult ADHD: Evaluating Impact on Daily Functioning and Well-Being*. American Psychological Association. doi:10.1037/12056-000

Reyes, C. Y. (2010). *What is psycho-education?* Retrieved from http://thepsychoeducationalteacher.blogspot.com/2010/10/what-is-psycho-education.html

Riggar, T. F., & Maki, D. R. (2003). *Handbook of Rehabilitation Counseling: Concepts and Paradigms*. Springer Publishing Company.

Sherwin, E. (2012). *The Oxford Handbook of Rehabilitation Psychology: A field in flux - The History of Rehabilitation Psychology*. Oxford University Press Inc.

The MTA Cooperative Group. (1999). A 14-month randomized clinical trial of treatment strategies for attention-deficit/hyperactivity disorder. Multimodal Treatment Study of Children with ADHD. *Archives of General Psychiatry*, *56*(12), 1073–1086. doi:10.1001/archpsyc.56.12.1073 PMID:10591283

Tuckman, A. (2009). *More attention, less deficit: success strategies for adults with ADHD*. Speciality Press, Inc.

Weiss, G., & Hechtman, L. (1993). *Hyperactive children grown up: ADHD in children, adolescents and adults*. Guildford Press.

Wender, P. H., & Tomb, D. A. (2017). *ADHD: A Guide to Understanding Symptoms, Causes, Diagnosis, Treatment and Changes over time in Children, Adolescents, and Adults, Treatment of the child with ADHD*. Oxford University Press.

Wilkes-gillan, S., Bundy, A., Cordier, R., Lincoln, M., & Chen, Y. W. (2016). A Randomised Controlled Trial of a Play-Based Intervention to Improve the Social Play Skills of Children with Attention Deficit Hyperactivity Disorder (ADHD). *PLoS One*, *11*(8), e0160558. doi:10.1371/journal.pone.0160558 PMID:27529693

Compilation of References

Aadil, M., Cosme, R. M., & Chernaik, J. (2017). Mindfulness-Based Cognitive Behavioral Therapy as an Adjunct Treatment of Attention Deficit Hyperactivity Disorder in Young Adults: A Literature Review. *Cureus*, *9*(5), e1269. doi:10.7759/cureus.1269 PMID:28775916

Abikoff, H., Hechtman, L., Klein, R. G., Weiss, G., Fleiss, K., Etcovitch, J., Cousins, L., Greenfield, B., Martin, D., & Pollack, S. (2004). Symptomatic improvement inchildren with ADHD treated with long-term methylphenidate and multimodal psychosocial treatment. *Journal of the American Academy of Child and Adolescent Psychiatry*, *43*(7), 802–811. doi:10.1097/01.chi.0000128791.10014.ac PMID:15213581

Abikoff, H., & Klein, R. (1992). Attention Deficit Hyperactivity and Conduct Disorders: Comorbidity and implications for treatment. *Journal of Consulting and Clinical Psychology*, *60*(6), 881–892. doi:10.1037/0022-006X.60.6.881 PMID:1360990

Able, S. L., Johnston, A. J., Adler, L. A., & Swindle, R. W. (2006). Functional and Psychological Impairment in Adults with Undiagnosed ADHD. *Psychological Medicine*, *37*(1), 97–107. doi:10.1017/S0033291706008713

Achenbach, T. M. (1991). *Integrative guide for the 1991 CBCL/4-18, YSR, and TRF profiles*. University of Vermont, Department of Psychiatry.

Adesman, A. R. (2001). The diagnosis and management of attention-deficit/hyperactivity disorder in pediatric patients. *The Journal of Clinical Psychiatry*, *3*(2), 66–77. doi:10.4088/pcc.v03n0204 PMID:15014618

ADHD Resource Center. (n.d.). *American Academy of Child & Adolescent Psychiatry website*. Available at http://www.aacap.org/AACAP/Families%5Fand%5FYouth/Resource%5FCenters/ADHD%5FResource%5FCenter/Home.aspx

Adler, L., & Cohen, J. (2004). Diagnosis and evaluation of adults with attention-deficit/hyperactivity disorder. *The Psychiatric Clinics of North America*, *27*(2), 187–201. doi:10.1016/j.psc.2003.12.003 PMID:15063992

Aida, S. A., Aili, H. H., Manveen, K. S., Salwina, W. I. W., Subash, K. P., Ng, C. G., & Muhsin, C. G. (2014). Prevalence of psychiatric disorders among juvenile offenders in Malaysian prisons and association with socio-demographic and personal factors. *International Journal of Prisoner Health*, *10*(2), 132–143. doi:10.1108/IJPH-06-2013-0029 PMID:25764076

Alderson, R. M., Rapport, M. D., & Kofler, M. J. (2007). Attention-Deficit/Hyperactivity disorder and behavioral inhibition: A meta-analytic review of the stop-signal paradigm. *Journal of Abnormal Child Psychology*, *35*(5), 745–758. doi:10.100710802-007-9131-6 PMID:17668315

Alessandri, S. M. (1992). Attention, play, and social behavior in ADHD preschoolers. *Journal of Abnormal Child Psychology*, *20*(3), 289–302. doi:10.1007/BF00916693 PMID:1619135

Alexander, G. K., Taylor, A. G., Innes, K. E., Kulbok, P., & Selfe, T. K. (2008). Contextualizing the effects of yoga therapy on diabetes management: A review of the social determinants of physical activity. *Family & Community Health, 31*(3), 228–239. doi:10.1097/01.FCH.0000324480.40459.20

Alexander, K. (2018). Integrative Review of the Relationship Between Mindfulness-Based Parenting Interventions and Depression Symptoms in Parents. *Journal of Obstetric, Gynecologic, and Neonatal Nursing, 47*(2), 184–190. doi:10.1016/j.jogn.2017.11.013 PMID:29294315

Algorta, P. G., Kragh, C. A., Arnold, L. E., Molina, B. S. G., Hinshaw, S. P., Swanson, J. M., Hechtman, L., Copley, L. M., Lowe, M., & Jensen, P. S. (2018). Maternal ADHD Symptoms, Personality, and Parenting Stress: Differences Between Mothers of Children With ADHD and Mothers of Comparison Children. *Journal of Attention Disorders, 22*(13), 1266–1277. doi:10.1177/1087054714561290 PMID:25525155

Almogbel, Y. S., Goyal, R., & Sansgiry, S. S. (2017). Association Between Parenting Stress and Functional Impairment Among Children Diagnosed with Neurodevelopmental Disorders. *Community Mental Health Journal, 53*(4), 405–414. doi:10.100710597-017-0096-9 PMID:28176211

Amen, D. G., Paldi, J. H., & Thisted, R. A. (1993). Brain SPECT imaging. *Journal of the American Academy of Child and Adolescent Psychiatry, 32*(5), 1080–1081. doi:10.1097/00004583-199309000-00036 PMID:8407758

America's Children and the Environment. 3rd Ed. (2015). Retrieved from the WWW on Friday August 2, 2019 From file:///E:/Clarion%20Folder/COUN %20591/ace3_neurodevelopmental.pdf

American Psychiatric Association. (1994). Diagnostic and Statistical Manual of Mental Disorders, 4th edition (DSM-IV). Washington DC.

American Psychiatric Association. (2000). Diagnostic and Statistical Manual of Mental Disorders (4th ed.). Washington DC: Author.

American Psychiatric Association. (2000). Diagnostic and Statistical Manual of Mental Disorders. APA.

American Psychiatric Association. (2013), Diagnostic and statistical manual of mental disorders (5th ed.; DSM–5). Washington, DC.

American Psychiatric Association. (2013). *Diagnostic and statistical manual of mental disorders* (5th ed.). American Psychiatric Publishing.

American Psychiatric Association. (2013). Diagnostic and statistical manual of mental disorders (5th ed.). Arlington, VA: American Psychiatric Publishing.

American Psychiatric Association. (2013). *Diagnostic and Statistical Manual of Mental Disorders* (5th ed.). Author.

American Psychiatric Association. (2013). *Diagnostic and Statistical Manual of Mental Disorders. 5*[th]. Author.

Ames, C. S., & White, S. J. (2011). Brief report: Are ADHD traits dissociable from the autistic profile? Links between cognition and behavior. *Journal of Autism and Developmental Disorders, 31*(3), 357–363. doi:10.100710803-010-1049-0 PMID:20585847

Anastopoulos, A. D., & Farley, S. E. (2003). A cognitive-behavioral training program for parents of children with attention-deficit/hyperactivity disorder. In A. E. Kazdin & J. R. Weisz (Eds.), *Evidence-based psychotherapies for children and adolescents*. Guilford Press.

Anastopoulos, A. D., Guevremont, D. C., Shelton, T. L., & DuPaul, G. J. (1992). Parenting stress among families of children with attention deficit hyperactivity disorder. *Journal of Abnormal Child Psychology*, *20*(5), 503–520. doi:10.1007/BF00916812 PMID:1487593

Anastopoulos, A. D., Shelton, T. L., DuPaul, G. J., & Guevremont, D. C. (1993). Parent training for attentiondeficit hyperactivity disorder: Its impact' of parent functioning. *Journal of Abnormal Child Psychology*, *21*(5), 581–596. doi:10.1007/BF00916320 PMID:8294653

Anckarsater, H., Stahlberg, O., Larsson, T., Hakansson, C., Jutblad, S. B., Niklasson, L., ... Rastam, M. (2006). The impact of ADHD and autism spectrum disorders on temperament character and personality development. *The American Journal of Psychiatry*, *163*(7), 1239–1244. doi:10.1176/ajp.2006.163.7.1239 PMID:16816230

Anderson, R., & Baldwin, S. (2000). What's in a name? Amphetamine and methylphenidate. *Journal of Substance Use*, *5*(2), 89–91. doi:10.3109/14659890009053070

Andrade, B. F., Brodeur, D. A., Waschbusch, D. A., Stewart, S. H., & McGee, R. (2009). Selective and sustained attention as predictors of social problems in children with typical and disordered attention abilities. *Journal of Attention Disorders*, *12*(4), 341–352. doi:10.1177/1087054708320440 PMID:18596299

Angold, A., Erkanli, A., Egger, H. L., & Costello, E. J. (2000). Stimulant treatment for children: A community perspective. *Journal of the American Academy of Child and Adolescent Psychiatry*, *39*(8), 975–984. doi:10.1097/00004583-200008000-00009

Anker, E., Bendiksen, B., & Heir, T. (2018). Comorbid psychiatric disorders in a clinical sample of adults with ADHD, and associations with education, work and social characteristics: A cross-sectional study. *BMJ Open*, *8*(3), e019700. doi:10.1136/bmjopen-2017-019700 PMID:29500213

Anker, E., Bendiksen, B., & Heir, T. (2018). Comorbid psychiatric disorders in a clinical sample of adults with ADHD, and associations with education, work and social characteristics: a cross-sectional study. *BMJ open*, *8*(3). Attention-deficit/hyperactivity disorder in adults: an overview. *Biological Psychiatry*, *48*(1), 9–20.

Ann, C. M. D., & Drugs, C. T. C. I.Treatment of Attention-Deficit/Hyperactivity Disorder. (2016). *Expert Opinion on Investigational Drugs*.

Antshel, K. M., Faraone, S. V., & Gordon, M. (2014). Cognitive behavioral treatment outcomes in adolescent ADHD. *Journal of Attention Disorders*, *18*(6), 483–495. doi:10.1177/1087054712443155 PMID:22628140

Antshel, K. M., & Remer, R. (2003). Social Skills Training in Children With Attention Deficit Hyperactivity Disorder: A Randomized Controlled Clinical Trial. *Journal of Clinical Child and Adolescent Psychology*, *32*(1), 153–165. doi:10.1207/S15374424JCCP3201_14 PMID:12611031

APA. (2013). Diagnostic and statistical manual of mental disorders-fifth edition (DSM-5). Arlington: American Psychiatric Publishing, Inc.

Appel, L. (2003). Lifestyle modification as a means to prevent and treat high blood pressure. *Journal of the American Society of Nephrology*, *14*(90002), S99–S102. doi:10.1097/01.ASN.0000070141.69483.5A

Arnold, E. H., O'Leary, S. G., & Edwards, G. H. (1997). Father involvement and self-report parenting of children with attention deficit-hyperactivity disorder. *Journal of Consulting and Clinical Psychology*, *65*(2), 337–342. doi:10.1037/0022-006X.65.2.337

Arnold, L. E., & DiSilvestro, R. A. (2005). Zinc in Attention-Deficit/ Hyperactivity Disorder. *Journal of Child and Adolescent Psychopharmacology*, *15*(4), 619–627. doi:10.1089/cap.2005.15.619 PMID:16190793

Arnold, L. E., Hodgkins, P., Kahle, J., Madhoo, M., & Kewley, G. (2020). Long -Term Outcomes of ADHD: Academic Achievement and Performance. *Journal of Attention Disorders*, *24*(1), 73–85. doi:10.1177/1087054714566076 PMID:25583985

Arnold, L. E., Roy, A., Taylor, E., Hetchman, L., Margaret, S., Swanson, J. M., ... Rohde, L. A. (2019). Predictive Utility of Childhood Diagnosis of ICD-10 HKD: Adult outcomes in MTA and Effect of Comorbidity. *European Child & Adolescent Psychiatry*, *28*, 557–570. doi:10.100700787-018-1222-0 PMID:30232561

Arnon, S., Shamai, S., & Ilatov, Z. (2008). Socialization agents and activities of young adolescents. *Adolescence*, *43*, 373–397. PMID:18689107

Asherson, P. J., Levy, F., &Faraone, S. V. (2011). Quantitative and moleculer genetic studies of attention-deficit hyperactivity disorder in adults. *ADHD in Adults*, 25.

Asherson, P., Buitelaar, J., Faraone, S. V., & Rohde, L. A. (2016). Adult attentiondeficit hyperactivity disorder: Key conceptual issues. *The Lancet. Psychiatry*, *3*(6), 568–578. doi:10.1016/S2215-0366(16)30032-3

Assessing adults with ADHD and comorbidities. (2009). *Primary care companion to the Journal of Clinical Psychiatry*, *11*(1), 25. doi:10.4088/pcc.7129bs4c

Atkinson, M., & Hollis, C. (2010). NICE guideline: Attention deficit hyperactivity disorder. *Archives of Disease in Childhood - Education and Practice*, *95*(1), 24–27. doi:10.1136/adc.2009.175943 PMID:20145015

Attention-deficit hyperactivity disorder (ADHD) in children and adolescents. (n.d.). EBSCO DynaMed Plus website. Available at: https://www.dynamed.com/topics/dmp~AN~T113926/Attention-deficit-hyperactivity-disorder-ADHD-in-children-and-adolescents

Ayuso, R., Maestu, F., & Gonzalez, M. J., RomoBarrientos, C., & Andrade, J. M. (2006). Executive Function in Attention Deficit Hyperactivity Disorder in Childhood. *Revista de Neurología*, *•••*, 265–271.

Azeredo, A., Moreira, D., & Barbosa, F. (2018, October). ADHD, CD, and ODD: Systematic review of genetic and environmental risk factors. *Research in Developmental Disabilities*, *82*, 10–19. doi:10.1016/j.ridd.2017.12.010 PMID:29361339

Babakhanian, M., Sayar, S., Babakhanian, M., & Mohammadi, G. (2016). Iranian Children With ADHD and Mental Health of Their Mothers: The Role of Stress. *Iranian Journal of Psychiatry and Behavioral Sciences*, *10*(1), e2026. doi:10.17795/ijpbs-2026 PMID:27284276

Babinski, D. E., Mazzant, J. R., Merrill, B. M., Waschbusch, D. A., Sibley, M. H., Gnagy, E. M., Molina, B. S. G., & Pelham, W. E. (2020). Lifetime caregiver strain among mothers of adolescents and young adults with attention-deficit/hyperactivity disorder. *Journal of Family Psychology*, *34*(3), 342–352. doi:10.1037/fam0000609 PMID:31750692

Bachmanna. (2017). Trends in ADHD medication use in children and adolescents in five western countries, 2005–2012. *European Neuropsychopharmacology, 27*(5), 484-493.

Bagwell, C. L., Molina, B. S., Pelham, W. E. Jr, & Hoza, B. (2001). Attention-deficit hyperactivity disorder and problems in peer relations: Predictions from childhood to adolescence. *Journal of the American Academy of Child and Adolescent Psychiatry*, *40*(11), 1285–1292. doi:10.1097/00004583-200111000-00008

Bai, G. N., Wang, Y. F., Yang, L., & Niu, W. Y. (2015). Effectiveness of a focused, brief psychoeducation program for parents of ADHD children: Improvement of medication adherence and symptoms. *Neuropsychiatric Disease and Treatment*, *11*, 2721–2735. PMID:26604761

Balazs, J., & Kereszteny, A. (2017). Attention-deficit/hyperactivity disorder and suicide: A systematic review. *World Journal of Psychiatry*, *7*(1), 44–59. doi:10.5498/wjp.v7.i1.44 PMID:28401048

Banaschewski, T., Roessner, V., Dittmann, R. W., Santosh, P. J., & Rothenberger, A. (2004). Non-stimulant medications in the treatment of ADHD. *European Child & Adolescent Psychiatry*, *13*(1), 102–116.

Bandura, A. (1977). *Social Learning Theory*. Prentice-Hall.

Banerjee, T. D., Middleton, F., & Faraone, S. V. (2007, September). Environmental risk factors for attention-deficit hyperactivity disorder. *Acta Paediatrica Nurturing the Child*, *96*(9), 1269–1274. doi:10.1111/j.1651-2227.2007.00430.x PMID:17718779

Banks, T., Ninowski, J. E., Mash, E. J., & Semple, D. L. (2008). Parenting behavior and cognitions in a community sample of mothers with and without symptoms of attention-deficit/hyperactivity disorder. *Journal of Child and Family Studies*, *17*(1), 28–43. doi:10.100710826-007-9139-0

Barbaresi, W. J., Colligan, R. C., Weaver, A. L., Voigt, R. G., Killian, J. M., & Katusic, S. K. (2013). Mortality, ADHD, and psychosocial adversity in adults with childhood ADHD: A prospective study. *Pediatrics*, *131*(4), 637–644. doi:10.1542/peds.2012-2354 PMID:23460687

Barbaresi, W. J., Katusic, S. K., Colligan, R. C., Weaver, A. L., & Jacobsen, S. J. (2007). Long-term school outcomes for children with attention-deficit/hyperactivity disorder: A population-based perspective. *Journal of Developmental and Behavioral Pediatrics*, *28*(4), 265–273. doi:10.1097/DBP.0b013e31811ff87d PMID:17700078

Barkley, R. A. (2002). *ADHD--Long-term course, adult outcome, and comorbid disorders*. Academic Press.

Barkley, R. A. (2006). Attention-deficit hyperactivity disorder: A handbook for diagnosis and treatment (3rd ed.). New York: Guilford.

Barkley, R. A., Fischer, M., Edelbrock, C. S., & Smallish, L. (1990). The adolescent outcome of hyperactive children diagnosed by research criteria: I. An 8-year prospective follow-up study. *Journal of the American Academy of Child and Adolescent Psychiatry, 29*(4), 546-57. doi: 00007 doi:10.1097/00004583- 199007000-

Barkley, R. A., Fischer, M., Edelbrock, C. S., Smallish, L. (1990). The adolescent outcome of hyperactive children diagnosed by research criteria: I. An 8-year prospective follow-up study. *Journal of the American Academy of Child and Adolescent Psychiatry, 29*(4), 546-557.

Barkley, R. A., Murphy, K. R., & Fischer, M. (2008). ADHD in adults: What the science says. New York: Guildford.

Barkley, R. (1997). Behavioral inhibition, sustained attention, and executive functions: Constructing a unifying theory of ADHD. *Psychological Bulletin*, *121*(1), 65–94. doi:10.1037/0033-2909.121.1.65 PMID:9000892

Barkley, R. (2004). Driving impairments in teens and adults with attention-deficit/hyperactivity disorder. *The Psychiatric Clinics of North America*, *27*(2), 233–260. doi:10.1016/S0193-953X(03)00091-1 PMID:15063996

Barkley, R. A. (1981). *Hyperactive children: A handbook for diagnosis and treatment*. Guilford.

Barkley, R. A. (1989). Hyperactive girls and boys: Stimulant drug effects on mother-child interactions. *Journal of Child Psychology and Psychiatry, and Allied Disciplines*, *30*(3), 379–390. doi:10.1111/j.1469-7610.1989.tb00253.x PMID:2663900

Barkley, R. A. (1990). *Attention Deficit Hyperactivity Disorder: A handbook for diagnosis and treatment*. Guilford Press.

Barkley, R. A. (1998). *Attention Deficit Hyperactivity Disorder: A Handbook for Diagnosis and Treatment*. Guilford Press.

Barkley, R. A. (1998). Attention-deficit hyperactivity disorder. *Scientific American*, *279*(3), 66–71. doi:10.1038cientificamerican0998-66 PMID:9725940

Barkley, R. A. (1998). Attention-deficit/hyperactivity disorder. In E. Mash & R. Barkley (Eds.), *Treatment of childhood disorders* (2nd ed., pp. 55–110). Guilford Press.

Barkley, R. A. (2002). Major Life Activity and Health Outcomes Associated with Attention Deficit/Hyperactivity Disorder. *The Journal of Clinical Psychiatry*, *63*, 10–15. PMID:12562056

Barkley, R. A. (2002). Major life activity and health outcomes associated with attention-deficit/ hyperactivity disorder. *The Journal of Clinical Psychiatry*, *63*(12), 10–15. PMID:12562056

Barkley, R. A. (2008). Classroom Accommodations for Children with ADHD. *The ADHD Report*, *16*(4), 7–10. doi:10.1521/adhd.2008.16.4.7

Barkley, R. A. (2010). Deficient emotional self-regulation is a core component of attention-deficit/hyperactivity disorder. *Journal of ADHD & Related Disorders*, *1*(2), 5–37.

Barkley, R. A. (2010). Deficient emotional self-regulation: A core component of attention-deficit/ hyperactivity disorder. *Journal of ADHD & Related Disorders*, (1), 1–30.

Barkley, R. A. (2015). History of ADHD. In R. A. Barkley (Ed.), *Attention-Deficit Hyperactivity Disorder: A Handbook for Diagnosis and Treatment* (4th ed., p. 6). Guilford.

Barkley, R. A. (2015b). Etiologies of ADHD. In R. A. Barkley (Ed.), *Attention-deficit hyperactivity disorder: A handbook for diagnosis and treatment* (4th ed., pp. 356–390). Guilford Press.

Barkley, R. A. (Ed.). (2014). *Attention-deficit hyperactivity disorder: A handbook for diagnosis and treatment*. Guilford Publications.

Barkley, R. A., Edwards, G., Laneri, M., Fletcher, K., & Metevia, L. (2001). The efficacy of problem-solving communication training alone, behavior management training alone, and their combination for parent– adolescent conflict in teenagers with ADHD and ODD. *Journal of Consulting and Clinical Psychology*, *69*(6), 926–941. doi:10.1037/0022-006X.69.6.926

Barkley, R. A., & Fischer, M. (2010). The unique contribution of emotional impulsiveness to impairment in major life activities in hyperactive children as adults. *Journal of the American Academy of Child and Adolescent Psychiatry*, *49*, 503–513. PMID:20431470

Barkley, R. A., Fischer, M., Edelbrock, C., & Smallish, L. (1991). The adolescent outcome of hyperactive children diagnosed by research criteria, III: Mother child interactions, family conflicts and maternal psychopathology. *Journal of Child Psychology and Psychiatry, and Allied Disciplines*, *32*(2), 233–255. doi:10.1111/j.1469-7610.1991.tb00304.x PMID:2033106

Barkley, R. A., Fischer, M., Smallish, L., & Fletcher, K. (2004). Young adult follow-up of hyperactive children: Antisocial activities and drug use. *Journal of Child Psychology and Psychiatry, and Allied Disciplines*, *45*(2), 195–211. doi:10.1111/j.1469-7610.2004.00214.x

Barkley, R. A., Guevremont, D. C., Anastopoulos, A. D., & Fletcher, K. E. (1992). A comparison of three family therapy programs for treating family conflicts in adolescents with attention-deficit hyperactivity disorder. *Journal of Consulting and Clinical Psychology*, *60*(3), 450–462. doi:10.1037/0022-006X.60.3.450 PMID:1619099

Barkley, R. A., Karlsson, J., & Pollard, S. (1985). Effects of age on the mother-child interactions of ADD-H and normal boys. *Journal of Abnormal Child Psychology*, *13*(4), 631–637. doi:10.1007/BF00923146 PMID:4078191

Barkley, R. A., Karlsson, J., & Pollard, S. (1985). Effects of age on the mother-child interactions of ADD-H and normal boys. *Journal of Child Psychology and Psychiatry, and Allied Disciplines*, *13*(4), 631–637. PMID:4078191

Barkley, R. A., & Murphy, K. R. (2006). *Attention Deficit Hyperactivity Disorder: A Clinical Workbook* (3rd ed.). Guilford Publications.

Barkley, R. A., & Murphy, K. R. (2010). Impairment in occupational functioning and adult ADHD: The predictive utility of executive function (EF) ratings versus EF tests. *Archives of Clinical Neuropsychology*, *25*(3), 157–173. doi:10.1093/arclin/acq014 PMID:20197297

Barkley, R. A., Murphy, K. R., & Fischer, M. (2010). *ADHD in Adults: What the Science Says*. Guilford Press.

Barkley, R. A., & Peters, H. (2012). The earliest references to ADHD in the medical literature? Melchior Adam Weikard's description in 1775 of "attention deficit" (Mangel Der Aufmerksamkeit, Attnentio Volubilis). *Journal of Attention Disorders*, *16*(8), 623–630. doi:10.1177/1087054711432309 PMID:22323122

Barkley, R., Fischer, M., Smallish, L., & Fletcher, K. (2002). The persistence of attention deficit hyperactivity disorder into young adulthood as a function of reporting source and definition of disorder. *Journal of Abnormal Psychology*, *111*(2), 279–289. doi:10.1037/0021-843X.111.2.279

Barkley, R., Fischer, M., Smallish, L., & Fletcher, K. (2006). Young adult outcome of hyperactive children: Adaptivefunctioning in major life activities. *Journal of the American Academy of Child and Adolescent Psychiatry*, *45*(2), 192–202. doi:10.1097/01.chi.0000189134.97436.e2

Barkley, R., Murphy, K., & Kwasnik, D. (1996). Psychological adjustment and adaptive impairments in young adults with ADHD. *Journal of Attention Disorders*, *1*(1), 41–54. doi:10.1177/108705479600100104

Barrett, J., & Fleming, A. S. (2011). Annual research review: All mothers are not created equal: Neural and psychobiological perspectives on mothering and the importance of individual differences. *Journal of Child Psychology and Psychiatry, and Allied Disciplines*, *52*(4), 368–397. doi:10.1111/j.1469-7610.2010.02306.x

Barroso, N. E., Mendez, L., Graziano, P. A., & Bagner, D. M. (2018). Parenting Stress through the Lens of Different Clinical Groups: A Systematic Review & Meta-Analysis. *Journal of Abnormal Child Psychology*, *46*(3), 449–461. doi:10.100710802-017-0313-6 PMID:28555335

Barry, R. J., Clarke, A. R., & Johnstone, S. J. (2003). A review of electrophysiology in attention-deficit/hyperactivity disorder: I. Qualitative and quantitative electroencephalography. *Clinical Neurophysiology*, *114*(2), 171–183. doi:10.1016/S1388-2457(02)00362-0 PMID:12559224

Barry, T., Lyman, R. D., & Klinger, L. G. (2002). Academic Underachievement and Attention Deficit Hyperactivity Disorder: The Negative Impact of Symptom Severity on School Performance. *Journal of School Psychology*, *40*(3), 259–283. doi:10.1016/S0022-4405(02)00100-0

Bauermeister, J. J., Matos, M., Reina, G., Salas, C. C., Martinez, J. V., Cumba, E., & Barkley, R. A. (2005). Comparison of the DSM-IV combined and inattentive types of ADHD in a school-based sample of Latino/Hispanic children. *Journal of Child Psychology and Psychiatry, and Allied Disciplines*, *46*(2), 166–179. doi:10.1111/j.1469-7610.2004.00343.x PMID:15679525

Bauml, J., Froböse, T., Kraemer, S., Rentrop, M., & Pitschel-Walz, G. (2006). Psychoeducation: A basic psychotherapeutic intervention for patients with schizophrenia and their families. *Schizophrenia Bulletin*, *32*(1), S1–S9. https://www.ncbi.nlm.nih.gov/pmc/articles/PMC2683741. doi:10.1093chbulbl017 PMID:16920788

Baumrind, D.(1971). Current patterns of parental authority. *Developmental Psychology Monographs, 4*(1-2).

Baumrind, D. (1991). Effective parenting during the early adolescent transition. In P. A. Cowan & E. M. Hetherington (Eds.), *Advances in family research* (Vol. 2). Erlbaum.

Baumrind, D. (1991). Effective parenting during the early adolescent transition. In P. A. Cowan & E. M. Hetherington (Eds.), *Family transitions* (pp. 111–163). Lawrence Erlbaum Associates.

Becker, S. J., Nargiso, J. E., Wolff, J. C., Uhl, K. M., Simon, V. A., Spirito, A., & Prinstein, M. J. (2012). Temporal relationship between substance use and delinquent behavior among young psychiatrically hospitalized adolescents. *Journal of Substance Abuse Treatment*, *43*(2), 251–259. doi:10.1016/j.jsat.2011.11.005 PMID:22197300

Becker, S. P., & Barley, R. A. (2019). *ADHD in Adolescents: Development, Assessment, and Treatment*. Guilford Publications.

Beck, J. S. (2011). *Cognitive behavior therapy: Basics and beyond* (2nd ed.). Guilford Press.

Behbahani, M., Zargar, F., Assarian, F., & Akbari, H. (2018). Effects of Mindful Parenting Training on Clinical Symptoms in Children with Attention Deficit Hyperactivity Disorder and Parenting Stress: Randomized Controlled Trial. *Iranian Journal of Medical Sciences*, *43*(6), 596–604. PMID:30510336

Bell. (2007). *Mindful Yoga, Mindful Life: A Guide for Everyday Practice*. Rodmell Press.

Ben Thabet, J., Sallemi, R., Hasïri, I., Zouari, L., Kamoun, F., Zouari, N., Triki, C., & Maâlej, M. (2013). Psycho-emotional impact of a child's disability on parents. *Archives of Pediatrics*, *20*(1), 9–16. doi:10.1016/j.arcped.2012.10.024 PMID:23266169

Ben-Naim, S., Gill, N., Laslo-Roth, R., & Einav, M. (2019). Parental Stress and Parental Self-Efficacy as Mediators of the Association Between Children's ADHD and Marital Satisfaction. *Journal of Attention Disorders*, *23*(5), 506–516. doi:10.1177/1087054718784659 PMID:29985090

Berenguer, C., Roselló, B., Colomer, C., Baixauli, I., & Miranda, A. (2018). Children with autism and attention deficit hyperactivity disorder. Relationships between symptoms and executive function, the theory of mind, and behavioral problems. *Research in Developmental Disabilities*, *83*, 260–269. doi:10.1016/j.ridd.2018.10.001 PMID:30368089

Besag, F., Gobbi, G., Aldenkamp, A., Caplan, R., Dunn, D. W., & Sillanpää, M. (2016). Psychiatric and Behavioural Disorders in Children with Epilepsy (ILAE Task Force Report): Behavioural and psychiatric disorders associated with childhood epilepsy syndromes. *Epileptic Disorders*. Advance online publication. doi:10.1684/epd.2016.0815 PMID:27184676

Bessler, C., Stiefel, D., Barra, S., Plattner, B., & Aebi, M. (2019). Mental disorders and criminal recidivism in male juvenile prisoners. *Zeitschrift fur Kinder- und Jugendpsychiatrie und Psychotherapie*, *47*(1), 73–88. doi:10.1024/1422-4917/a000612 PMID:30156463

Bethancourt, J. A., Camarena, Z. Z., & Britton, G. B. (2009). Exposure to oral methylphenidate from adolescence through young adulthood produces transient effects on hippocampal-sensitive memory in rats. *Behavioural Brain Research*, *202*(1), 50–57. doi:10.1016/j.bbr.2009.03.015 PMID:19447280

Bhatia, M. S., Choudry, S., & Sidhana, A. (1998). Attention Deficit hyperactive disorder among Psychiatric patients. *Indian Pediatrics*, *36*, 583–587. PMID:10736588

Bhide, S., Sciberras, E., Anderson, V., Hazell, P., & Nicholson, J. M. (2016). Association between parenting style and socio-emotional and academic functioning in children with and without ADHD: A community based study. *Journal of Attention Disorders*, *23*(5), 463–474. doi:10.1177/1087054716661420 PMID:27474160

Bickman, L., Foster, E. M., & Lambert, E. W. (1996). Who gets hospitalized in a continuum of care? *Journal of the American Academy of Child and Adolescent Psychiatry*, *35*(1), 74–80. doi:10.1097/00004583-199601000-00015 PMID:8567616

Biederman, J., Spencer, T., & Wilens, T. (2004). Evidence based pharmacotherapy for attention deficit hyperactivity disorder. *International Journal of Neuropharmocotherapy*, *7*, 77-97

Biederman, J., & Faraone, S. V. (2005). Attention-deficit hyperactivity disorder. *Lancet*, *366*(9481), 237–248. doi:10.1016/S0140-6736(05)66915-2 PMID:16023516

Biederman, J., Faraone, S. V., & Lapey, K. (1992). Comorbidity of diagnosis in attention deficit hyperactivity disorder. *Child and Adolescent Psychiatric Clinics of North America*, *1*(2), 335–360. doi:10.1016/S1056-4993(18)30591-1

Biederman, J., Faraone, S. V., Mick, E., Spencer, T., Wilens, T., Kiely, K., ... Warburton, R. (1995). High risk for attention deficit hyperactivity disorder among children of parents with childhood onset of the disorder: A pilot study. *The American Journal of Psychiatry*, *152*(3), 431–435. doi:10.1176/ajp.152.3.431 PMID:7864271

Biederman, J., Faraone, S. V., & Monuteaux, M. C. (2002). Impact of exposure to parental attention-deficit hyperactivity disorder on clinical features and dysfunction in the offspring. *Psychological Medicine*, *32*(5), 817–827. doi:10.1017/S0033291702005652 PMID:12171376

Biederman, J., Faraone, S. V., Spencer, T. J., Mick, E., Monuteaux, M. C., & Aleardi, M. (2006). Functional impairments in adults with self-reports of diagnosed ADHD: A controlled study of 1001 adults in the community. *The Journal of Clinical Psychiatry*, *67*(4), 524–540. doi:10.4088/JCP.v67n0403 PMID:16669717

Biederman, J., Faraone, S. V., Spencer, T., Wilens, T., Mick, E., & Lapey, K. A. (1994). Gender differences in a sample of adults with Attention Deficit Hyperactivity Disorder. *Psychiatry Research*, *53*(1), 13–29. doi:10.1016/0165-1781(94)90092-2

Biederman, J., Faraone, S., Milberger, S., Curtis, S., Chen, L., Marrs, A., Ouellette, C., Moore, P., & Spencer, T. (1996). Predictors of persistence and remission of ADHD into adolescence: Results from a four-year prospective follow-up study. *Journal of the American Academy of Child and Adolescent Psychiatry*, *35*(3), 343–351. doi:10.1097/00004583-199603000-00016 PMID:8714323

Biederman, J., Faroane, S. V., Spencer, T., Wilens, T., Norman, D., Lapey, K. A., & … . (1993). Patterns of psychiatric comorbidity, cognition, and psychosocial functioning in adults with Attention Deficit Hyperactivity Disorder. *The American Journal of Psychiatry*, *150*(12), 1792–1798. doi:10.1176/ajp.150.12.1792

Biederman, J., Monuteaux, M. C., Mick, E., Spencer, T., Wilens, T. E., Silva, W. J., Snyder, L. E., & Faraone, S. V. (2006). Young adult outcome of attention deficit hyperactivity disorder: A controlled 10-year follow-up study. *Psychological Medicine*, *36*(2), 167–179. doi:10.1017/S0033291705006410 PMID:16420713

Biederman, J., Monuteaux, M. C., Mick, E., Wilens, T. E., Fontanella, J. A., Poetzl, K. M., Kirk, T., Masse, J., & Faraone, S. V. (2006). Is cigarette smoking a gateway to alcohol and illicit drug use disorders? A study of youths with and without attention deficit hyperactivity disorder. *Biological Psychiatry*, *59*(3), 258–264. doi:10.1016/j.biopsych.2005.07.009 PMID:16154546

Biederman, J., Monuteaux, M., Doyle, A., Seidman, L., Wilens, T., Ferrero, F., Morgan, C. L., & Faraone, S. V. (2004). Impact of executive function deficits and attention-deficit/hyperactivity disorder (ADHD) on academic outcomes in children. *Journal of Consulting and Clinical Psychology*, *72*(5), 757–766. doi:10.1037/0022-006X.72.5.757 PMID:15482034

Biederman, J., Newcorn, J., & Sprich, S. (1991). Comorbidity of attention deficit hyperactivity disorder with conduct, depressive, anxiety, and other disorders. *The American Journal of Psychiatry*, *148*(5), 564–577. doi:10.1176/ajp.148.5.564 PMID:2018156

Biederman, J., Petty, C. R., Clarke, A., Lomedico, A., & Faraone, S. V. (2011). Predictors of persistent ADHD: An 11-year follow-up study. *Journal of Psychiatric Research*, *45*(2), 150–155. doi:10.1016/j.jpsychires.2010.06.009 PMID:20656298

Biederman, J., Petty, C. R., Dolan, C., Hughes, S., Mick, E., Monuteaux, M. C., & Faraone, S. V. (2008). The long-term longitudinal course of oppositional defiant disorder and conduct disorder in ADHD boys: Findings from a controlled 10-year prospective longitudinal follow-up study. *Psychological Medicine*, *38*(7), 1027–1036. doi:10.1017/S0033291707002668 PMID:18205967

Biederman, J., Petty, C. R., Evans, M., Small, J., & Faraone, S. V. (2010). How persistent is ADHD? A controlled 10-year follow-up study of boys with ADHD. *Psychiatry Research*, *177*(3), 299–304. doi:10.1016/j.psychres.2009.12.010 PMID:20452063

Biederman, J., Petty, C. R., Monuteaux, M. C., Fried, R., Byrne, D., Mirto, T., Spencer, T., Wilens, T. E., & Faraone, S. V. (2010). Adult psychiatric outcomes of girls with attention deficit hyperactivitydisorder:11-year follow-up in a longitudinal case-control study. *The American Journal of Psychiatry*, *167*(4), 409–417. doi:10.1176/appi.ajp.2009.09050736 PMID:20080984

Biederman, J., Petty, C. R., Monuteaux, M.C., Fried, R., Byrne, D., & Mirto, T.,….Faraone, S. V. (2010). Adult Psychiatric Outcomes of Girls With Attention Deficit Hyperactivity Disorder: 11-Year Follow-Up in a Longitudinal Case-Control Study. *Journal of Psychiatry*, *167*(4), 409–417. PMID:20080984

Biederman, J., Petty, C. R., Woodworth, K. Y., Lomedico, A., Hyder, L. L., & Faraone, S. V. (2012). Adult outcome of attention-deficit/hyperactivity disorder: A controlled 16-year follow-up study. *The Journal of Clinical Psychiatry*, *73*(7), 941–950. doi:10.4088/JCP.11m07529

Biederman, J., Wilens, T. E., Mick, E., Faraone, S. V., & Spencer, T. (1998). Does attention-deficit hyperactivity disorder impact the developmental course of drug and alcohol abuse and dependence? *Biological Psychiatry*, *44*(4), 269–273. doi:10.1016/S0006-3223(97)00406-X PMID:9715358

Biederman, J., Wilens, T., Mick, E., Milberger, S., Spencer, T. J., & Faraone, S. V. (1995, November). Psychoactive substance use disorders in adults with attention deficit hyperactivity disorder (ADHD): Effects of ADHD and psychiatric comorbidity. *The American Journal of Psychiatry*, *152*(11), 1652–1658. doi:10.1176/ajp.152.11.1652 PMID:7485630

Bijlenga, D., van der Heijden, K. B., Breuk, M., van Someren, E. J., Lie, M. E., Boonstra, A. M., Swaab, H. J., & Kooij, J. J. (2013). Associations between sleep characteristics, seasonal depressive symptoms, lifestyle, and ADHD symptoms in adults. *Journal of Attention Disorders*, *17*(3), 261–275. doi:10.1177/1087054711428965

Bilkey, T., Surman, C., & Weintraub, K. (2014). ADHD grows up. *Scientific American Mind*, *25*(1), 64–69. doi:10.10 38cientificamericanmind0114-64

Billstedt, E., Anckarsäter, H., Wallinius, M., & Hofvander, B. (2017). Neurodevelopmental disorders in young violent offenders: Overlap and background characteristics. *Psychiatry Research*, *252*, 234–241. doi:10.1016/j.psychres.2017.03.004 PMID:28285251

Bird, H. R., Shaffer, D., Fisher, P., & Gould, M. S. (1993). The Columbia impairment scale (CIS): Pilot findings on a measure of global impairment for children and adolescents. *International Journal of Methods in Psychiatric Research*, *3*, 167–176.

Bjornstad, G., & Montgomery, P. (2005). Family therapy for attention-deficit disorder or attention-deficit/hyperactivity disorder in children and adolescents. *Cochrane Database of Systematic Reviews*, *18*(2). Advance online publication. doi:10.1002/14651858.CD005042.pub2 PMID:15846741

Black Rhonda. (n.d.). *Special Education: Behavioral Terms*. Retrieved from https://www.studyblue.com/notes/note/n/behavioral-terms/deck/17764131

Bockting, C. L., Spinhoven, P., Koeter, M. W., Wouters, L. F., & Schene, A. H. (2006). Prediction of recurrence in recurrent depression and the influence of consecutive episodes on vulnerability for depression: A 2-year prospective study. *The Journal of Clinical Psychiatry*, *67*(5), 747–755. doi:10.4088/JCP.v67n0508 PMID:16841624

Bögels, S., Hoogstad, B., van Dun, L., de Schutter, S., & Restifo, K. (2008). Mindfulness training for adolescents with externalizing disorders and their parents. *Behavioural and Cognitive Psychotherapy*, *36*(2), 193–209. doi:10.1017/S1352465808004190

Bonifacci, P., Massi, L., Pignataro, V., Zocco, S., & Chiodo, S. (2019). Parenting Stress and Broader Phenotype in Parents of Children with Attention Deficit Hyperactivity Disorder, Dyslexia or Typical Development. *International Journal of Environmental Research and Public Health*, *16*(11), 1878. doi:10.3390/ijerph16111878 PMID:31141931

Boomsma, D. I., Saviouk, V., Hottenga, J. J., Distel, M. A., de Moor, M. H., Vink, J. M., Geels, L. M., van Beek, J. H. D. A., Bartels, M., de Geus, E. J. C., & Willemsen, G. (2010). Genetic epidemiology of attention deficit hyperactivity disorder (ADHD index) in adults. *PLoS One*, *5*(5), e10621. doi:10.1371/journal.pone.0010621 PMID:20485550

Borawski, E. A., Ievers-Landis, C. E., Lovegreen, L. D., & Trapl, E. S. (2003). Parental monitoring, negotiated unsupervised time, and parental trust: The role of perceived parenting practices in adolescent health risk behaviors. *The Journal of Adolescent Health*, *33*(2), 60–70. doi:10.1016/S1054-139X(03)00100-9

Borrill, J. (2000). *All About ADHD*. Mental Health Foundation.

Bostic, J. Q., Biederman, J., Spencer, T. J., Wilens, T. E., Prince, J. B., Monuteaux, M. C., Sienna, M., Polisner, D. A., & Hatch, M. (2000). Pemoline treatment of adolescents with attention deficit hyperactivity disorder: A short-term controlled trial. *Journal of Child and Adolescent Psychopharmacology*, *10*(3), 205–216. doi:10.1089/10445460050167313 PMID:11052410

Bradley, C. (1937). The behavior of children receiving benzedrine. *The American Journal of Psychiatry*, *94*(3), 577–585. doi:10.1176/ajp.94.3.577

Brahmbhatt, K., Hilty, D. M., Hah, M., Han, J., Angkustsiri, M. D., & Schweitzer, J. (2016). Diagnosis and Treatment of ADHD during Adolescence in the Primary care setting: Review and Future Directions. *The Journal of Adolescent Health*, *59*(2), 135–143. doi:10.1016/j.jadohealth.2016.03.025

Bramham, J., Young, S. J., Morris, R. G., Asherson, P., & Toone, B. K. (2005). *Behavioural symptoms and cognitive deficits in adults with ADHD: do they improve with age?* Paper presented at the Division of Clinical Psychology, British Psychological Society Conference.

Breen, M. J., & Barkley, R. A. (1988). Child psychopathology and parenting stress in girls and boys having attention deficit disorder with hyperactivity. *Journal of Pediatric Psychology*, *13*(2), 265–280. doi:10.1093/jpepsy/13.2.265 PMID:3171819

Breggin, P. (2001). *Talking back to Ritalin: What doctors aren't telling you about stimulants and ADHD*. Perseus Books Group.

Breslau, J., Miller, E., Breslau, N., Bohnert, K., Lucia, V., & Schweitzer, J. (2009). The impact of early behavior disturbances on academic achievement in high school. *Pediatrics*, *123*(6), 1472–1476. doi:10.1542/peds.2008-1406

Bresnahan, S. M., Anderson, J. W., & Barry, R. J. (1999). Age-related changes in quantitative EEG in attention-deficit/hyperactivity disorder. *Biological Psychiatry*, *46*(12), 1690–1697. doi:10.1016/S0006-3223(99)00042-6 PMID:10624551

Bresnahan, S. M., Barry, R. J., Clarke, A. R., & Johnstone, S. J. (2006). Quantitative EEG analysis in dexamphetamine-responsive adults with attention-deficit/hyperactivity disorder. *Psychiatry Research*, *141*(2), 151–159. doi:10.1016/j.psychres.2005.09.002 PMID:16343642

Brikell, I., Ghirardi, L., D'Onofrio, B. M., Dunn, D. W., Almqvist, C., Dalsgaard, S., Kuja-Halkola, R., & Larsson, H. (2018). Familial Liability to Epilepsy and Attention-Deficit/Hyperactivity Disorder: A Nationwide Cohort Study. *Biological Psychiatry*, *83*(2), 173–180. doi:10.1016/j.biopsych.2017.08.006 PMID:28950988

Brookes, K. J., Mill, J., Guindalini, C., Curran, S., Xu, X., Knight, J., Chen, C.-K., Huang, Y.-S., Sethna, V., Taylor, E., Chen, W., Breen, G., & Asherson, P. (2006). A common haplotype of the dopamine transporter gene associated with attention-deficit/hyperactivity disorder and interacting with maternal use of alcohol during pregnancy. *Archives of General Psychiatry*, *63*(1), 74–81. doi:10.1001/archpsyc.63.1.74 PMID:16389200

Brook, R. D., Appel, L. J., Rubenfire, M., Ogedegbe, G., Bisognano, J. D., Elliott, W. J., Fuchs, F. D., Hughes, J. W., Lackland, D. T., Staffileno, B. A., Townsend, R. R., & Rajagopalan, S. (2013). Beyond medications and diet. Alternative approaches to lowering blood pressure. A Scientific Statement from American Heart Association. *Hypertension*, *61*(6), 1360–1363. doi:10.1161/HYP.0b013e318293645f

Brook, U., & Boaz, M. (2005). Attention deficit and hyperactivity disorder/learning disabilities (ADHD/LD): Parental characterization and perception. *Patient Education and Counseling*, *57*(1), 96–100. doi:10.1016/j.pec.2004.03.018 PMID:15797157

Brown, N. M., Brown, S. N., Briggs, R. D., Germán, M., Belamarich, P. F., & Oyeku, S. O. (2017). Associations between adverse childhood experiences and ADHD diagnosis and severity. *Academic Pediatrics*, *17*(4), 349–355. doi:10.1016/j.acap.2016.08.013 PMID:28477799

Brown, R. T., & Pacini, J. N. (1989). Perceived family functioning, marital status, and depression in parents of boys with attention deficit disorder. *Journal of Learning Disabilities*, *22*(9), 581–587. doi:10.1177/002221948902200911 PMID:2809411

Brown, T. (2005). *Attention deficit disorder: The unfocused mind in children and adults*. Yale University Press.

Brown, T. (2009, March). ADD/ADHD and impaired executive function in clinical practice. *Current Attention Disorders Reports*, *1*(1), 37–41. doi:10.100712618-009-0006-3

Brown, T. E. (2013). *A new understanding of ADHD in children and adults: Executive function impairments*. Routledge. doi:10.4324/9780203067536

Buitelaar, J. K., Van der Wees, M., Swaab-Barneveld, H., & Van der Gaag, R. J. (1999). Verbal memory and performance IQ predict theory of mind and emotion recognition ability in children with autistic spectrum disorders and in psychiatric control children. *Journal of Child Psychology and Psychiatry, and Allied Disciplines*, *40*(6), 869–881. doi:10.1111/1469-7610.00505 PMID:10509882

Bukstein, O. G. (2012). Attention Deficit Hyperactivity Disorder and Substance Use Disorders. In C. Stanford & R. Tannock (Eds.), *Behavioral Neuroscience of Attention Deficit Hyperactivity Disorder and Its Treatment, Current Topics in Behavioral Neurosciences 9* (pp. 145–172). Springer-Verlag Berlin Heidelberg.

Bunford, N., Evans, S. W., & Langberg, J. M. (2014). Emotion Dysregulation Is Associated with Social Impairment Among Young Adolescents With ADHD. *Journal of Attention Disorders*, *22*(1), 66–82. doi:10.1177/1087054714527793 PMID:24681899

Burden, M. J., Jacobson, J. L., Westerlund, A., Lundahl, L. H., Morrison, A., Dodge, N. C., & Jacobson, S. W. (2010). An Event-Related Potential Study of Response Inhibition in ADHD With and Without Prenatal Alcohol Exposure. *Alcoholism, Clinical and Experimental Research*, *34*(4), 617–627. doi:10.1111/j.1530-0277.2009.01130.x PMID:20102568

Burgdorf, V., Szabó, M., & Abbott, M. J. (2019). The Effect of Mindfulness Interventions for Parents on Parenting Stress and Youth Psychological Outcomes: A Systematic Review and Meta-Analysis. *Frontiers in Psychology*, *10*, 1336. doi:10.3389/fpsyg.2019.01336 PMID:31244732

Burton, K., Rogathe, J., Hunter, E., Burton, M., Swai, M., Todd, J., Neville, B., Walker, R., & Newton, C. (2011). Behavioural comorbidity in Tanzanian children with epilepsy: A community-based case-control study. *Developmental Medicine and Child Neurology*, *53*(12), 1135–1142. doi:10.1111/j.1469-8749.2011.04109.x PMID:22092080

Bussing, R., Fernandez, M., Harwood, M., & Hou, W. (2008). Parent and teacher SNAP-IV ratings of attention deficit hyperactivity disorder symptoms: Psychometric properties and normative ratings from a school district sample. *Assessment*, *15*(3), 317–328. doi:10.1177/1073191107313888 PMID:18310593

Bussing, R., Mason, D. M., Bell, L., Porter, P., & Garvan, C. (2010). Adolescent outcomes of childhood attention-deficit/hyperactivity disorder in a diverse community sample. *Journal of the American Academy of Child and Adolescent Psychiatry*, *49*(6), 595–605. doi:10.1016/j.jaac.2010.03.006 PMID:20494269

Bussing, R., Meyer, J., Zima, B. T., Mason, D. M., Gary, F. A., & Garvan, C. W. (2015). Childhood ADHD Symptoms: Association with Parental Social Networks and Mental Health Service Use during Adolescence. *International Journal of Environmental Research and Public Health*, *12*(9), 11893–11909. doi:10.3390/ijerph120911893 PMID:26402692

Butcher, J., Mineka, S., & Hooley, J. (2013). *Abnormal psychology* (15th ed.). Pearson.

Calam, R., Bolten, C., & Roberts, J. (2002). Maternal expressed emotion, attributions and depression and entry into therapy for children with behaviour problems. *British Journal of Clinical Psychology*, *41*(2), 213–216. doi:10.1348/014466502163985 PMID:12034007

Campbell, W. (2015). *Eight limbs of yoga*. Retrieved from https://www.wendycampbellyoga.com/newsposts/2015/9/13/7-practical-tips-for-yoga-beginners

Campbell, S. B. (1975). Mother-child interaction: A comparison of hyperactive, learning disabled, and normal boys. *The American Journal of Orthopsychiatry*, *45*(1), 51–57. doi:10.1111/j.1939-0025.1975.tb01165.x PMID:1111300

Campbell, S. B., Breaux, A. M., Ewing, L. J., & Szumowski, E. K. (1986). Correlates and predictors of hyperactivity and aggression: A longitudinal study of parent – referred problem preschoolers. *Journal of Abnormal Child Psychology*, *14*(2), 217–234. doi:10.1007/BF00915442 PMID:3722619

Cantwell, D. P. (1972). Psychiatric illness in the families of hyperactive children. *Archives of General Psychiatry*, *27*(3), 414–417. doi:10.1001/archpsyc.1972.01750270114018 PMID:5051632

Cantwell, D. P. (1996). Attention deficit disorder: A review of the past 10 years. *Journal of the American Academy of Child and Adolescent Psychiatry*, *35*(8), 978–987. doi:10.1097/00004583-199608000-00008 PMID:8755794

Canu, W. H., & Carlson, C. L. (2003). Differences in heterosocial behavior and outcomes of ADHD- symptomatic subtypes in a college sample. *Journal of Attention Disorders*, *6*(3), 123–133. doi:10.1177/108705470300600304

Canu, W., & Carlson, C. (2007). Rejection sensitivity and social outcomes of young adult men with ADHD. *Journal of Attention Disorders*, *10*(3), 261–275. doi:10.1177/1087054706288106

Canu, W., Newman, M., Morrow, T., & Pope, D. (2008). Social appraisal of adult ADHD: Stigma and influences of the beholder's big five personality traits. *Journal of Attention Disorders*, *11*(6), 700–710. doi:10.1177/1087054707305090

Cappe, E., Bolduc, M., Rougé, M. C., Saiag, M. C., & Delorme, R. (2017). Quality of life, psychological characteristics, and adjustment in parents of children with Attention-Deficit/Hyperactivity Disorder. *Quality of Life Research: An International Journal of Quality of Life Aspects of Treatment, Care and Rehabilitation*, *26*(5), 1283–1294. doi:10.100711136-016-1446-8 PMID:27798755

Capusan, A. J., Bendtsen, P., Marteinsdottir, I., Kuja-Halkola, R., & Larsson, H. (2015). Genetic and environmental contributions to the association between attention deficit hyperactivity disorder and alcohol dependence in adulthood: A large population-based twin study. *Neuropsychiatric Genetics*, Part *B* of the *American Journal* of Medical. *Genetics*, *168*, 414–422. PMID:25711682

Carabellese, F., La Tegola, D., Margari, L., Craig, F., Ostuni, A., Scardaccione, E., Perrini, F., & Margari, F. (2016). ADHD and illegal conduct: A survey in Juvenile Justice Services in Puglia. *Rivista di Psichiatria*, *51*(4), 156–163. doi:10.1708/2342.25122 PMID:27727266

Carabellese, F., Tegola, D. L., Margari, L., Craig, F., & Ostuni, A. (2017). Scardaccione,E., Francesca Perrini,F., & Margari,F. (2017). Comorbidities and Correlates of Conduct Disorder Among Male Juvenile Detainees in South Korea. *Child and Adolescent Psychiatry and Mental Health*, *11*(1), 44. doi:10.118613034-017-0182-3 PMID:28924450

Cardiovascular Diseases (CVDs). (2017). Retrieved from https://www.who.int/news-room/fact-sheets/detail/cardiovascular-diseases-(cvds)

Carlson, C. L., & Bunner, M. R. (1993). Effects of methylphenidate on the academic performance of children with attention deficit hyperactivity disorder and learning disabilities. *School Psychology Review*, *22*(2), 184–198.

Carpenter, R. E., Loo, S. K., Yang, M., Dang, J., & Smalley, S. L. (2009). Social Functioning Difficulties in ADHD: Association with PDD Risk. *Clinical Child Psychology and Psychiatry*, *14*(3), 329–344. doi:10.1177/1359104508100890 PMID:19515751

Carr, A. (2015). *The handbook of child and adolescent clinical psychology: a contextual approach* (3rd ed.). Routledge. doi:10.4324/9781315744230

Carrellas, N., Wilens, T. E., & Anselmo, R. (2016). Treatment of comorbid substance use disorders and ADHD in youth. *Current Treatment Options in Psychiatry*, *3*(1), 15–27. doi:10.100740501-016-0072-y

Carroll, K. M., & Rounsaville, B. J. (1993). History and significance of childhood attention deficit disorder in treatment-seeking cocaine abusers. *Comprehensive Psychiatry*, *34*(2), 75–82. doi:10.1016/0010-440X(93)90050-E PMID:8485984

Carter, J. D., & Swanson, H. L. (1995). The relationship between intelligence and vigilance in children at risk. *Journal of Abnormal Child Psychology*, *23*(2), 201–220. doi:10.1007/BF01447089 PMID:7642834

Casey, B. J., & Jones, R. M. (2010). Neurobiology of the adolescent brain and behavior: Implications for substance use disorders. *Journal of the American Academy of Child and Adolescent Psychiatry*, *49*(12), 1189–1201. doi:10.1097/00004583-201012000-00005 PMID:21093769

Caspi, A., Block, J., Block, J. H., Klopp, B., Lynam, D., Moffitt, T. E., & Stouthamer-Loeber, M. (1992). A" common-language" version of the California Child Q-Set for personality assessment. *Psychological Assessment*, *4*(4), 512–523. doi:10.1037/1040-3590.4.4.512

Cassone, A. R. (2015). Mindfulness training as an adjunct to evidence-based treatment for ADHD within families. *Journal of Attention Disorders*, *19*(2), 147–157. doi:10.1177/1087054713488438 PMID:23704114

Catalá-López, F., Hutton, B., Núñez-Beltrán, A., Mayhew, A. D., Page, M. J., Ridao, M., Tobías, A., Catalá, M. A., Tabarés-Seisdedos, R., & Moher, D. (2017). The pharmacological and non-pharmacological treatment of attention deficit hyperactivity disorder in children and adolescents: Protocol for a systematic review and network meta-analysis of randomised controlled trials. *Systematic Reviews*, *4*(1), 19. doi:10.118613643-015-0005-7 PMID:25875125

Catherine, T. G., Robert, N. G., Mala, K. K., Kanniammal, C., & Arullapan, J. (2019). Assessment of prevalence of attention deficit hyperactivity disorder among schoolchildren in selected schools. *Indian Journal of Psychiatry*, (61), 232–237. PMID:31142899

Cavelti, M., Corbisiero, S., Bitto, H., Moerstedt, B., Newwark, P., Faschina, S., ... Stieglitz, R. D. (2019). A Comparison of Self Reported Emotion Regulation Skills in Adults with Attention Deficit Hyperactivity Disorder and Borderline Personality Disorder. *Journal of Attention Disorders*, *23*(12), 1396–1406. doi:10.1177/1087054717698814 PMID:28367706

Caye, A., Spadini, A. V., Karam, R. G., Grevet, E. H., Rovaris, D. L., Bau, C. H., Rohde, L. A., & Kieling, C. (2016). Predictors of persistence of ADHD into adulthood: A systematic review of the literature and meta-analysis. *European Child & Adolescent Psychiatry*, *25*(11), 1151–1159. doi:10.100700787-016-0831-8

Center for Disease Control. (2003). *Mental health in the United States: prevalence of diagnosis and medication treatment for attention-deficit/hyperactivity disorder - United States*. Author.

Centers for Disease Control and Prevention (CDC). (2019, October 8). *Treatment of ADHD*. https://www.cdc.gov/ncbddd/adhd/treatment.html

Chabot, R. J., & Serfontein, G. (1996). Quantitative electroencephalographic profiles of children with attention deficit disorder. *Biological Psychiatry*, *40*(10), 951–963. doi:10.1016/0006-3223(95)00576-5 PMID:8915554

CHADD ADHD Weekly. (2018). Retrieved from https://chadd.org/adhd-weekly/yoga-could-benefit-children-with-adhd/

Chang, C. C., Chen, Y. M., Liu, T. L., Hsiao, R. C., Chou, W. J., & Yen, C. F. (2020). Affiliate Stigma and Related Factors in Family Caregivers of Children with Attention-Deficit/Hyperactivity Disorder. *International Journal of Environmental Research and Public Health*, *17*(2), 576. doi:10.3390/ijerph17020576 PMID:31963190

Chang, Y. K., Liu, S., Yu, H. H., & Lee, Y. H. (2012). Effect of acute exercise on executive function in children with attention deficit hyperactivity disorder. *Archives of Clinical Neuropsychology*, *27*(2), 225–237. doi:10.1093/arclin/acr094 PMID:22306962

Chang, Z., Lichtenstein, P., & Larsson, H. (2012). The effects of childhood ADHD symptoms on early-onset substance Use: A Swedish twin study. *Journal of Abnormal Child Psychology*, *40*(3), 425–435. doi:10.100710802-011-9575-6 PMID:21947618

Charach, A., Carson, P., Fox, S., Ali, M. U., Beckett, J., & Lim, C. G. (2013). Interventions for preschool children at high risk for ADHD: A comparative effectiveness review. *Paediatrics*, *131*(5), 1–21. doi:10.1542/peds.2012-0974 PMID:23545375

Charach, A., Yeung, E., Climans, T., & Lillie, E. (2011). Childhood attention-deficit/hyperactivity disorder and future substance use disorders: Comparative meta-analyses. *Journal of the American Academy of Child and Adolescent Psychiatry*, *50*(1), 9–21. doi:10.1016/j.jaac.2010.09.019 PMID:21156266

Chatterjee, S., & Mondal, S. (2017). Effect of combined yoga programme on blood levels of thyroid hormones: a quasi-experimental study. *Indian Journal of Traditional Knowledge*, *16*, S9-S16.

Cheng, X., & Qi, Y. (2010). Variations of eddy kinetic energy in the South China Sea. *Journal of Oceanography*, *66*(1), 85–94. doi:10.100710872-010-0007-y

Chen, W. L., Tsai, S. T., & Chou, F. H. (2015). Depression and Related Factors in Mothers of School-Aged Children With Attention-Deficit Hyperactivity Disorder. *Hu Li Za Zhi*, *62*(1), 39–49. doi:10.6224/JN.62.1.39 PMID:25631183

Chen, Y. C., Hwang-Gu, S. L., Ni, H. C., Liang, S. H., Lin, H. Y., Lin, C. F., Tseng, Y. H., & Gau, S. S. F. (2017). Relationship between parenting stress and informant discrepancies on symptoms of ADHD/ODD and internalizing behaviors in preschool children. *PLoS One*, *12*(10), e0183467. doi:10.1371/journal.pone.0183467 PMID:29016602

Cherry, K. (2020, March 13). *How Behavioral Therapy Is Used in Psychology*. Verywell Mind. https://www.verywellmind.com/what-is-behavioral-therapy-2795998

Chess, S. (1960). Diagnosis and treatment of the hyperactive child. *New York State Journal of Medicine*, *60*, 2379–2385. PMID:13809736

Chidi, I. R., Chidi, N. A., Ebele, A. A., & Chinyelu, O. N. (2014). Co-Morbidity of attention deficit Hyperactivity Disorder (ADHD) and epilepsy In children seen In University of Nigeria Teaching Hospital Enugu: Prevalence, Clinical and social correlates. *The Nigerian Postgraduate Medical Journal*, *21*, 273–278. PMID:25633443

Children and Adults with Attention-Deficit/Hyperactivity Disorder (CHADD). (n.d.). *Relationships and Social Skills*. Retrieved from https://chadd.org/for-adults/relationships-social-skills/

Childress, A. C. (2015). A critical appraisal of atomoxetine in the management of ADHD. *Therapeutics and Clinical Risk Management*, *12*, 27–39. doi:10.2147/TCRM.S59270 PMID:26730199

Chiodo, L. M., Jacobson, S. W., & Jacobson, J. L. (2004). Neurodevelopmental effects of postnatal lead exposure at very low levels. *Neurotoxicology and Teratology*, *26*(3), 359–371. doi:10.1016/j.ntt.2004.01.010 PMID:15113598

Chou, C.C., & Huang, C.J. (2017). Effects of an 8-week yoga program on sustained attention and discrimination function in children with attention deficit hyperactivity disorder. *PeerJ.com*, *5*, e2883. doi:10.7717/peerj.2883

Chou,W.J., Hsiao, R.C., Ni, H.C., Liang, S.H., Lin, C.F., Chan, H.L., Hsieh, Y.H., Wang, L.J., Lee, M.J., Hu, H.F., & Yen, C.F.(2019). Self-Reported and Parent-Reported School Bullying in Adolescents with High Functioning Autism Spectrum Disorder: The Roles of Autistic Social Impairment, Attention-Deficit/Hyperactivity and Oppositional Defiant Disorder Symptoms. *International Journal of Environmental Research* and *Public Health, 16*(7). pii: E1117. doi: . doi:10.3390/ijerph16071117

Chou, W. J., Liu, T. L., Yang, P., Yen, C. F., & Hu, H. F. (2018). Bullying Victimization and Perpetration and Their Correlates in Adolescents Clinically Diagnosed With ADHD. *Journal of Attention Disorders*, *22*(1), 25–34. doi:10.1177/1087054714558874 PMID:25403369

Christian, L., & Bachmanna, J. (2017, May). Trends in ADHD medication use in children and adolescents in five western countries, 2005–2012. *European Neuropsychopharmacology*, *27*(5), 484–493. doi:10.1016/j.euroneuro.2017.03.002 PMID:28336088

Chronis, A. M., Chacko, A., Fabiano, G. A., Wymbs, B. T., & Pelham, W. E. Jr. (2004). Enhancements to the Behavioural Parent Training Paradigm for Families of Children with ADHD: Review and Future Directions. *Clinical Child and Family Psychology Review*, *7*(1), 1–27. doi:10.1023/B:CCFP.0000020190.60808.a4 PMID:15119686

Chronis-Tuscano, A., Raggi, V. L., Clarke, T. L., Rooney, M. E., Diaz, Y., & Pian, J. (2008). Associations between maternal attention-deficit/hyperactivity disorder symptoms and parenting. *Journal of Abnormal Child Psychology*, *36*(8), 1237–1250. doi:10.100710802-008-9246-4 PMID:18553132

Chronis-Tuscano, A., Wang, C. H., Woods, K. E., Strickland, J., & Stein, M. A. (2017). Parent ADHD and evidence-based treatment for their children: Review and directions for future research. *Journal of Abnormal Child Psychology, 45*(3), 501–517. doi:10.100710802-016-0238-5 PMID:28025755

Chung, K. M., Ebesutani, C., Bang, H. M., Kim, J., Chorpita, B. F., Weisz, J. R., Suh, D., & Byun, H. (2013). Parenting stress and child behavior problems among clinic-referred youth: Cross-cultural differences across the US and Korea. *Child Psychiatry and Human Development, 44*(3), 460–468. doi:10.100710578-012-0340-z PMID:23073610

Clark, D. B., & Cornelius, J. (2004). Childhood psychopathology and adolescent cigarette smoking: A prospective survival analysis in children at high risk for substance use disorders. *Addictive Behaviors, 29*(4), 837–841. doi:10.1016/j.addbeh.2004.02.019 PMID:15135569

Clarke, A. R., Barry, R. J., Heaven, P. C., McCarthy, R., Selikowitz, M., & Byrne, M. K. (2008). EEG in adults with attention-deficit/hyperactivity disorder. *International Journal of Psychophysiology: Official Journal of the International Organization of Psychophysiology, 70*(3), 176–183.

Clarke, A. R., Barry, R. J., Dupuy, F. E., Heckel, L. D., McCarthy, R., Selikowitz, M., & Johnstone, S. J. (2011). Behavioural differences between EEG-defined subgroups of children with attention-deficit/hyperactivity disorder. *Clinical Neurophysiology, 122*(7), 1333–1341. doi:10.1016/j.clinph.2010.12.038 PMID:21247797

Clarke, A. R., Barry, R. J., Heaven, P. C. L., McCarthy, R., Selikowitz, M., & Byrne, M. K. (2008). EEG in adults with attention-deficit/hyperactivity disorder. *International Journal of Psychophysiology, 70*(3), 176–183. doi:10.1016/j.ijpsycho.2008.07.001 PMID:18662727

Coghill, D. R., Seth, S., & Matthews, K. (2014). A comprehensive assessment of memory, delay aversion, timing, inhibition, decision making, and variability in attention deficit hyperactivity disorder: Advancing beyond the three-pathway models. *Psychological Medicine, 44*(9), 1989–2001. doi:10.1017/S0033291713002547 PMID:24176104

Coghill, D., Soutullo, C., d'Aubuisson, C., Preuss, U., Lindback, T., Silverberg, M., & Buitelaar, J. (2008). Impact of attention-deficit/hyperactivity disorder on the patient and family: Results from a European survey. *Child and Adolescent Psychiatry and Mental Health, 2*(31), 31. doi:10.1186/1753-2000-2-31 PMID:18957105

Cohen, J. A., & Mannarino, A. P. (2008). Trauma-focused cognitive behavioral therapy for children and parents. *Child and Adolescent Mental Health, 13*(4), 158–162. doi:10.1111/j.1475-3588.2008.00502.x

Cohen, J. A., Mannarino, A. P., & Deblinger, E. (2006). *Treating trauma and traumatic grief in children and adolescents.* Guilford Press.

Collins, W. A., Hennighausen, K. C., Schmit, D. T., & Sroufe, L. A. (1997). Developmental precursors of romantic relationships: A longitudinal analysis. *New Directions for Child and Adolescent Development, 78*(78), 69–84. doi:10.1002/cd.23219977807

Comings, D. E., Gade-Andavolu, R., Gonzalez, N., Wu, S., Muhleman, D., Blake, H., ... MacMurray, J. P. (2000). Comparison of the role of dopamine, serotonin, and noradrenaline genes in ADHD, ODD and conduct disorder: Multivariate regression analysis of 20 genes. *Clinical Genetics, 57*(3), 178–196. doi:10.1034/j.1399-0004.2000.570304.x PMID:10782925

Conners, C. K. (2008). *Conners* (3rd edition: manual). Multi-Health Systems.

Connor, D. F. (2011, August 11). Problems of overdiagnosis and overprescribing in ADHD. *The Psychiatric Times.*

Connor, D. F. (2017). Disruptive Behavior Disorders in Children and Adolescents. In B. J. Sadock, V. A. Sadock, & P. Ruiz (Eds.), *Kaplan & Sadock's comprehensive textbook of psychiatry* (10th ed., Vol. 2, p. 3618). Wolters Kluwer.

Cooper, J. O., Heron, T. E., & Heward, W. L. (2007). *Applied behavior analysis* (2nd ed.). Pearson Merrill Prentice Hall.

Copur, M., Turkcan, A., & Erdogmus, M. (2005). Substance Abuse, Conduct Disorder and Crime: Assessment in a Juvenile Detention House in Istanbul, Turkey. *Psychiatry and Clinical Neurosciences*, *59*(2), 151–154. doi:10.1111/j.1440-1819.2005.01350.x PMID:15823160

Corey, G. (2017). *Theory and practice of counseling and psychotherapy*. Nelson Education.

Cornelius, C., Fedewa, A. L., & Ahn, S. (2017, January). The Effect Of Physical Activity on Children with ADHD: A Quantitative Review of the Literature. *Journal of Applied School Psychology*, *33*(2), 136–170. doi:10.1080/15377903.2016.1265622

Craig, F., Operto, F. F., De Giacomo, A., Margari, L., Frolli, A., Conson, M., Ivagnes, S., Monaco, M., & Margari, F. (2016). Parenting stress among parents of children with Neurodevelopmental Disorders. *Journal of Psychiatric Research*, *242*, 121–129. doi:10.1016/j.psychres.2016.05.016 PMID:27280521

Craig, F., Savino, R., Fanizza, I., Lucarelli, E., Russo, L., & Trabacca, A. (2020). A systematic review of coping strategies in parents of children with attention deficit hyperactivity disorder (ADHD). *Research in Developmental Disabilities*, *98*, 103571. doi:10.1016/j.ridd.2020.103571 PMID:31931455

Crick, N. R., & Dodge, K. A. (1994). A review and reformulation of social information-processing mechanisms in children's social adjustment. *Psychological Bulletin*, *115*(1), 74–101. doi:10.1037/0033-2909.115.1.74

Crocker, N., Vaurio, L., Riley, E. P., & Mattson, S. N. (2009). Comparison of Adaptive Behavior in Children With Heavy Prenatal Alcohol Exposure or Attention-Deficit/Hyperactivity Disorder. *Alcoholism, Clinical and Experimental Research*, *33*(11), 2015–2023. doi:10.1111/j.1530-0277.2009.01040.x PMID:19719794

Cunningham, C. E., & Barkley, R. A. (1979). The interactions of normal and hyperactive children with their mothers in free play and structured tasks. *Child Development*, *50*(1), 217–224. doi:10.2307/1129059 PMID:446207

Cunningham, C. E., Benness, B. B., & Siegel, L. S. (1988). Family functioning, time allocation, and parental depression in the families of normal and ADHD children. *Journal of Clinical Child Psychology*, *17*(2), 169–177. doi:10.120715374424jccp1702_10

Cunningham, C. E., & Boyle, M. H. (2002). Pre-schoolers at risk for attention-deficit hyperactivity disorder and oppositional defiant disorder: Family, parenting, and behavioural correlates. *Journal of Abnormal Child Psychology*, *30*(6), 555–569. doi:10.1023/A:1020855429085 PMID:12481971

Curatolo, P., D'Agati, E., & Moavero, R. (2010). The neurobiological basis of ADHD. *Italian Journal of Pediatrics*, *36*(1), 79. doi:10.1186/1824-7288-36-79 PMID:21176172

D'Agati, E., Curatolo, P., & Mazzone, L. (2019). Comorbidity between ADHD and anxiety disorders across the lifespan. *International Journal of Psychiatry in Clinical Practice*, *23*(4), 238–244. doi:10.1080/13651501.2019.1628277 PMID:31232613

Dalsgaard, S., Mortensen, P. B., Frydenberg, M., & Thomsen, P. H. (2002). Conduct problems, gender and adult psychiatric outcome of children with attention-deficit hyperactivity disorder. *The British Journal of Psychiatry*, *181*(5), 416–421. doi:10.1192/bjp.181.5.416 PMID:12411268

Dalsgaard, S., Østergaard, S. D., Leckman, J. F., Mortensen, P. B., & Pedersen, M. G. (2015). stergaard SD, Leckman JF, Mortensen PB, Pedersen MG. Mortality in children, adolescents, and adults with attention deficit hyperactivity disorder: A nationwide cohort study. *Lancet*, *385*(9983), 2190–2196. doi:10.1016/S0140-6736(14)61684-6 PMID:25726514

Daly, B. P., Creed, T., Xanthopoulos, M., & Brown, R. T. (2007). Psychosocial treatments for children with attention deficit/hyperactivity disorder. *Neuropsychology Review*, *17*(1), 73–89. doi:10.100711065-006-9018-2

Daly, B. P., Hildenbrand, A. K., & Brown, R. T. (2015). *ADHD in Children and Adolescents*. Hogrefe Publishing.

Darke, S., Baker, A., Dixon, J., Wodak, A., & Heather, N. (1992). Drug use and HIV risk taking behaviour among clients in methadone maintenance treatment. *Drug and Alcohol Dependence*, *29*(3), 263–268. doi:10.1016/0376-8716(92)90101-H PMID:1559433

Darling, K. A., Eggleston, M., Retallick-Brown, H., & Rucklidge, J. J. (2019, November). Mineral-Vitamin Treatment Associated with Remission in Attention-Deficit/Hyperactivity Disorder Symptoms and Related Problems: 1-Year Naturalistic Outcomes of a 10-Week Randomized Placebo-Controlled Trial. *Journal of Child and Adolescent Psychopharmacology*, *29*(9), 688–704. doi:10.1089/cap.2019.0036 PMID:31343273

Darling, N., & Steinberg, L. (1993). Parenting style as context: An integrative model. *Psychological Bulletin*, *113*(3), 487–496. doi:10.1037/0033-2909.113.3.487

Datta, S. S., Premkumar, T. S., Fielding, S., Chandy, S., Kumar, S., Eagles, J., & Cherian, A. (2006). Impact of pediatric epilepsy on Indian families: Influence of psychopathology and seizure related variables. *Epilepsy & Behavior*, *9*(1), 145–151. doi:10.1016/j.yebeh.2006.04.011 PMID:16725375

Davids, E., & Gastpar, M. (2003). Attention-deficit/hyperactivity disorder and substance abuse. *Psychiatrische Praxis*, *30*(4), 182–186. doi:10.1055-2003-39496 PMID:12768521

Davis, J. M., Cheung, S. F., Takahashi, T., Shinoda, H., & Lindstrom, W. A. (2011). Cross-national invariance of attention-deficit/hyperactivity disorder factors in Japanese and U.S. university students. *Research in Developmental Disabilities*, *32*(6), 2972–2980. doi:10.1016/j.ridd.2011.05.004 PMID:21624817

Dawson, P., & Guare, R. (2010). *Executive skills in children and adolescents: A practical guide to assessment and intervention (2nd ed.)*. Guilford.

De Boo, G. M., & Prins, P. J. (2007). Social incompetence in children with ADHD: Possible moderators and mediators in social-skills training. *Clinical Psychology Review*, *27*(1), 78–97. doi:10.1016/j.cpr.2006.03.006 PMID:16814435

Deater-Deckard, K., Sewell, M. D., Petrill, S. A., & Thompson, L. A. (2010). Maternal working memory and reactive negativity in parenting. *Psychological Science*, *21*(1), 75–79. doi:10.1177/0956797609354073

DeFries, J. C., & Fulker, D. W. (1985). Multiple regression analysis of twin data. *Behavior Genetics*, *15*(5), 467–473. doi:10.1007/BF01066239

DeFries, J. C., & Fulker, D. W. (1988). Multiple regression analysis of twin data: Etiology of deviant scores versus individual differences. *ActaGeneticaeMedicaeetGemellologiae*, *37*, 205–216.

Del Campo, N., Chamberlain, S. R., Sahakian, B. J., & Robbins, T. W. (2011). The roles of dopamine and noradrenaline in the pathophysiology and treatment of attention-deficit/hyperactivity disorder. *Biological Psychiatry*, *69*(12), e145–e157. doi:10.1016/j.biopsych.2011.02.036

dela Peña, I., Jeon, S. J., Lee, E., Ryu, J. H., Shin, C. Y., Noh, M., & Cheong, J. H. (2013). Neuronal development genes are key elements mediating the reinforcing effects of methamphetamine, amphetamine, and methylphenidate. *Psychopharmacology*, *230*(3), 399–413. doi:10.100700213-013-3168-8 PMID:23783774

Denckla, M. B., Barquero, L. A., Lindstrom, E. R., Benedict, S. L., & Wilson, L. M. (2013). Attention-deficit/hyperactivity disorder, executive function and reading comprehension: Different but related. In Handbook of learning disabilities (2nd ed.). New York, NY: Guilford.

Dennis, M., Godley, S. H., Diamond, G., Tims, F. M., Babor, T., Donaldson, J., Liddle, H., Titus, J. C., Kaminer, Y., Webb, C., Hamilton, N., & Funk, R. (2004). The Cannabis Youth Treatment (CYT) Study: Main findings from two randomized trials. *Journal of Substance Abuse Treatment, 27*(3), 197–213. doi:10.1016/j.jsat.2003.09.005 PMID:15501373

DeRubeis, R. J., Gelfand, L. A., Tang, T. Z., & Simons, A. D. (1999). Medications versus cognitive behavior therapy for severely depressed outpatients: Mega-analysis of four randomized comparisons. *The American Journal of Psychiatry, 156*(7), 1007–1013. PMID:10401443

Dhawan, A., Pattanayak, R. D., Chpra, A., Tikko, V. K., & Kumar, R. (2017). Pattern and profile of children using substances in India: Insights and recommendations. *The National Medical Journal of India, 30*(4), 224–229. doi:10.4103/0970-258X.218679 PMID:29162759

Diagnostic and Statistical Manual of Mental Disorders. (2013). *American Psychiatric Association* (5th ed.). American Psychiatric Publishing.

Diamantopoulou, S., Henricsson, L., & Rydell, A. (2005). ADHD symptoms and peer relations of children in a community sample: Examining associated problems, self-perceptions, and gender differences. *International Journal of Behavioral Development, 29*(5), 388–398. doi:10.1177/01650250500172756

Dinis-Oliveira, R. J. (2017). Metabolomics of methylphenidate and ethylphenidate: Implications in pharmacological and toxicological effects. *European Journal of Drug Metabolism and Pharmacokinetics, 42*(1), 11–16. doi:10.100713318-016-0362-1 PMID:27438788

Dirks, H., Scherbaum, N., Kis, B., & Mette, C. (2017). ADHD in Adults and Comorbid Substance Use Disorder: Prevalence, Clinical Diagnostics and Integrated Therapy. *Fortschritte der Neurologie-Psychiatrie, 85*(6), 336–344. doi:10.1055-0043-100763 PMID:28645126

Dixon, D. R., Vogel, T., & Tarbox, J. (2012). A brief history of functional analysis and applied behavior analysis. In J. L. Matson (Ed.), *Autism and Child Psychopathology Series* (pp. 3–24). doi:10.1007/978-1-4614-3037-7_2

Dixon, E. B. (1995). Impact of adult ADD on the family. In K. Nadeau (Ed.), *A comprehensive guide to attention deficit disorder in adults: Research, diagnosis, and treatment* (pp. 236–259). Bruner/Mazel.

Doernberg, E., & Hollander, E. (2016). Neurodevelopmental Disorders (ASD and ADHD): DSM-5, ICD-10, and ICD-11. *CNS Spectrums, 21*(4), 295–299. doi:10.1017/S1092852916000262 PMID:27364515

Dongre, A., Deshmukh, P., Murali, N., & Garg, B. (2008). Tobacco consumption among adolescents in rural Wardha: Where and how tobacco control should focus its attention? *Indian Journal of Cancer, 45*(3), 100–106. doi:10.4103/0019-509X.44065 PMID:19018113

Doulabi, M. A., Sajedi, F., Vameghi, R., Mazaheri, M. A., Baghban, A. A., & Afraz, F. (2019). Marital Satisfaction and Depression in Mothers of 3-4 Year Old Children with Developmental Delay in Comparison with Mothers of Normal Children. *Iranian Journal of Child Neurology, 13*(4), 91–108. PMID:31645870

Ducharme, J. M., Atkinson, L., & Poulton, L. (2000). Success-based, Non-coercive treatment of oppositional behaviour in children from violent homes. *Journal of the American Academy of Child and Adolescent Psychiatry, 39*(8), 995–1004. doi:10.1097/00004583-200008000-00014 PMID:10939227

Dulcan, M. (1997). Practice parameters for the assessment and treatment of children, adolescents, and adults with attention-deficit/hyperactivity disorder. *Journal of the American Academy of Child and Adolescent Psychiatry, 36*(10), 85S–121S. doi:10.1097/00004583-199710001-00007 PMID:9334567

Dumas, M. C. (1998). The risk of social interaction problems among adolescents with ADHD. *Education & Treatment of Children*, 447–460.

Dunn, D. W., & Kronenberger, W. G. (2005). Childhood epilepsy, attention problems, and ADHD: Review and practical considerations. *Seminars in Pediatric Neurology*, *12*(4), 222–228. doi:10.1016/j.spen.2005.12.004 PMID:16780293

Dupar, L. (2017). *ADDitude, Expert eBook*. ADHD Medication & Treatment.

DuPaul, G. J. (2001). Preschool children with attention-deficit/hyperactivity disorder: impairments in behavioral, social, and school functioning. *Journal of American Academy of Child and Adolescent Psychiatry. 40*(5), 508-515.

DuPaul, G. J., Barkley, R. A., & McMurray, M. B. (1994). Response of children with ADHD to methylphenidate: Interaction with internalizing symptoms. *Journal of the American Academy of Child and Adolescent Psychiatry*, *33*(6), 894–903. doi:10.1097/00004583-199407000-00016 PMID:8083147

DuPaul, G. J., & Eckert, T. L. (1997). The effects of school-based interventions for attention deficit hyperactivity disorder: A meta-analysis. *School Psychology Review*, *26*, 5–27.

DuPaul, G. J., Eckert, T. L., & Vilardo, B. (2012). The effects of school-based interventions for attention deficit hyperactivity disorder: A meta-analysis 1996-2010. *School Psychology Review*, *41*, 387–412.

DuPaul, G. J., & Ervin, R. A. (1996). Functional assessment of behaviours related to attention-deficit/hyperactivity disorder: Linking assessment to intervention design. *Behavior Therapy*, *27*(4), 601–622. doi:10.1016/S0005-7894(96)80046-3

Dupaul, G. J., Gormley, M. J., & Laracy, S. D. (2012). Comorbidity of LD and ADHD: Implications of DSM-5 for assessment and treatment. *Journal of Learning Disabilities*. Advance online publication. doi:10.1177/0022219412464351 PMID:23144063

DuPaul, G. J., Power, T. J., Anastopoulos, A. D., & Reid, R. (1998). *ADHD rating scale–IV (for children and adolescents): Checklists, norms, and clinical interpretation*. Guilford.

DuPaul, G., McGoey, K., Eckert, T., & VanBrakle, J. (2001). Preschool children with attention-deficit/hyperactivity disorder: Impairments in behavioral, social, and school functioning. *Journal of the American Academy of Child and Adolescent Psychiatry*, *40*(5), 508–515. doi:10.1097/00004583-200105000-00009 PMID:11349694

Dyson, L. L. (1993). Response to the presence of a child with disabilities: Parental stress and Family functioning over time. *American Journal of Mental Retardation*, *98*, 207–218. PMID:7691096

Eakin, L., Minde, K., Hechtman, L., Ochs, E., Krane, E., Bouffard, R., Greenfield, B., & Looper, K. (2004). The marital and family functioning of adults with ADHD and their spouses. *Journal of Attention Disorders*, *8*(1), 1–10. doi:10.1177/108705470400800101 PMID:15669597

Education for All Handicapped Children Act of 1975, Pub. L. No. 94-142.

Edwards, M., Gardner, E., Chelonis, J., Schulz, E., Flake, R., & Diaz, P. (2007). Estimates of the validity and utility of the Conners' continuous performance test in the assessment of inattentive and/or hyperactive-impulsive behaviors in children. *Journal of Abnormal Child Psychology*, *35*(3), 393–404. doi:10.100710802-007-9098-3 PMID:17295064

Egeland, J. (2012). Cutting Corners: Neuropsychological Research into the Energetics of ADHD. In *Contemporary Trends in ADHD Research*. InTech. Available from: http://www.intechopen.com/books/contemporary-trends-in-adhd-research/cutting-corners- neuropsychological-research-into-the-energetics-of-adhd

Ehringer, M. A., Rhee, S. H., Young, S., Corley, R., & Hewitt, J. K. (2006). Genetic and environmental contributions to common psychopathologies of childhood and adolescence: A study of twins and their siblings. *Journal of Abnormal Child Psychology, 34*(1), 1–17. doi:10.100710802-005-9000-0 PMID:16465480

Eilertsen, E. M., Gjerde, L. C., Reichborn-Kjennerud, T., Ørstavik, R. E., Knudsen, G. P., Knudsen, C., ... Ystrom, E. (2017). Maternal alcohol use during pregnancy and offspring attention-deficit hyperactivity disorder (ADHD): A prospective sibling control study. *International Journal of Epidemiology, 46*(5), 1633–1640. doi:10.1093/ije/dyx067 PMID:28449133

Elaine Klaus-Taylor & Dempster Diane. (2016). *Parenting ADHD Now! Easy Intervention Strategies to Empower Kids with ADHD* (1st ed.). Althea Press.

Elbaz, F., Zahra, S., & Hanafy, H. (2017). Magnesium, Zinc and Copper estimation in children with attention deficit hyperactivity disorder (ADHD). *The Egyptian Journal of Medical Human Genetics, 18*(2), 153–163. doi:10.1016/j.ejmhg.2016.04.009

Elia, J., Ambrosini, P., & Berrettini, W. (2008). ADHD characteristics: I. Concurrent co-morbidity patterns in children and adolescents. *Child and Adolescent Psychiatry and Mental Health, 2*(1), 15. doi:10.1186/1753-2000-2-15

Elia, J., & Devoto, M. (2007). ADHD genetics: 2007 update. *Current Psychiatry Reports, 9*(5), 434–439. doi:10.100711920-007-0057-z PMID:17915085

Elkins, I. J., Saunders, G. R. B., Malone, S. M., Keyes, M. A., Samek, D. R., McGue, M., & Iacono, W. G. (2018). Increased Risk of Smoking in Female Adolescents Who Had Childhood ADHD. *The American Journal of Psychiatry, 175*(1), 63–70. doi:10.1176/appi.ajp.2017.17010009 PMID:28838251

Emilsson, B., Gudjonsson, G., Sigurdsson, J. F., Baldursson, G., Einarsson, E., Ofafsdottir, H., & Young, S. (2011). Cognitive behaviour therapy in medication-treated adults with ADHD and persistent symptoms: A randomized controlled trial. *BMC Psychiatry, 11*(1), 116. doi:10.1186/1471-244X-11-116

Emser, T. S., Johnston, B. A., Steele, J. D., Kooij, S., Thorell, L., & Christiansen, H. (2018). Assessing ADHD symptoms in children and adults: Evaluating the role of objective measures. *Behavioral and Brain Functions, 14*(1), 11. doi:10.118612993-018-0143-x PMID:29776429

Engel-Yeger, B., & Ziv-On, D. (2011). The relationship between sensory processing difficulties and leisure activity preference of children with different types of ADHD. *Research in Developmental Disabilities, 32*(3), 1154–1162. doi:10.1016/j.ridd.2011.01.008 PMID:21324640

Engert, V., & Pruessner, J. C. (2008). Dopaminergic and noradrenergic contributions to functionality in ADHD: The role of methylphenidate. *Current Neuropharmacology, 6*(4), 322–328. doi:10.2174/157015908787386069 PMID:19587853

Epstein, J. N., Langberg, J. M., Lichtenstein, P. K., Mainwaring, B. A., Luzader, C. P., & Stark, L. J. (2008). Community-wide intervention to improve the attention-deficit/hyperactivity disorder assessment and treatment practices of community physicians. *Pediatrics, 122*(1), 19–27. doi:10.1542/peds.2007-2704

Epstein, J. N., & Loren, R. E. (2013, October). Changes in the Definition of ADHD in DSM-5: Subtle but Important. *HHS Public Access: Neuropsychiatry (London), 3*(5), 455–458. doi:10.2217/npy.13.59 PMID:24644516

Epstein-Ngo, Q. M., McCabe, S. E., Veliz, P. T., Stoddard, S. A., Austic, E. A., & Boyd, C. J. (2016). Diversion of ADHD Stimulants and Victimization Among Adolescents. *Journal of Pediatric Psychology, 41*(7), 786–798. doi:10.1093/jpepsy/jsv105 PMID:26590265

Erhardt, D., & Hinshaw, S. P. (1994). Initial sociometric impressions of attention-deficit hyperactivity disorder and comparison boys: Predictions from social behaviors and from nonbehavioral variables. *Journal of Consulting and Clinical Psychology*, *62*(4), 833–842. doi:10.1037/0022-006X.62.4.833 PMID:7962888

Erskine, H. E., Norman, R. E., Ferrari, A. J., Chan, G. C., Copeland, W. E., Whiteford, H. A., & Scott, J. G. (2016). Long-term outcomes of attention-deficit/hyperactivity disorder and conduct disorder: A systematic review and meta-analysis. *Journal of the American Academy of Child and Adolescent Psychiatry*, *55*(10), 841–850. doi:10.1016/j.jaac.2016.06.016 PMID:27663939

Ervin, R. A., Kern, L., Clarke, S., DuPaul, G. J., Dunlap, G., & Friman, P. C. (2000). Evaluating assessment-based intervention strategies for students with ADHD and comorbid disorders within the natural classroom context. *Behavioral Disorders*, *25*(4), 344–358. doi:10.1177/019874290002500403

Escobar, R., Hervas, A., Soutullo, C., Mardomingo, M. J., Uruñuela, A., & Gilaberte, I. (2008). Attention deficit/hyperactivity disorder: Burden of the disease according to subtypes in recently diagnosed children. *Actas Españolas de Psiquiatría*, *36*(5), 285–294. PMID:18830848

Esparham. A., Evans, R.G., Wagner, L.E., & Drisko, J.A. (2014). Pediatric integrative medicine approaches to attention deficit hyperactivity disorder (ADHD) Children. *mdpi.com*, *1*, 186–207. doi:10.3390/children1020186

Estévez, N., Dey, M., Eich-Höchli, D., Foster, S., Gmel, G., & Mohler-Kuo, M. (2016). Adult attention-deficit/hyperactivity disorder and its association with substance use and substance use disorders in young men. *Epidemiology and Psychiatric Sciences*, *25*(3), 255–266. doi:10.1017/S2045796015000360 PMID:25989844

Evans-Lacko, S., Brohan, E., Mojtabai, R., & Thornicroft, G. (2012). Association between public views of mental illness and self-stigma among individuals with mental illness in 14 European countries. *Psychological Medicine*, *42*(8), 1741–1752. doi:10.1017/S0033291711002558 PMID:22085422

Evans, S. W., Owens, J. S., & Bunford, N. (2014). Evidence-based psychosocial treatments for children and adolescents with attention-deficit/hyperactivity disorder. *Journal of Clinical Child and Adolescent Psychology*, *43*(4), 527–551. doi:10.1080/15374416.2013.850700

Evans, S. W., Pelham, W. E., Smith, B. H., Bukstein, O., Gnagy, E. M., Greiner, A. R., Altenderfer, L., & Baron-Myak, C. (2001). Dose-response effects of methylphenidate on ecologically valid measures of academic performance and classroom behavior in adolescents with ADHD. *Experimental and Clinical Psychopharmacology*, *9*(2), 163–175. doi:10.1037/1064-1297.9.2.163

Evans, S., Ling, M., Hill, B., Rinehart, N., Austin, D., & Sciberras, E. (2018). Systematic review of meditation-based interventions for children with ADHD. *European Child & Adolescent Psychiatry*, *27*(1), 9–27. doi:10.100700787-017-1008-9 PMID:28547119

Everyday Health. (2011). *7 ADHD stress reduction techniques*. Retrieved from https://www.everydayhealth.com/adhd-pictures/adhd-stress-reduction-techniques.aspx

Everyday Times. (2013). *ADHD kids: Benefit from Yoga*. Retrieved from https://www.everydayhealth.com/adhd/bending-energy-adhd-kids-benefit-from-yoga.aspx

Evren, C. (2018). Comorbidity of attention deficit-hyperactivity disorder and substance use disorder. *Dusunen Adam The Journal of Psychiatry and Neurological Sciences*, *31*, 115–124. doi:10.5350/DAJPN20183102001

Evren, C., Dalbudak, E., Evren, B., Can, Y., & Umut, G. (2014). The severity of attention deficit hyperactivity symptoms and its relationship with lifetime substance use and psychological variables among 10th grade students in Istanbul. *Comprehensive Psychiatry*, *55*(7), 1665–1670. doi:10.1016/j.comppsych.2014.06.002 PMID:25015303

Fabiano, G. A., Schatz, N. K., Aloe, A. M., Chacko, A., & Chronis-Tuscano, A. (2015). A systematic review of meta-analyses of psychosocial treatment for attention- deficit/hyperactivity disorder. *Clinical Child and Family Psychology Review*, *18*(1), 77–97. doi:10.100710567-015-0178-6 PMID:25691358

Fang, X., Massetti, G. M., Ouyang, L., Grosse, S. D., & Mercy, J. A. (2010). Attention-deficit/hyperactivity disorder, conduct disorder, and young adult intimate partner violence. *Archives of General Psychiatry*, *67*(11), 1179–1186. doi:10.1001/archgenpsychiatry.2010.137 PMID:21041619

Faraone, S. V., & Biederman, J. (1997). Do attention deficit hyperactivity disorder and major depression share familial risk factors? *The Journal of Nervous and Mental Disease*, *185*(9), 533–541. doi:10.1097/00005053-199709000-00001 PMID:9307614

Faraone, S. V., Biederman, J., & Friedman, D. (2000). Validity of DSM-IV subtypes of attention-deficit/hyperactivity disorder: A family study perspective. *Journal of the American Academy of Child and Adolescent Psychiatry*, *39*(3), 300–307. doi:10.1097/00004583-200003000-00011 PMID:10714049

Faraone, S. V., Biederman, J., & Mick, E. (2006). The age-dependent decline of attention deficit hyperactivity disorder: A meta-analysis of follow-up studies. *Psychological Medicine*, *36*(2), 159–165. doi:10.1017/S003329170500471X PMID:16420712

Faraone, S. V., Biederman, J., & Monuteaux, M. C. (2001). A psychometric measure of learning disability predicts educational failure four years later in boys with ADHD. *Journal of Attention Disorders*, 220–230. doi:10.1177/108705470100400404

Faraone, S. V., Biederman, J., Spencer, T., Wilens, T., Seidman, L. J., Mick, E., & Doyle, A. E. (2000). Attention-deficit/hyperactivity disorder in adults: An overview. *Biological Psychiatry*, *48*(1), 9–20. doi:10.1016/S0006-3223(00)00889-1 PMID:10913503

Faraone, S. V., & Buitelaar, J. (2010). Comparing the efficacy of stimulants for ADHD in children and adolescents using meta-analysis. *European Child & Adolescent Psychiatry*, *19*(4), 353–364. doi:10.100700787-009-0054-3 PMID:19763664

Faraone, S. V., & Glatt, S. J. (2010). A comparison of the efficacy of medications for adult attention-deficit/hyperactivity disorder using meta-analysis of effect sizes. *The Journal of Clinical Psychiatry*, *71*(6), 754–763. doi:10.4088/JCP.08m04902pur PMID:20051220

Faraone, S. V., Rostain, L., Blader, J., Busch, B., Childress, A. C., Connor, D. F., & Newcorn, J. H. (2019). Practitioner Review: Emotional Dysregulation in Attention Deficit/ Hyperactive Disorder- Implications For Clinical Recognition and Intervention. *Journal of Child Psychology and Psychiatry, and Allied Disciplines*, *60*(2), 133–150. doi:10.1111/jcpp.12899 PMID:29624671

Faraone, S., Sergeant, J., Gillberg, C., & Biederman, J. (2005). The worldwide prevalence of ADHD: Is it an American condition? *World Psychiatry; Official Journal of the World Psychiatric Association (WPA)*, *2*(2), 104–113. PMID:16946911

Farley, J., Risko, E., & Kingstone, A. (2013). Everyday attention and lecture retention: The effects of time,fidgeting and mind wandering. *Frontiers in Psychology*, *4*, 619. PMID:24065933

Farokhzadi, F., Mohammadi, M. R., Alipour, A., Rostami, R., & Dehestani, M. (2012). Substance abuse disorders in the parents of ADHD children, and parents of normal children. *Acta Medica Iranica*, *50*(5), 319–327. PMID:22837085

Farrington, D. P. (1995). The development of offending and antisocial behaviour from childhood: Key findings from the Cambridge study in delinquent development. *Journal of Child Psychology and Psychiatry, and Allied Disciplines*, *36*(6), 929–964. doi:10.1111/j.1469-7610.1995.tb01342.x PMID:7593403

Feeney, T., & Ylvisaker, M. (2006). Context-sensitive cognitive-behavioural supports for young children with TBI: A replication study. *Brain Injury*, *20*(6), 629–645. doi:10.1080/02699050600744194 PMID:16754288

Feldman, R. (2010). Middle Childhood. In Discovering The Life Span (p. 209). Pearson.

Ferguson, J. H. (2000). National Institutes of Health Consensus Development Conference Statement: Diagnosis and Treatment of Attention-Deficit/Hyperactivity Disorder (ADHD) (2000). *Journal of the American Academy of Child and Adolescent Psychiatry*, *39*(2), 182–193. doi:10.1097/00004583-200002000-00018 PMID:10673829

Fergusson, D. M., Horwood, L. J., & Lynskey, M. T. (1993). The effects of conduct disorder and Attention Deficit in middle childhood on offending and scholastic ability at age 13. *Journal of Child Psychology and Psychiatry, and Allied Disciplines*, *34*(6), 899–916. doi:10.1111/j.1469-7610.1993.tb01097.x PMID:8408374

Fernandez, T. V., Gupta, A., & Hoffman, E. H. (2017). Assessing risk: gene discovery. In A. Martin, F. R. Volkmar, & M. H. Bloch (Eds.), *Lewis's Child and Adolescent Psychiatry: A Comprehensive Textbook* (pp. 246–261). Wolters Kluwer Health.

Feuerstein, G. (2003). *The Deeper Dimensions of Yoga: Theory and Practice*. Shambhala Publications.

Findling, R. L., & Dogin, J. W. (1998). Psychopharmacology of ADHD: Children and adolescents. *The Journal of Clinical Psychiatry*, *59*(7), 42–49. PMID:9680052

Fischer, M., Barkley, R. A., Smallish, L., & Fletcher, K. (2002). Young adult follow-up of hyperactive children: Self-reported psychiatric disorders, comorbidity, and the role of childhood conduct problems and teen CD. *Journal of Abnormal Child Psychology*, *30*(5), 463–475. doi:10.1023/A:1019864813776

Fitzgerald, C., Dalsgaard, S., Nordentoft, M., & Erlangsen, A. (2019). Suicidal behaviour among persons with attention-deficit hyperactivity disorder. *The British Journal of Psychiatry*, *215*(4), 615–620. doi:10.1192/bjp.2019.128 PMID:31172893

Fitzgerald, M. M., & Cohen, J. A. (2012). Trauma-focused cognitive behavior therapy for school psychologists. *Journal of Applied School Psychology*, *28*(3), 294–315. doi:10.1080/15377903.2012.696037

Fletcher, J., & Wolfe, B. (2009). Long-term consequences of childhood ADHD on criminal activities. *The Journal of Mental Health Policy and Economics*, *12*(3), 119–138. PMID:19996475

Flicek, M. (1992). Social status of boys with both academic problems and attention-deficit hyperactivity disorder. *Journal of Abnormal Child Psychology*, *20*(4), 353–366. doi:10.1007/BF00918981 PMID:1527277

Fliers, E., Rommelse, N., Vermeulen, S. H. H. M., Altink, M., Buschgens, C. J. M., Faraone, S. V., Sergeant, J. A., Franke, B., & Buitelaar, J. K. (2008). Motor coordination problems in children and adolescents with ADHD rated by parents and teachers: Effects of age and gender. *Journal of Neural Transmission (Vienna, Austria)*, *115*(2), 211–220. doi:10.100700702-007-0827-0 PMID:17994185

Flory, K., Molina, B., Pelham, W. Jr, Gnagy, E., & Smith, B. (2006). Childhood ADHD Predicts Risky Sexual Behaviorin Young Adulthood. *Journal of Clinical Child and Adolescent Psychology*, *35*(4), 571–577. doi:10.120715374424jccp3504_8

Fogleman, N. D., Leaberry, K. D., Rosen, P. J., Walerius, D. M., & Slaughter, K. E. (2018). Relation between internalizing behaviors, externalizing behaviors, and peer victimization among children with and without ADHD. *Attention Deficit and Hyperactivity Disorders*, *10*(3), 209–222. doi:10.100712402-018-0248-y PMID:29330700

Folkman, S., & Lazarus, R. S. (1985). If it changes it must be a process: Study of emotion and coping during three stages of a college examination. *Journal of Personality and Social Psychology*, *48*(1), 150–170. doi:10.1037/0022-3514.48.1.150 PMID:2980281

Folkman, S., & Lazarus, R. S. (1988). Coping as a mediator of emotion. *Journal of Personality and Social Psychology, 54*(3), 466–475. doi:10.1037/0022-3514.54.3.466 PMID:3361419

Fond, G., Loundou, A., Guillaume, S., Quantin, X., Macgregor, A., Lopez, R., Courtet, P., Bernard, P., Bailly, D., Abbar, M., Leboyer, M., & Boyer, L. (2014). Smoking behavior characteristics of non-selected smokers with childhood attention-deficit/hyperactivity disorder (AD/HD) history: A systematic review and meta-analysis. *European Archives of Psychiatry and Clinical Neuroscience, 264*(5), 379–389. doi:10.100700406-014-0497-5 PMID:24619241

Fone, K. C., & Nutt, D. J. (2005). Stimulants: Use and abuse in the treatment of attention deficit hyperactivity disorder. *Current Opinion in Pharmacology, 5*(1), 87–93. doi:10.1016/j.coph.2004.10.001 PMID:15661631

Ford-Jones, P. C. (2015). Misdiagnosis of attention deficit hyperactivity disorder: 'Normal behaviour' and relative maturity. *Paediatrics & Child Health, 20*(4), 200–202. doi:10.1093/pch/20.4.200 PMID:26038639

Ford, T., Goodman, R., & Meltzer, H. (2003). The British Child and Adolescent Mental Health Survey 1999: The prevalence of DSM-IV disorders. *Journal of the American Academy of Child and Adolescent Psychiatry, 42*(10), 1203–1211. doi:10.1097/00004583-200310000-00011 PMID:14560170

Forness, S. R., & Kavale, K. A. (2001). ADHD and a return to the medical model of special education. *Education & Treatment of Children*, 224–247.

Foster, E. M., Saunders, R. C., & Summerfelt, W. T. (1996). A comparison of multiple methods of predicting level of care in mental health services. *Evaluation and Program Planning, 19*, 143–153. doi:10.1016/0149-7189(96)00005-5

Franke, B., Faraone, S. V., Asherson, P., Buitelaar, J., Bau, C. H., Ramos-Quiroga, J. A., ... Lesch, K. P. (2012). International Multicentre persistent ADHD CollaboraTion. The genetics of attention deficit/hyperactivity disorder in adults, a review. *Molecular Psychiatry, 17*(10), 960–987. doi:10.1038/mp.2011.138 PMID:22105624

Franke, B., Neale, B. M., & Faraone, S. V. (2009). Genome-wide association studies in ADHD. *Human Genetics, 126*(1), 13–50. doi:10.100700439-009-0663-4 PMID:19384554

Frankel, F., & Feinberg, D. (2002). Social Problems Associated with ADHD Vs. ODD in Children Referred For Friendship Problems. *Child Psychiatry and Human Development, 33*(2), 125–146. doi:10.1023/A:1020730224907 PMID:12462351

Frazier, J. A., Biederman, J., Bellordre, C. A., Garfield, S. B., Geller, D. A., Coffey, B. J., & Faraone, S. V. (2001). Should the diagnosis of attention-deficit/hyperactivity disorder be considered in children with a pervasive developmental disorder? *Journal of Attention Disorders, 4*(4), 203–211. doi:10.1177/108705470100400402

Frazier, T., Youngstrom, E., Glutting, J., & Watkins, M. (2007). ADHD and achievement: Meta-analysis of the child, adolescent, and adult literatures and a concomitant study with college students. *Journal of Learning Disabilities, 40*(1), 49–65. doi:10.1177/00222194070400010401 PMID:17274547

Freeman, R. (2007). Tic disorder and ADHD: Answeres from a world-wide clinical dataset on Tourette syndrome. *European Child & Adolescent Psychiatry, 16*(S1), 15–23. doi:10.100700787-007-1003-7 PMID:17665279

Freeman, R. B. (1996). Why do so many young American men commit crimes and what might we do about it? *The Journal of Economic Perspectives, 10*(1), 25–42. doi:10.1257/jep.10.1.25

Freitag, C. M., Hänig, S., Schneider, A., Seitz, C., Palmason, H., Retz, W., & Meyer, J. (2011). Biological and psychosocial environmental risk factors influence symptom severity and psychiatric comorbidity in children with ADHD. *Journal of Neural Transmission (Vienna, Austria), 119*(1), 81–94. doi:10.100700702-011-0659-9 PMID:21626412

French, W. P. (2015). Assessment and treatment of attention-deðcit/hyperactivity disorder part 1. *Pediatric Annals, 44*(3), 114–120. doi:10.3928/00904481-20150313-13 PMID:25806728

Friedrichs, B., Igl, W., Larsson, H., & Larsson, J.-O. (2012). Coexisting psychiatric problems and stressful life events in adults with symptoms of ADHD–a large Swedish population-based study of twins. *Journal of Attention Disorders, 16*(1), 13–22. doi:10.1177/1087054710376909 PMID:20686099

Friesen, B. J. (1989). National study of parents whose children have serious emotional disorders. In A. Algarin, R. Friedman, A. Duchnowski, K. Kutash, S. Silver, & M. Johnson (Eds.), *Children's mental health service and policy. Building a research base*. University of South Florida Research and Training Centre for Children's Mental Health.

Frodl, T. (2010). Comorbidity of ADHD and Substance Use Disorder (SUD): A neuroimaging perspective. *Journal of Attention Disorders, 14*(2), 109–120. doi:10.1177/1087054710365054 PMID:20495160

Froehlich, T.E., Lanphear, B.P., Epstein, J.N., Barbaresi, W.J., Katusic, S.K., & Kahn, R.S. (n.d.). Prevalence, recognition, and treatment of attention-deficit/hyperactivity disorder in a national sample of US children. Archives of Pediatrics & Adolescent Medicine, 161(9), 857–864. PubMed doi:10.1001/archpedi.161.9.857

Froehlich, T. E., Anixt, J. S., Loe, I. M., Chirdkiatgumchai, V., Kuan, L., & Gilman, R. C. (2011). Update on environmental risk factors for attention-deficit/hyperactivity disorder. *Current Psychiatry Reports, 13*(5), 333–344. doi:10.100711920-011-0221-3 PMID:21779823

Froehlich, T. E., Lanphear, B. P., Auinger, P., Hornung, R., Epstein, J. N., Braun, J., & Kahn, R. S. (2009). Association of tobacco and lead exposures with attention-deficit/hyperactivity disorder. *Pediatrics, 124*(6), e1054–e1063. doi:10.1542/peds.2009-0738 PMID:19933729

Furman, L. M. (2008). Attention-deficit hyperactivity disorder (ADHD): Does new research support old concepts? *Journal of Child Neurology, 23*(7), 775–784. doi:10.1177/0883073808318059 PMID:18658077

Gable, R. A., Hester, P. H., Rock, M. L., & Hughes, K. G. (2009). Back to basics: Rules, praise, ignoring, and reprimands revisited. *Intervention in School and Clinic, 44*(4), 195–205. doi:10.1177/1053451208328831

Galéra, C., Côté, S. M., & Bouvard, M. P. (2011). Early risk factors for hyperactivity-impulsivity and inattention trajectories from age 17 months to 8 years. *Archives of General Psychiatry, 68*(12), 1267–1275. doi:10.1001/archgenpsychiatry.2011.138 PMID:22147844

Galera, C., Pingault, J., Fombonne, E., Michel, G., Lagarde, E., Bouvard, M.-P., & Melchior, M. (2013). Attention problems in childhood and adult substance use. *The Journal of Pediatrics, 163*(6), 1677–1683.e1. Advance online publication. doi:10.1016/j.jpeds.2013.07.008 PMID:23972646

Galland, D., Tisserant, I., & Notardonato, L. (2017). Attention deficit hyperactivity disorder in forensic psychiatry: A review. *L'Encéphale, 43*(3), 268–272. doi:10.1016/j.encep.2016.04.012 PMID:27637873

Gardner, D. M., & Gerdes, A. C. (2015). A Review of Peer Relationships and Friendships in Youth With ADHD. *Journal of Attention Disorders, 19*(10), 844–855. doi:10.1177/1087054713501552 PMID:24062277

Gaub, M., & Carlson, C. L. (1997). Gender Differences in ADHD: A Meta-Analysis and a Critical Review. *Journal of the American Academy of Child and Adolescent Psychiatry, 36*(8), 1136–1139. doi:10.1097/00004583-199708000-00023 PMID:9256583

Gaviria, M., & Smith, M. (Producers). (2001). Frontline: Medicating kids [Television broadcast]. Alexandria, VA: Public Broadcasting Service.

Geddes, J. R., & Andreasen, N. C. (2020). *New Oxford Textbook of Psychiatry* (3rd ed.). Oxford University Press. doi:10.1093/med/9780198713005.001.0001

Geffen, J. & Forster, K. (2018). Treatment of adult ADHD: A clinical perspective. *Therapeutic Advances in Psychopharmacology, 8*(1), 25-32. doi: / doi:10.1177/2045125317734977

Gelder, M., Mayou, R., & Cowen, P. (2001). *Shorter Oxford Textbook of Psychiatry* (4th ed.). Oxford University Press.

Gentschel, D. A., & McLaughlin, T. F. (2000). Attention deficit hyperactivity disorder as a social disability: Characteristics and suggested methods of treatment. *Journal of Developmental and Physical Disabilities, 12*(4), 333–347. doi:10.1023/A:1009432130076

Germanò, E., Gagliano, A., & Curatolo, P. (2010). Comorbidity of ADHD and dyslexia. *Developmental Neuropsychology, 35*(5), 475–493. doi:10.1080/87565641.2010.494748 PMID:20721770

Ghanizadeh, A. (2011). Sensory processing problems in children with ADHD, a systematic review. *Psychiatry Investigation, 8*(2), 89. doi:10.4306/pi.2011.8.2.89 PMID:21852983

Ghaziuddin, M., Weidmer-Mikhail, E., & Ghaziuddin, N. (1998). Comorbidity of Asperger syndrome: A preliminary report. *Journal of Intellectual Disability Research, 42*(4), 279–283. doi:10.1111/j.1365-2788.1998.tb01647.x PMID:9786442

Ghriwati, N. A., Langberg, J. M., Gardner, W., Peugh, J., Kelleher, K. J., Baum, R., ... Epstein, J. N. (2017). Impact of comorbid conditions on the community-based pediatric treatment and outcomes of children with ADHD. *Journal of Developmental and Behavioral Pediatrics, 38*(1), 20–28. doi:10.1097/DBP.0000000000000359 PMID:27902542

Giannakopoulos, G., Assimopoulos, H., Petanidou, D., Tzavara, C., Kolaitis, G., & Tsiantis, J. (2012). Effectiveness of a school-based intervention for enhancing adolescents' positive attitudes towards people with mental illness. *Mental Illness, 4*(2), e16. doi:10.4081/mi.2012.e16 PMID:25478117

Giannotta, F., & Rydell, A. (2016). The Prospective Links Between Hyperactive/Impulsive, Inattentive, and Oppositional-Defiant Behaviors in Childhood and Antisocial Behavior in Adolescence: The Moderating Influence of Gender and the Parent-Child Relationship Quality. *Child Psychiatry and Human Development, 47*(6), 857–870. doi:10.100710578-015-0617-0 PMID:26680210

Gillberg, C., Carlstrom, G., & Rasmussen, P. (1983). Hyperkinetic disorders in seven-year-old children with perceptual, motor and attention deficits. *Journal of Child Psychology and Psychiatry, and Allied Disciplines, 24*(2), 233–246. doi:10.1111/j.1469-7610.1983.tb00572.x PMID:6841509

Gillig, P. M., Gentile, J. P., & Atiq, R. (2005). Attention-deficit hyperactivity disorder in adults. *Hospital Physician, 9*(2), 1–11. PMID:15737940

Gill, K. E., Pierre, P. J., Daunais, J., Bennett, A. J., Martelle, S., Gage, H. D., Swanson, J. M., Nader, M. A., & Porrino, L. J. (2012). Chronic treatment with extended release methylphenidate does not alter dopamine systems or increase vulnerability for cocaine self-administration: A study in nonhuman primates. *Neuropsychopharmacology, 37*(12), 2555–2565. doi:10.1038/npp.2012.117 PMID:22805600

Ginsberg, Y., Quintero, J., Anand, E., Casillas, M., & Upadhyaya, H. P. (2014). Underdiagnosis of attention-deficit/hyperactivity disorder in adult patients: A review of the literature. *The Primary Care Companion for CNS Disorders, 16*(3), PCC.13r01600. doi:10.4088/PCC.13r01600

Girard, R., & Joober, R. (2017). Treatment of ADHD in patients with bipolar disorder. *Journal of psychiatry & neuroscience. JPN, 42*(6), E11–E12. doi:10.1503/jpn.170097 PMID:29083298

Gizer, I., Ficks, C., & Waldman, I. (2009). Candidate gene studies of ADHD: A meta-analytic review. *Human Genetics, 126*(1), 51–90. doi:10.100700439-009-0694-x

Gnanavel, S., Sharma, P., Kaushal, P., & Hussain, S. (2019). Attention deficit hyperactivity disorder and comorbidity: A review of literature. *World Journal of Clinical Cases*, *7*(17), 2420–2426. doi:10.12998/wjcc.v7.i17.2420 PMID:31559278

Gohari, Z., Dehghani, F., Rajabi, G., & Mahmoudi-Gharaei, J. (2012). Parenting Self Efficacy in Mothers of Children with Attention Deficit Hyperactivity Disorder vs. Normal Children. *Iranian Journal of Psychiatry*, *7*(2), 57–60. PMID:22952546

Gokten, E. (2016). Effects of attention-deficit/hyperactivity disorder on child abuse and neglect. *Child Abuse & Neglect*, *62*, 1–9. doi:10.1016/j.chiabu.2016.10.007 PMID:27770673

Goldin, R. L., Matson, J. L., Tureck, K., Cervantes, P. E., & Jang, J. (2013). A comparison of tantrum behavior profiles in children with ASD, ADHD and comorbid ASD and ADHD. *Research in Developmental Disabilities*, *34*(9), 2669–2675. doi:10.1016/j.ridd.2013.04.022 PMID:23764824

Goldstein, S. (2009). Current literature in ADHD summarized by Sam Goldstein. *Journal of Attention Disorders*, *12*(4), 386–388. doi:10.1177/1087054708328266

Goldstein, S., Naglieri, J. A., Princoitta, D., & Otero, T. M. (2014). Introduction: A History of executive functioning as a theoretical and clinical construct. In S. Goldstein & J. A. Naglieri (Eds.), *Handbook of executive functioning* (pp. 3–12). Springer. doi:10.1007/978-1-4614-8106-5_1

Gomez, K. M., & Cole, C. L. (1991). Attention deficit hyperactivity disorder: A review of treatment alternatives. *Elementary School Guidance & Counseling*, *26*(2), 106–114.

Gomez, R., Vance, A., Watson, S., & Stavropoulos, V. (2019). *ROC Analysis of Relevant Conners' 3 - Short Forms, CBCL and TRF Scales for Screening ADHD and ODD*. Sage Journals., doi:10.1177/1073191119876023

Gonzalez, J., Dodds, A., Whitney, J., MacMillan, C., Waber, D., Faraone, S. V., ... Biederman, J. (2007). Psychiatric disorders and behavioral characteristics of pediatric patients with both epilepsy and attention deficit hyperactivity disoredr. *Epilepsy & Behavior*, *10*(3), 384–388. doi:10.1016/j.yebeh.2007.01.010 PMID:17368109

Goodman, R. (1997). The Strengths and Difficulties Questionnaire: A Research Note. *Journal of Child Psychology and Psychiatry, and Allied Disciplines*, *38*(5), 581–586. doi:10.1111/j.1469-7610.1997.tb01545.x PMID:9255702

Goodwin, G. M. (2009). Evidence-based guidelines for treating bipolar disorder: Revised second edition recommendations from the British Association of Psychopharmacology. Journal of Psychopharmacology, 4, 346– 388.

Gopalan, R. T., Oomme, A., Srinath, S., & Kapur, M. (2006). *Clinic based multimodal intervention for children with Attention Deficit Hyperactivity Disorder* (PhD Thesis). National Institute of Mental Health and Neuro Sciences, Bengaluru, India.

Gordon, C. T., & Hinshaw, S. P. (2017). Parenting Stress and Youth Symptoms among Girls with and without ADHD. *Parenting, Science and Practice*, *17*(1), 11–29. doi:10.1080/15295192.2016.1262178 PMID:29308056

Gordon, C. T., & Hinshaw, S. P. (2017). Parenting Stress as a Mediator Between Childhood ADHD and Early Adult Female Outcomes. *Journal of Clinical Child and Adolescent Psychology*, *46*(4), 588–599. doi:10.1080/15374416.2015.1041595 PMID:26042524

Gordon, L., Morrison, E. Y., McGrowder, D., Penas, Y. E., Zamoraz, E. M., Garwood, D., Alexander-Lindo, R., & Irving, R. (2008). Effect of yoga and traditional physical exercise on hormones and percentage insulin binding receptor in patients with type 2 diabetes. *American Journal of Biotechnology & Biochemistry*, *4*(1), 35–42. doi:10.3844/ajbbsp.2008.35.42

Gottlieb, B. H. (1981). *Social networks and social support*. Sage Publications.

Gozal, D., & Molfese, D. L. (2005). *Attention Deficit Hyperactivity Disorder*. Humana Press. doi:10.1385/1592598919

Grassmann, V., Alves, M. V., Santos-Galduróz, R. F., & Galduróz, J. C. F. (2017). Possible cognitive benefits of acute physical exercise in children with ADHD: A systematic review. *Journal of Attention Disorders*, *21*(5), 367–371. doi:10.1177/1087054714526041 PMID:24621460

Greene, R. W., Biederman, J., Faraone, S. V., Wilens, T. E., Mick, E., & Blier, H. K. (1999). Further validation of social impairment as a predictor of substance use disorders: Findings from a sample of siblings of boys with and without ADHD. *Journal of Clinical Child Psychology*, *28*(3), 349–354. doi:10.1207/S15374424jccp280307 PMID:10446684

Greenway, C. (2018). The Efficacy of Social Stories in the Classroom to Reduce Disruptive Behaviors in Children with ADHD. *Acta Psychopathologica, 4*.

Grenblatt, J. M., & Delane, D. D. (2017). Micronutrient Deficiencies in ADHD: AGlobal Research Consensus. *Journal of Orthomolecular Medicine*, *32*(6).

Gresham, F. M., & Elliot, S. N. (1990). *Social skills rating system manual*. American Guidance Service.

Griggs, M. S., & Mikami, A. Y. (2011). The role of maternal and child ADHD symptoms in shaping interpersonal relationships. *Journal of Abnormal Child Psychology*, *39*(3), 437–449. doi:10.100710802-010-9464-4 PMID:20931275

Grizenko, N., Fortier, M. E., & Zadorozny, C. (2012). Maternal stress during pregnancy, ADHD symptomatology in children and genotype: Gene-environment interaction. *Journal of the Canadian Academy of Child and Adolescent Psychiatry*, *21*, 9–15. PMID:22299010

Grizenko, N., Shayan, Y. R., & Polotskaia, A. (2008). Relation of maternal stress during pregnancy to symptom severity and response to treatment in children with ADHD. *Journal of Psychiatry & Neuroscience*, *33*, 10–16. PMID:18197267

Groen-Blokhuis, M. M., Middeldorp, C. M., Van Beijsterveldt, C. E., & Boomsma, D. I. (2011). Evidence for a causal association of low birth weight and attention problems. *Journal oftheAmericanAcademy of Child &. Adolescent Psychiatry*, *50*(12), 1247–1254. doi:10.1016/j.jaac.2011.09.007

Groenman, A. P., Janssen, T. W. P., & Oosterlaan, J. (2017). Childhood Psychiatric Disorders as Risk Factor for Subsequent Substance Abuse: A Meta-Analysis. *Journal of the American Academy of Child and Adolescent Psychiatry*, *56*(7), 556–569. doi:10.1016/j.jaac.2017.05.004 PMID:28647007

Groenman, A. P., Oosterlaan, J., Rommelse, N., Franke, B., Roeyers, H., Oades, R. D., Sergeant, J. A., Buitelaar, J. K., & Faraone, S. V. (2013). Substance use disorders in adolescents with attention deficit hyperactivity disorder: A 4-year follow-up study. *Addiction (Abingdon, England)*, *108*(8), 1503–1511. doi:10.1111/add.12188 PMID:23506232

Grogan, M., & Weitzman, J. (2015). Using the 12-steps as a Parenting intervention with ADHD Adolescents. *The American Journal of Family Therapy*, *43*(4), 364–377. doi:10.1080/01926187.2015.1051904

Grohol, J. (2020). Causes & Risk Factors of Childhood ADHD. *Psych Central*. Retrieved on May 3, 2020, from https://psychcentral.com/childhood-adhd/causes-risk-factors-of-childhood-adhd/

Grund, T., Lehmann, K., Bock, N., Rothenberger, A., & Teuchert-Noodt, G. (2006). Influence of methylphenidate on brain development–an update of recent animal experiments. *Behavioral and Brain Functions*, *2*(1), 2. doi:10.1186/1744-9081-2-2 PMID:16403217

Gul, H., Solmaz, Y. Y., Gul, E., & Oner, O. (2018). Facebook overuse and addiction among Turkish adolescents: Are ADHD and ADHD-related problems risk factors? *Psychiatry and Clinical Psychopharmacology*, *28*(1), 80–90. doi:10.1080/24750573.2017.1383706

Gunter, T. D., Arndt, S., Riggins-Caspers, K., Wenman, G., & Cadoret, R. J. (2006). Adult outcomes of attention deficit hyperactivity disorder and conduct disorder: Are the risks independent or additive? *Annals of Clinical Psychiatry*, *18*(4), 233–237. doi:10.1080/10401230600948415 PMID:17162622

Hafner, H., & An Der, H. W. (1997). Epidemiology of Schizophrenia. *Canadian Journal of Psychiatry*, *42*(2), 139–151. doi:10.1177/070674379704200204

Hah, M., & Chang, K. (2005). Atomoxetine for the treatment of attention-deficit/hyperactivity disorder in children and adolescent with bipolar disorders. *Journal of Child and Adolescent Psychopharmacology*, *15*(6), 996–1004. doi:10.1089/cap.2005.15.996 PMID:16379520

Hales, C. M., Kit, B. K., Gu, Q., & Ogden, C. L. (2007). Trends in prescription medication use among children and adolescents—United States, 1999-2014. *Journal of the American Medical Association*, *319*(19), 2009–2020.

Hale, T. S., Bookheimer, S., McGough, J. J., Phillips, J. M., & McCracken, J. T. (2007). Atypical brain activation during simple & complex levels of processing in adult ADHD: An fMRI study. *Journal of Attention Disorders*, *11*(2), 125–140. doi:10.1177/1087054706294101 PMID:17494829

Halperin, J. M., & Healey, D. M. (2011). The influences of environmental enrichment, cognitive enhancement, and physical exercise on brain development: Can we alter the developmental trajectory of ADHD? *Neuroscience and Biobehavioral Reviews*, *35*(3), 621–634. doi:10.1016/j.neubiorev.2010.07.006 PMID:20691725

Halverstadt, J. (1998). *A.D.D. and romance: Finding fulfilment in love, sex, and relationships*. Taylor Publishing Company.

Hamblen, J. L., Gibson, L. E., Mueser, K. T., & Norris, F. H. (2006). Cognitive behavioral therapy for prolonged post-disaster distress. *Journal of Clinical Psychology*, *62*(8), 1043–1052. doi:10.1002/jclp.20288 PMID:16700022

Harpin, V. A. (2005). The effect of ADHD on the life of an individual, their family, and community from preschool to adult life. *Archives of Disease in Childhood*, *90*(suppl 1), i2–i7. doi:10.1136/adc.2004.059006 PMID:15665153

Harpin, V., Mazzone, L., Raynaud, J. P., Kahle, J., & Hodgkins, P. (2013). Long-Term Outcomes of ADHD: A Systematic Review of Self-Esteem and Social Function. *Journal of Attention Disorders*.

Harris, K. R., Graham, S., & Mason, L. H. (2003). Self-regulated strategy development in the classroom: Part of a balanced approach to writing instruction for students with disabilities. *Focus on Exceptional Children*, *35*, 1–16.

Harrison, L., Manocha, R., & Rubia, K. (2004). Sahaja yoga meditation as a family treatment programme for children with attention deficits-hyperactivity disorder. *Clinical Child Psychology and Psychiatry*, *9*(4), 479–497. doi:10.1177/1359104504046155

Harstad, E. B., Weaver, A. L., Katusic, S. K., Colligan, R. C., Kumar, S., Chan, E., Voigt, R. G., & Barbaresi, W. J. (2014). ADHD, stimulant treatment, and growth: A longitudinal study. *Pediatrics*, *134*(4), e935–e944. doi:10.1542/peds.2014-0428 PMID:25180281

Hartman, R., Stage, S., & Webster-Stratton, C. A. (2003). Growth curve analysis of parent training outcomes: Examining the influence of child risk factors (inattention, impulsivity, and hyperactivity problems), parental and family risk factors. *Journal of Child Psychology and Psychiatry, and Allied Disciplines*, *44*(3), 388–398. doi:10.1111/1469-7610.00129 PMID:12635968

Harvey, W. J., & Reid, G. (2003). Attention-deficit/hyperactivity disorder: A review of research on movement skill performance and physical fitness. *Adapted Physical Activity Quarterly; APAQ*, *20*(1), 1–25. doi:10.1123/apaq.20.1.1

Harwell, J. M., & Jackson, R. W. (2008). *The complete learning disabilities handbook: Ready-to-use strategies and activities for teaching students with learning disabilities*. John Wiley & Sons.

Hasson-Ohayon, I., Ben-Pazi, A., Silberg, T., Pijnenborg, G. H. M., & Goldzweig, G. (2019). The mediating role of parental satisfaction between marital satisfaction and perceived family burden among parents of children with psychiatric disorders. *Journal of Psychiatric Research, 271*, 105–110. doi:10.1016/j.psychres.2018.11.037 PMID:30472503

Hawkins, N. E., & Singer, G. H. S. (1989). A skills training approach from assisting parents to cope with stress. In G.H.S. Singer & L.K Irwin (Eds.), Support for caregiving families: Enabling positive adaptation to disability. Baltimore, MD: Paul Brookes.

Haworth, C. M. A., Wright, M. J., Luciano, M., Martin, N. G., de Geus, E. J. C., van Beijsterveldt, C. E. M., Bartels, M., Posthuma, D., Boomsma, D. I., Davis, O. S. P., Kovas, Y., Corley, R. P., DeFries, J. C., Hewitt, J. K., Olson, R. K., Rhea, S.-A., Wadsworth, S. J., Iacono, W. G., McGue, M., ... Plomin, R. (2010). The herita- bility of general cognitive ability increases linearly from childhood to young adulthood. *Molecular Psychiatry, 15*(11), 1112–1120. doi:10.1038/mp.2009.55 PMID:19488046

Hayes, M., & Chase, S. (2010). Prescribing Yoga. *Primary Care, 37*(1), 31–47.

Hazell, P. (2007). Pharmacological management of attention-deficit hyper activity disorder in adolescents. *CNS Drugs, 21*(1), 37–46. doi:10.2165/00023210-200721010-00004 PMID:17190528

Heal, D. J., Smith, S. L., & Findling, R. L. (2012). ADHD: Current and future therapeutics. *Current Topics in Behavioral Neurosciences, 9*, 361–390. doi:10.1007/7854_2011_125

Healthline. (2017). *A review by Daniel Murrell, '6 common thyroid disorders and problems'*. Retrieved from https://www.healthline.com/health/common-thyroid-disorders

Hechtman, L., Swanson, J. M., Sibley, M. H., Stehli, A., Owens, E. B., Mitchell, J. T., Arnold, L. E., Molina, B. S. G., Hinshaw, S. P., Jensen, P. S., Abikoff, H. B., Perez Algorta, G., Howard, A. L., Hoza, B., Etcovitch, J., Houssais, S., Lakes, K. D., Nichols, J. Q., Vitiello, B., ... Stern, K. (2016). Functional Adult Outcomes 16 Years After Childhood Diagnosis of Attention-Deficit/Hyperactivity Disorder: MTA Results. *Journal of the American Academy of Child and Adolescent Psychiatry, 55*(11), 945–952.e2. doi:10.1016/j.jaac.2016.07.774 PMID:27806862

Hechtman, L., Weiss, G., Finklestein, J., Werner, A., & Benn, R. (1976). Hyperactives as young adults: Preliminary report. *Canadian Medical Association Journal, 115*(7), 625–630. PMID:974949

Hechtman, L., Weiss, G., & Perlman, T. (1984). Hyperactives as young adults: Past and current substance abuse and antisocial behavior. *The American Journal of Orthopsychiatry, 54*(3), 415–442. doi:10.1111/j.1939-0025.1984.tb01507.x PMID:6331769

Hegde, V. (2007). *The science of stress and The Art of managing it.* Mind Tree Consulting.

Heiman, T. (2005). An examination of peer relationships of children with and without attention deficit hyperactivity disorder. *School Psychology International, 26*(3), 330–339. doi:10.1177/0143034305055977

Heinonen, K., Räikkönen, K., Pesonen, A. K., Andersson, S., Kajantie, E., Eriksson, J. G., Wolke, D., & Lano, A. (2010). Behavioural symptoms of attention deficit/hyperactivity disorder in preterm and term children born small and appropriate for gestational age: A longitudinal study. *BMC Pediatrics, 10*(1), 91. doi:10.1186/1471-2431-10-91 PMID:21159164

Hellström, L. (2019). A Systematic Review of Polyvictimization among Children with Attention Deficit Hyperactivity or Autism Spectrum Disorder. *International Journal of Environmental Research* and *Public Health, 16*(13). pii: E2280. doi:10.3390/ijerph16132280

Henderson, T. A., & Hartman, K. (2004). Aggression, mania and hypomania induction associated with atomoxetine. *Pediatrics, 114*(3), 895–896. doi:10.1542/peds.2004-1140 PMID:15342872

Hennig, T., Schramm, S. A., Linderkamp, F., & Koglin, U. (2016). Mediation and moderation of outcome in a training intervention for adolescents with attention-deficit/hyperactivity disorder. *Journal of Cognitive Education and Psychology, 15*(3), 412–427. doi:10.1891/1945-8959.15.3.412

Herbert, J. D., & Forman, E. M. (2012). Mindfulness and Acceptance Techniques. In D. J. A. Dozois (Ed.), *Cognitive Behavioral Therapy: A Complete Reference Guide*. John Wiley.

Hernandez, E., Smith, C. L., Day, K. L., Neal, A., & Dunsmore, J. C. (2018). Patterns of parental emotion-related discourse and links with children's problem behaviours: A person-centred approach. *Developmental Psychology, 54*(11), 2077–2089. doi:10.1037/dev0000602 PMID:30284881

Hesson, J., & Fowler, K. (2018). Prevalence and correlates of self-reported ADD/ADHD in a large national sample of Canadian adults. *Journal of Attention Disorders, 22*(2), 191–200. doi:10.1177/1087054715573992 PMID:25749874

Hickey, G., & Fricker, P. (1999). Attention deficit hyperactivity disorder, CNS stimulants and sport. *Sports Medicine (Auckland, N.Z.), 27*(1), 11–21. doi:10.2165/00007256-199927010-00002 PMID:10028130

Hillman, C. H., Erickson, K. I., & Kramer, A. F. (2008). Be smart, exercise your heart: Exercise effects on brain and cognition. *Nature Reviews. Neuroscience, 9*(1), 58–65. doi:10.1038/nrn2298 PMID:18094706

Hinshaw, S. P. (1992). Academic underachievement, attention deficits, and aggression: Comorbidity and implications for intervention. *Journal of Consulting and Clinical Psychology, 60*(6), 893–903. doi:10.1037/0022-006X.60.6.893 PMID:1460150

Hinshaw, S. P. (2017). Developmental psychopathology as a scientific discipline: A 21st-century perspective. In T. P. Beauchaine & S. P. Hinshaw (Eds.), *Child and adolescent psychopathology* (3rd ed., pp. 3–32). Wiley.

Hinshaw, S. P., Zupan, B. A., Simmel, C., Nigg, J. T., & Melnick, S. (1997). Peer status in boys with and without attention-deficit hyperactivity disorder: Predictions from overt and covert antisocial behavior, social isolation, and authoritative parenting beliefs. *Child Development, 68*(5), 880–896. doi:10.2307/1132039 PMID:29106718

Hirisave, U., Oommen, A., & Kapur, M. (2002). *Psychological Assessment of Children in the clinical setting*. Published at NIMHANS.

Hjern, A., Weitoft, G. R., & Lindblad, F. (2010). Social adversity predicts ADHD-medication in school children–a national cohort study. *Acta Paediatrica (Oslo, Norway), 99*(6), 920–924. doi:10.1111/j.1651-2227.2009.01638.x PMID:20002622

Hodgkins, P., Arnold, L. E., Shaw, M., Caci, H., Kahle, J., Woods, A. G., & Young, S. (2012). A systematic review of global publication trends regarding long-term outcomes of ADHD. *Frontiers in Psychiatry, 2*, 84. doi:10.3389/fpsyt.2011.00084 PMID:22279437

Hodgson, K., Hutchingson, A. D., & Denson, L. (2014, May). Nonpharmacological Treatments for ADHD: A Meta-Analytic Review. *Journal of Attention Disorders, 18*(4), 275–282. doi:10.1177/1087054712444732 PMID:22647288

Hofmann, S. G., Asnaani, A., Vonk, I. J., Sawyer, A. T., & Fang, A. (2012). The Efficacy of Cognitive Behavioral Therapy: A Review of Meta-analyses. *Cognitive Therapy and Research, 36*(5), 427–440. doi:10.100710608-012-9476-1 PMID:23459093

Hofvander, B., Bering, S., Tärnhäll, A., Wallinius, M., & Billstedt, E. (2019). Few Differences in the Externalizing and Criminal History of Young Violent Offenders With and Without Autism Spectrum Disorders. *Front Psychiatry, 17*(10), 911. doi: . doi:10.3389/fpsyt.2019.00911

Holmes, J., Hilton, K. A., Place, M., Alloway, T. P., Elliott, J. G., & Gathercole, S. E. (2014). Children with low working memory and children with ADHD: Same or different? *Frontiers in Human Neuroscience*, *8*, 976. doi:10.3389/fnhum.2014.00976 PMID:25538599

Honos-Webb, L. (2010). The Gift of ADHD. *New Harbinger Publications.*, *ISBN-13*, 978–1572248502.

Hoogman, M., Bralten, J., Hibar, D., Mennes, M., Zweirs, M. P., Shweren, L. S., ... Franke, B. (2017, April). Subcortical brain volume differences in participants with attention deficit hyperactivity disorder in children and adults: A cross-sectional mega-analysis. *The Lancet. Psychiatry*, *4*(4), 310–319. doi:10.1016/S2215-0366(17)30049-4 PMID:28219628

Horner, R. H. (1994). Functional assessment: Contributions and future directions. *Journal of Applied Behavior Analysis*, *27*(2), 401–404. doi:10.1901/jaba.1994.27-401 PMID:16795831

Houck, G., Kendall, J., Miller, A., Morrell, P., & Wiebe, G. (2010). Self concept in children and adolescents with ADHD. *Journal of Pediatric Nursing*, *26*(3), 239–247. doi:10.1016/j.pedn.2010.02.004 PMID:21601148

Hoza, B. (2007). Peer functioning in children with ADHD. *Ambulatory Pediatrics*, *7*(1), 101–106. doi:10.1016/j.ambp.2006.04.011 PMID:17261489

Hoza, B. (2007). Peer functioning in children with ADHD. *Journal of Pediatric Psychology*, *32*(6), 655–663. doi:10.1093/jpepsy/jsm024 PMID:17556400

Hoza, B., Martin, C. P., Pirog, A., & Shoulberg, E. K. (2016). Using physical activity to manage ADHD symptoms: The state of the evidence. *Current Psychiatry Reports*, *18*(12), 113. doi:10.100711920-016-0749-3 PMID:27807701

Huang, L., Wang, Y., Zhang, L., Zheng, Z., Zhu, T., Qu, Y., & Mu, D. (2017). Maternal Smoking and Attention-Deficit/Hyperactivity Disorder in Offspring: A Meta-analysis. *Pediatrics, 141*(1). doi:10.1542/peds

Hubbard, J. A., & Newcomb, A. F. (1991). Initial dyadic peer interaction of attention deficit-hyperactivity disorder and normal boys. *Journal of Abnormal Child Psychology*, *19*(2), 179–195. doi:10.1007/BF00909977 PMID:2056162

Hughes, S. M. (2017). *Coaching parents of children with ADHD: A Western Australian study*. Retrieved from https://ro.ecu.edu.au/ theses/2031

Hughes, C. W., Emslie, G. J., Crismon, M. L., Posner, K., Birmaher, B., Ryan, N., Jensen, P., Curry, J., Vitiello, B., Lopez, M., Shon, S. P., Pliszka, S. R., & Trivedi, M. H.Texas Consensus Conference Panel on Medication Treatment of Childhood Major Depressive Disorder. (2007). Texas Children's Medication Algorithm Project. Update from Texas Consensus Conference Panel on Medication Treatment of Childhood Major Depressive Disorder. *Journal of the American Academy of Child and Adolescent Psychiatry*, *46*(6), 667–686. doi:10.1097/chi.0b013e31804a859b PMID:17513980

Huh, S. Y., Kim, S. G., Lee, J. S., Jung, W. Y., Choi, B. S., & Kim, J. H. (2019). A study on the school violence experience of children with attention-deficit hyperactivity disorder in the context of bullying. *Asia-Pacific Psychiatry*, *11*(3), e12353. doi:10.1111/appy.12353 PMID:30941893

Hultman, C. M., Torrång, A., Tuvblad, C., Cnattingius, S., Larsson, J. O., & Lichtenstein, P. (2007). Birth weight and attention-deficit/hyperactivity symptoms in childhood and early adolescence: A prospective Swedish twin study. *Journal of the American Academy of Child and Adolescent Psychiatry*, *46*(3), 370–377. doi:10.1097/01.chi.0000246059.62706.22 PMID:17314723

Hunsucker, G. (1988). *Attention Deficit Disorder: A common but often overlooked disorder of children*. Forrest Publishing.

Hunter, S. B., Miles, J. N., Pedersen, E. R., Ewing, B. A., & D'Amico, E. J. (2014). Temporal associations between substance use and delinquency among youth with a first time offense. *Addictive Behaviors*, *39*(6), 1081–1086. doi:10.1016/j.addbeh.2014.03.002 PMID:24656642

Hutchison, S. L., Ghuman, J. K., Ghuman, H. S., Karpov, I., & Schuster, J. M. (2016). Efficacy of atomoxetine in the treatment of attention-deficit hyperactivity disorder in patients with common comorbidities in children, adolescents and adults: A review. *Therapeutic Advances in Psychopharmacology*, *6*(5), 317–334. doi:10.1177/2045125316647686 PMID:27721971

Individuals with Disabilities Education Act, 20 U.S.C. § 1400 (2004).

Infante, M. A., Moore, E. M., Nguyen, T. T., Fourligas, N., Mattson, S. N., & Riley, E. P. (2015). Objective assessment of ADHD core symptoms in children with heavy prenatal alcohol exposure. *Physiology & Behavior*, *148*, 45–50. doi:10.1016/j.physbeh.2014.10.014 PMID:25447751

Iyengar, B. K. S. (1979). *Light on Yoga: Yoga Dipika*. Thorsons.

Jacob, C. P., Nguyen, T. T., Dempfle, A., Heine, M., Windemuth-Kieselbach, C., Baumann, K., Jacob, F., Prechtl, J., Wittlich, M., Herrmann, M. J., Gross-Lesch, S., Lesch, K.-P., & Reif, A. (2010). A gene-environment investigation on personality traits in two independent clinical sets of adult patients with personality disorder and attention deficit/hyperactive disorder. *European Archives of Psychiatry and Clinical Neuroscience*, *260*(4), 317–326. doi:10.100700406-009-0079-0 PMID:19894072

Jacob, L., Haro, J. M., & Koyanagi, A. (2018). Relationship between attention-deficit hyperactivity disorder symptoms and problem gambling: A mediation analysis of influential factors among 7,403 individuals from the UK. *Journal of Behavioral Addictions*, *7*(3), 781–791. doi:10.1556/2006.7.2018.72 PMID:30238788

Jaffe, P. (1995). History and overview of adulthood ADD. In K. G. Nadeau (Ed.), *A Comprehensive Guide to Attention Deficit Disorder in Adults: Research, Diagnosis, and Treatment*. Brunner/Mazel.

Jansen, D., Petry, K., Ceulemans, E., van der Oord, S., Noens, I., & Baeyens, D. (2017). Functioning and participation problems of students with ADHD in higher education: Which reasonable accommodations are effective? *European Journal of Special Needs Education*, *32*(1), 35–53. doi:10.1080/08856257.2016.1254965

Jarrett, M. A., Wolff, J. C., Davis, T. E. III, Cowart, M. J., & Ollendick, T. H. (2016). Characteristics of children with ADHD and comorbid anxiety. *Journal of Attention Disorders*, *20*(7), 636–644. doi:10.1177/1087054712452914 PMID:22863769

Jensen, P. S., Hinshaw, S. P., Swanson, J. M., Greenhill, L. L., Conners, C. K., Arnold, L. E., Abikoff, H. B., Elliott, G., Hechtman, L., Hoza, B., March, J. S., Newcorn, J. H., Severe, J. B., Vitiello, B., Wells, K., & Wigal, T. (2001). Findings from the NIMH multimodal treatment study of ADHD (MTA): Implications and applications for primary care providers. *Journal of Developmental and Behavioral Pediatrics*, *22*(1), 60–73. doi:10.1097/00004703-200102000-00008 PMID:11265923

Jensen, P. S., Martin, D., & Cantwell, D. P. (1997). Comorbidity in ADHD: Implications for future research, practice and DSM-IV. *Journal of the American Academy of Child and Adolescent Psychiatry*, *36*(8), 1065–1079. doi:10.1097/00004583-199708000-00014 PMID:9256586

Jepsen, J., Fagerlund, B., & Mortensen, E. L. (2009). Do Attention Deficits Influence IQ Assessment in Children and Adolescents with ADHD? *Journal of Attention Disorders*, *12*(6), 551–562. doi:10.1177/1087054708322996 PMID:18815437

Jester, J. M., Nigg, J. T., Adams, K., Fitzgerald, H. E., Puttler, L. I., Wong, M. M., & Zucker, R. A. (2005). Inattention/hyperactivity and aggression from early childhood to adolescence: Heterogeneity of trajectories and differential influence of family environment characteristics. *Development and Psychopathology*, *17*(1), 99–125. doi:10.1017/S0954579405050066 PMID:15971762

Johnson, M. H. (2012). Executive function and developmental disorders: The flip side of the coin. *Trends in Cognitive Sciences*, *16*(9), 454–457. doi:10.1016/j.tics.2012.07.001 PMID:22835639

Johnston, C., & Mash, E. J. (2001). Families of children with attention-deficit/hyperactivity disorder: Review and recommendations for future research. *Clinical Child and Family Psychology Review*, *4*(3), 183–207. doi:10.1023/A:1017592030434 PMID:11783738

Johnston, C., Mash, E. J., Miller, N., & Ninowski, J. E. (2012). Parenting in adults with attention-deficit/hyperactivity disorder (ADHD). *Clinical Psychology Review*, *32*(4), 215–228. doi:10.1016/j.cpr.2012.01.007

Jokela, M., Power, C., & Kivimäki, M. (2009). Childhood problem behaviors and injury risk over the life course. *Journal of Child Psychology and Psychiatry, and Allied Disciplines*, *50*(12), 1541–1549. doi:10.1111/j.1469-7610.2009.02122.x

Joseph, J., & Robert, R. (2011). Overcoming Executive Function Deficits With Students With ADHD. *Theory into Practice*, *50*(1), 61–67. doi:10.1080/00405841.2010.534942

Joseph, S., & Linley, P. A. (2004). Positive therapy: A positive psychological theory of Therapeutic practice. In P. A. Linley & S. Joseph (Eds.), *Positive psychology in practice* (pp. 354–368). John Wiley. doi:10.1002/9780470939338.ch22

Jouriles, E. N., Murphy, C. M., & O'Leary, K. D. (1989). Effects of maternal mood on Mother-son interaction patterns. *Journal of Abnormal Child Psychology*, *17*(5), 513–525. doi:10.1007/BF00916510 PMID:2808944

Kachooei, H., Daneshmand, R., Dolatshahi, B., Samadi, R., & Samiei, M. (2016). Attention-Deficit/Hyperactivity Disorder and Martial Satisfaction: The Preliminary Roles of Employment and Income. *Iranian Journal of Psychiatry and Behavioral Sciences*, *10*(2), e4012. doi:10.17795/ijpbs-4012 PMID:27803722

Kadden, R. M., Cooney, N. L., Getter, H., & Litt, M. D. (1989). Matching alcoholics to coping skills or interactional therapies: Posttreatment results. *Journal of Consulting and Clinical Psychology*, *57*(6), 698–704. doi:10.1037/0022-006X.57.6.698 PMID:2557364

Kadden, R. M., Litt, M. D., Kabela-Cormier, E., & Petry, N. M. (2007). Abstinence rates following behavioral treatments for marijuana dependence. *Addictive Behaviors*, *32*(6), 1220–1236. doi:10.1016/j.addbeh.2006.08.009 PMID:16996224

Kahn, R. S., Khoury, J., Nichols, W. C., & Lanphear, B. P. (2003). Role of dopamine transporter genotype and maternal prenatal smoking in childhood hyperactive-impulsive, inattentive, and oppositional behaviors. *The Journal of Pediatrics*, *143*(1), 104–110. doi:10.1016/S0022-3476(03)00208-7 PMID:12915833

Kaiser, N. M., & Pfiffner, L. J. (2011). Evidence-based psychosocial treatments for childhood ADHD. *Psychiatric Annals*, *41*(1), 9–15. doi:10.3928/00485713-20101221-03

Kaplan & Sadock. (2007). *Kaplan & Sadock's Synopsis of Psychiatry: Behavioral Sciences/clinical Psychiatry* (10th ed.). Wolter Kluwer/Lippincott Williams & Wilkins.

Kapner, D. A. (2003). *Recreational use of Ritalin on college campuses. Info Fact Resources*. U.S. Department of Justice.

Karmananda S. (1983). *Yogic management of common diseases*. Yoga Publication Trust.

Katya, R. (2018). Cognitive neuroscience of attention deficit hyperactivity disorder (ADHD) and its clinical translation. *Frontiers in Human Neuroscience*, *12*, 100-123. doi:10.3389/fnhum.2018.00100

Katzman, M. A., Bilkey, T. S., Chokka, P. R., Fallu, A., & Klassen, L. J. (2017). Adult ADHD and comorbid disorders: Clinical implications of a dimensional approach. *BMC Psychiatry*, *17*(1), 302. doi:10.118612888-017-1463-3 PMID:28830387

Kaufman, J., Birmaher, B., Brent, D., Rao, U., & Ryan, N. (1996). *Kiddie-Sads-present and Lifetime version (K-SADS-PL)*. University of Pittsburgh, School of Medicine.

Kaunhoven, R. J., & Dorjee, D. (2017). How does mindfulness modulate self-regulation in pre-adolescent children? An integrative neurocognitive review. *Neuroscience and Biobehavioral Reviews*, *74*, 163–184. doi:10.1016/j.neubiorev.2017.01.007

Kavale, K. A., Mathur, S. R., Forness, S. R., Rutherford, R. B., & Quinn, M. M. (1997). Effectiveness of social skills training for students with behavior disorders: A meta-analysis. *Advances in Learning and Behavioral Disabilities*, *11*, 1–26.

Kazdin, A. (1997). Parent management training: Evidence, outcomes, and issues. *Journal of the American Academy of Child and Adolescent Psychiatry*, *36*(10), 1349–1356. doi:10.1097/00004583-199710000-00016 PMID:9334547

Kazdin, A. E., & Wassell, G. (2000). Therapeutic changes in children, parents and families resulting from treatment of children with conduct problems. *Journal of the American Academy of Child and Adolescent Psychiatry*, *39*(4), 414–420. doi:10.1097/00004583-200004000-00009 PMID:10761342

Keeley, L. M., Makol, B. G., Qasmieh, N., Deros, D. E., Karp, J. N., Lipton, M. F., Augenstein, T. M., Truong, M. L., Racz, S. J., & Reyes, A. D. L. (2018). Validity of Adolescent and Parent Reports on the Six-Item ADHD Self Report Scale (ASRS-6) in Clinical Assessments of Adolescent Social Anxiety. *Journal of Child and Family Studies*, *27*(4), 1041–1053. doi:10.100710826-017-0950-y

Keilow, M., Holm, A., & Fallesen, P. (2018). Medical treatment of Attention Deficit/Hyperactivity Disorder (ADHD) and children's academic performance. *PLoS One*, *13*(11), e0207905. doi:10.1371/journal.pone.0207905 PMID:30496240

Kelly, T. M., Cornelius, J. R., & Clark, D. B. (2004). Psychiatric disorders and attempted suicide among adolescents with substance use disorders. *Drug and Alcohol Dependence*, *73*(1), 87–97. doi:10.1016/j.drugalcdep.2003.10.004 PMID:14687963

Kendall, J. (1999). Sibling accounts of attention deficit hyperactivity disorder (ADHD). *Family Process*, *38*(1), 117–136. doi:10.1111/j.1545-5300.1999.00117.x PMID:10207714

Keng, S. L., Smoski, M. J., & Robins, C. J. (2011). Effects of mindfulness on psychological health: A review of empirical studies. *Clinical Psychology Review*, *31*(6), 1041–1056. doi:10.1016/j.cpr.2011.04.006 PMID:21802619

Kent, K. M., Pelham, W. E., Molina, B. S. G., Waschbusch, D. A., Yu, J., Sibley, M. H., & … . (in press). The academic-experience of male high school students with ADHD. Paper submitted for publication. *Journal of Abnormal Child Psychology*.

Kern, J. K., Geier, D. A., Sykes, L. K., Geier, M. R., & Deth, R. C. (2015). Are ASD and ADHD a continuum? A comparison of pathophysiological similarities between the disorders. *Journal of Attention Disorders*, *19*(9), 805–827. doi:10.1177/1087054712459886 PMID:23074304

Kerr, M. M., & Nelson, C. M. (2010). *Strategies for addressing behavior problems in the classroom* (6th ed.). Pearson.

Kessler, R.C., Adler, L., Barkley, R., Biederman, J., Conners, C. K., Demler, O., … Zaslavsky, A.M. (2006).The prevalence and correlates of adult ADHD in the United States: results from the National Comorbidity Survey Replication. *American Journal of Psychiatry, 163*(4), 716–23.

Kessler, R., Adler, L., Barkley, R., Biederman, J., Conners, C., Demler, O., Faraone, S. V., Greenhill, L. L., Howes, M. J., Secnik, K., Spencer, T., Ustun, T. B., Walters, E. E., & Zaslavsky, A. M. (2006). The prevalence and correlates of adult ADHD in the United States: Results from the national comorbidity survey replication. *The American Journal of Psychiatry*, *163*(4), 716–723. doi:10.1176/ajp.2006.163.4.716 PMID:16585449

Ketzer, C. R., Gallois, C., Martinez, A. L., Rohde, L. A., & Schmitz, M. (2012). Is there an association between perinatal complications and attention-deficit/hyperactivity disorder-inattentive type in children and adolescents? *Revista Brasileira de Psiquiatria (Sao Paulo, Brazil)*, *34*(3), 321–328. doi:10.1016/j.rbp.2012.01.001 PMID:23429778

Kilpatrick, D. G., Ruggiero, K. J., Acierno, R., Saunders, B. E., Resnick, H. S., & Best, C. L. (2003). Violence and risk of PTSD, major depression, substance abuse/dependence, and comorbidity: Results from the National Survey of Adolescents. *Journal of Consulting and Clinical Psychology*, *71*(4), 692–700. doi:10.1037/0022-006X.71.4.692 PMID:12924674

Kim, H. W., Cho, S. C., Kim, B. N., Kim, J. W., Shin, M. S., & Kim, Y. (2009). Perinatal and familial risk factors are associated with full syndrome and subthreshold attention-deficit hyperactivity disorder in a Korean community sample. *Psychiatry Investigation*, *6*(4), 278–285. doi:10.4306/pi.2009.6.4.278 PMID:20140126

Klassen, A. F., Miller, A., & Fine, S. (2004). Health-related quality of life in children and adolescents who have a diagnosis of attention-deficit/hyperactivity disorder. *Pediatrics*, *114*(5), e541–e547. doi:10.1542/peds.2004-0844 PMID:15520087

Klein, R. G., & Abikoff, H. (1997, July). Behaviour therapy and methyphanidate in treatment of children with ADHD. *Journal of Attention Disorders*, *2*(2), 89–114. doi:10.1177/108705479700200203

Klein, R. G., Mannuzza, S., Olazagasti, M. A., Roizen, E., Hutchison, J. A., Lashua, E. C., & Castellanos, F. X. (2012). Clinical and functional outcome of childhood attention-deficit/hyperactivity disorder 33 years later. *Archives of General Psychiatry*, *69*(12), 1295–1303. doi:10.1001/archgenpsychiatry.2012.271

Klimowicz, A., Janicic, A., & IsHak, W. W. (2017). Sex and chronic psychiatric illness. In *The Textbook of Clinical Sexual Medicine* (pp. 507-524). Springer.

Knopik, V. S., Sparrow, E. P., Madden, P. A., Bucholz, K. K., Hudziak, J. J., Reich, W., Slutske, W. S., Grant, J. D., McLAUGHLIN, T. L., Todorov, A., Todd, R. D., & Heath, A. C. (2005). Contributions of parental alcoholism, prenatal substance exposure, and genetic transmission to child ADHD risk: A female twin study. *Psychological Medicine*, *35*(5), 625–635. doi:10.1017/S0033291704004155 PMID:15918339

Knouse, L. E. & Safren, S. A. (2010). Current statusof cognitive behavioural therapy for adult attention deficit hyperactivity disorder. *Psychiatric Clinic of North America, 33*(3), 497-509.

Knouse, L. E., & Safren, S. A. (2013). Psychosocial treatment for adult ADHD. In *ADHD in adults* (pp. 119–136). Humana Press. doi:10.1007/978-1-62703-248-3_7

Koehler, S., Lauer, P., Schreppel, T., Jacob, C., Heine, M., Boreatti-Hümmer, A., … Herrmann, M. J. (2009). Increased EEG power density in alpha and theta bands in adult ADHD patients. *Journal of Neural Transmission, 116*(1), 97–104.

Koemans, R. G., van Vroenhoven, S., Karreman, A., & Bekker, M. H. J. (2015). Attachment and autonomy problems in adults with ADHD. *Journal of Attention Disorders*, *19*(5), 435–446. doi:10.1177/1087054712453170

Kohrt, B.A., Turner, E.L., Rai, S., Bhardwaj,A., Sikkema,K.J., Adelekun,A., Dhakal,M., Luitel,N.P, Lund,C., Patel,V., & Jordans, M. (in press). Reducing mental illness stigma in healthcare settings: Proof of concept for a social contact intervention to address what matters most for primary care providers. *Social Science & Medicine*, *250*, 112852. doi:10.1016/j.socscimed.2020.112852

Koisaari, T., Michelsson, K., Holopainen, J. M., Maksimainen, R., Päivänsalo, J., Rantala, K., & Tervo, T. (2015). Traffic and criminal behavior of adults with attention deficit–hyperactivity with a prospective follow-up from birth to the age of 40 years. *Traffic Injury Prevention*, *16*(8), 824–830. doi:10.1080/15389588.2015.1029068 PMID:25837647

Kolkman, M., Hoijtink, H. J. A., Kroesbergen, E. H., & Leseman, P. P. M. (2013). The role of executive functions in numerical magnitude skills. *Learning and Individual Differences*, *24*, 145–151. doi:10.1016/j.lindif.2013.01.004

Kolla, N. J., van der Maas, M., Erickson, P. G., Mann, R. E., Seeley, J., & Vingilis, E. (2018). Attention deficit hyperactivity disorder and arrest history: Differential association of clinical characteristics by sex. *International Journal of Law and Psychiatry*, *58*, 150–156. doi:10.1016/j.ijlp.2018.04.006 PMID:29853005

Konrad, K., Gunther, T., Hanisch, C., & Herpertz-Dahlmann, B. (2004). Differential effects of methylphenidate on attentional functions in children with attention-deficit /hyperactivity disorder. *Journal of the American Academy of Child and Adolescent Psychiatry*, *43*(2), 191–198. doi:10.1097/00004583-200402000-00015 PMID:14726726

Konstenius, M., Jayaram-Lindström, N., Beck, O., & Franck, J. (2010). Sustained release methylphenidate for the treatment of ADHD in amphetamine abusers: A pilot study. *Drug and Alcohol Dependence*, *108*(1-2), 130–133. doi:10.1016/j.drugalcdep.2009.11.006 PMID:20015599

Kooij, S. J. J., Bejerot, S., Blackwell, A., Caci, H., Casas-Brugué, M., Carpentier, P. J., … Fayyad, J. (2010). European consensus statement on diagnosis and treatment of adult ADHD: The european network adult ADHD. *BMC Psychiatry, 67.* Retrieved from https://www.biomedcentral.com/1471-244X/10/67

Kooij, J. J. S. (2012). *Adult ADHD: Diagnostic assessment and Treatment* (3rd ed.). Springer.

Kooij, J. S. (2012). *Adult ADHD: Diagnostic assessment and treatment.* Springer Science & Business Media.

Kopko, K. (2007). *Parenting Styles and Adolescents.* Retrieved from: http://www.parenting.cit.cornell.edu

Koposov, R. A., Ruchkin, V. V., Eisemann, M., & Sidorov, P. I. (2005). Alcohol abuse in Russian delinquent adolescents. Associations with comorbid psychopathology, personality and parenting. *European Child & Adolescent Psychiatry*, *14*(5), 254–261. doi:10.100700787-005-0463-x PMID:15981137

Koumoula, A. (2012). The Course of Attention Deficit Hyperactivity Disorder (ADHD) Over the Life Span. *Psychiatriki*, *23*(S1), 49-59.

Kousha, M., & Abbasi Kakrodi, M. (2019). Can Parents Improve the Quality of Life of Their Children with Attention Deficit Hyperactivity Disorder? *Iranian Journal of Psychiatry*, *14*(2), 154–159. doi:10.18502/ijps.v14i2.995 PMID:31440297

Kousha, M., Shahrivar, Z., & Alaghband-Rad, J. (2012). Substance use disorder and ADHD: Is ADHD a particularly "specific" risk factor? *Journal of Attention Disorders*, *16*(4), 325–332. doi:10.1177/1087054710387265 PMID:22127397

Kovács, I., Demeter, I., Janka, Z., Demetrovics, Z., Maraz, A., & Andó, B. (2020). Different aspects of impulsivity in chronic alcohol use disorder with and without comorbid problem gambling. *PLoS One*, *15*(1), e0227645. doi:10.1371/journal.pone.0227645 PMID:31999707

Kovacs, M. (1995). *Manual: The Children's Depression Inventory*. Multi-Health Systems.

Kowatch, R. A., Fristad, M., Birmaher, B., Wagner, K. D., Findling, R. L., & Hellander, M. (2005). Treatment guidelines for children and adolescents with bipolar disorders. *Journal of the American Academy of Child and Adolescent Psychiatry*, *44*(3), 213–235. doi:10.1097/00004583-200503000-00006 PMID:15725966

Kraemer, M., Uekermann, J., Wiltfang, J., & Kis, B. (2010). Methylphenidate-induced psychosis in adult attention-deficit/hyperactivity disorder: Report of 3 new cases and review of the literature. *Clinical Neuropharmacology*, *33*(4), 204–206. doi:10.1097/WNF.0b013e3181e29174 PMID:20571380

Kratochvil, C. J., Michelson, D., Newcorn, J. H., Weiss, M. D., Busner, J., Moore, R. J., Ruff, D. D., Ramsey, J., Dickson, R., Turgay, A., Saylor, K., Luber, S., Vaughan, B., & Allen, A. J. (2007). High-dose atomoxetine treatment of ADHD in youths with limited response to standard doses. *Journal of the American Academy of Child and Adolescent Psychiatry*, *46*(9), 1128–1137. doi:10.1097/chi.0b013e318074eeb3 PMID:17712236

Kratochvil, C. J., Vaughan, B. S., Barker, A., Corr, L., Wheeler, A., & Madaan, V. (2009, March). Review of pediatric attention deficit/hyperactivity disorder for the general psychiatrist. *The Psychiatric Clinics of North America*, *32*(1), 39–56. doi:10.1016/j.psc.2008.10.001 PMID:19248915

Krauss, M. W. (1993). Child-related and parenting stress: Similarities and differences between mothers and fathers of children with disabilities. *American Journal of Mental Retardation*, *97*, 393–404. PMID:8427694

Krisanaprakornkit, T., Ngamjarus, C., Witoonchart, C., & Piyavhatkul, N. (2010). Meditation therapies for attention-deficit/hyperactivity disorder (ADHD). *Cochrane Database of Systematic Reviews*, (6), CD006507. doi:10.1002/14651858.CD006507.pub2 PMID:20556767

Kuppa, A., & Maysun, A. (2019). Risk of Alcohol Abuse in Humans with Attention-deficit/Hyperactivity Disorder Symptoms. *Cureus*, *11*(10), e5996. doi:10.7759/cureus.5996 PMID:31807384

La Forge, R. (1997). Mind–body fitness: Encouraging prospects for primary and secondary prevention. *The Journal of Cardiovascular Nursing*, *11*(3), 53–65. doi:10.1097/00005082-199704000-00006

Labuhn, A. S., Zimmerman, B. J., & Hasselhorn, M. (2010). Enhancing students' self-regulation and mathematics performance: The influence of feedback and self-evaluative standards. *Metacognition and Learning*, *5*(2), 173–194. doi:10.100711409-010-9056-2

Lahey, B. B., Pelham, W. E., Schaughency, E. A., Atkins, M. S., Murphy, H. A., Hynd, G. W., Russo, M., Hartdagen, S., & Lorys-Vernon, A. (1988). Dimensions and types of Attention Deficit Disorder with Hyperactivity children. A factor analytic and cluster analytic approach. *Journal of the American Academy of Child and Adolescent Psychiatry*, *27*(3), 330–335. doi:10.1097/00004583-198805000-00011 PMID:3379015

Lambert, N. M., & Hartsough, C. S. (1998). Prospective study of tobacco smoking and substance dependencies among samples of ADHD and non-ADHD participants. *Journal of Learning Disabilities*, *31*(6), 533–544. doi:10.1177/002221949803100603 PMID:9813951

Landau, S., & Moore, L. A. (1991). Social skill deficits in children with attention-deficit hyperactivity disorder. *School Psychology Review*, *20*(2), 235–251.

Langberg, J. M., Epstein, J. N., Altaye, M., Molina, B. S., Arnold, L. E., & Vitiello, B. (2008). The transition to middle school is associated with changes in the developmental trajectory of ADHD symptomatology in young adolescents with ADHD. *Journal of Clinical Child and Adolescent Psychology*, *37*(3), 651–663. doi:10.1080/15374410802148095 PMID:18645755

Lange, K. W., Hauser, J., Lange, K. M., Makulska-Gertruda, E., Nakamura, Y., Reissmann, A., Sakaue, Y., Takano, T., & Takeuchi, Y. (2017). The Role of Nutritional Supplements in the Treatment of ADHD: What the Evidence Says. *Current Psychiatry Reports*, *19*(2), 8. doi:10.100711920-017-0762-1 PMID:28168597

Lange, K. W., Reichl, S., Lange, K. M., Tucha, L., & Tucha, O. (2010). The History of Attention Deficit Hyperactive Disorder. *ADHD Attention Deficit Hyperactivity Disorders*, *2*(4), 241–255. doi:10.100712402-010-0045-8 PMID:21258430

Langer, N., Benjamin, C., Becker, B., & Gaab, N. (2015, June). Comorbidity of reading disabilities and ADHD: Structural and functional brain characteristics. *Human Brain Mapping*, *40*(9), 2677–2698. doi:10.1002/hbm.24552 PMID:30784139

Langley, K., Holmans, P. A., van den Bree, M. B., & Thapar, A. (2007). Effects of low birth weight, maternal smoking in pregnancy and social class on the phenotypic manifestation of attention deficit hyperactivity disorder and associated antisocial behaviour: Investigation in a clinical sample. *BMC Psychiatry*, *7*(1), 26. doi:10.1186/1471-244X-7-26 PMID:17584500

Lang, R., O'Reilly, M., Healy, O., Rispoli, M., Lydon, H., Streusand, W., ... Didden, R. (2012). Sensory integration therapy for autism spectrum disorders: A systematic review. *Research in Autism Spectrum Disorders*, *6*(3), 1004–1018. doi:10.1016/j.rasd.2012.01.006

Lara, C., Fayyad, J., De Graaf, R., Kessler, R. C., Aguilar-Gaxiola, S., Angermeyer, M., Demytteneare, K., de Girolamo, G., Haro, J. M., Jin, R., Karam, E. G., Lépine, J.-P., Mora, M. E. M., Ormel, J., Posada-Villa, J., & Sampson, N. (2009). Childhood predictors of adult attention-deficit/hyperactivity disorder: Results from the World Health Organization World Mental Health Survey Initiative. *Biological Psychiatry*, *65*(1), 46–54. doi:10.1016/j.biopsych.2008.10.005 PMID:19006789

Larsson, H., Chang, Z., D'Onofrio, B. M., & Lichtenstein, P. (2014). The heritability of clinically diagnosed attention deficit hyperactivity disorder across the lifespan. *Psychological Medicine*, *44*(10), 2223–2229. doi:10.1017/S0033291713002493 PMID:24107258

Lasky-Su, J., Anney, R. J., Neale, B. M., Franke, B., Zhou, K., Maller, J. B., ... Faraone, S. V. (2008). Genome-wide association scan of the time to onset of attention deficit hyperactivity disorder. *American Journal of Medical Genetics. Part B, Neuropsychiatric Genetics: The Official Publication of the International Society of Psychiatric Genetics*, *147B*(8), 1355–1358.

Laufer, M. W., Denhoff, E., & Solomons, G. (1957). Hyperkinetic Impulse Disorder in children's behaviour problems. *Psychosomatic Medicine*, *19*(1), 38–49. doi:10.1097/00006842-195701000-00005 PMID:13400991

Laufer, M., & Denhoff, E. (1957). Hyperkinetic behaviour syndrome in children. *The Journal of Pediatrics*, *50*(4), 463–473. doi:10.1016/S0022-3476(57)80257-1 PMID:13406705

Laugesen, B., & Groenkjaer, M. (2015). Parenting experiences of living with a child with attention deficit hyperactivity disorder: A systematic review of qualitative evidence. *JBI Database of Systematic Reviews and Implementation Reports*, *13*(11), 169–234. doi:10.11124/jbisrir-2015-2449 PMID:26657468

Lavoie, R. (2010). *Motivating the Child with Attention Deficit Disorder*. Retrieved from http://www.ldonline.org/article/19975

Lawrence, V., Houghton, S., Douglas, G., Durkin, K., Whiting, K., & Tannock, R. (2004). Executive Function and ADHD: A comparison of children's performance during neuropsychological testing and real-world activities. *Journal of Attention Disorders*, *7*(3), 137–149. doi:10.1177/108705470400700302 PMID:15260171

Lazarus, R. S. (1993). Coping theory and research: Past, present and future. *Psychosomatic Medicine*, *55*(3), 234–247. doi:10.1097/00006842-199305000-00002 PMID:8346332

Lazarus, R. S., & Launier, R. (1978). Stress-Related Transactions between Person and Environment. In L. A. Pervin & M. Lewis (Eds.), *Perspectives in Interactional Psychology* (pp. 287–327). Plenum. doi:10.1007/978-1-4613-3997-7_12

Lecendreux, M., Konofal, E., & Faraone, S. V. (2011). Prevalence of attention deficit hyperactivity disorder and associated features among children in France. *Journal of Attention Disorders*, *15*(6), 516–524. doi:10.1177/1087054710372491 PMID:20679156

Lee, C. S. C., Ma, M. T., Ho, H. Y., Tsang, K. K., Zheng, Y. Y., & Wu, Z. Y. (2017). The Effectiveness of Mindfulness-Based Intervention in Attention on Individuals with ADHD: A Systematic Review. *Hong Kong Journal of Occupational Therapy*, *30*(1), 33–41. doi:10.1016/j.hkjot.2017.05.001 PMID:30186078

Lee, P. C., Niew, W., Yang, H., Chen, V. C., & Lin, K. (2012). A Meta-analysis: Behavioural Parent Training for Children with Attention Deficit Hyperactive Disorder. *Research in Developmental Disabilities*, *33*(6), 2040–2049. doi:10.1016/j.ridd.2012.05.011 PMID:22750360

Lee, S. I., Schachar, R. J., Chen, S. X., Orstein, T. J., Charach, A., Barr, C., & Ickwoicz, A. (2008). Predictive Validity of DSM-IV and ICD-10 Criteria for ADHD and Hyperkinetic Disorder. *Journal of Child Psychology and Psychiatry, and Allied Disciplines*, *49*(1), 70–78. doi:10.1111/j.1469-7610.2007.01784.x PMID:17979965

Lee, S. S., Humphreys, K. L., Flory, K., Liu, R., & Glass, K. (2011). Prospective association of childhood attention-deficit/hyperactivity disorder (adhd) and substance use and abuse/dependence: A meta analytic review. *Clinical Psychology Review*, *31*(3), 328–341. doi:10.1016/j.cpr.2011.01.006 PMID:21382538

Leeth, C. D., Villarreal, V., & Styck, K. M. (2019). Mindfulness Interventions for Children and Adolescents with ADHD: A Review of Objectives and Skills. *Journal of Creativity in Mental Health*, *14*(4), 436–446. doi:10.1080/15401383.2019.1625840

LeFever, G. B., Arcona, A. P., & Antonuccio, D. O. (2003). ADHD among American schoolchildren: Evidence of overdiagnosis and overuse of medication. *The Scientific Review of Mental Health Practice*, *2*, 49–60.

LeFevre, J.-A., Berrigan, L., Vendetti, C., Kamawar, D., Bisanz, J., Skwarchuk, S.-L., & Smith-Chant, B. L. (2012). The role of executive attention in the acquisition of mathematical skills for children in grades 2 through 4. *Journal of Experimental Child Psychology*, *114*(2), 243–261. doi:10.1016/j.jecp.2012.10.005 PMID:23168083

Leitch, S., Scriberras, E., Post, B., Gerner, B., Rinehart, N., Nicholson, J. M., & Evans, S. (2019). Experience of stress in parents of children with ADHD: A qualitative study. *International Journal of Qualitative Studies on Health and Well-being*, *14*(1), 1690091. Advance online publication. doi:10.1080/17482631.2019.1690091 PMID:31713473

Leitner, Y. (2014). The co-occurrence of autism and attention deficit hyperactivity disorder in children–what do we know? *Frontiers in Human Neuroscience*, *8*, 268. doi:10.3389/fnhum.2014.00268 PMID:24808851

Leo, I. M., & Feldman, H. M. (2007). Academic and educational outcomes of children with ADHD [Special issue]. *Journal of Pediatric Psychology*, *32*(6), 643–654. doi:10.1093/jpepsy/jsl054 PMID:17569716

Levin, F. R., & Kleber, H. D. (1995). Attention-deficit hyperactivity disorder and substance abuse: Relationships and implications for treatment. *Harvard Review of Psychiatry*, *2*(5), 246–258. doi:10.3109/10673229509017144 PMID:9384909

Lewis, M. (2002). *Child and Adolescent Psychiatry: A Comprehensive Textbook* (3rd ed.). Lippincott Williams & Wilkins.

Liberman, R. P. (Ed.). (1988). *Psychiatric rehabilitation of chronic mental patients*. American Psychiatric Pub.

Linden, C. B., Zalenski, J. R., & Newman, R. L. (1989). *Pay attention*. Transact Health Systems.

Linnet, K. M., Dalsgaard, S., Obel, C., Wisborg, K., Henriksen, T. B., Rodriguez, A., Kotimaa, A., Moilanen, I., Thomsen, P. H., Olsen, J., & Jarvelin, M. R. (2003). Maternal Lifestyle Factors in Pregnancy Risk of Attention Deficit Hyperactivity Disorder and Associated Behaviors: Review of the Current Evidence. *The American Journal of Psychiatry*, *160*(6), 1028–1040. doi:10.1176/appi.ajp.160.6.1028 PMID:12777257

Lin, Y. F., & Chung, H. H. (2002). Parenting stress and parents' willingness to accept treatment in relation to behavioral problems of children with attention-deficit hyperactive disorder. *The Journal of Nursing Research*, *10*(1), 43–56. doi:10.1097/01.JNR.0000347582.54962.04 PMID:11923900

Lionel, A. C., Tammimies, K., Vaags, A. K., Rosenfeld, J. A., Ahn, J. W., Merico, D., & Gazzellone, M. J. (2014). Disruption of the ASTN2/TRIM32 locus at 9q33. 1 is a risk factor in males for autism spectrum disorders, ADHD and other neurodevelopmental phenotypes. *Human Molecular Genetics*, *23*(10), 2752–2768. doi:10.1093/hmg/ddt669 PMID:24381304

Little, L. M., Dean, E., Tomchek, S., & Dunn, W. (2018). Sensory processing patterns in autism, attention deficit hyperactivity disorder, and typical development. *Physical & Occupational Therapy in Pediatrics*, *38*(3), 243–254. doi:10.1080/01942638.2017.1390809 PMID:29240517

Loe, I.M., & Feldman, H.M. (2007).Academic and educational outcomes of children with ADHD. *Ambulatory Pediatrics: The Official Journal of the Ambulatory Pediatric Association, 7*(1), 82–90.

Lopez-Williams, A., Chacko, A., Wymbs, B. T., Fabiano, G. A., Seymour, K. E., Gnagy, E. M., Chronis, A. M., Burrows-Maclean, L., Pelham, W. E. Jr, & Morris, T. L. (2005). Athletic performance and social behavior as predictors of peer acceptance in children diagnosed with attention-deficit/hyperactivity disorder. *Journal of Emotional and Behavioral Disorders*, *13*(3), 173–180. doi:10.1177/10634266050130030501

Lorch, E. P., Milich, R., Sanchez, R. P., van den Broek, P., Baer, S., Hooks, K., Hartung, C., & Welsh, R. (2000). Comprehension of televised stories in boys with attention deficit/hyperactivity disorder and nonreferred boys. *Journal of Abnormal Psychology*, *109*(2), 321–330. doi:10.1037/0021-843X.109.2.321 PMID:10895570

Loureiro-Vieira, S., Costa, V. M., Lourdes Bastos, M., Carvalho, F., & Capela, J. P. (2017, August). Methylphenidate effects in the young brain: Friend or foe? *International Journal of Developmental Neuroscience*, *60*(1), 34–47. doi:10.1016/j.ijdevneu.2017.04.002 PMID:28412445

Lovecky, D. (1999). *Gifted Children with ADHD*. Program of the 11th Annual CHADD International. Conference, Washington, DC. Retrieved from https://australiangiftedsupport.com/ccmword/wp-content/uploads/2014/12/1352289425.pdf

Lugoboni, F., Levin, F. R., Pieri, M. C., Manfredini, M., Zamboni, L., Somaini, L., Gerra, G., & Gics, G. S.Gruppo InterSert Collaborazione Scientifica (GICS). (2017). Co-occurring Attention Deficit Hyperactivity Disorder symptoms in adults affected by heroin dependence: Patients characteristics and treatment needs. *Psychiatry Research*, *250*, 210–216. doi:10.1016/j.psychres.2017.01.052 PMID:28473157

Lunsky, Y. P., Hastings, R., Weiss, J. A. M., Palucka, A., Hutton, S., & White, K. (2017). Comparative Effects of Mindfulness and Support and Information Group Interventions for Parents of Adults with Autism Spectrum Disorder and Other Developmental Disabilities. *Journal of Autism and Developmental Disorders*, *47*(6), 1769–1779. doi:10.100710803-017-3099-z PMID:28374207

Luoni, C., Balottin, U., Zaccagnino, M., Brembilla, L., Livetti, G., & Termine, C. (2013). Reading difficulties and attention deficit hyperactivity behaviours: Evidence of an early association in a non-clinical sample. *Journal of Research in Reading*, *38*(1), 73–90. doi:10.1111/j.1467-9817.2013.01555.x

Lynn, D. E., Lubke, G., Yang, M., McCracken, J. T., McGough, J. J., Ishii, J., ... Nelson, S. F. (2005). Temperament and character profiles and the dopamine D4 receptor gene in ADHD. [Doi]. *The American Journal of Psychiatry*, *162*(5), 906–913. doi:10.1176/appi.ajp.162.5.906 PMID:15863792

Macey, K. D. (2003). Conners' Adult ADHD Rating Scales (CAARS). *Archives of Clinical Neuropsychology*, *18*(4), 431–437. doi:10.1016/S0887-6177(03)00021-0

Madhiraju, P. (2001). R.I.P. Ritalinin proportion! The Eighth Circuit's restriction on a parent's right to have schools accommodate the needs of their disabled children: Debord and Davis. *Northwestern University Law Review*, *95*, 1661–1697.

Magnus, W., Nazir, S., Arayamparambil, C., Kumar, A., & Shaban, K. (2019). *Attention Deficit Hyperactivity Disorder (ADHD)*. Retrieved from: https://www.ncbi.nlm.nih.gov/books/NBK441838

Maki, D. R., & Tarvydas, V. M. (2012). The Professional Practice of Rehabilitation Counseling: Concepts and Paradigms in Rehabilitation Counseling. Academic Press.

Maldonado, R. (2013). Comparison of the pharmacokinetics and clinical efficacy of new extended-release formulations of methylphenidate. *Expert Opinion on Drug Metabolism & Toxicology*, *9*(8), 1001–1014. doi:10.1517/17425255.2013.786041 PMID:23611637

Mandal, A. M. (2019, February 26). *ADHD Causes and Risk factors. News-Medical.* Retrieved on May 03, 2020 from https://www.news-medical.net/health/ADHD-Causes-and-Risk-factors.aspx

Mangle, L., Phillips, P., Pitts, M., & Laver-Bradbury, C. (2014). Implementation of independent nurse prescribing in UK mental health settings: Focus on attention-deficit/hyperactivity disorder. *ADHD Attention Deficit and Hyperactivity Disorders*, *6*(4), 269–279. doi:10.100712402-014-0138-x PMID:24744052

Manley, M. R. S. (2000). Psychiatric interview, history, and mental status examination. In B. J. Sadock & V. A. Sadock (Eds.), *Kaplan & Sadock's Comprehensive Textbook of Psychiatry* (7th ed., pp. 1426–1455). Lippincott.

Mannuzza, S., & Klein, R. G. (2000). Long-term prognosis in attention-deficit/hyperactivity disorder. *Child and Adolescent Psychiatric Clinics of North America*, *9*(3), 711–726. doi:10.1016/S1056-4993(18)30114-7 PMID:10944664

Mannuzza, S., Klein, R. G., Bessler, A., Malloy, P., & LaPadula, M. (1993). Adult outcome of hyperactive boys: Educational achievement, occupational rank, and psychiatric status. *Archives of General Psychiatry*, *50*(7), 565–576. doi:10.1001/archpsyc.1993.01820190067007 PMID:8317950

Mannuzza, S., Klein, R. G., Bessler, A., Malloy, P., & LaPadula, M. (1998). Adult psychiatric status of hyperactive boys grown up. *The American Journal of Psychiatry*, *155*(4), 493–498. doi:10.1176/ajp.155.4.493 PMID:9545994

Mansour, R., Dovi, A. T., Lane, D. M., Loveland, K. A., & Pearson, D. A. (2017). ADHD severity as it relates to comorbid psychiatric symptomatology in children with autism spectrum disorders (ASD). *Research in Developmental Disabilities*, *60*, 52–64. doi:10.1016/j.ridd.2016.11.009 PMID:27889487

Mao, A. R., & Findling, R. L. (2014). Comorbidities in adult attention-deficit/hyperactivity disorder: A practical guide to diagnosis in primary care. *Postgraduate Medicine*, *126*(5), 42–51. doi:10.3810/pgm.2014.09.2799 PMID:25295649

March, J. S., Parker, J. D. A., Sullivan, K., Stallings, P., & Conners, K. (1997). The multidimensional anxiety scale for children (MASC): Factor structure, reliability, and validity. *Journal of the American Academy of Child and Adolescent Psychiatry*, *36*(4), 554–565. doi:10.1097/00004583-199704000-00019

March, J. S., Swanson, J. M., Arnold, L. E., Hoza, B., Conners, C. K., Hinshaw, S. P., Hechtman, L., Kraemer, H. C., Greenhill, L. L., Abikoff, H. B., Elliott, L. G., Jensen, P. S., Newcorn, J. H., Vitiello, B., Severe, J., Wells, K. C., & Pelham, W. E. (2000). Anxiety as a predictor and outcome variable in the multimodal treatment study of children with ADHD (MTA). *Journal of Abnormal Child Psychology*, *28*(6), 527–541. doi:10.1023/A:1005179014321 PMID:11104315

Markowitz, J. S., & Patrick, K. S. (2017). The clinical pharmacokinetics of amphetamines utilized in the treatment of attention-deficit/hyperactivity disorder. *Journal of Child and Adolescent Psychopharmacology*, *27*(8), 678–689. doi:10.1089/cap.2017.0071 PMID:28910145

Marshal, M. P., Molina, B. S., & Pelham, W. E. Jr. (2003). Childhood ADHD and adolescent substance use: An examination of deviant peer group affiliation as a risk factor. *Psychology of Addictive Behaviors*, *17*(4), 293–302. doi:10.1037/0893-164X.17.4.293 PMID:14640825

Marsh, L. E., Norvilitis, J. M., Ingersoll, T. S., & Li, B. (2015). ADHD symptomatology, fear of intimacy, and sexual anxiety and behavior among college students in China and the Unites States. *Journal of Attention Disorders*, *19*(3), 211–221. doi:10.1177/1087054712453483

Marsh, P. J., & Williams, L. M. (2004). An investigation of individual typologies of AttentionDeficit Hyperactivity Disorder using cluster analysis of DSM-IV criteria. *Personality and Individual Differences*, *36*(5), 1187–1195. doi:10.1016/S0191-8869(03)00210-1

Martel, M. M., Nikolas, M., Jernigan, K., Friderici, K., Waldman, I., & Nigg, J. T. (2011). The dopamine receptor D4 gene (DRD4) moderates family environmental effects on ADHD. *Journal of Abnormal Child Psychology*, *39*(1), 1–10. doi:10.100710802-010-9439-5 PMID:20644990

Martin, C. A., Papadopoulos, N., Chellew, T., Rinehart, N. J., & Sciberras, E. (2019). Associations between parenting stress, parent mental health and child sleep problems for children with ADHD and ASD: Systematic review. *Research in Developmental Disabilities*, *93*, 103463. doi:10.1016/j.ridd.2019.103463 PMID:31446370

Martínez-Zambrano, F., García-Morales, E., García-Franco, M., Miguel, J., Villellas, R., Pascual, G., Arenas, O., & Ochoa, S. (2013). Intervention for reducing stigma: Assessing the influence of gender and knowledge. *World Journal of Psychiatry*, *3*(2), 18–24. doi:10.5498/wjp.v3.i2.18 PMID:24175182

Martin, N., Scourfield, J., & McGuffin, P. (2002). Observer effects and heritability of childhood attention-deficit hyperactivity disorder symptoms. *The British Journal of Psychiatry*, *180*(3), 260–265. doi:10.1192/bjp.180.3.260 PMID:11872519

Mash, E, J., & Johnston, C., (1982). A comparison of the mother-child interactions of younger and older hyperactive and normal children. *Journal of Child Development,* (53), 1371-1381.

Mash, E. J., & Johnston, C. (1983b). Parental perceptions of child behaviour problems, parenting self-esteem, and mothers' reported stress in younger and older hyperactive and normal children. *Journal of Consulting and Clinical Psychology*, *51*(1), 86–99. doi:10.1037/0022-006X.51.1.86 PMID:6826870

Mash, E. J., & Johnston, C. (1990). Determinants of parenting stress: Illustrations from families of hyperactive children and families of physically abused children. *Journal of Clinical Child Psychology*, *19*(4), 313–328. doi:10.120715374424jccp1904_3

Mash, E. J., & Sc Johnston, C. (1983a). Sibling interactions of hyperactive and normal children and their relationship to reports of maternal stress and self-esteem. *Journal of Clinical Child Psychology*, *12*(1), 91–99. doi:10.1080/15374418309533116

Maske, U., & Barnwal, S. (2016). Effect of hatha yogic practices on the level of triiodothyronine (T3) in patients of hyperthyroidism. *International Journal of Applied Research*, *2*(7), 754–757.

Mason, W. A., & Windle, M. (2002). Reciprocal relations between adolescent substance use and delinquency: A longitudinal latent variable analysis. *Journal of Abnormal Psychology*, *111*(1), 63–76. doi:10.1037/0021-843X.111.1.63 PMID:11866180

Mastronardi, C. A., Pillai, E., Pineda, D. A., Martinez, A. F., Lopera, F., Velez, J. I., Palacio, J. D., Patel, H., Easteal, S., Acosta, M. T., Castellanos, F. X., Muenke, M., & Arcos-Burgos, M. (2016). Linkage and association analysis of ADHD endophenotypes in extended and multigenerational pedigrees from a genetic isolate. *Molecular Psychiatry*, *21*(10), 1434–1440. doi:10.1038/mp.2015.172 PMID:26598068

Masuch, T. V., Bea, M., Alm, B., Deibler, P., & Sobanski, E. (2019). Internalized stigma, anticipated discrimination and perceived public stigma in adults with ADHD. *ADHD Attention Deficit and Hyperactivity Disorders*, *11*(2), 211–220. doi:10.100712402-018-0274-9 PMID:30341693

Matos, M., Bauermeister, J. J., & Bernal, G. (2009). Parent-Child Interaction Therapy for Puerto Rican Preschool Children with ADHD and Behaviour Problems: A Pilot Efficacy Study. *Family Process*, *48*(2), 232–252. doi:10.1111/j.1545-5300.2009.01279.x PMID:19579907

Matthews, M., Nigg, J. T., & Fair, D. A. (2014). Attention deficit hyperactivity disorder. *Current Topics in Behavioral Neurosciences*, *16*, 235–266. doi:10.1007/978-3-662-45758-0_249 PMID:24214656

Mayes, R., & Rafalovich, A. (2008). Suffer the restless children: The evolution of ADHD and paediatric stimulant use, 1900–80. *History of Psychiatry*, *18*(72), 435–457. doi:10.1177/0957154X06075782 PMID:18590022

Mayes, S. D., Calhoun, S. L., Baweja, R., Feldman, L., Syed, E., Gorman, A. A., & Siddiqui, F. (2015). Suicide ideation and attempts are associated with co-occurring oppositional defiant disorder and sadness in children and adolescents with ADHD. *Journal of Psychopathology and Behavioral Assessment*, *37*(2), 274–282. doi:10.100710862-014-9451-0

Mayes, S. D., Waschbusch, D. A., Calhoun, S. L., & Mattison, R. E. (2019). How Common are Academic Overachievement and Underachievement in Children with Autism or ADHD? *Journal of Developmental and Physical Disabilities*. Advance online publication. doi:10.100710882-019-09719-8

McBride, B. A., Shoppe, S. J., & Rane, T. R. (2002). Child characteristics, parenting stress and parental involvement: Fathers Vs mothers. *Journal of Marriage and the Family*, *64*(4), 998–1011. doi:10.1111/j.1741-3737.2002.00998.x

McClafferty, H. (2011). (in Review). Complementary, holistic and integrative medicine. *Pediatrics*, *32*, 201–203. doi:10.1542/pir.32-5-201

McCoach, D. B., Siegle, D., & Rubenstein, L. D. (2020). Pay Attention to Innatention: Exploring ADHD Symptoms In A Sample Of Underachieving Gifted Students. *Gifted Child Quarterly*, *64*(2), 100–116. doi:10.1177/0016986219901320

McConaughy, S. H., Ivanova, M. Y., Antshel, K., Eiraldi, R. B., & Dumenci, L. Standardized observational assessment of attention deficit hyperactivity disorder combined and predominantly inattentive subtypes. II. Classroom observations. *School Psychology Review*, 38(3), 362–381. Retrieved from https://www.ncbi.nlm.nih.gov/pmc/articles/PMC2929014/

Mccracken, J. T. (2000). Attention-deficit disorders. In B. J. Sadock & V. A. Sadock (Eds.), *Kaplan & Sadock's Comprehensive Textbook of Psychiatry* (7th ed., pp. 5540–5541). Lippincott.

McGough, J. J. (2017). Adult Manifestations of Attention-Deficit/Hyperactivity Disorder. In B. J. Sadock, V. A. Sadock, & P. Ruiz (Eds.), *Kaplan & Sadock's comprehensive textbook of psychiatry* (10th ed., Vol. 2, p. 3601). Wolters Kluwer.

McGough, J. J., Smalley, S. L., McCracken, J. T., Yang, M., Del'Homme, M., Lynn, D. E., & Loo, S. (2005). Psychiatric comorbidity in adult attention deficit hyperactivity disorder: Findings from multiplex families. *The American Journal of Psychiatry*, *162*(9), 1621–1627. doi:10.1176/appi.ajp.162.9.1621 PMID:16135620

McGrath, L. M., & Stoodley, C. J. (2019). Are there shared neural correlates between dyslexia and ADHD? A meta-analysis of voxel-based morphometry studies. *Journal of Neurodevelopmental Disorders*, *11*(1), 31. doi:10.118611689-019-9287-8 PMID:31752659

McKee, T. E., Harvey, E., Danforth, J. S., Ulaszek, W. R., & Friedman, J. L. (2004). The relation between parental coping styles and parent-child interactions before and after treatment for children with ADHD and oppositional behavior. *Journal of Clinical Child and Adolescent Psychology*, *33*(1), 158–168. doi:10.1207/S15374424JCCP3301_15 PMID:15028550

McLean, A., Dawson, J., Toone, B., Young, S., Bazanis, E., Robbins, T. W., & Sahakian, B. J. (2004). Characteristic neurocognitive profile associated with adult attention-deficit/hyperactivity disorder. *Psychological Medicine*, *34*(4), 681–692. doi:10.1017/S0033291703001296

McMahan, I. (2009). *Adolescence*. Pearson Education.

Mehta, M.A., Owen, A.M., Sahakain, B.J., Mavaddat, N., Pickard, J.D., & Robbins, T.W. (2000). Methylphenidate enhances working memory by modulating discretefrontal and parietal lobe regions in thehuman brain. *J Neurosci, 20*, 1-6.

Meichenbaum, D. H., & Goodman, J. (1971). Training impulsive children to talk to themselves: A means of developing self-control. *Journal of Abnormal Psychology*, *77*(2), 115–126. doi:10.1037/h0030773 PMID:5550424

Meltzer, L. (2007). Executive function difficulties and learning disabilities: Understandings and misunderstandings. In L. Meltzer (Ed.), *Executive function in education: From theory to practice* (pp. 77–105). Guilford.

Meltzer, L., Pollica, L., & Barzillai, M. (2007). Executive function in the classroom: Embedding strategy instruction into daily teaching practice. In L. Meltzer (Ed.), *Executive function in education: From theory to practice* (pp. 165–193).

Mercer, C. D., Mercer, A. R., & Pullen, P. C. (2011). *Teaching Students With Learning Problems* (8th ed.). Pearson.

Merrell, K. W., & Wolfe, T. M. (1998). The relationship of teacher-rated social skills deficits and ADHD characteristics among kindergarten-age children. *Psychology in the Schools*, *35*(2), 101–110. doi:10.1002/(SICI)1520-6807(199804)35:2<101::AID-PITS1>3.0.CO;2-S

Merrill, B. M., Molina, B. S. G., Coxe, S., Gnagy, E. M., Altszuler, A. R., Macphee, F. L., Morrow, A. S., Trucco, E. M., & Pelham, W. E. (2020). Functional Outcomes of Young Adults with Childhood ADHD: A Latent Profile Analysis. *Journal of Clinical Child and Adolescent Psychology*, *49*(2), 215–228. doi:10.1080/15374416.2018.1547968 PMID:30689405

Merzenich, M., van Vleet, T. M., & Nahum, M. (2014). Brain plasticity-based therapeutics. *Frontiers in Human Neuroscience*, *8*, 385-401. Doi:10.3389/fnhum.2014.00385

Meyers, J. E., & Meyers, K. R. (1995). *Rey complex figure test and recognition trial*. Psychological Assessment Resources.

Mick, E., Biederman, J., Faraone, S. V., Sayer, J., & Kleinman, S. (2002). Case-control study of attention-deficit hyperactivity disorder and maternal smoking, alcohol use, and drug use during pregnancy. *Journal of the American Academy of Child and Adolescent Psychiatry*, *41*(4), 378–385. doi:10.1097/00004583-200204000-00009 PMID:11931593

Mikami, A. Y. (2010). The importance of friendship for youth with attention-deficit/hyperactivity disorder. *Clinical Child and Family Psychology Review*, *13*(2), 181–198. doi:10.100710567-010-0067-y

Mikami, A. Y., Chong, G. K., Saporito, J. M., & Na, J. J. (2015). Implications of parental affiliate stigma in families of children with ADHD. *Journal of Clinical Child and Adolescent Psychology*, *44*(4), 595–603. doi:10.1080/15374416.2014.888665 PMID:24697640

Mikami, A. Y., Cox, D. J., Davis, M. T., Wilson, H. K., Merkel, R. L., & Burket, R. (2009). Sex differences in effectiveness of extended-release stimulant medication among adolescents with attention-deficit/hyperactivity disorder. *Journal of Clinical Psychology in Medical Settings*, *16*(3), 233–242. doi:10.100710880-009-9165-8 PMID:19418208

Mikami, A. Y., Huang-Pollock, C. L., Pfiffner, L. J., McBurnett, K., & Hangai, D. (2007). Social skills differences among attention-deficit/hyperactivity disorder types in a chat room assessment task. *Journal of Abnormal Child Psychology*, *35*(4), 509–521. doi:10.100710802-007-9108-5 PMID:17354064

Mikami, A. Y., Smit, S., & Khalis, A. (2017). Social Skills Training and ADHD-What Works? *Current Psychiatry Reports*, *19*(12), 93. doi:10.100711920-017-0850-2 PMID:29082428

Milberger, S., Biederman, J., Faraone, S. V., Chen, L., & Jones, J. (1997). ADHD Is Associated With Early Initiation of Cigarette Smoking in Children and Adolescents. *Journal of the American Academy of Child and Adolescent Psychiatry*, *36*(1), 37–44. doi:10.1097/00004583-199701000-00015 PMID:9000779

Milich, R., & Dodge, K. A. (1984). Social information processing in child psychiatric populations. *Journal of Abnormal Child Psychology*, *12*(3), 471–489. doi:10.1007/BF00910660 PMID:6747124

Milich, R., Whitten, P., Landau, S., & Kilby, G. (1982). Preschool peer perceptions of the behavior of hyperactive and aggressive children. *Journal of Abnormal Child Psychology*, *10*(4), 497–510. doi:10.1007/BF00920750 PMID:7161441

Miller, C. J., Newcorn, J. H., & Halperin, J. M. (2010). Fading memories: Retrospective recall inaccuracies in ADHD. *Journal of Attention Disorders*, *14*(1), 7–14. doi:10.1177/1087054709347189

Miller, L. J. (2006). *Sensational Kids: Help and Hope for Children with Sensory Processing Disorder*. Putnam.

Miller, L. J., Nielsen, D. M., Schoen, S. A., & Brett-Green, B. A. (2009). Perspectives on sensory processing disorder: A call for translational research. *Frontiers in Integrative Neuroscience*, *3*, 22. doi:10.3389/neuro.07.022.2009 PMID:19826493

Mill, J., & Petronis, A. (2008). Pre- and Peri-natal environmental risks for attention-deficit hyperactivity disorder (ADHD): The potential role of epigenetic processes in mediating susceptibility. *Journal of Child Psychology and Psychiatry, and Allied Disciplines*, *49*(10), 1020–1030. doi:10.1111/j.1469-7610.2008.01909.x PMID:18492038

Miltenberger, R. G. (2008). *Behavior Modification: Principles and Procedures* (4th ed.). Thomas Learning Inc.

Mirzaiyan, M., Kunwar, P. S., Uzayisenga, R., & Rashidi, S. (2018). Transcranial Direct Current Stimulation for Treatment of ADHD: A Review of the Mechanisms of Action. *Current Psychiatry Reviews, 14*(4), 215-220.

Mitchison, G. M., & Njardvik, U. (2019). Prevalence and Gender Difference of ODD, Anxiety and Depression in a Sample of Children with ADHD. *Journal of Attention Disorders*, *23*(11), 1339–1345. doi:10.1177/1087054715608442 PMID:26443719

Mochrie, K. D., Whited, M. C., Cellucci, T., Freeman, T., & Corson, A. T. (2020). ADHD, Depression and substance abuse risk among beginning college students. *Journal of American College Health*, *68*(1), 6–10. doi:10.1080/07448481.2018.1515754 PMID:30257141

Modesto-Lowe, V., Chaplin, M., Godsay, V., & Soovajian, V. (2014). Parenting teens with attention-deficit/hyperactivity disorder: Challenges and opportunities. *Clinical Pediatrics*, *53*(10), 943–948. doi:10.1177/0009922814540984 PMID:24982442

Modesto-Lowe, V., Danforth, J. S., Neering, C., & Easton, C. (2010). Can We Prevent Smoking in Children With ADHD: A Review of the Literature. *Connecticut Medicine*, *74*(4), 229–236. PMID:20441004

Modesto-Lowe, V., Farahmand, P., Chaplin, M., & Sarro, L. (2015). Does mindfulness meditation improve attention in attention deficit hyperactivity disorder? *World Journal of Psychiatry*, *5*(4), 397–403. doi:10.5498/wjp.v5.i4.397 PMID:26740931

Mofokeng, M., & van der Wath, A. E. (2017). Challenges experienced by parents living with a child with attention deficit hyperactivity disorder. *Journal of Child and Adolescent Mental Health*, *29*(2), 137–145. doi:10.2989/17280583.2017.1364253 PMID:28974169

Mohammadi, M. R., Farokhzadi, F., Alipour, A., Rostami, R., Dehestani, M., & Salmanian, M. (2012). Marital Satisfaction amongst Parents of Children with Attention Deficit Hyperactivity Disorder and Normal Children. *Iranian Journal of Psychiatry*, *7*(3), 120–125. PMID:23139693

Mohr-Jensen, C., Müller Bisgaard, C., Boldsen, S. K., & Steinhausen, H. C. (2019). Attention-Deficit/Hyperactivity Disorder in Childhood and Adolescence and the Risk of Crime in Young Adulthood in a Danish Nationwide Study. *Journal of the American Academy of Child and Adolescent Psychiatry*, *58*(4), 443–452. doi:10.1016/j.jaac.2018.11.016 PMID:30768385

Mohr-Jensen, C., & Steinhausen, H. C. (2016). A meta-analysis and systematic review of the risks associated with childhood attention-deficit hyperactivity disorder on long-term outcome of arrests, convictions, and incarcerations. *Clinical Psychology Review*, *48*, 32–42. doi:10.1016/j.cpr.2016.05.002 PMID:27390061

Mokrova, I., O'Brien, M., Calkins, S., & Keane, S. (2010). Parental ADHD symptomology and ineffective parenting: The connecting link of home chaos. *Parenting, Science and Practice*, *10*(2), 119–135. doi:10.1080/15295190903212844

Molina, B. S. G., Howard, A. L., Swanson, J. M., Stehli, A., Mitchell, J. T., Kennedy, T. M., Epstein, J. N., Arnold, L. E., Hechtman, L., Vitiello, B., & Hoza, B. (2018). Substance use through adolescence into early adulthood after childhood-diagnosed ADHD: Findings from the MTA longitudinal study. *Journal of Child Psychology and Psychiatry, and Allied Disciplines*, *59*(6), 692–702. doi:10.1111/jcpp.12855 PMID:29315559

Molina, B. S. G., & Pelham, W. E. (2003). Childhood predictors of adolescent substance use in a longitudinal study of children with ADHD. *Journal of Abnormal Psychology*, *112*(3), 497–507. doi:10.1037/0021-843X.112.3.497 PMID:12943028

Molina, B. S. G., Pelham, W. E., Gnagy, E. M., Thompson, A. L., & Marshal, M. P. (2007). Attention-deficit/hyperactivitydisorder risk for heavy drinking and alcohol use disorder is age specific. *Alcoholism, Clinical and Experimental Research*, *31*, 643–654.

Molina, B., Hinshaw, S., Swanson, J., Arnold, L., Vitiello, B., Jensen, P., Epstein, J. N., Hoza, B., Hechtman, L., Abikoff, H. B., Elliott, G. R., Greenhill, L. L., Newcorn, J. H., Wells, K. C., Wigal, T., Gibbons, R. D., Hur, K., & Houck, P. R.MTA Cooperative Group. (2009). The MTA at 8 years: Prospective follow-up of children treated for combined-type ADHD in a multi-site study. *Journal of the American Academy of Child and Adolescent Psychiatry*, *48*(5), 484–500. doi:10.1097/CHI.0b013e31819c23d0 PMID:19318991

Monastra, V. J., Monastra, D. M., & George, S. (2002). The effects of stimulant therapy, EEG biofeedback, and parenting style on the primary symptoms of attention-deficit/ hyperactivity disorder. *Applied Psychophysiology and Biofeedback*, *27*(4), 231–249. doi:10.1023/A:1021018700609 PMID:12557451

Mondal, S., Kundu, B., & Saha, S. (2018). Yoga as therapeutic intervention for the management of type 2 diabetes mellitus. *International Journal of Yoga*, *11*(2), 129–138. doi:10.4103/ijoy.IJOY_74_16

Mongia, M., & Hechtman, L. (2016). Attention-deficit hyperactivity disorder across the lifespan: Review of literature on cognitive behavior therapy. *Current Developmental Disorders Reports*, *3*(1), 7–14. doi:10.100740474-016-0072-z

Montoya, A., Colom, F., & Ferrin, M. (2011). Is psychoeducation for parents and teachers of children and adolescents with ADHD efficacious? A systematic literature review. *European Psychiatry*, *26*(3), 166–175. doi:10.1016/j.eurpsy.2010.10.005 PMID:21292454

Montoya, A., Quail, D., Anand, E., Cardo, E., Alda, J. A., & Escobar, R. (2014). Prognostic factors of improvement in health-related quality of life in atomoxetine-treated children and adolescents with attention-deficit/hyperactivity disorder, based on a pooled analysis. *Attention Deficit and Hyperactivity Disorders*, *6*(1), 25–34. doi:10.100712402-013-0119-5 PMID:24142305

Moore, E., Sunjic, S., Kaye, S., Archer, V., & Indig, D. (2016). Adult ADHD among NSW prisoners: Prevalence and psychiatric comorbidity. *Journal of Attention Disorders*, *20*(11), 958–967. doi:10.1177/1087054713506263 PMID:24134874

Mordre, M., Groholt, B., Kjelsberg, E., Sandstad, B., & Myhre, A. M. (2011). The impact of ADHD and conduct disorder in childhood on adult delinquency: A 30 years follow-up study using official crime records. *BMC Psychiatry*, *11*(1), 57. doi:10.1186/1471-244X-11-57 PMID:21481227

Morgan, C. T., King, R. A., Weisz, J. R., & Scholper, J. (1993). *Introduction to psychology* (7th ed.). Tata McGraw-Hill.

Morris, J. (1998). *Facing AD/HD: A Survival Guide for Parents of Children with Attention Deficit/Hyperactivity Disorder*. Research Press.

Morrison, G. S. & Merrill, E. (1978). *Parent involvement in the home, school and community.* Academic Press.

Morrison, J. R., & Stewart, M. A. (1971). A family study of the hyperactive child syndrome. *Biological Psychiatry, 3*(3), 189–195. PMID:5163807

Morton, W. A., & Stockton, G. G. (2000). Methylphenidate abuse and psychiatric side effects. *Primary Care Companion to the Journal of Clinical Psychiatry, 2*(5), 159–164. doi:10.4088/PCC.v02n0502 PMID:15014637

Motlagh, M. G., Katsovich, L., Thompson, N., Lin, H., Kim, Y., Scahill, L., Lombroso, P. J., King, R. A., Peterson, B. S., & Leckman, J. F. (2010). Severe psychosocial stress and heavy cigarette smoking during pregnancy: An examination of the pre- and perinatal risk factors associated with ADHD and Tourette syndrome. *European Child & Adolescent Psychiatry, 19*(10), 755–764. doi:10.100700787-010-0115-7 PMID:20532931

Mrug, S., Hoza, B., & Gerdes, A. C. (2001). Children with attention-deficit/hyperactivity disorder: Peer relationships and peer-oriented interventions. *New Directions for Child and Adolescent Development, 2001*(91), 51–78. doi:10.1002/cd.5 PMID:11280014

Mrug, S., Molina, B. S., Hoza, B., Gerdes, A. C., Hinshaw, S. P., Hechtman, L., & Arnold, L. E. (2012). Peer rejection and friendships in children with attention-deficit/hyperactivity disorder: Contributions to long-term outcomes. *Journal of Abnormal Child Psychology, 40*(6), 1013–1026. doi:10.100710802-012-9610-2

MTA Cooperative Group. (2004). National Institute of Mental Health Multimodal Treatment study of ADHD follow-up: Changes in effectiveness and growth after the end of treatment. *Pediatrics, 113*(4), 762–769. doi:10.1542/peds.113.4.762 PMID:15060225

Mueller, A. K., Fuermaier, A. B., Koerts, J., & Tucha, L. (2012). Stigma in attention deficit hyperactivity disorder. *Attention Deficit and Hyperactivity Disorders, 4*(3), 101–114. doi:10.100712402-012-0085-3 PMID:22773377

Muktibodhananda, S. (1998). *Hatha Yoga Pradipika.* Yoga Publication Trust.

Muñoz-Silva, A., Lago-Urbano, R., Sanchez-Garcia, M., & Carmona-Márquez, J. (2017). Child/Adolescent's ADHD and Parenting Stress: The Mediating Role of Family Impact and Conduct Problems. *Frontiers in Psychology, 8*, 2252. doi:10.3389/fpsyg.2017.02252 PMID:29312090

Murphy, D. A., Pelham, W. E., & Lang, A. R. (1992). Aggression in boys with attention deficit-hyperactivity disorder: Methylphenidate effects on naturalistically observed aggression, response to provocation, and social information processing. *Journal of Abnormal Child Psychology, 20*(5), 451–466. doi:10.1007/BF00916809 PMID:1487590

Murphy, K. R., & Barkley, R. A. (1996). Attention Deficit Hyperactivity Disorder in adults. *Comprehensive Psychiatry, 37*(6), 393–401. doi:10.1016/S0010-440X(96)90022-X

Murray, C., & Johnston, C. (2006). Parenting in mothers with and without attention-deficit/ hyperactivity disorder. *Journal of Abnormal Psychology, 115*(1), 52–61. doi:10.1037/0021-843X.115.1.52

Murray-Close, D., Hoza, B., Hinshaw, S. P., Arnold, L. E., Swanson, J., Jensen, P. S., ... Wells, K. (2010, November). Developmental Process in Peer Problems of Children with Attention-Deficit/ Hyperactivity Disorder in The Multimodal Treatment Study of Children with ADHD. *Development and Psychopathology, 22*(4), 785–802. doi:10.1017/S0954579410000465 PMID:20883582

Murray, D. W., Lawrence, J. R., & LaForett, D. R. (2018). The Incredible Years® Programs for ADHD in young children: A critical review of the evidence. *Journal of Emotional and Behavioral Disorders, 26*(4), 195–208. doi:10.1177/1063426617717740

Nabors, L. (2020). Substance abuse and anxiety in children. In Anxiety management in children with Mental and Physical health problems. Springer. doi:10.1007/978-3-030-35606-4_4

Naddar, T. S., Silberg, J. L., Eaves, L. J., Maes, H. H., & Meyer, J. M. (1998). Genetic Effects on ADHD Symptomatology in 7-to-13 Year-Old Twins: Results From Telephone Survey. *Behavior Genetics, 28*(2), 83–99. doi:10.1023/A:1021686906396 PMID:9583234

Nadeau, K. (1999). *Understanding girls with ADHD*. Advantage Books.

NairM. K. C.RussellP. (2019). *Parenting*. Retrieved from www.noblevision.in

Najavits, L. M., & Weiss, R. D. (1994). The role of psychotherapy in the treatment of substance-use disorders. *Harvard Review of Psychiatry, 2*(2), 84–96. doi:10.3109/10673229409017121 PMID:9384886

Narkunam, N. (2012). Stress among parents of children with attention deficit hyperactivity disorder, a Malaysian experience. *Journal Asia-Pacific Psychiatry,* 1-10.

Neuman, R. J., Lobos, E., Reich, W., Henderson, C. A., Sun, L.-W., & Todd, R. D. (2007). Prenatal smoking exposure and dopaminergic genotypes interact to cause a severe ADHD subtype. *Biological Psychiatry, 61*(12), 1320–1328. doi:10.1016/j.biopsych.2006.08.049 PMID:17157268

Newcorn, J. H., Kratochvil, C. J., Allen, A. J., Casat, C. D., Ruff, D. D., Moore, R. J., & Michelson, D. (2008). Atomoxetine/Methylphenidate Comparative Study Group: Atomoxetine and osmotically released methylphenidate for the treatment of attention deficit hyperactivity disorder: acute comparison and differential response. *The American Journal of Psychiatry, 165*(6), 721–730. doi:10.1176/appi.ajp.2007.05091676 PMID:18281409

Newcorn, J. H., Weiss, M., & Stein, M. A. (2007). The complexity of ADHD: Diagnosis and treatment of the adult patient with comorbidities. *CNS Spectrums, 12*(S12), 1–16. doi:10.1017/S1092852900026158 PMID:17667893

Newton-Howes, G. (2004). What happens when children with attention deficit/hyperactivity disorder grow up? *Journal of the Royal Society of Medicine, 97*(11), 531–535. PMID:15520147

Ngo, Q. M., Veliz, P. T., Kusunoki, Y., Stein, S. F., & Boyd, C. J. (2018). Adolescent sexual violence: Prevalence, adolescent risks, and violence characteristics. *Preventive Medicine, 116*, 68–74. doi:10.1016/j.ypmed.2018.08.032 PMID:30194960

NICE. (2018). *Attention deficit hyperactivity disorder: diagnosis and management*. Available from: https://www.nice.org.uk/guidance/ng87

Nichols, J. Q. V. A., Shoulberg, E. K., Garner, A. A., Hoza, B., Burt, K. B., Close, D. M., & Arnold, L. E. (2017). Exploration of the Factor Structure of ADHD in Adolescence through Self, Parent, and Teacher Reports of Symptomatology. *Journal of Abnormal Child Psychology, 45*(3), 625–641. doi:10.100710802-016-0183-3

Nigg, J. T. (2001). Is ADHD a disinhibitory disorder? *Psychological Bulletin, 127*(5), 571–598. doi:10.1037/0033-2909.127.5.571 PMID:11548968

Nigg, J. T. (2013). Attention-deficit/hyperactivity disorder and adverse health outcomes. *Clinical Psychology Review, 33*(2), 215–228. doi:10.1016/j.cpr.2012.11.005 PMID:23298633

Nigg, J. T., & Holton, K. (2014, October). Restiction and Elimination Diets in ADHD treatment. *Child & Adolescent Psychiatric Clinics, 23*(4), 937–953. doi:10.1016/j.chc.2014.05.010 PMID:25220094

Nigg, J. T., & Huang-Pollock, C. L. (2003). An early-onset model of the role of executive functions and intelligence in conduct disorder/delinquency. In B. B. Lahey, T. E. Moffitt, & A. Caspi (Eds.), *Cause of conduct disorder and juvenile delinquency* (pp. 227–253). Guilford Press.

Nigg, J., & Nikolas, M. (2008). Attention- deficit /hyperactivity disorder. In T. P. Beauchaine & S. P. Hinshaw (Eds.), *Child and Adolescent Psychopathology* (pp. 323–325). John Wiley.

Nikolas, M., Friderici, K., Waldman, I., Jernigan, K., & Nigg, J. T. (2010). Gene x environment interactions for ADHD: Synergistic effect of 5HTTLPR genotype and youth appraisals of inter-parental conflict. *Behavioral and Brain Functions*, *6*(1), 23. doi:10.1186/1744-9081-6-23 PMID:20398347

NIMH. (2016). *Attention Deficit/ Hyperactivity Disorder (ADHD): The Basics*. NIH Publication.

Ningombam, S., Hutin, Y., & Murhekar, M. V. (2011). Prevalence and pattern of substance use among the higher secondary school students of Imphal, Manipur, India. *The National Medical Journal of India*, *24*(1), 11–15. PMID:21608351

Noordermeer, S. D., Luman, M., Weeda, W. D., Buitelaar, J. K., Richards, J. S., Hartman, C. A., Hoekstra, P. J., Franke, B., Heslenfeld, D. J., & Oosterlaan, J. (2017). Risk factors for comorbid oppositional defiant disorder in attention-deficit/hyperactivity disorder. *European Child & Adolescent Psychiatry*, *26*(10), 1155–1164. doi:10.100700787-017-0972-4 PMID:28283834

Normand, S., Schneider, B. H., Lee, M. D., Maisonneuve, M. F., Kuehn, S. M., & Robaey, P. (2011). How do children with ADHD (mis) manage their real-life dyadic friendships? A multi-method investigation. *Journal of Abnormal Child Psychology*, *39*(2), 293–305. doi:10.100710802-010-9450-x PMID:20824323

Novotni, M. (1999). *What does everybody else know that I don't? Social skills help for adults with attention-deficit hyperactivity disorder (ADHD)*. Speciality Press.

O'Driscoll, C., Heary, C., Hennessy, E., & McKeague, L. (2012). Explicit and implicit stigma towards peers with mental health problems in childhood and adolescence. *Journal of Child Psychology and Psychiatry, and Allied Disciplines*, *53*(10), 1054–1062. doi:10.1111/j.1469-7610.2012.02580.x PMID:22823158

O'Leary, P. A. (1957). Dermatohistopathology of various types of scleroderma. *A.M.A. Archives of Dermatology*, *75*(1), 78–87. doi:10.1001/archderm.1957.01550130080008 PMID:13381197

Oh, W. O., Park, E. S., Suk, M. H., Song, D. H., & Im, Y. (2012). Parenting of children with ADHD in South Korea: The role of socio-emotional development of children with ADHD. *Journal of Clinical Nursing*, *21*(13-14), 1932–1942. doi:10.1111/j.1365-2702.2011.03968.x PMID:22340017

Olfson, M., King, M., & Schoenbaum, M. (2015). Treatment of young people with antipsychotic medications in the United States. *JAMA Psychiatry*, *72*(9), 867–874. doi:10.1001/jamapsychiatry.2015.0500 PMID:26132724

Oliveira, C. T., & Dias, A. C. G. (2018). Psychoeducation for Attention Deðcit/Hyperactivity Disorder: What, How and Who Shall We Inform? *Trends in Psychology/TemasemPsicologia, 26*(1), 263-281.

Osland, S.T., Steeves, T.D.L., & Pringsheim, T. (2018). Pharmacological treatment for attention deficit hyperactivity disorder (ADHD) in children with comorbid tic disorders. *Cochrane Database of Systematic Reviews, 6*.

Ostrander, R., & Herman, K. C. (2006). Potential cognitive, parenting, and developmental mediators of the relationship between ADHD and depression. *Journal of Consulting and Clinical Psychology*, *74*(1), 89–98. doi:10.1037/0022-006X.74.1.89 PMID:16551146

Otto, M. W. (2000). Stories and metaphors in cognitive-behavioral therapy. *Cognitive and Behavioral Practice*, *7*(2), 172–177. doi:10.1016/S1077-7229(00)80027-9

Owens, E., Cardoos, S., & Hinshaw, S. (2014). Developemental Progression and Differences among Individuals with ADHD. In Attention deficit Hyperactive Disorder: A Handbook for Diagnosis and Treatment, (4th ed., pp. 223-255). New York, NY: Guilford Press.

Owens, E. B., & Hinshaw, S. P. (2016). Childhood conduct problems and young adult outcomes among women with childhood attention-deficit/hyperactivity disorder (ADHD). *Journal of Abnormal Psychology*, *125*(2), 220–232. doi:10.1037/abn0000084 PMID:26854507

Pagán, C. N. (n.d.). *ADHD and Risky Behavior in Adults*. https://www.webmd.com/add-adhd/features/adhd-dangerous-risky-behavior#1

Pagnin, D., Grecco, M. L., & Furtado, E. F. (2018). Prenatal alcohol use as a risk for attention-deficit/hyperactivity disorder. *European Archives of Psychiatry and Clinical Neuroscience*. Advance online publication. doi:10.100700406-018-0946-7 PMID:30353263

Palaniappan, P., Seshadri, S., Girimaji, S., & Srinath, S. (2013). Pattern of comorbidities in indian children and adolescents with attention deficit hyperactivity disorder. *European Psychiatry*, *28*, 1. doi:10.1016/S0924-9338(13)77398-X

Pal, R., Singh, S. N., Chatterjee, A., & Saha, M. (2014). Age-related changes in cardiovascular system, autonomic functions, and levels of BDNF of healthy active males: Role of yogic practice. *Age (Dordrecht, Netherlands)*, *36*(4), 9683. doi:10.100711357-014-9683-7

Pan, C. Y., Tsai, C. L., Chu, C. H., Sung, M. C., Huang, C. Y., & Ma, W. Y. (2019). Effects of physical exercise intervention on motor skills and executive functions in children with ADHD: A pilot study. *Journal of Attention Disorders*, *23*(4), 384–397. doi:10.1177/1087054715569282 PMID:25646023

Paris, J., Bhat, V., & Thombs, B. (2015). Is adult attention-deficit hyperactivity disorder being over diagnosed? *Canadian Journal of Psychiatry*, *60*(7), 324–328. doi:10.1177/070674371506000705 PMID:26175391

Parker, J. G., & Asher, S. R. (1987). Peer relations and later personal adjustment: Are low-accepted children at risk? *Psychological Bulletin*, *102*(3), 357–389. doi:10.1037/0033-2909.102.3.357 PMID:3317467

Park, M. J., Paul Mulye, T., Adams, S. H., Brindis, C. D., & Irwin, C. E. Jr. (2006). The health status of young adults in the United States. *The Journal of Adolescent Health*, *39*(3), 305–317. doi:10.1016/j.jadohealth.2006.04.017

Pasamanick, B., Rogers, M. E., & Lilienfeld, A. M. (1956). Pregnancy experience and the development of behaviour disorder in children. *The American Journal of Psychiatry*, *112*(8), 613–618. doi:10.1176/ajp.112.8.613 PMID:13292548

Pasini, A., Paloscia, C., Alessandrelli, R., Porfirio, M. C., & Curatolo, P. (2007). Attention and executive functions profile in drug naive ADHD subtypes. *Brain & Development*, *29*(7), 400–408. doi:10.1016/j.braindev.2006.11.010 PMID:17207595

Patros, C. H., Hudec, K. L., Alderson, R. M., Kasper, L. J., Davidson, C., & Wingate, L. R. (2013). Symptoms of attention-deficit/hyperactivity disorder (ADHD) moderate suicidal behaviors in college students with depressed mood. *Journal of Clinical Psychology*, *69*(9), 980–993. doi:10.1002/jclp.21994

Patterson, G.R. (1980). Mothers: The unacknowledged victims. *Monographs of the Society for Research in Child Development*, *45*(5).

Patterson, T. G., & Joseph, S. (2007). Person-centered personality theory: Support from self-determination theory and positive psychology. *Journal of Humanistic Psychology*, *47*(1), 117–139. doi:10.1177/0022167806293008

Pearson, G. S., & Crowley, A. A. (2013). Attention deficit hyperactivity disorder (ADHD). *Child and Adolescent Behavioral Health*, 139-152. doi:10.1002/9781118704660.ch7

Peck, H., Kehle, T., Bray, M., & Theodore, L. (2005). Yoga as an intervention for children with attention problems. *School Psychology Review*, *34*, 415–424.

Pejović-Milovancević, M., Lecić-Tosevski, D., Tenjović, L., Popović-Deusić, S., & Draganić-Gajić, S. (2009). Changing attitudes of high school students towards peers with mental health problems. *Psychiatria Danubina*, *21*(2), 213–219. PMID:19556951

Pelham, W. E., Jr., &Hoza, B. (1996). *Intensive treatment: A summer treatment program for children with ADHD*. Academic Press.

Pelham, W. E. Jr, Fabiano, G. A., & Massetti, G. M. (2005). Evidence-based assessment of attention deficit hyperactivity disorder in children and adolescents. *Journal of Clinical Child and Adolescent Psychology*, *34*(3), 449–476. doi:10.120715374424jccp3403_5 PMID:16026214

Pennington, B. F. (2006). From single to multiple deficit models of developmental disorders. *Cognition*, *101*(2), 385–413. doi:10.1016/j.cognition.2006.04.008 PMID:16844106

Pennington, B. F., & Ozonoff, S. (1996). Executive functions and developmental psychopathology. *Journal of Child Psychology and Psychiatry, and Allied Disciplines*, *37*(1), 51–87. doi:10.1111/j.1469-7610.1996.tb01380.x

Perera, F. P., Wheelock, K., Wang, Y., Tang, D., Margolis, A. E., Badia, G., Cowell, W., Miller, R. L., Rauh, V., Wang, S., & Herbstman, J. B. (2018). Combined effects of prenatal exposure to polycyclic aromatic hydrocarbons and material hardship on child ADHD behavior problems. *Environmental Research*, *160*, 506–513. doi:10.1016/j.envres.2017.09.002 PMID:28987706

Pettersson, E., Anckarsäter, H., Gillberg, C., & Lichtenstein, P. (2013). Different neurodevelopmental symptoms have a common genetic etiology. *Journal of Child Psychology and Psychiatry, and Allied Disciplines*, *54*(12), 1356–1365. doi:10.1111/jcpp.12113 PMID:24127638

Pettersson, R., Soderstrom, S., Edlund-Soderstrom, K., & Nilsson, K. W. (2017). Internet-based cognitive behavioral therapy for adults with ADHD in outpatient psychiatric care: A randomized trial. *Journal of Attention Disorders*, *21*(6), 508–521. doi:10.1177/1087054714539998

Pfiffner, L. J., Barkley, R. A., & DuPaul, G. J. (2006). Treatment of ADHD in school settings. *Attention deficit hyperactivity disorder: A handbook for diagnosis and treatment*, *3*, 547-589.

Pfiffner, L., & Kaiser, N. (2010). Behavioral parent training, Dulcan's textbook of child and adolescent psychiatry. American Psychiatric Association.

Pheula, G. F., Rohde, L. A., & Schmitz, M. (2011). Are family variables associated with ADHD, inattentive type? A case-control study in schools. *European Child & Adolescent Psychiatry*, *20*(3), 137–145. doi:10.100700787-011-0158-4 PMID:21290154

Philip, J., Patil, N. M., & Kamate, M. (2016). Attention-deficit hyperactivity disorder in children with idiopathic epilepsy: A cross-sectional study. *Indian Journal of Health Sciences and Biomedical Research*, *9*(1), 31–34. doi:10.4103/2349-5006.183682

Philipp-Wiegmann, F., Rösler, M., Clasen, O., Zinnow, T., Retz-Junginger, P., & Retz, W. (2018). ADHD modulates the course of delinquency: A 15-year follow-up study of young incarcerated man. *European Archives of Psychiatry and Clinical Neuroscience*, *268*(4), 391–399. doi:10.100700406-017-0816-8 PMID:28612143

Pingali, S., & Sunderajan, J. (2014). A study of comorbidities in attention deficit hyperactivity disorder: A retrospective analysis of case records. *Andhra Pradesh Journal of Psychological Medicine*, *15*(2), 206–210.

Pingault, J. B., Côté, S. M., Lacourse, E., Galéra, C., Vitaro, F., & Tremblay, R. E. (2013). Childhood hyperactivity, physical aggression and criminality: A 19-year prospective population-based study. *PLoS One*, *8*(5), e62594. doi:10.1371/journal.pone.0062594 PMID:23658752

Plantation, F. L., (1993). *Children & Adults with Attention Deficit Disorders (CHADD). The disability named ADD.* Academic Press.

Pliszka, S. (2007). Practice parameter for the assessment and treatment of the children and adolescents with attention deficit/ hyperactivity disorder. *Journal of the American Academy of Child and Adolescent Psychiatry*, *46*(7), 894–921. doi:10.1097/chi.0b013e318054e724 PMID:17581453

Podolski, C. L., & Nigg, J. T. (2001). Parent stress and coping in relation to child ADHD severity and associated child disruptive behavior problems. *Journal of Clinical Child Psychology*, *30*(4), 503–513. doi:10.1207/S15374424JCCP3004_07 PMID:11708238

Pohlabeln, H., Rach, S., De Henauw, S., Eiben, G., Gwozdz, W., & Pigeot, I. (2017). Further evidence for the role of pregnancy-induced hypertension and other early life influences in the development of ADHD: Results from the IDEFICS study. *European Child & Adolescent Psychiatry*, *26*(8), 957–967. doi:10.100700787-017-0966-2 PMID:28258320

Polanczyk, G. V., Willcutt, E. G., Salum, G. A., Kieling, C., & Rohde, L. A. (2014). ADHD prevalence estimates across three decades: An updated systematic review and meta-regression analysis. *International Journal of Epidemiology*, *43*(2), 434–442. doi:10.1093/ije/dyt261 PMID:24464188

Polanczyk, G., Lima, M., Horta, B. L., Biederman, J., & Rohde, L. A. (2007). The Worldwide Prevalence of ADHD: A Systematic Review and Metaregression Analysis. *The American Journal of Psychiatry*, *164*(6), 942–948. doi:10.1176/ajp.2007.164.6.942 PMID:17541055

Poulton, A. (2005). Growth on stimulant medication; clarifying the confusion: A review. *Archives of Disease in Childhood*, *90*(8), 801–806. doi:10.1136/adc.2004.056952 PMID:16040876

Preston, J., O'Neal, J. H., & Talaga, M. C. (2017). *Handbook of clinical psychopharmacology for therapists.* New Harbinger Publications.

Prinstein, M. J., Boergers, J., & Vernberg, E. M. (2001). Overt and relational aggression in adolescents: Social-psychological adjustment of aggressors and victims. *Journal of Clinical Child Psychology*, *30*(4), 479–491. doi:10.1207/S15374424JCCP3004_05 PMID:11708236

Psychoeducation: Definition, goals and methods. (2014). Retrieved from http://www.aipc.net.au/articles/psychoeducation-definition-goals-and-methods

Psychogiou, L., Daley, D. M., Thompson, M. J., & Sonuga-Barke, E. J. (2008). Do maternal attention-deficit/hyperactivity disorder symptoms exacerbate or ameliorate the negative effect of child attention-deficit/hyperactivity disorder symptoms on parenting? *Development and Psychopathology*, *20*(1), 121–137. doi:10.1017/S0954579408000060 PMID:18211731

Purdie, N., Hattie, J., & Carroll, A. (2002). A review of the research on interventions for attention deficit hyperactivity disorder: What works best? *Review of Educational Research*, *72*(1), 61–99. doi:10.3102/00346543072001061

Quinlan, D. M. (2000). Assessment of attention-deficit/hyperactivity disorder and comorbidities. In T. E. Brown (Ed.), *Attention-deficit disorders and comorbidities in children, adolescents, and adults* (pp. 455–508). American Psychiatric Press.

Rafalovich, A. (2001). The conceptual history of attention deficit hyperactivity disorder: Idiocy, imbecility, encephalitis and the child deviant, 1877–1929. *Deviant Behavior*, *22*(2), 93–115. doi:10.1080/016396201750065009

Ramsay, J. R. (2017). Assessment and monitoring of treatment response in adult ADHD patients: Current perspectives. *Neuropsychiatric Disease and Treatment, 13*, 221–232. doi:10.2147/NDT.S104706 PMID:28184164

Ramsay, J. R., & Rostain, A. L. (2005). Adapting psychotherapy to meet the needs of adults with attention-deficit/hyperactivity disorder. *Psychotherapy (Chicago, Ill.), 42*(1), 72–84. doi:10.1037/0033-3204.42.1.72

Ramsay, R. J. (2010). *Nonmedication Treatments for Adult ADHD: Evaluating Impact on Daily Functioning and Well-Being*. American Psychological Association. doi:10.1037/12056-000

Rasmussen, P. D., Storebø, O. J., Shmueli-Goetz, Y., Bojesen, A. B., Simonsen, E., & Bilenberg, N. (2018). Childhood ADHD and treatment outcome: The role of maternal functioning. *Child and Adolescent Psychiatry and Mental Health, 12*(1), 31. doi:10.118613034-018-0234-3 PMID:29983736

Rasmussen, P., & Gillberg, C. (2000). Natural outcome of ADHD with developmental coordination disorder at age 22 years: A controlled, longitudinal, community-based study. *Journal of the American Academy of Child and Adolescent Psychiatry, 39*(11), 1424–1431. doi:10.1097/00004583-200011000-00017 PMID:11068898

Rau, S., Skapek, M. F., Tiplady, K., Seese, S., Burns, A., Armour, A. C., & Kenworthy, L. (2020). Identifying comorbid ADHD in autism: Attending to the inattentive presentation. *Research in Autism Spectrum Disorders, 69*, 101468. doi:10.1016/j.rasd.2019.101468

Rayan, A., & Ahmad, M. (2018). Mindfulness and parenting distress among parents of children with disabilities: A literature review. *Perspectives in Psychiatric Care, 54*(2), 324–330. doi:10.1111/ppc.12217 PMID:28247409

Reale, L., Bartoli, B., Cartabia, M., Zanetti, M., Costantino, M. P., Canevini, M. P., Termine, C., & Bonati, M.Lombardy ADHHD Group. (2017). Comobidity, Prevalence & Treatment Outcome in Children and Adolescents with ADHD. *European Child & Adolescent Psychiatry, 26*(12), 1443–1457. doi:10.100700787-017-1005-z PMID:28527021

Reardon & Naglieri. (1992). PASS cognitive processing characteristics of normal and ADHD males. *Journal of School Psychology, 30*(2).

Reed, G. M., First, M. B., Kogan, C. S., Hyman, S. E., Gureje, O., Gaebel, W., Maj, M., Stein, D. J., Maercker, A., Tyrer, P., Claudino, A., Garralda, E., Salvador-Carulla, L., Ray, R., Saunders, J. B., Dua, T., Poznyak, V., Medina-Mora, M. E., Pike, K. M., ... Saxena, S. (2019). Innovations and changes in the ICD-11 classification of mental, behavioural and neurodevelopmental disorders. *World Psychiatry; Official Journal of the World Psychiatric Association (WPA), 18*(1), 3–19. doi:10.1002/wps.20611 PMID:30600616

Reich, W. (2000). Diagnostic Interview for Children and Adolescents (DICA). *Journal of the American Academy of Child and Adolescent Psychiatry, 39*(1), 59–66. doi:10.1097/00004583-200001000-00017

Reid, R. (1996). Self-monitoring for students with learning disabilities: The present, the prospects, the pitfalls. *Journal of Learning Disabilities, 29*(3), 317–331. doi:10.1177/002221949602900311 PMID:8732894

Reid, R., & Lienemann, T. O. (2006a). *Strategy in- struction for students with learning disabilities*. Guilford.

Reimherr, F. W., Marchant, B. K., Strong, R. E., Hedges, D. W., Adler, L., Spencer, T. J., West, S. A., & Soni, P. (2005). Emotional dysregulation in adult ADHD and response to atomoxetine. *Biological Psychiatry, 58*(2), 125–131. doi:10.1016/j.biopsych.2005.04.040 PMID:16038683

Reinhardt, M. C., & Reinhardt, C. A. (2013). Attention deficit-hyperactivity disorder, comorbidities, and risk situations. *The Journal of Pediatrics, 89*(2), 124–130. doi:10.1016/j.jped.2013.03.015 PMID:23642421

Rejani, T. G., Oommen, A., Srinath, S., & Kapur, M. (2012). Efficacy of Multimodal Intervention for Children with Attention Deficit Hyperactivity Disorder (ADHD)- An Indian Study. *Journal of Behavioral and Brain Science*, *2*(01), 117–127. doi:10.4236/jbbs.2012.21014

Resnick, R. J. (2005). Attention deficit hyperactivity disorder in teens and adults: They don't all outgrow it. *Journal of Clinical Psychology*, *61*(5), 529–533. doi:10.1002/jclp.20117

Retz, W., Freitag, C. M., Retz-Junginger, P., Wenzler, D., Schneider, M., Kissling, C., Thome, J., & Rösler, M. (2008). A functional serotonin transporter promoter gene polymorphism increases ADHD symptoms in delinquents: Interaction with adverse childhood environment. *Psychiatry Research*, *158*(2), 123–131. doi:10.1016/j.psychres.2007.05.004 PMID:18155777

Reyes, C. Y. (2010). *What is psycho-education?* Retrieved from http://thepsychoeducationalteacher.blogspot.com/2010/10/what-is-psycho-education.html

Reynolds, C. R., & Kamphaus, R. W. (2015). *Behavior Assessment System for Children. 3*. Pearson.

Rhee, S. H., Waldman, I. D., Hay, D. A., & Levy, F. (1999). Sex differences in genetic and environmental influences on DSM–III–R attention-deficit/hyperactivity disorder. *Journal of Abnormal Psychology*, *108*(1), 24–41. doi:10.1037/0021-843X.108.1.24 PMID:10066990

Riccio, C. A., Wolfe, M., Davis, B., Romine, C., George, C., & Lee, D. (2005). Attention deficit hyperactivity disorder: Manifestation in adulthood. *Archives of Clinical Neuropsychology*, *20*(2), 249–269. doi:10.1016/j.acn.2004.07.005 PMID:15708734

Richters, J.E., Arnold, L.E., Jensen, P.S., Abikoff, H., & Conners, C.K. (1995). IMH collaborative multisite multi-modal treatment study of children with ADHD: I. Background andrationale. *Journal of the American Academy of Child and Adolescent Psychiatry, 34*, 987-1000.

Rief, S. F. (2016). *How to reach and teach children and teens with ADD/ADHD*. Jossey-Bass.

Riggar, T. F., & Maki, D. R. (2003). *Handbook of Rehabilitation Counseling: Concepts and Paradigms*. Springer Publishing Company.

Riggs, P. D., Winhusen, T., Davies, R. D., Leimberger, J. D., Mikulich-Gilbertson, S., Klein, C., Macdonald, M., Lohman, M., Bailey, G. L., Haynes, L., Jaffee, W. B., Haminton, N., Hodgkins, C., Whitmore, E., Trello-Rishel, K., Tamm, L., Acosta, M. C., Royer-Malvestuto, C., Subramaniam, G., ... Liu, D. (2011). Randomized controlled trial of osmotic-release methylphenidate with cognitive-behavioral therapy in adolescents with attention-deficit/ hyperactivity disorder and substance-use disorders. *Journal of the American Academy of Child and Adolescent Psychiatry*, *50*(9), 903–914. doi:10.1016/j.jaac.2011.06.010 PMID:21871372

Ringer, N., Wilder, J., Scheja, M., & Gustavsson, A. (2019). Managing children with challenging behaviours. Parents' meaning-making processes in relation to their children's ADHD diagnosis. *International Journal of Disability Development and Education*. Advance online publication. doi:10.1080/1034912X.2019.1596228

Rivera-Flores, G. W. (2015). Self-instructional cognitive training to reduce impulsive cognitive style in children with Attention Deficit with Hyperactivity Disorder. *Electronic Journal of Research in Educational Psychology*, *13*(1), 27–46.

Rivero, O., Selten, M. M., Sich, S., Popp, S., Bacmeister, L., Amendola, E., ... Schmitt, A. G. (2015). Cadherin-13, a risk gene for ADHD and comorbid disorders, impacts GABAergic function in hippocampus and cognition. *Translational Psychiatry*, *5*(10), e655. doi:10.1038/tp.2015.152 PMID:26460479

Robbins, C. A. (2005). ADHD couple and family relationships: Enhancing communication and understanding through imago relationship therapy. *Journal of Clinical Psychology*, *61*(5), 567–577. doi:10.1002/jclp.20120

Roberts, S. (n.d.). *Patanjali's Eightfold path of yoga*. Retrieved from https://yoga.sherry-roberts.com/patanjali-and-his-eightfold-path-of-yoga/

Robin, A., Koepke, T., Moye, A., & Gerhardstein, R. (2009). Assessment of the parent-adolescent relationship in teens with ADHD. *The ADHD Report*, *17*(5), 1–6. doi:10.1521/adhd.2009.17.5.1

Robin, A., & Payson, E. (2000). Can your marriage survive ADHD? Presented at the *Children and Adults with ADD (CHADD) National Conference*, Chicago, IL.

Rockhill, C., Violette, H., Vander Stoep, A., Grover, S., & Myers, K. (2013). Caregivers' distress: Youth with attention-deficit/hyperactivity disorder and comorbid disorders assessed via telemental health. *Journal of Child and Adolescent Psychopharmacology*, *23*(6), 379–385. doi:10.1089/cap.2013.0019 PMID:23952184

Roelofs, J., Meesters, C., ter Huurne, M., Bamelis, L., & Muris, P. (2006). On the links between attachment style, parental rearing behaviours, and internalizing and externalizing problems in non-clinical children. *Journal of Child and Family Studies*, *15*(3), 331–345. doi:10.100710826-006-9025-1

Rogers, C. R. (1940). The processes of therapy. *Journal of Consulting Psychology*, *4*(5), 161–164. doi:10.1037/h0062536

Rogers, M. A., Wiener, J., Marton, I., & Tannock, R. (2009). Parental involvement in children's learning: Comparing parents of children with and without Attention-Deficit/Hyperactivity Disorder (ADHD). *Journal of School Psychology*, *47*(3), 167–185. doi:10.1016/j.jsp.2009.02.001 PMID:19328285

Rogers, M. A., Wiener, J., Marton, I., & Tannock, R. (2009). Supportive and controlling parental involvement as predictors of children' academic achievement: Relations to children's ADHD symptoms and parenting stress. *School Mental Health*, *1*(2), 89–102. doi:10.100712310-009-9010-0

Rokeach, A., & Wiener, J. (2014). The romantic relationships of adolescents with ADHD. *Journal of Attention Disorders*, 1–11.

Román-Ithier, J. C., González, R. A., Vélez-Pastrana, M. C., González-Tejera, G. M., & Albizu-García, C. E. (2017). Attention deficit hyperactivity disorder symptoms, type of offending and recidivism in a prison population: The role of substance dependence. *Criminal Behaviour and Mental Health*, *27*(5), 443–456. doi:10.1002/cbm.2009 PMID:27455899

Romero-Martínez, Á., Lila, M., & Moya-Albiol, L. (2019). The importance of impulsivity and attention switching deficits in perpetrators convicted for intimate partner violence. *Aggressive Behavior*, *45*(2), 129–138. doi:10.1002/ab.21802 PMID:30474120

Rommelse, N. N., Oosterlaan, J., Buitelaar, J., Faraone, S. V., & Sergeant, J. A. (2007). Time reproduction in children with ADHD and their nonaffected siblings. *Journal of the American Academy of Child and Adolescent Psychiatry*, *46*(5), 582–590. doi:10.1097/CHI.0b013e3180335af7 PMID:17450049

Rommelse, N. N., Van der Stigchel, S., Witlox, J., Geldof, C., Deijen, J. B., Theeuwes, J., Oosterlaan, J., & Sergeant, J. A. (2008). Deficits in visuo-spatial working memory, inhibition and oculomotor control in boys with ADHD and their non-affected brothers. *Journal of Neural Transmission (Vienna, Austria)*, *115*(2), 249–260. doi:10.100700702-007-0865-7 PMID:18253811

Roskam, I., Stievenart, M., Meunier, J.-C., & Noël, M.-P. (2014). The development of children's inhibition: Does parenting matter? *Journal of Experimental Child Psychology*, *122*, 166–182. doi:10.1016/j.jecp.2014.01.003 PMID:24607865

Ros, R., & Graziano, P. A. (2018). Social functioning in children with or at risk for attention deficit/hyperactivity disorder: A meta-analytic review. *Journal of Clinical Child and Adolescent Psychology*, *47*(2), 213–235. doi:10.1080/15374416.2016.1266644 PMID:28128989

Ross, A., & Thomas, S. (2010). The health benefits of yoga and exercise: A review of comparison studies. *Journal of Alternative and Complementary Medicine (New York, N.Y.)*, *16*(1), 3–12. doi:10.1089/acm.2009.0044

Rothbaum, F., & Weisz, J. R. (1994). Parental caregiving and child externalizing behaviour in nonclinical samples: A meta-analysis. *Psychological Bulletin*, *116*(1), 55–74. doi:10.1037/0033-2909.116.1.55

Rowland, A. S., Skipper, B. J., Rabiner, D. L., Qeadan, F., Campbell, R. A., Naftel, A. J., & Umbach, D. M. (2018). Attention-deficit/hyperactivity disorder (ADHD): Interaction between socioeconomic status and parental history of ADHD determines prevalence. *Journal of Child Psychology and Psychiatry, and Allied Disciplines*, *59*(3), 213–222. doi:10.1111/jcpp.12775 PMID:28801917

Rubia, K., Smith, A., & Taylor, E. (2007). Performance of children with Attention Deficit Hyperactivity Disorder (ADHD) on a test battery of impulsiveness. *Child Neuropsychology*, *13*(3), 276–304. doi:10.1080/09297040600770761 PMID:17453834

Rubin, K. H., Chen, X., McDougall, P., Bowker, A., & McKinnon, J. (1995). The Waterloo Longitudinal Project: Predicting internalizing and externalizing problems in adolescence. *Development and Psychopathology*, *7*(4), 751–764. doi:10.1017/S0954579400006829

Rucklidge, J. J., Downs-Woolley, M., Taylor, M., Brown, J. A., & Harrow, S. E. (2016). Psychiatric comorbidities in a New Zealand sample of adults with ADHD. *Journal of Attention Disorders*, *20*(12), 1030–1038. doi:10.1177/1087054714529457 PMID:24743977

Runnheim, V. A., Frankenberger, W. R., & Hazelkorn, M. N. (1996). Medicating students with emotional and behavioral disorders and ADHD: A state survey. *Behavioral Disorders*, *21*(4), 306–314. doi:10.1177/019874299602100405

Russell, A. E., Ford, T., & Russell, G. (2015). Socioeconomic associations with ADHD: Findings from a mediation analysis. *PLoS One*, *10*(6), e0128248. doi:10.1371/journal.pone.0128248 PMID:26030626

Rutter, M. (2005). Environmentally mediated risks for psychopathology: Research strategies and findings. *Journal of Child Psychology and Psychiatry, and Allied Disciplines*, *44*(1), 3–18.

Sadati, A. K., Salehzade, H., Hemmati, S., Darvish, M., Heydari, S. T., & Tabrizi, R. (2015). The Causal Factors Associated with the Loving Care of the Mothers of Children with Multiple Disabilities. *International Journal of Community Based Nursing and Midwifery*, *3*(4), 309–317. PMID:26448958

Sadock, B. J., Kaplan, H. I., & Sadock, V. A. (2007). *Kaplan &Sadock's synopsis of psychiatry: Behavioral sciences/clinical psychiatry* (10th ed.). Wolter Kluwer.

Sadock, B. J., Sadock, V. A., & Ruiz, P. (2015). *Kaplan & Sadock's synopsis of psychiatry: Behavioral sciences/clinical psychiatry* (11th ed.). Wolters Kluwer.

Safer, D. (1997). Central stimulant treatment of childhood attention deficit hyperactivity disorder: Issues and recommendations from a US perspective. *CNS Drugs*, *7*(4), 264–272. doi:10.2165/00023210-199707040-00002 PMID:27520752

Safren, S. A., Otto, M. W., Sprich, S., Winett, C. L., Wilens, T. E., & Biederman, J. (2005). Cognitive-behavioral therapy for ADHD in medication-treated adults with continued symptoms. *Behaviour Research and Therapy*, *43*(7), 831–842. doi:10.1016/j.brat.2004.07.001 PMID:15896281

Safren, S. A., Perlman, C. A., Sprich, S. E., & Otto, M. W. (2005). *Mastering your adult ADHD: A cognitive behavioral treatment program, therapist guide*. Oxford University Press.

Safren, S. A., Sprich, S., & Mimiaga, M. J. (2010). Cognitive behavioral therapy vs relaxation with educational support for medicationtreated adults with ADHD and persistent symptoms: A randomized controlled trial. *Journal of the American Medical Association*, *304*(8), 875–880. doi:10.1001/jama.2010.1192 PMID:20736471

Sagiv, S. K., Epstein, J. N., Bellinger, D. C., & Korrick, S. A. (2012). Pre- and postnatal risk factors for ADHD in a nonclinical pediatric population. *Journal of Attention Disorders*, *17*(1), 47–57. doi:10.1177/1087054711427563 PMID:22298092

Sagvolden, T., Johansen, E. B., Aase, H., & Russell, V. A. (2005). A dynamic developmental theory of attention-deficit/hyperactivity disorder (ADHD) predominantly hyperactive/impulsive and combined subtypes. *Behavioral and Brain Sciences*, *28*(3), 397–419. doi:10.1017/S0140525X05000075

Sakellari, E., Lehtonen, K., Sourander, A., Kalokerinou-Anagnostopoulou, A., & Leino-Kilpi, H. (2014). Greek adolescents' views of people with mental illness through drawings: Mental health education's impact. *Nursing & Health Sciences*, *16*(3), 358–364. doi:10.1111/nhs.12113 PMID:24382318

Sakellari, E., Leino-Kilpi, H., & Kalokerinou-Anagnostopoulou, A. (2011). Educational interventions in secondary education aiming to affect pupils' attitudes towards mental illness: A review of the literature. *Journal of Psychiatric and Mental Health Nursing*, *18*(2), 166–176. doi:10.1111/j.1365-2850.2010.01644.x PMID:21299729

Salehinejad, M. A., & Nejati, V. (2019). Cognition-engaging physical exercise for improving cognitive impairments in attention-deficit hyperactivity disorder: A behavioral medicine approach. *Heart and Mind*, *3*(2), 73. doi:10.4103/hm.hm_54_19

Salmivalli, C., Kaukiainen, A., & Lagerspetz, K. (2000). Aggression and sociometric status among peers: Do gender and type of aggression matter? *Scandinavian Journal of Psychology*, *41*(1), 17–24. doi:10.1111/1467-9450.00166 PMID:10731839

Saluja, B. S., Grover, S., Irpati, S. R., Mattoo, S. K., & Basu, D. (2004). Drug dependence in adolescents 1978-2003: A clinical –based observation from north India. *Indian Journal of Pediatrics*, *74*(5), 455–458. doi:10.100712098-007-0077-z PMID:17526956

Salvatore, J. E., Kuo, S., Steele, R. D., Simpson, J. A., & Collins, W. (2011). Recovering from conflict in romantic relationships: A developmental perspective. *Psychological Science*, *22*(3), 376–383. doi:10.1177/0956797610397055

Samiei, M., Daneshmand, R., Keramatfar, R., Khooshabi, K., Amiri, N., Farhadi, Y., Farzadfard, S. Z., Kachooi, H., & Samadi, R. (2015). Attention Deficit Hyper Activity Disorder (ADHD) and Stress: A Mutual Relationship between Children and Mothers. *Basic and Clinical Neuroscience*, *6*(2), 113–121. PMID:27307956

Sánchez, M., Lavigne, R., Romero, J. F., & Elósegui, E. (2019). Emotion regulation in participants diagnosed with attention deficit hyperactivity disorder, before and after an emotion regulation intervention. *Frontiers in Psychology*, *10*, 10. doi:10.3389/fpsyg.2019.01092 PMID:31178779

Sánchez-Mora, C., Richarte, V., & Garcia-Martínez, I. (2015). Dopamine receptor DRD4 gene and stressful life events in persistent attention deficit hyperactivity disorder. *Neuropsychiatric Genetics, Part B of the American Journal of Medical Genetics*, *168*, 480-491.

Sanctis, V. A. D., Trampush, J. W., Harty, S. C., Marks, D. J., Newcorn, J. H., Miller, C., & Halperin, J. M. (2008). Childhood Maltreatment and Conduct Disorder: Independent Predictors of Adolescent Substance Use Disorders in Youth With Attention Deficit/Hyperactivity Disorder. *Journal of Clinical Child and Adolescent Psychology*, *37*(4), 785–793. doi:10.1080/15374410802359650 PMID:18991129

Sander, J. W., & Shorvon, S. D. (1996). Epidemiology of the epilepsies. *Journal of Neurology, Neurosurgery, and Psychiatry, 61*(5), 433–443. doi:10.1136/jnnp.61.5.433 PMID:8965090

Sangal, R. B., Owens, J., Allen, A. J., Sutton, V., Schuh, K., & Kelsey, D. (2006). Effects of atomoxetine and methylphenidate on sleep in children with ADHD. *Sleep, 29*(12), 1573–1585. doi:10.1093leep/29.12.1573 PMID:17252888

Santosh, P. J., Taylor, E., Swanson, J., Wigal, T., Chuang, S., & Davies, M. (2005). Refining the diagnoses of inattention and over activity syndromes: A reanalysis of the Multimodal Treatment study of attention deficit hyperactivity disorder (ADHD) based on ICD-10 criteria for hyperkinetic disorder. *Clinical Neuroscience Research*, (5), 295–306.

Saraswati, S. S. (1969). *Asana Pranayama Mudra Bandha. Yoga Publication Trust.*

Satchitananda, S. (2011). Meditation. Internal Yoga Publication.

Sauer, J. M., Ring, B. J., & Witcher, J. W. (2005). Clinical pharmacokinetics of atomoxetine. *Clinical Pharmacokinetics, 44*(6), 571–590. doi:10.2165/00003088-200544060-00002 PMID:15910008

Saules, K. K., Pomerleau, C. S., & Schubiner, H. (2003). Patterns of inattentive and hyperactive symptomatology in cocaine-addicted and non-cocaine-addicted smokers diagnosed with adult attention deficit hyperactivity disorder. *Journal of Addictive Diseases, 22*(2), 71–78. doi:10.1300/J069v22n02_06 PMID:12703670

Sayal, K., Washbrook, E., & Propper, C. (2015). Childhood behavior problems and academic outcomes in adolescence: Longitudinal population-based study. *Journal of the American Academy of Child and Adolescent Psychiatry, 54*(5), 360–8.e2. doi:10.1016/j.jaac.2015.02.007 PMID:25901772

Saylor, K. E., & Amann, B. H. (2016). Impulsive aggression as a comorbidity of attention-deficit/hyperactivity disorder in children and adolescents. *Journal of Child and Adolescent Psychopharmacology, 26*(1), 19–25. doi:10.1089/cap.2015.0126 PMID:26744906

Schachar, R., & Ickowicz, A. (2003). Attention-deficit hyperkinetic disorders in childhood and adolescence. In M. G. Gelder, J. J. Lopez-Ibor, N. Andreasen, & J. J. Lopez-Idor (Eds.), *New Oxford Textbook of Psychiatry* (pp. 1365–1366). Oxford University Press.

Schachar, R., Mota, V. L., Logan, G. D., Tannock, R., & Klim, P. (2000). Confirmation of an inhibitory control deficit in attention-deficit/hyperactivity disorder. *Journal of Abnormal Child Psychology, 28*(3), 227–235. doi:10.1023/A:1005140103162 PMID:10885681

Schachar, R., Taylor, E., Wieselberg, M., Thorley, G., & Rutter, M. (1987). Changes in family function and relationships in children who respond to Methylphenidate. *Journal of the American Academy of Child and Adolescent Psychiatry, 26*(5), 728–732. doi:10.1097/00004583-198709000-00019 PMID:3667503

Schaughency, E. A., & Lahey, B. B. (1985). Mothers' and Fathers' perceptions of child deviance: Roles of child behaviour, parental depression and marital satisfaction. *Journal of Consulting and Clinical Psychology, 53*(5), 718–723. doi:10.1037/0022-006X.53.5.718 PMID:4056189

Schmidt, S., & Petermann, F. (2009). Developmental psychopathology: Attention deficit hyperactivity disorder (ADHD). *BMC Psychiatry, 9*(1), 58. doi:10.1186/1471-244X-9-58 PMID:19761584

Schmiedeler, S. (2015). Mindfulness-based intervention in attention-deficit-/hyperactivity disorder (ADHD. *Zeitschrift fur Kinder- und Jugendpsychiatrie und Psychotherapie, 43*(2), 123–131. doi:10.1024/1422-4917/a000341 PMID:25769764

Schnabel, W. (2005). Nicotine use in suicides: A case–control study Barbara Schneider Axel. *European Psychiatry, 20*(2), 129–136. doi:10.1016/j.eurpsy.2004.04.016 PMID:15797697

Schredl, M., Alm, B., & Sobanski, E. (2007). Sleep quality in adult patients with attention deficit hyperactivity disorder (ADHD). *European Archives of Psychiatry and Clinical Neuroscience, 257*(3), 164–168. doi:10.100700406-006-0703-1 PMID:17131215

Schroeder, R. D., & Mowen, T. J. (2014). Parenting style transitions and delinquency. *Youth & Society, 46*(2), 228–254. doi:10.1177/0044118X12469041

Schubiner, H., Tzelepis, A., Milberger, S., Lockhart, N., Kruger, M., Kelley, B. J., & Schoener, E. P. (2000). Prevalence of attention-deficit/hyperactivity disorder and conduct disorder among substance abusers. *The Journal of Clinical Psychiatry, 61*(4), 244–251. doi:10.4088/JCP.v61n0402 PMID:10830144

Schunk, D. (1990). Goal setting and self-efficacy dur- ing self-regulated learning. *Educational Psychologist, 25*(1), 71–86. doi:10.120715326985ep2501_6

Sciberras, E., Mulraney, M., Silva, D., & Coghill, D. (2017). Prenatal risk factors and the etiology of ADHD—Review of existing evidence. *Current Psychiatry Reports, 19*(1), 1. Advance online publication. doi:10.100711920-017-0753-2 PMID:28091799

Scime, M., & Norvilitis, J. M. (2006). Task perfor- mance and response to frustration in children with attention deficit hyperactivity disorder. *Psychology in the Schools, 43*(3), 377–386. doi:10.1002/pits.20151

Scott, J. G., & Schoenberg, M. R. (2011). Frontal lobe/executive functioning. In The little black book of neuropsychology (pp. 219-248). Springer.

Scuitto, M., & Eisenberg, M. (2007). Evaluating the evidence for and against the overdiagnosis of ADHD. *Journal of Attention Disorders, 11*(2), 106–113. doi:10.1177/1087054707300094 PMID:17709814

Seiffge-Krenke, I. (2003). Testing theories of romantic development from adolescence to young adulthood: Evidence of a developmental sequence. *International Journal of Behavioral Development, 27*(6), 519–531. doi:10.1080/01650250344000145

Seligman, L. D., & Ollendick, T. H. (2011). Cognitive behavioral therapy for anxiety disorders in youth. *Child and Adolescent Psychiatric Clinics of North America, 20*(2), 217–238. doi:10.1016/j.chc.2011.01.003 PMID:21440852

Seligman, L., & Reichenberg, L. W. (2016). *Selecting effective treatments: A comprehensive, systematic guide to treating mental disorders* (5th ed.). John Wiley & Sons.

Seltzer, M. M., Greenberg, J. S., Floyd, F. J., Pettee, Y., & Hong, J. (2001). Life course impacts of parenting a child with a disability. *American Journal of Mental Retardation, 106*(3), 265–286. doi:10.1352/0895-8017(2001)106<0265:LCIOPA>2.0.CO;2 PMID:11389667

Selye, H. (1956). *The stress of life*. McGraw-Hill.

Sergeant, J. A., Geurts, H., Huijbregts, S., Scheres, A., & Oosterlaan, J. (2003). The top and the bottom of ADHD: A neuropsychological perspective. *Neuroscience and Biobehavioral Reviews, 27*(7), 583–592. doi:10.1016/j.neubiorev.2003.08.004 PMID:14624803

Shah, R., Grover, S., & Avasthi, A. (2019). Clinical practice guidelines for the assessment and management of attention deficit/hyperactivity disorder. *Indian Journal of Psychiatry, 61*(8), 176–193. doi:10.4103/psychiatry.IndianJPsychiatry_543_18 PMID:30745695

Shapiro, E., & Derr, T. (1987). School Interventions for Aggression. *Special Services in the Schools, 3*(4), 5-19. doi: / doi:10.1300/j008v03n03_02

Sharp, C. (2002). Sex Differences in Antisocial Behaviour: Conduct Disorder, Delinquency and Violence in the Dunedin Longitudinal Study. By T. Moffitt, A. Caspi, M. Rutter and P. Silva.(Pp. 278;£ 14.95/$21.95.) Cambridge University Press: Cambridge. 2001. *Psychological Medicine*, *32*(8), 1475–1478. doi:10.1017/S0033291702216670

Shaw, P., Stringaris, A., Nigg, J., & Leinbenluft, E. (2014, March). Emotion Dysregulation in Attention-Deficit/Hyperactivity Disorder. *The American Journal of Psychiatry*, *171*(3), 276–293. doi:10.1176/appi.ajp.2013.13070966 PMID:24480998

Shaywitz, S. E., & Shaywitz, B. A. (1984). (in Review). Evaluation and treatment of children with attention deficit disorders. *Pediatrics*, *6*(4), 99–109.

Sheir, A. C., Reichenbacher, T., Ghuman, H. S., & Ghuman, J. K. (2012). Pharmacological Treatment of Attention Deficit Hyperactivity Disorder in Children and Adolescents: Clinical Strategies. *Journal of Central Nervous System Disease*, *5*, 1–17. doi:10.4137/JCNSD.S6691 PMID:23650474

Sherwin, E. (2012). *The Oxford Handbook of Rehabilitation Psychology: A field in flux - The History of Rehabilitation Psychology*. Oxford University Press Inc.

Shmueli-Goetz, Y., Target, M., Fonagy, P., & Datta, A. (2008). The Child Attachment Interview: A psychometric study of reliability and discriminant validity. *Developmental Psychology*, *44*(4), 939–956. doi:10.1037/0012-1649.44.4.939 PMID:18605826

Sibley, M. H., Comer, J. S., & Gonazalez, J. (2017). Delivering Parent-Teen Therapy for ADHD through Videoconferencing: A preliminary investigation. *Journal of Psychopathology and Behavioral Assessment*, *39*(3), 467–485. doi:10.100710862-017-9598-6

Sibley, M. H., Evans, S. W., & Serpell, Z. N. (2010). Social cognition and interpersonal impairment in young adolescents with ADHD. *Journal of Psychopathology and Behavioral Assessment*, *32*(2), 193–202. doi:10.100710862-009-9152-2

Sibley, M. H., Kuriyan, A. B., Evans, S. W., Waxmonsky, J. G., & Smith, B. H. (2014). Pharmacological and psychosocial treatments for adolescents with ADHD: An updated systematic review of the literature. *Clinical Psychology Review*, *34*(3), 218–232. doi:10.1016/j.cpr.2014.02.001

Sibley, M. H., Pelham, E. M., Molina, B. S. G., Gnaggy, E. M., Waschbusch, D. A., Garefino, A. C., & … . (2012). Diagnosing ADHD in Adolescence. *Journal of Consulting and Clinical Psychology*, *80*(1), 139–150. doi:10.1037/a0026577

Sibley, M. H., Pelham, W. E., Molina, B. S. G., Gnagy, E. M., Waschbusch, D. A., Biswas, A., MacLean, M. G., Babinski, D. E., & Karch, K. M. (2011). TheDelinquency Outcomes of Boys with ADHD with and without comorbidity. *Journal of Abnormal Child Psychology*, *39*(1), 21–32. doi:10.100710802-010-9443-9

Sibley, M. H., & Yeguez, C. E. (2018). The Impact of DSM-5 A-Criteria on Parent Ratings of ADHD in Adolescents. *Journal of Attention Disorders*, *22*(1), 83–91. doi:10.1177/1087054714526040 PMID:24626330

Siev, J., & Chambless, D. L. (2007). Specificity of treatment effects: Cognitive therapy and relaxation for generalized anxiety and panic disorders. *Journal of Consulting and Clinical Psychology*, *75*(4), 513–522. doi:10.1037/0022-006X.75.4.513 PMID:17663606

Silverstein, M. J., Faraone, S. V., Leon, T. L., Biederman, J., Spencer, T. J., & Adler, L. A. (2018). The Relationship Between Executive Function Deficits and DSM-5 Defined ADHD Symptoms. *Journal of Attention Disorders*, *24*(1), 41–51. doi:10.1177/1087054718804347 PMID:30296883

Simon, A. (2016). Prenatal, Perinatal and Postnatal Risk Facotrs for Attention Deficit Hyperactivity Disorder in India- A Retrospective Analysis. *Indian Journal of Applied Research*, *6*(4).

Simon, V., Czobor, P., Bálint, S., Mészáros, A., & Bitter, I. (2009). Prevalence and correlates of adult attention-deficit hyperactivity disorder: Meta-analysis. *The British Journal of Psychiatry*, *194*(3), 204–211. doi:10.1192/bjp.bp.107.048827 PMID:19252145

Sinfield, J. (2019, August 11). *How Is ADHD Treated for Children and Adults?* Verywell Mind. https://www.verywellmind.com/adhd-treatment-4157278

Singh, N. N. (1995). In search of unity: Some thoughts on the family- professional relationships in service delivery systems. *Journal of Child and Family Studies*, *4*(1), 3–18. doi:10.1007/BF02233951

Sinha, R., & O'Malley, S. S. (2000). Alcohol and Eating Disorders: Implications for Alcohol Treatment and Health Services Research. *Alcoholism, Clinical and Experimental Research*, *24*(8), 1312–1319. doi:10.1111/j.1530-0277.2000.tb02097.x PMID:10968671

Sinzig, J., Morsch, D., & Lehmkuhl, G. (2008). Do hyperactivity, impulsivity inattention have an impact on the ability of facial affect recognition in children with autism and ADHD? *European Child & Adolescent Psychiatry*, *17*(2), 63–72. doi:10.100700787-007-0637-9 PMID:17896119

Siregar, J., & Wimbarti, S. (2018). Screening for the hyperkinetic disorder by using strength and difficulties questionnaire teacher report (SDQ-TR) in Indonesia school-aged children. *Global Journal of Psychology Research: New Trends and Current Issues*, *8*(2), 76–87. doi:10.18844/gjpr.v8i2.3490

Sitnick, S. L., Galán, C. A., & Shaw, D. S. (2019). Early childhood predictors of boys' antisocial and violent behavior in early adulthood. *Infant Mental Health Journal*, *40*(1), 67–83. doi:10.1002/imhj.21754 PMID:30576588

Skirrow, C., Hosang, G. M., Farmer, A. E., & Asherson, P. (2012). An update on the debated association between ADHD and bipolar disorder across the lifespan. *Journal of Affective Disorders*, *141*(2-3), 143–149. doi:10.1016/j.jad.2012.04.003 PMID:22633181

Skogheima, T. S., Villangera, G. D., Vegard, K., Weydea, S. M., Engelb, P. S., Øiec, M. G., ... Aasea, H. (2020). Prenatal exposure to perfluoroalkyl substances and associations with symptoms of attention-deficit/hyperactivity disorder and cognitive functions in preschool children. *International Journal of Hygiene and Environmental Health*, 223. PMID:31653559

Slesnick, N., Kaminer, Y., & Kelly, J. (2008). Most common psychosocial intervention for adolescent use disorder. In Y. Kaminer & O. G. Bukstien (Eds.), *Adolescent substance abuse: psychiatric comorbidity and high risk behaviors*. Routledge, Taylor, and Francis Group.

Slobodin, O., & Crunelle, C. L. (2019). Mini review: Socio-cultural influences on the link between ADHD and SUD. *Frontiers in Public Health*, *7*, 173–186. doi:10.3389/fpubh.2019.00173 PMID:31294015

Smith, A. L., Hoza, B., Linnea, K., McQuade, J. D., Tomb, M., Vaughn, A. J., Shoulberg, E. K., & Hook, H. (2013). Pilot physical activity intervention reduces severity of ADHD symptoms in young children. *Journal of Attention Disorders*, *17*(1), 70–82. doi:10.1177/1087054711417395 PMID:21868587

Smith, B. H., Pelham, W. E. Jr, Gnagy, E., Molina, B., & Evans, S. (2000). The reliability, validity, and unique contributions of self-report by adolescents receiving treatment for attention-deficit/hyperactivity disorder. *Journal of Consulting and Clinical Psychology*, *68*(3), 489–499. doi:10.1037/0022-006X.68.3.489

Smith, T. E., & Martel, M. M. (2019). Trait-Based Profiles of ADHD in Adolescents and Young Adults. *Journal of Clinical Child and Adolescent Psychology*, *48*(3), 440–454. doi:10.1080/15374416.2018.1491004

Sobob, M. P., Ashbourne, D. T., Earn, B. M., & Cunningham, C. E. (1989). ' Parents' attributions for achieving compliance from attention-deficit-disordered children. *Journal of Abnormal Child Psychology*, *17*(3), 359–369. doi:10.1007/BF00917405 PMID:2754118

Sodano, S. M., Tamulonis, J. P., Fabiano, G. A., Caserta, A. M., Hulme, K. F., Hulme, K. L., Stephan, G. R., & Tronci, F. (2019). Interpersonal Problems of Young Adults With and Without Attention-Deficit/Hyperactivity Disorder. *Journal of Attention Disorders*. doi:10.1177/1087054718821728 PMID:30614417

Solanto, M. (2011). *Cognitive-Behavioral Therapy for Adult ADHD: Targeting Executive Dysfunction*. Guilford Press.

Solanto, M., Abikoff, H., Sonuga-Barke, E., Schachar, R., Logan, G. D., Wigal, T., Hechtman, L., Hinshaw, S., & Turkel, E. (2001). The ecological validity of delay aversion and response inhibition as measures of impulsivity in ADHD: A supplement to the NIMH multi-modal treatment study of AD/HD. *Journal of Abnormal Child Psychology*, *29*(3), 215–228. doi:10.1023/A:1010329714819 PMID:11411784

Sontag, T. A., Tucha, O., Walitza, S., & Lange, K. W. (2010). Animal models of attention deficit/hyperactivity disorder (ADHD): A critical review. *ADHD Attention Deficit and Hyperactivity Disorders*, *2*(1), 1–20. doi:10.100712402-010-0019-x PMID:21432586

Sonuga-Barke, E., Dalen, L., & Remington, B. (2003). Do executive deficits and delay aversion make independent contributions to preschool Attention Deficit/Hyperactivity Disorder symptoms? *Journal of the American Academy of Child & Adolescent Psychiatrists*, *42*(11), 1335–1342. doi:10.1097/01.chi.0000087564.34977.21 PMID:14566171

Sonuga-Barke, E., Daley, D., Thompson, M., Laver-Bradbury, C., & Weeks, A. (2001). Parent-based therapies for preschool attention-deficit/hyperactivity disorder: A randomized, controlled trial with a community sample. *Journal of the American Academy of Child and Adolescent Psychiatry*, *40*(4), 402–408. doi:10.1097/00004583-200104000-00008 PMID:11314565

Sorensen, L., Plessen, K. J., Nicholas, J., & Lundervold, A. J. (2011). Is behavioral regulation in children with ADHD aggravated by comorbid anxiety disorders? *Journal of Attention Disorders*, *15*(1), 56–66. doi:10.1177/1087054709356931 PMID:20071639

Sparrow, E. P., & Erhardt, D. (2014). *Essentials of ADHD Assessment for Children and Adolescents*. John Wiley & Sons.

Spencer, T. J. (2004). ADHD treatment across the life cycle. *The Journal of Clinical Psychiatry*, *65*(3), 22–26.

Spencer, T. J. (2006). ADHD and comorbidity in childhood. *The Journal of Clinical Psychiatry*, *67*(8), 27–31. PMID:16961427

Spencer, T., Biederman, J., Wilens, T., & Faraone, S. (1994). Is attention deficit hyperactivity disorder in adults a valid disorder? *Harvard Review of Psychiatry*, *1*(6), 326–335. doi:10.3109/10673229409017099 PMID:9384867

Sprich, S. E., Safren, S. A., Finkelstein, D., Remmert, J. E., & Hammerness, P. (2016). A randomized controlled trial of cognitive behavioral therapy for ADHD in medication treated adolescents. *Journal of Child Psychology and Psychiatry, and Allied Disciplines*, *57*(11), 1218–1226. doi:10.1111/jcpp.12549

Srinivasaraghavan, R., Mahadevan, S., & Kattimani, S. (2013). Impact of Comorbidity on Three Month Follow-up Outcome of Children with ADHD in a Child Guidance Clinic: Preliminary Report. *Indian Journal of Psychological Medicine*, *35*(4), 346–351. doi:10.4103/0253-7176.122223 PMID:24379493

Stahl, S. M. (n.d.). *Stahl's Essential Psychopharmacology Neuroscientific Basis and Practical Application* (4th ed.). Cambridge University Press.

Ståhlberg, O., Boman, S., Robertsson, C., Kerekes, N., Anckarsäter, H., & Nilsson, T. (2017). A 3-year follow-up study of Swedish youths committed to juvenile institutions: Frequent occurrence of criminality and health care use regardless of drug abuse. *International Journal of Law and Psychiatry*, *50*, 52–60. doi:10.1016/j.ijlp.2016.09.004 PMID:27745884

Stamler, J., Rose, G., Stamler, R., Elliott, P., Dyer, A., & Marmot, M. (1989). INTERSALT study findings. Public health and medical care implications. *Hypertension*, *14*(5), 570–577. doi:10.1161/01.HYP.14.5.570

Steinhausen, H.-C. (2009). The heterogeneity of causes and courses of attention-deficit hyperactivity disorder. *Acta Psychiatrica Scandinavica*, *120*(5), 392–399. doi:10.1111/j.1600-0447.2009.01446.x

Stergiakouli, E., & Thapar, A. (2010). Fitting the pieces together: Current research on the genetic basis of attention-deficit/hyperactivity disorder (ADHD). *Journal of Neuropsychiatric Disease and Treatment*, *6*, 551–560. doi:10.2147/NDT.S11322

Stevenson, C. S., Whitmont, S., Bornholt, L., Livesey, D., & Stevenson, R. J. (2002). A cognitive remediation programme for adults with Attention Deficit Hyperactivity Disorder. *The Australian and New Zealand Journal of Psychiatry*, *36*(5), 610–616. doi:10.1046/j.1440-1614.2002.01052.x PMID:12225443

Stickley, A., Koposov, R., Koyanagi, A., Inoue, Y., & Ruchkin, V. (2019). ADHD and depressive symptoms in adolescents: The role of community violence exposure. *Social Psychiatry and Psychiatric Epidemiology*, *54*(6), 683–691. doi:10.100700127-019-01662-5 PMID:30706080

Still, G. F. (1902). The Coulsonian lectures on some abnormal physical conditions in children. *Lancet*, *I*, 1008–1012, 1077–1082, 1163–1168.

Storebø, O. J., Gluud, C., Winkel, P., & Simonsen, E. (2012). Social-skills and parental training plus standard treatment versus standard treatment for children with ADHD–the randomised SOSTRA trial. *PLoS One*, *7*(6), e37280. doi:10.1371/journal.pone.0037280 PMID:22745657

Storebø, O. J., Pedersen, N., Ramstad, E., Kielsholm, M. I., Nielsen, S. S., Krogh, H. B., & … . (2018). Methylpheidate for attention deficit hyperactivity disorder (ADHD) in children and adolescents – assessment of possible adverse events in non-randomised studies. *Cochrane Database of Systematic Reviews*, *5*, CD012069. PMID:29744873

Storebø, O. J., Ramstad, E., Krogh, H. B., Nilausen, T. D., Skoog, M., Holmskov, M., & … . (2015). Methyphenidate for children and adolescents with attention deficit hyperactivity disorder (ADHD). *Cochrane Database of Systematic Reviews*, *1*, CD009885. PMID:26599576

Storebö, O. J., & Simonsen, E. (2016). The Association between ADHD and Antisocial Personality Disorder (ASPD): A Review. *Journal of Attention Disorders*, *20*(10), 815–824. doi:10.1177/1087054713512150 PMID:24284138

Stormont, M. (2001). Social outcomes of children with AD/HD: Contributing factors and implications for practice. *Psychology in the Schools*, *38*(6), 521–531. doi:10.1002/pits.1040

Stormont-Spurgin, M., & Zentall, S. S. (1996). Child-rearing practices associated with aggression in youth with and without ADHD: An Exploratory Study. *International Journal of Disability Development and Education*, *43*(2), 135–146. doi:10.1080/0156655960430204

Strang, J. F., Kenworthy, L., Dominska, A., Sokoloff, J., Kenealy, L. E., Berl, M., Walsh, K., Menvielle, E., Slesaransky-Poe, G., Kim, K.-E., Luong-Tran, C., Meagher, H., & Wallace, G. L. (2014). Increased gender variance in autism spectrum disorders and attention deficit hyperactivity disorder. *Archives of Sexual Behavior*, *43*(8), 1525–1533. doi:10.100710508-014-0285-3

Strattera® (atomoxetine capsules) [strattera summary of product characteristics]. (2015). Eli Lilly and Company Ltd.

Strauss, A. A., & Lehtinen, L. E. (1947). *Psychopathology and Education of the Brain-Injured Child*. Grune and Stratton.

Stroop, J. R. (1935). Studies of interference in serial verbal reactions. *Journal of Experimental Psychology*, *18*(6), 643–662. doi:10.1037/h0054651

Stubbs, A. (2014). Reducing mental illness stigma in health care students and professionals: A review of the literature. *Australasian Psychiatry*, *22*(6), 579–584. doi:10.1177/1039856214556324 PMID:25371444

Substance Abuse and Mental Health Services Administration. (2016). *Co-occurring disorders*. Received from www.samhsa.gov/disorders/co-occurring

Sucksdorff, M., Brown, A. S., Chudal, R., Surcel, H. M., Salomaki, S. H., Postava, K. C., ... Sourander, A. (2019). Maternal Vitamin D Levels and the Risk of Offspring Attention-Deficit/ Hyperactivity Disorder. *Journal of the American Academy of Child and Adolescent Psychiatry*. Advance online publication. doi:10.1016/j.jaac.2019.11.021 PMID:31863882

Sultan, R. S., Wang, S., Crystal, S., & Olfson, M. (2019). Antipsychotic Treatment Among Youths With Attention-Deficit/ Hyperactivity Disorder. *JAMA Network Open*, *2*(7), e197850. doi:10.1001/jamanetworkopen.2019.7850 PMID:31348506

Surkan, P. J., Zhang, A., Trachtenberg, F., Daniel, D., McKinlay, S., & Bellinger, D. (2007). Neuropsychological function in children with blood lead levels <10 microg/dL. *Neurotoxicology*, *28*(6), 1170–1177. doi:10.1016/j.neuro.2007.07.007 PMID:17868887

Swanson, J. M., Schuck, S., Mann, M., Carlson, C., Hartman, K., Sergeant, J. A., & Wigal, T. (2001). *Categorical and dimensional definitions and evaluations of symptoms of ADHD: the SNAP and SWAN ratings scales*. Academic Press.

Swanson, J. M., Kinsbourne, M., Nigg, J., Lanphear, B., Stephanatos, G. A., Volkow, N., ... Wadhwa, P. D. (2007). Etiological Subtypes of Attention Deficit/Hyperactivity Disorder: Brain Imaging, Molecular Genetic & Environmental Factors and the Dopamine Hypothesis. *Neuropsychology Review*, *17*(1), 39–59. doi:10.100711065-007-9019-9 PMID:17318414

Swanson, J., Gupta, S., Guinta, D., Flynn, D., Agler, D., Lerner, M., Williams, L., Shoulson, I., & Wigal, S. (1999). Acute tolerance to methylphenidate in the treatment of attention deficit hyperactivity disorder in children. *Clinical Pharmacology and Therapeutics*, *66*(3), 295–305. doi:10.1016/S0009-9236(99)70038-X PMID:10511066

Swendsen, J. D., & Merikangas, K. R. (2000). The comorbidity of depression and substance use disorders. *Clinical Psychology Review*, *20*(2), 173–189. doi:10.1016/S0272-7358(99)00026-4 PMID:10721496

Szatmari, P. (1992). The epidemiology of attention-deficit hyperactivity disorders. In G. Weiss (Ed.), *Child and adolescent psychiatry clinics of North America: Attention deficit disorder* (pp. 361–372). W. B. Saunders.

Szobot, C. M., Rohde, L. A., Bukstein, O., Molina, B. S. G., Martins, C., Ruaro, P., & Pechansky, F. (2007). Is attention-deficit/hyperactivity disorder associated with illicit substance use disorders in male adolescents? A community-based case-control study. *Addiction (Abingdon, England)*, *102*(7), 1122–1130. doi:10.1111/j.1360-0443.2007.01850.x PMID:17567400

Takahashi, K., Miyawaki, D., Suzuki, F., Mamoto, A., Matsushima, N., Tsuji, H., Horino, A., Ballas, P. A., & Kiriike, N. (2007). Hyperactivity and comorbidity in Japanese children with attention-deficit/ hyperactivity disorder. *Psychiatry and Clinical Neurosciences*, *61*(3), 255–262. doi:10.1111/j.1440-1819.2007.01651.x PMID:17472593

Tallmadge, J. M., Paternite, C. E., & Gordon, M. (1989). *Hyperactivity and aggression in parent-child interaction: Test of a two-factor theory*. Paper presented at the meeting of the Society for Research in Child Development, Kanas City, MO.

Tallmadge, J., & Barkley, R. A. (1983). The interactions of hyperactive and normal boys' with their fathers and mothers. *Journal of Child Psychology and Psychiatry, and Allied Disciplines*, *11*(4), 565–580. PMID:6655156

Tannock, T., & Schachar, L. G. D. (1995). Methylphenidate and cognitive flexibility: dissociated dose effects in hyperactive children. *Journal of Abnormal Child Psychology, 23*, 235-267.

Tarver, J., Daley, D., & Sayal, K. (2014). Attention-deficit hyperactivity disorder (ADHD): An updated review of the essential facts. *Child: Care, Health and Development*, *40*(6), 762–774. doi:10.1111/cch.12139 PMID:24725022

Taşkıran, S., Mutluer, T., Tufan, A. E., & Semerci, B. (2017). Understanding the associations between psychosocial factors and severity of crime in juvenile delinquency: A cross-sectional study. *Neuropsychiatric Disease and Treatment*, *18*(13), 1359–1366. doi:10.2147/NDT.S129517 PMID:28572731

Taurines, R., Schmitt, J., Renner, T., Conner, A. C., Warnke, A., & Romanos, M. (2010). Developmental comorbidity in attention-deficit/hyperactivity disorder. *Attention Deficit and Hyperactivity Disorders*, *2*(4), 267–289. doi:10.100712402-010-0040-0 PMID:21432612

Taylor, F. B., & Russo, J. (2000). Efficacy of modafinil compared to dextroamphetamine for the treatment of attention deficit hyperactivity disorder in adults. *Journal of Child and Adolescent Psychopharmacology*, *10*(4), 311–320. doi:10.1089/cap.2000.10.311 PMID:11191692

Teichner, G. (2016). *Attention-Deficit/Hyperactivity Disorder in Children and Adolescents: A DSM-5 Handbook for Medical and Mental Health Professionals*. Momentum Press.

Teixeira, M. C., Marino, R. L., & Carreiro, L. R. (2015). Associations between Inadequate Parenting Practices and Behavioral Problems in Children and Adolescents with Attention Deficit Hyperactivity Disorder. *The Scientific World Journal*, *683062*. Advance online publication. doi:10.1155/2015/683062 PMID:26844292

Telman, L. G. E., van Steensel, F. J. A., Maric, M., & Bögels, S. M. (2017). Are Anxiety Disorders in Children and Adolescents Less Impairing Than ADHD and Autism Spectrum Disorders? Associations with Child Quality of Life and Parental Stress and Psychopathology. *Child Psychiatry and Human Development*, *48*(6), 891–902. doi:10.100710578-017-0712-5 PMID:28176178

Thapar, A., & Cooper, M. (2016). Attention deficit hyperactivity disorder. *Lancet*, *387*(10024), 1240–1250. doi:10.1016/S0140-6736(15)00238-X PMID:26386541

Thapar, A., Cooper, M., Jefferies, R., & Stergiakouli, E. (2012). What causes attention deficit hyperactivity disorder? *Archives of Disease in Childhood*, *97*(3), 260–265. doi:10.1136/archdischild-2011-300482 PMID:21903599

Thapar, A., Fowler, T., Rice, F., Scourfield, J., van den Bree, M., Thomas, H., Harold, G., & Hay, D. (2003). Maternal smoking during pregnancy and attention deficit hyperactivity disorder symptoms in offspring. *The American Journal of Psychiatry*, *160*(11), 1985–1989. doi:10.1176/appi.ajp.160.11.1985 PMID:14594745

Thapar, A., Harrington, R., & McGuffin, P. (2001). Examining the comorbidity of ADHD-related behaviours and conduct problems using a twin study design. *The British Journal of Psychiatry*, *179*(3), 224–229. doi:10.1192/bjp.179.3.224

Thapar, A., van den Bree, M., Fowler, T., Langley, K., & Whittinger, N. (2006). Predictors of antisocial behaviour in children with attention deficit hyperactivity disorder. *European Child & Adolescent Psychiatry*, *15*(2), 118–125. doi:10.100700787-006-0511-1

The MTA Cooperative Group. (1999). A 14-month randomized clinical trial of treatment strategies for attention-deficit/hyperactivity disorder. Multimodal Treatment Study of Children with ADHD. *Archives of General Psychiatry*, *56*(12), 1073–1086. doi:10.1001/archpsyc.56.12.1073 PMID:10591283

Theriault, S. W., & Holmberg, D. (2001). Impulsive, but violent? Are components of the attention deficit-hyperactivity syndrome associated with aggression in relationship? *Violence Against Women*, *7*(12), 1464–1489. doi:10.1177/10778010122183946

Thirthalli, J., & Benegal, V. (2006). Addictive disorders Psychosis among substance users. *Current Opinion in Psychiatry*, *19*(3), 239–245. doi:10.1097/01.yco.0000218593.08313.fd PMID:16612208

Thompson, A., Molina, B., Pelham, W., & Gnagy, E. (2007). Risky driving in adolescents and young adults withchildhood ADHD. *Journal of Pediatric Psychology*, *32*(7), 745–759. doi:10.1093/jpepsy/jsm002

Timothy, W. e. (1997). Attention Deficit Hyperactivity Disorder (ADHD) is Associated with Early Onset Substance Use Disorders. *The Journal of Nervous and Mental Disease*, *185*(8), 475–482. doi:10.1097/00005053-199708000-00001 PMID:9284860

Tole, F., Kopf, J., Schröter, K., Palladino, V. S., Jacob, C. P., Reif, A., & Kittel-Schneider, S. (2019). The role of pre-, peri-, and postnatal risk factors in bipolar disorder and adult ADHD. *Journal of Neural Transmission (Vienna, Austria)*, *126*(9), 1117–1126. doi:10.100700702-019-01983-4 PMID:30758784

Toplak, M. E., Dockstader, C., & Tannock, R. (2006). Temporal information processing in ADHD: Findings to date and new methods. *Journal of Neuroscience Methods*, *151*(1), 15–29. doi:10.1016/j.jneumeth.2005.09.018 PMID:16378641

Toplak, M. E., West, R. F., & Stanovich, K. E. (2013). Practitioner review: Do performance based measures and ratings of executive function assess the same construct? *Journal of Child Psychology and Psychiatry, and Allied Disciplines*, *54*(2), 131–143. doi:10.1111/jcpp.12001 PMID:23057693

Tosto, M.G., Momi, S.K., Asherson, P., & Malki, K. (2015). A Systematic Review of Attention Deficit Hyperactivity Disorder (ADHD) and Mathematical Ability: Current Findings and Future Implications. *BMC Medicine, 27*(13), 204. doi: . doi:10.118612916-015-0414-4

Townshend, K., Jordan, Z., Stephenson, M., & Tsey, K. (2016). The effectiveness of mindful parenting programs in promoting parents' and children's wellbeing: A systematic review. *JBI Database of Systematic Reviews and Implementation Reports*, *14*(3), 139–180. doi:10.11124/JBISRIR-2016-2314 PMID:27532143

Tredgold, A. F. (1908). *Mental Deficiency (Amentia)*. Wood.

Triparthi, B. M., & Lal, R. (1999). Substance abuse in children and adolescents. *Indian Journal of Pediatrics*, *66*(4), 269–575. PMID:10798113

Tripp, G., Luk, S. L., Schaughency, E. A., & Singh, R. (1999). DSM-IV and ICD-10: A Comparison of The Correlates of ADHD and Hyperkinetic Disorder. *Journal of the American Academy of Child and Adolescent Psychiatry*, *38*(2), 156–164. doi:10.1097/00004583-199902000-00014 PMID:9951214

Tripp, G., & Wickens, J. R. (2009). Neurobiology of ADHD. *Neuropharmacology*, *57*(7-8), 579–589. doi:10.1016/j.neuropharm.2009.07.026 PMID:19627998

Trites, R. L., Dugas, F., Lynch, G., & Ferguson, H. B. (1979). Prevalence of hyperactivity. *Journal of Pediatric Psychology*, *4*(2), 179–188. doi:10.1093/jpepsy/4.2.179

Tuckman, A. (2009). *More attention, less deficit: success strategies for adults with ADHD*. Speciality Press, Inc.

Tur-Kaspa, H., & Michal, Y. (2003). *Social information-processing skills of students with ADHD*. Poster presented at the Society for Research in Child Development Conference, Tampa, FL.

Turnbull, H. R., & Turnbull, A. (1998). *Free appropriate public education: The law and children with disabilities* (5th ed.). Love.

Understanding, A. D. H. D. (n.d.). *Information for parents. Healthy Children—American Academy of Pediatrics website.* Available at: https://www.healthychildren.org/English/health-issues/conditions/adhd/Pages/Understanding-ADHD.aspx

Upadhyaya, H. P. (2008). Substance use disorders in children and adolescents with attention- deficit/hyperactivity disorder: Implications for treatment and the role of the primary care physician. *Primary Care Companion to the Journal of Clinical Psychiatry, 10*(3), 211–221. doi:10.4088/PCC.v10n0306 PMID:18615170

Vaidya, C.J., Austin, G., Kirkorian, G., Ridlehuber, H.W., Desmond, J.E., Glorer, G.H., & Gabrieli, J.D. (1998). Selective effects of methylphenidate in attention deficit hyperactivity disorder: a functional magnetic resonance study. *Proceedings of the National Academy of Science USA, 95*, 14491-14499.

Vaidya, C. J. (2012). Neurodevelopmental abnormalities in ADHD. *Current Topics in Behavioral Neurosciences, 9*, 49–66. doi:10.1007/7854_2011_138 PMID:21541845

Valera, E. M., Faraone, S. V., Biederman, J., Poldrack, R. A., & Seidman, L. J. (2005). Functional neuroanatomy of working memory in adults with attention-deficit/hyperactivity disorder. *Biological Psychiatry, 57*(5), 439–447. doi:10.1016/j.biopsych.2004.11.034 PMID:15737657

Valero, S., Bosch, R., Corominas, M., Barrau, V., Ramos-Quiroga, J. A., & Casas, M. (2018). Remittance or persistence of attention deficit-hyperactivity disorder (ADHD) and its impact on recidivism in risky driving behaviors. *Traffic Injury Prevention, 19*(7), 701–707. doi:10.1080/15389588.2018.1505043 PMID:30485128

Van Apeldoorn, F. J., Van Hout, W. J., Mersch, P. P., Huisman, M., Slaap, B. R., Hale, W. W., Visser, S., van Dyck, R., & den Boer, J. A. (2008). Is a combined therapy more effective than either CBT or SSRI alone? Results of a multicenter trial on panic disorder with or without agoraphobia. *Acta Psychiatrica Scandinavica, 117*(4), 260–270. doi:10.1111/j.1600-0447.2008.01157.x PMID:18307586

van de Glind, G., Konstenius, M., Koeter, M. W. J., van Emmerik-van Oortmerssen, K., Carpentier, P.-J., Kaye, S., Degenhardt, L., Skutle, A., Franck, J., Bu, E.-T., Moggi, F., Dom, G., Verspreet, S., Demetrovics, Z., Kapitány-Fövény, M., Fatséas, M., Auriacombe, M., Schillinger, A., Møller, M., ... van den Brink, W. (2014). Variability in the prevalence of adult ADHD in treatment seeking substance use disorder patients: Results from an international multi-center study exploring DSM-IV and DSM-5 criteria. *Drug and Alcohol Dependence, 134*, 158–166. doi:10.1016/j.drugalcdep.2013.09.026 PMID:24156882

Van der Ende, J., & Verhulst, F.C. (2005). Informant, gender and age differences in ratings of adolescent problem behaviour. *European Child* and *Adolescent Psychiatry, 14*, 117–126.

Van der Marel, K., Bouet, V., Meerhoff, G. F., Freret, T., Boulouard, M., Dauphin, F., & Reneman, L. (2015). Effects of long-term methylphenidate treatment in adolescent and adult rats on hippocampal shape, functional connectivity and adult neurogenesis. *Neuroscience, 309*, 243–258. doi:10.1016/j.neuroscience.2015.04.044 PMID:25934041

Van der Oord, S., Ponsioen, A. J. G. B., Geurts, H. M., Brink, E. L. T., & Prins, P. J. M. (2014). A pilot study of the efficacy of a computerized executive functioning remediation training with game elements for children with ADHD in an outpatient setting: Outcome on parentand teacher-rated executive functioning and ADHD behavior. *Journal of Attention Disorders, 18*(8), 699–712. doi:10.1177/1087054712453167

Van der Oord, S., Prins, P. J., Oosterlaan, J., & Emmelkamp, P. M. (2008). Efficacy of methylphenidate, psychosocial treatments and their combination in school-aged children with ADHD: A meta-analysis. *Clinical Psychology Review, 28*(5), 783–800. doi:10.1016/j.cpr.2007.10.007 PMID:18068284

Van Doren, J., Arns, M., Heinrich, H., Vollebreat, M. A., Strehl, U., & Loo, S. K. (2019). Sustained effects of neurofeedback in ADHD: A systematic review and meta-analysis. *European Child & Adolescent Psychiatry*, *28*, 293–305. doi:10.100700787-018-1121-4 PMID:29445867

van Emmerik-van Oortmerssen, K., van de Glind, G., Koeter, M. W., Allsop, S., Auriacombe, M., Barta, C., Bu, E. T. H., Burren, Y., Carpentier, P.-J., Carruthers, S., Casas, M., Demetrovics, Z., Dom, G., Faraone, S. V., Fatseas, M., Franck, J., Johnson, B., Kapitány-Fövény, M., Kaye, S., ... Schoevers, R. A. (2014). Psychiatric comorbidity in treatment-seeking substance use disorder patients with and without attention deficit hyperactivity disorder: Results of the IASP study. *Addiction (Abingdon, England)*, *109*(2), 262–272. doi:10.1111/add.12370 PMID:24118292

Van Emmerik-van Oortmerssen, K., van de Glind, G., van den Brink, W., Smit, F., Crunelle, C. L., Swets, M., & Schoevers, R. A. (2012). Prevalence of attention-deficit hyperactivity disorder in substance use disorder patients: A meta-analysis and meta-regression analysis. *Drug and Alcohol Dependence*, *122*(1-2), 11–19. doi:10.1016/j.drugalcdep.2011.12.007 PMID:22209385

Van Emmerik-van Oortmerssen, K., Vedel, E., van den Brink, W., & Schoevers, R. A. (2015). Integrated cognitive behavioral therapy for patients with substance use disorder and comorbid ADHD: Two case presentations. *Addictive Behaviors*, *45*, 214–217. doi:10.1016/j.addbeh.2015.01.040 PMID:25706067

Van Mil, N. H., Steegers-Theunissen, R. P., Motazedi, E., Jansen, P. W., Jaddoe, V. W., Steegers, E. A., Verhulst, F. C., & Tiemeier, H. (2015). Low and high birth weight and the risk of child attention problems. *The Journal of Pediatrics*, *166*(4), 862–869.e3. doi:10.1016/j.jpeds.2014.12.075 PMID:25681197

Van Steijn, D. J., Oerlemans, A. M., de Ruiter, S. W., van Aken, M. A., Buitelaar, J. K., & Rommelse, N. N. (2013). Are parental autism spectrum disorder and/or attention-deficit/Hyperactivity disorder symptoms related to parenting stylesin families with ASD (+ADHD) affected children? *European Child & Adolescent Psychiatry*, *22*(11), 671–681. doi:10.100700787-013-0408-8

Van Veen, M. M., Kooij, J. J., Boonstra, A. M., Gordijn, M. C., & van Someren, E. J. (2010). Delayed circadian rhythm in adults with attention-deficit/hyperactivity disorder and chronic sleep-onset insomnia. *Biological Psychiatry*, *67*(11), 1091–1096. doi:10.1016/j.biopsych.2009.12.032

Vance, A. L. A., & Luk, E. S. L. (2000). Attention Deficit Hyperactivity Disorder: Current progress and controversies. *The Australian and New Zealand Journal of Psychiatry*, *34*(5), 719–730. doi:10.1080/j.1440-1614.2000.00809.x PMID:11037357

Venkatesh, C., Andal, A., Ravikumar, T., & Virudhagirinathan, B. (2012). Attention-deficit/Hyperactivity disorder in children: Clinical profile and Co-morbidity. *Indian Journal of Psychological Medicine*, *34*(1), 34. doi:10.4103/0253-7176.96155 PMID:22661805

Verma, R., Balhara, Y. P., & Mathur, S. (2011). Management of attention-deficit hyperactivity disorder. *Journal of Pediatric Neurosciences*, *6*(1), 13–18. doi:10.4103/1817-1745.84400

Vernhet, C., Dellapiazza, F., Blanc, N., Cousson-Gélie, F., Miot, S., Roeyers, H., & Baghdadli, A. (2019). Coping strategies of parents of children with autism spectrum disorder: A systematic review. *European Child & Adolescent Psychiatry*, *28*(6), 747–758. doi:10.100700787-018-1183-3 PMID:29915911

Verret, C., Guay, M. C., Berthiaume, C., Gardiner, P., & Béliveau, L. (2012). A physical activity program improves behavior and cognitive functions in children with ADHD: An exploratory study. *Journal of Attention Disorders*, *16*(1), 71–80. doi:10.1177/1087054710379735 PMID:20837978

Vickers, M. Z. (2010). *Accommodating College Students with Learning Disabilities: ADD, ADHD, and Dyslexia.* John William Pope Center for Higher Education Policy (NJ1).

Vila-Badia, R., Martínez-Zambrano, F., Arenas, O., Casas-Anguera, E., García-Morales, E., Villellas, R., Martín, J. R., Pérez-Franco, M. B., Valduciel, T., Casellas, D., García Franco, M., Miguel, J., Balsera, J., Pascual, G., Julia, E., & Ochoa, S. (2016). Effectiveness of an intervention for reducing social stigma towards mental illness in adolescents. *World Journal of Psychiatry*, *6*(2), 239–247. doi:10.5498/wjp.v6.i2.239 PMID:27354967

Visser, S. N., Danielson, M. L., Bitsko, R. H., Holbrook, J. R., Kogan, M. D., Ghandour, R. M., & Blumberg, S. J. (2014). Trends in the parent-report of health care provider-diagnosed and medicated attention-deficit/hyperactivity disorder: United states, 2003– 2011. *Journal of the American Academy of Child and Adolescent Psychiatry*, *53*(1), 34–46. doi:10.1016/j.jaac.2013.09.001

Vitaro, F., Tremblay, R. E., Gagnon, C., & Pelletier, D. (1994). Predictive accuracy of behavioral and sociometric assessments of high-risk kindergarten children. *Journal of Clinical Child Psychology*, *23*(3), 272–282. doi:10.120715374424jccp2303_5

Vokina, V. A., & Sosedova, L. M. (2018). Correlation between behavioural and eeg components of prenatal hypoxed rats. *GISAP: Medical Science Pharmacology*, (11), 30–32.

Volkow, N. D., Ding, Y. S., Fowler, J. S., Wang, G. J., Logan, J., Gatley, J. S., ... Wolf, A. P. (1995). Is Methylphenidate Like Cocaine? *Archives of General Psychiatry*, *52*(6), 456–463. doi:10.1001/archpsyc.1995.03950180042006 PMID:7771915

Volkow, N. D., Wang, G. J., Gatley, S. J., Fowler, J. S., Ding, Y.-S., Logan, J., Volkow, N. D., Hitzemann, R., Angrist, B., & Lieberman, J. (1996). Temporal relationships between the pharmacokinetics of methylphenidate in the human brain and its behavioral and cardiovascular effects. *Psychopharmacology*, *123*(1), 26–33. doi:10.1007/BF02246277 PMID:8741951

Vrijsen, J. N., Tendolkar, I., Onnik, M., Hoogman, M., Schene, A. H., & Fernández, G. (2018). ADHD symptoms in healthy adults are associated with stressful life events and negative memory bias. *Attention Deficit and Hyperactivity Disorders*, *10*(2), 151–160. doi:10.100712402-017-0241-x PMID:29081022

Wahler, R. G., & Afton, A. D. (1980). Attentional processes in insular and non-insular mothers. Some differences in their summary reports about child problem behaviours. *Child Behaviour Therapy*, *2*, 25–41. doi:10.1300/J473V02N02_02

Wang, C. H., Mazursky-Horowitz, H., & Chronis-Tuscano, A. (2014). Delivering evidence-based treatments for child attention-deficit/hyperactivity disorder (ADHD) in the context of parental ADHD. *Current Psychiatry Reports*, *16*(10), 474. doi:10.100711920-014-0474-8 PMID:25135774

Wang, M., Zhao, Q., Kang, H., & Zhu, S. (2019). Attention deficit hyperactivity disorder (ADHD) in children with epilepsy. *Irish Journal of Medical Science*. Advance online publication. doi:10.100711845-019-02042-3 PMID:31187336

Ware, A. L., Glass, L., Crocker, N., Deweese, B. N., Coles, C. D., Kable, J. A., May, P. A., Kalberg, W. O., Sowell, E. R., Jones, K. L., Riley, E. P., & Mattson, S. N. (2014). Effects of Prenatal Alcohol Exposure and Attention-Deficit/ Hyperactivity Disorder on Adaptive Functioning. *Alcoholism, Clinical and Experimental Research*, *38*(5), 1439–1447. doi:10.1111/acer.12376 PMID:24655090

Warner, D. O., Zaccariello, M. J., Katusic, S. K., Schroeder, D. R., Hanson, A. C., Schulte, P. J., ... Hu, D. (2018). Neuropsychological and behavioral outcomes after exposure of young children to procedures requiring general anesthesia: The MASK study. *Anesthesiology*, *129*(1), 89–105. doi:10.1097/ALN.0000000000002232 PMID:29672337

Watson, G.R.A., & Morin, L.L. (2016). The Role of Executive Functions in Classroom Instruction of Students with Learning Disabilities. *International Journal of School Cognitive Psychology, 3*, 167. doi:10.4172/2469-9837.1000167

Watts, S. J. (2018). ADHD Symptomatology and Criminal Behavior During Adolescence: Exploring the Mediating Role of School Factors. *International Journal of Offender Therapy and Comparative Criminology*, *62*(1), 3–23. doi:10.1177/0306624X16639970 PMID:27056790

Webster-Stratton, C., Reid, M. J., & Hammond, M. (2001). Preventing conduct problems, promoting social competence: A parent and teacher training partnership in Head Start. *Journal of Clinical Child Psychology*, *30*(3), 283–302. doi:10.1207/S15374424JCCP3003_2 PMID:11501247

Wechsler, D. (1992). *Wechsler individual achievement test: Manual*. Psychological Corp.

Wechsler, D. (2004). *WISC-IV: Wechsler Intelligence Scale for Children, Integrated: Technical and interpretive manual*. Harcourt Brace.

Wehmeier, P. M., Schacht, A., & Barkley, R. A. (2010). Social and emotional impairment in children and adolescents with ADHD and the impact on quality of life. *The Journal of Adolescent Health*, *46*(3), 209–217. doi:10.1016/j.jadohealth.2009.09.009 PMID:20159496

Weinberger, K. A., Gardner, D. M., & Gerdes, A. C. (2018). Maternal Functioning Differences Based on ADHD Subtype. *Journal of Attention Disorders*, *22*(13), 218–1223. doi:10.1177/1087054714567132 PMID:25589371

Weinberg, S. L., & Richardon, M. S. (1981). Dimensions of Stress in early parenting. *Journal of Consulting and Clinical Psychology*, *49*(5), 686–693. doi:10.1037/0022-006X.49.5.686 PMID:7287978

Weiner, A. L. (2000). Emerging drugs of abuse in Connecticut. *Connecticut Medicine*, *64*(1), 19–23. PMID:10697361

Weiss, G. S., & Hechtman, L. T. (1986). Hyperactive children grown up: Empirical findings and theoretical considerations. New York: Guilford Press.

Weiss, G., & Hechtman, L. (1993). *Hyperactive Children Grow Up* (2nd ed.). Guilford.

Weiss, G., & Hechtman, L. (1993). *Hyperactive children grown up: ADHD in children, adolescents and adults*. Guildford Press.

Weiss, G., & Hechtman, L. T. (1993). *Hyperactive children grown up: ADHD in children, adolescents, and adults*. Guilford Press.

Weiss, M., Hechtman, L., & Weiss, G. (1999). *ADHD in adulthood: A guide to current theory, diagnosis, and treatment*. The John Hopkins University Press.

Weiss, M., & Murray, C. (2003). Assessment and management of attention-deficit hyperactivity disorder in adults. *Canadian Medical Association Journal*, *168*(6), 715–722. PMID:12642429

Wells, K. C., Epstein, J. N., Hinshaw, S. P., Conners, C. K., Klaric, J., Abikoff, H. B., Abramowitz, A., Arnold, L. E., Elliott, G., Greenhill, L. L., Hechtman, L., Hoza, B., Jensen, P. S., March, J. S., Pelham, W. Jr, Pfiffner, L., Severe, J., Swanson, J. M., Vitiello, B., & Wigal, T. (2000). Parenting and family stress treatment outcomes in attention deficit hyperactivity disorder (ADHD): An empirical analysis in the MTA study. *Journal of Abnormal Child Psychology*, *28*(6), 543–553. doi:10.1023/A:1005131131159 PMID:11104316

Wender, P. H. (1995). *Attention-Deficit Hyperactivity Disorder in Adults*. Oxford University Press.

Wender, P. H. (1995). *Attention-deficit hyperactivity disorders in adulthood*. Oxford University Press.

Wender, P. H., Reimherr, F. W., Wood, D., & Ward, M. (1985). A controlled study of methylphenidate in the treatment of attention deficit disorder, residual type, in adults. *The American Journal of Psychiatry*, *142*(5), 547–552. doi:10.1176/ajp.142.5.547 PMID:3885760

Wender, P. H., & Tomb, D. A. (2017). *ADHD: A Guide to Understanding Symptoms, Causes, Diagnosis, Treatment and Changes over time in Children, Adolescents, and Adults, Treatment of the child with ADHD*. Oxford University Press.

Werner, O., Wallace, R. K., Charles, B., Janssen, G., Stryker, T., & Chalmers, R. A. (1986). Long-term endocrinologic changes in subjects practicing the transcendental meditation and TM sidhi program. *Psychosomatic Medicine*, *48*(1-2), 59–65. doi:10.1097/00006842-198601000-00004

Wernicke, J. F., Adler, L., Spencer, T., West, S. A., Allen, A. J., Heiligenstein, J., Milton, D., Ruff, D., Brown, W. J., Kelsey, D., & Michelson, D. (2004). Changes in symptoms and adverse events after discontinuation of atomoxetine in children and adults with attention deficit/hyperactivity disorder: A prospective, placebo-controlled assessment. *Journal of Clinical Psychopharmacology*, *24*(1), 30–35. doi:10.1097/01.jcp.0000104907.75206.c2 PMID:14709944

Westwood, S., Radua, J., & Rubia, K. (2019). Non-invasive brain stimulation as an alternative treatment for ADHD: A systematic review and meta-analysis. *Brain Stimulation*, *12*(2), 502. doi:10.1016/j.brs.2018.12.644

Whalen, C. K., & Henker, B. (1985). The social worlds of hyperactive (ADDH) children. *Clinical Psychology Review*, *5*(5), 447–478. doi:10.1016/0272-7358(85)90004-2

Whitesell, M., Bachand, A., Peel, J., & Brown, M. (2013). Familial, social, and individual factors contributing to risk for adolescent substance abuse. *Journal of Addiction*, *2013*, 1–9. Advance online publication. doi:10.1155/2013/579310 PMID:24826363

Wiener, J., Biondic, D., Grimbos, T., & Herbert, M. (2016). Parenting Stress of Parents of Adolescents with Attention-Deficit Hyperactivity Disorder. *Journal of Abnormal Child Psychology*, *44*(3), 561–574. doi:10.100710802-015-0050-7 PMID:26183609

Wilcox, C. E., Washburn, R., & Patel, V. (2007). Seeking help for attention deficit hyperactivity disorder in developing countries: A study of parental explanatory models in Goa, India. *Social Science & Medicine*, *64*(8), 1600–1610. doi:10.1016/j.socscimed.2006.11.032 PMID:17267087

Wilens, T. E. (2004). Attention deficit/hyperactivity disorder and the substance use disorders: The nature of the relationship, subtypes at risk, and treatment issues. *The Psychiatric Clinics of North America*, *27*(2), 283–301. doi:10.1016/S0193-953X(03)00113-8 PMID:15063998

Wilens, T. E., & Biederman, J. (2006). Alcohol, drugs, and attention-deficit/ hyperactivity disorder: A model for the study of addictions in youth. *Journal of Psychopharmacology (Oxford, England)*, *20*(4), 580–588. doi:10.1177/0269881105058776 PMID:16174669

Wilens, T. E., Biederman, J., & Spencer, T. J. (2002). Attention deficit/hyperactivity disorder across the lifespan. *Annual Review of Medicine*, *53*(1), 113–131. doi:10.1146/annurev.med.53.082901.103945 PMID:11818466

Wilens, T. E., Hammerness, P., Utzinger, L., Schillinger, M., Georgiopoulous, A., Doyle, R. L., Martelon, M. K., & Brodziak, K. (2009). An open study of adjunct OROS-methylphenidate in children and adolescents who are atomoxetine partial responders: I. Effectiveness. *Journal of Child and Adolescent Psychopharmacology*, *19*(5), 485–492. doi:10.1089/cap.2008.0125 PMID:19877972

Wilens, T. E., Martelon, M., Joshi, G., Bateman, C., Fried, R., Petty, C., & Biederman, J. (2011). Does ADHD predict substance-use disorders? A 10-year follow-up study of young adults with ADHD. *Journal of the American Academy of Child and Adolescent Psychiatry*, *50*(6), 543–553. doi:10.1016/j.jaac.2011.01.021 PMID:21621138

Wilens, T. E., & Morrison, N. R. (2012). Substance-use disorders in adolescents and adults with ADHD: Focus on treatment. *Neuropsychiatry*, *2*(4), 301–312. doi:10.2217/npy.12.39 PMID:23105949

Wilens, T. E., & Spencer, T. J. (2010). Understanding attention-deficit/hyperactivity disorder from childhood to adulthood. *Postgraduate Medical Journal, 122*(5), 97–109. doi:10.3810/pgm.2010.09.2206 PMID:20861593

Wilens, T., Nierenberg, A. A., Rostain, A., & Spencer, T. J. (2008). Adult attention-deficit hyperactivity disorder and the role of depression. *CNS Spectrums, 13*(5), 2–17.

Wilhelm, H., Brandon, S., & Alan, B. (2012, March). Executive functions and self-regulation. *Trends in Cognitive Sciences, 16*(3). PMID:22336729

Wilkes-gillan, S., Bundy, A., Cordier, R., Lincoln, M., & Chen, Y. W. (2016). A Randomised Controlled Trial of a Play-Based Intervention to Improve the Social Play Skills of Children with Attention Deficit Hyperactivity Disorder (ADHD). *PLoS One, 11*(8), e0160558. doi:10.1371/journal.pone.0160558 PMID:27529693

Willcutt, E. G. (2012). The prevalence of DSM-IV attention-deficit/hyperactivity disorder: A meta-analytic review. *Neurotherapeutics; the Journal of the American Society for Experimental NeuroTherapeutics, 9*(3), 490–499. doi:10.100713311-012-0135-8

Willcutt, E. G., Betjemann, R. S., McGrath, L. M., Chhabildas, N. A., Olson, R. K., DeFries, J. C., & Pennington, B. F. (2010). Etiology and neuropsychology of comorbidity between RD and ADHD: The case for multiple-deficit models. *Cortex, 46*(10), 1345–1361. doi:10.1016/j.cortex.2010.06.009

Willcutt, E. G., Betjemann, R. S., Pennington, B. F., Olson, R. K., DeFries, J. C., & Wadsworth, S. J. (2007). Longitudinal study of reading disability and attentiondeficit/hyperactivity disorder: Implications for education. *Mind, Brain and Education: the Official Journal of the International Mind, Brain, and Education Society, 4*(4), 181–192. doi:10.1111/j.1751-228X.2007.00019.x

Willcutt, E. G., Pennington, B. F., Duncan, L., Smith, S. D., Keenan, J. M., Wadsworth, S. J., DeFries, J. C., & Olson, R. K. (2010). Understanding the complex etiology of developmental disorders: Behavioral and molecular genetic approaches. *Journal of Developmental and Behavioral Pediatrics, 31*(7), 533–544. doi:10.1097/DBP.0b013e3181ef42a1

Williamson, D., & Johnston, C. (2019). Maternal ADHD Symptoms and Parenting Stress: The Roles of Parenting Self-Efficacy Beliefs and Neuroticism. *Journal of Attention Disorders, 23*(5), 493–505. doi:10.1177/1087054717693373 PMID:28201945

Wilson, M. (2002). Six views of embodied cognition. *Psychonomic Bulletin & Review, 9*(4), 625–636. doi:10.3758/BF03196322 PMID:12613670

Wolf, R. C., Plichta, M. M., Sambataro, F., Fallgatter, A. J., Jacob, C., Lesch, K. P., Herrmann, M. J., Schönfeldt-Lecuona, C., Connemann, B. J., Grön, G., & Vasic, N. (2009). Regional brain activation changes and abnormal functional connectivity of the ventrolateral prefrontal cortex during working memory processing in adults with attention-deficit/hyperactivity disorder. *Human Brain Mapping, 30*(7), 2252–2266. doi:10.1002/hbm.20665 PMID:19107748

Wolraich, M. L., & Doffing, M. A. (2004). Pharmacokinetic considerations in the treatment of attention-deficit hyperactivity disorder with methylphenidate. *CNS Drugs, 18*(4), 243–250. doi:10.2165/00023210-200418040-00004 PMID:15015904

Wolraich, M. L., Wibbelsman, C. J., & Brown, T. E. (2005). Attention-deficit/hyperactivity disorder among adolescents: A review of the diagnosis, treatment, and clinical implications. *Pediatrics, 115*(6), 1734–1746. doi:10.1542/peds.2004-1959

Wolraich, M., Brown, L., Brown, R. T., DuPaul, G., Earls, M., Feldman, H. M., Ganiats, T. G., Kaplanek, B., Meyer, B., Perrin, J., Pierce, K., Reiff, M., Stein, M. T., & Visser, S. (2011). Subcommittee on attention-deðcit/ hyperactivity disorder; Steering Committee on quality improvement and management. ADHD: Clinical practice guideline for the diagnosis, evaluation, and treatment of attention-deðcit/hyperactivity disorder in children and adolescents. *Pediatrics, 128*(5), 1007–1022. doi:10.1542/peds.2011-2654 PMID:22003063

Wolraich, M., Lambert, W., Doffing, M., Bickman, L., Simmons, L., & Worley, K. (2003). Psychometric Properties of the Vanderbilt ADHD Diagnostic Parent Rating Scale in a Referred Population. *Journal of Pediatric Psychology*, *28*(8), 559–568. doi:10.1093/jpepsy/jsg046 PMID:14602846

Wood, D. R., Reimherr, F. W., Wender, P. H., & Johnson, G. E. (1976). Diagnosis and treatment of minimal brain dysfunction in adults: A preliminary report. *Archives of General Psychiatry*, *33*(12), 1453–1460. doi:10.1001/archpsyc.1976.01770120057005 PMID:793563

Wood, J. J., McLeod, B. D., Sigman, M., Hwang, W.-C., & Chu, B. C. (2003). Parenting and childhood anxiety: Theory, empirical findings, and future directions. *Journal of Child Psychology and Psychiatry, and Allied Disciplines*, *44*(1), 134–151. doi:10.1111/1469-7610.00106 PMID:12553416

Wood, L., Egger, M., Gluud, L. L., Schulz, K. F., Jüni, P., Altman, D. G., Gluud, C., Martin, R. M., Wood, A. J. G., & Sterne, J. A. (2008). Empirical evidence of bias in treatment effect estimates in controlled trials with different interventions and outcomes: Meta-epidemiological study. *BMJ (Clinical Research Ed.)*, *336*(7644), 601–605. doi:10.1136/bmj.39465.451748.AD PMID:18316340

World Health Organization. (1992). *International Statistical Classification of Diseases and Related Health Problems. 10th Revision (ICD-10) edition*. Geneva: World Health Organization.

World Health Organization. (1992). *The ICD10 Classification of Mental and Behavioural Disorders: Clinical descriptions and diagnostic guidelines*. Author.

World Health Organization. (2004). *The ICD 10 classification of mental and behavioural disorder: Clinical descriptions and diagnostic guidelines*. https://www.who.int/classifications/icd/en/bluebook.pdf

World Health Organization. (2004). *The ICD-10 Classification of mental and behavioral disorders*. WHO.

Wymbs, B. T., Dawson, A. E., Egan, T. E., Sacchetti, G. M., Tams, S. T., & Wymbs, F. A. (2017). ADHD and Depression Symptoms in Parent Couples Predict Response to Child ADHD and ODD Behavior. *Journal of Abnormal Child Psychology*, *45*(3), 471–484. doi:10.100710802-016-0220-2 PMID:27796690

Wymbs, B. T., Dawson, A. E., Suhr, J. A., Bunford, N., & Gidycz, C. A. (2017). ADHD Symptoms as Risk Factors for Intimate Partner Violence Perpetration and Victimization. *Journal of Interpersonal Violence*, *32*(5), 659–681. doi:10.1177/0886260515586371 PMID:26025345

Wymbs, B., Molina, B., Pelham, W., Cheong, J., Gnagy, E., Belendiuk, K., Walther, C., Babinski, D., & Waschbusch, D. (2012). Risk of intimate partner violence among young adult males with childhood ADHD. *Journal of Attention Disorders*, *16*(5), 373–383. doi:10.1177/1087054710389987

Xu, G., Strathearn, L., Liu, B., Yang, B., & Bao, W. (2018). Twenty-year trends in diagnosed attention-deficit/hyperactivity disorder among US children and adolescents, 1997-2016. *JAMA Network Open*, *1*(4), e181471–e181471. doi:10.1001/jamanetworkopen.2018.1471 PMID:30646132

Yamaguchi, S., Mino, Y., & Uddin, S. (2011). Strategies and future attempts to reduce stigmatization and increase awareness of mental health problems among young people: A narrative review of educational interventions. *Psychiatry Journal of Clinical Neuroscience*, *65*(5), 405–415. doi:10.1111/j.1440-1819.2011.02239.x PMID:21851449

Yang, P., Jong, Y. J., Hsu, H. Y., & Tsai, J. H. (2007). Psychiatric features and parenting stress profiles of subtypes of attention-deficit/hyperactivity disorder: Results from a clinically referred Taiwanese sample. *Journal of Developmental and Behavioral Pediatrics*, *28*(5), 369–375. doi:10.1097/DBP.0b013e3181131f8e PMID:18049319

Yogananda, P. (2014). Autobiography of a yogi (13th ed.). Self Realization Fellowship.

Yogananda, P. (2005). *The Essence of Kriya Yoga* (1st ed.). Alight Publications.

Yoshimasu, K. (2016). Substance-Related and Addictive Disorders as a Risk Factor of Suicide and Homicide among Patients with ADHD: A Mini Review. *Current Drug Abuse Reviews*, *9*(2), 80–86. doi:10.2174/1874473709666160802112215 PMID:27492359

Yoshimasu, K., Barbaresi, W. J., Colligan, R. C., Voigt, R. G., Killian, J. M., Weaver, A. L., & Katusic, S. K. (2012). Childhood ADHD is strongly associated with a broad range of psychiatric disorders during adolescence: A population-based birth cohort study. *Journal of Child Psychology and Psychiatry, and Allied Disciplines*, *53*(10), 1036–1043. doi:10.1111/j.1469-7610.2012.02567.x PMID:22647074

Yoshimasu, K., Barbaresi, W. J., Colligan, R. C., Voigt, R. G., Killian, J. M., Weaver, A. L., & Katusic, S. K. (2019). Psychiatric comorbidities modify the association between childhood ADHD and risk for suicidality: A population-based longitudinal study. *Journal of Attention Disorders*, *23*(8), 777–786. doi:10.1177/1087054717718264 PMID:28689473

Young, S. (2005). Coping strategies used by adults with ADHD. *Personality and Individual Differences*, *38*(4), 809–816. doi:10.1016/j.paid.2004.06.005

Young, S., & Bramhan, J. (2012). *Cognitive-Behavioural Therapy for ADHD in Adolescents and Adults: A Psychological Guide to Practice* (2nd ed.). John Wiley & Sons. doi:10.1002/9781119943440

Young, S., González, R. A., Mullens, H., Mutch, L., Malet-Lambert, I., & Gudjonsson, G. H. (2018). Neurodevelopmental disorders in prison inmates: Comorbidity and combined associations with psychiatric symptoms and behavioural disturbance. *Psychiatry Research*, *261*, 109–115. doi:10.1016/j.psychres.2017.12.036 PMID:29291476

Young, S., Wells, J., & Gudjonsson, G. H. (2011). Predictors of offending among prisoners: The role of attention-deficit hyperactivity disorder and substance use. *Journal of Psychopharmacology (Oxford, England)*, *25*(11), 1524–1532. doi:10.1177/0269881110370502 PMID:20558498

Zappitelli, M., Pinto, T., & Grizenko, N. (2001). Pre-, peri-, and postnatal trauma in subjects with attention-deficit hyperactivity disorder. *Canadian Journal of Psychiatry*, *46*(6), 542–548. doi:10.1177/070674370104600609 PMID:11526811

Zeanah, C. H., Berlin, L. J., & Boris, N. W. (2011). Practitioner Review: Clinical applications of attachment theory and research for infants and young children. *Journal of Child Psychology and Psychiatry, and Allied Disciplines*, *52*(8), 819–833. doi:10.1111/j.1469-7610.2011.02399.x PMID:21554304

Zentall, S. S., Cassady, J. C., & Javorsky, J. (2001). Social comprehension of children with hyperactivity. *Journal of Attention Disorders*, *5*(1), 11–24. doi:10.1177/108705470100500102

Zhang, W., Fan, L., & Jiang, Y. P. (2016). Memory Updating Deficit in Attention Deficit Hyperactivity Disorder (ADHD) Children. *Medicine and Biopharmaceutical*, 3-11. doi:10.1142/9789814719810_0001

Zhou, K., Dempfle, A., Arcos-Burgos, M., Bakker, S. C., Banaschewski, T., Biederman, J., … Asherson, P. (2008). Meta-analysis of genome-wide linkage scans of attention deficit hyperactivity disorder. *American Journal of Medical Genetics. Part B, Neuropsychiatric Genetics: The Official Publication of the International Society of Psychiatric Genetics, 147B*(8), 1392–1398.

Zulauf, C. A., Sprich, S. E., Safren, S. A., & Wilens, T. E. (2014). The Complicated Relationship Between Attention Deficit/Hyperactivity Disorder and Substance Use Disorders. *Current Psychiatry Reports*, *16*(3), 436. doi:10.100711920-013-0436-6 PMID:24526271

Zwi, M., Jones, H., Thorgaard, C., York, A., & Dennis, J. A. (2011). Parent training interventions for Attention Deficit Hyperactivity Disorder (ADHD) in children aged 5 to 18 years. *Cochrane Database of Systematic Reviews*, 12. doi:10.1002/14651858.CD003018.pub3 PMID:22161373

Zylowska, L., Ackerman, D. L., Yang, M. H., Futrell, L., Horton, N. L., Hale, T. S., Pataki, C., & Smalley, S. L. (2008). Mindfulness meditation training in adults and adolescents with ADHD: A feasibility study. *Journal of Attention Disorders*, *11*(6), 737–746. doi:10.1177/1087054707308502 PMID:18025249

About the Contributors

Rejani Thudalikunnil Gopalan is an Academician and registered Clinical Psychologist who has closer to two decades work experience in mental health area. Currently she is working as Professor and Head, Department of Clinical Psychology, Mahatma Gandhi Medical College and Hospital, Rajasthan, Jaipur, India. She has received many awards for her academic excellence and contribution to mental health area and research. Recently she was awarded Fellow by International Institute of Organisational Psychological Medicine, USA. Her specialized services extended to clinical consultation and therapeutic remedies for the group including adults and children with mental illness in Prison and juvenile homes along with court related disputes. Research Area: Traumas and abuses, especially sexual abuse; childhood mental health issues, school mental health, forensic, neuro psychological and mental health issues among convicted adult and juvenile offenders.

* * *

Vaishali Chaudhari is a RCI registered Clinical Psychologist. She has done M.Phil in Clinical Psychology from Gujarat Forensic Sciences University, Gandhinagar. At present, she is working as a Clinical Psychologist at General Hospital, Bharuch, Gujarat, India. She has been working in this field since last 4 years. She has worked with different types of population suffering from different mental health related problems. She interested in working with children with special needs and childhood disorders. She is doing different types of psychological assessment and doing psychotherapies for intervention of the psychological disorders. Her research interest lies in examining the effect of different alternative therapies in children and old age on mental health.

Sandamita Choudhury is a Licensed Clinical Psychologist serving in 151 Army Base hospital, Guwahati, Assam. She has been associated with the field of mental health since 2013 as a professional catering her services to the special needs children, individuals with psychiatric issues, helping students, adults to deal with minor and major issues related to transitional phase. She has been using various psychological approaches and therapies; for the identification, diagnosis and treatment of psychiatric disorders in a wide range of clinical cases. She has completed her M.Phil. (Clinical Psychology) from Gujarat Forensic Sciences University, Gandhinagar in 2016, MSc. (Clinical Psychology) from Jain University, Bangalore in 2013 and B.A. (hons) Psychology from Delhi University. She has served as a visiting faculty for the under graduate and post graduate level courses in psychology in Cotton University, Tata Institute of Social Sciences, Composite Regional Centre and Army Institute of Nursing, Guwahati. Her research areas lies in understanding of HIV Pregnant women, intellectually disabled and their rehabilitation, Caregivers of Mentally ill and Adolescents, Mental health of prisoners, Homeless Youth, Addiction among armed forces.

Dorothy Deka is working as a Clinical Psychologist in Sarvodaya Healthcare in Guwahati. She did her Mphil from Gujarat Forensic Sciences University and did her Graduation and Post Graduation from Maharaja Sayajirao University of Baroda. She also did her Diploma in Clinical and Applied Hypnosis from Maharaja Sayajirao University of Baroda.

Aastha Dhingra Hasija is the Director & Co founder at AD Executive Training And Coaching Pvt Ltd. She is an Assistant Professor with SGT University Gurugram. She is a clinical psychologist with Polaris hospital and Jeewan Multispeciality Hospital gurugram. She has been former psychologist on the panel of juvenile justice board Gurugram. She has around 20 papers to her credit in national and international journals

Aarzoo Gupta completed her Graduation and Post-Graduation in Psychology in 2001 and 2003 respectively from Panjab University, Chandigarh; Diploma in Clinical Applied Hypnosis in 2004 from MSU, Baroda. After having worked as a tele-Counsellor in a Suicide Prevention Helpline and Lecturer in General Psychology, she then did her MPhil in Clinical Psychology, 2-years regular program recognized by the Rehabilitation Council of India from SRMC&RI, Chennai. She has been in a clinical setting since 2007 working in areas of adult psychiatry; children having an intellectual disability, autism, and ADHD. She has been involved as a CP in Psychosexual Clinic of the Dept. since 2012. She has been in-charge of the Behaviour Therapy Unit of the Department since January 2017. She has been involved in work with Juveniles in Observation Home, Children's Home thru Child Welfare Committee and various other activities of Dept of Social Welfare. To her credit, she has; 9 published, 7 submitted, 5 papers in preparation. She has supervised 11 thesis of MPhil CP (10) and MD Psychiatry(1) till date since December 2016. She is a Reviewer for 2 National peer-reviewed Journals of Psychiatry. She has been resource person for 45 invites including lectures or talks or workshops or training programs. She has made 28 presentations at National or International Conferences.

Tsuyoshi Imasaka has completed Bachelor (B.Sc) and Honours degree majoring in psychology, and Master of Education in Applied Behaviour Analysis at Monash University, Melbourne, Australia. He joined the team at Sunrise Behavioural Health as a behaviour support practitioner in 2019. He has completed the requirements of supervised independent fieldwork hours toward his professional certification as a Board Certified Behaviour Analyst (BCBA). He hopes to gain the BCBA credential soon. Tsuyoshi has keen research interests in developing and implementing behavioural intervention strategies in supporting individuals with ASD, ADHD and other mental health disabilities. He has published research in a peer-reviewed journal and intends to expand his research interest in evaluating and optimising clinical outcomes at Sunrise Behavioural Health.

Aneesha Jose is currently pursuing her M.Phil in Clinical Psychology from SRM University, Chennai. She completed her MSc in Psychology from Montfort College, Bangalore and BA from Sophia College, Mumbai. Psychology is a subject that she is passionate about and she enjoys working with people. She is interested in research and in topics surrounding areas of neuropsychology, developmental disorders among children and social cognition. She is a keen learner and is open to new approaches that are constantly being developed in the field of study. She has presented papers at multiple scientific conferences and has a paper published in the International Journal of Psychosocial Research in the year 2015 on issues faced by the LGBT community. During her years working as a special educator she has learnt to work with differently abled children with patience and empathy.

Archana Kashyap completed her Graduation and Post Graduation in Psychology in 2012 and 2014 respectively and completed her M.Phil in Clinical psychology, a 2-years regular program recognized by the Rehabilitation Council of India from the Department of Psychiatry, GMCH. She has been working as a Clinical Psychologist since 2017. She has the experience of working with children having an Intellectual Disability, Autism, ADHD as well as behavioral problems. She has been working in the Behaviour Therapy Unit of the Department since October, 2018. She has been involved in assessment and psychotherapy in children as well as adults having psychiatric as well as non-psychiatric issues. She did her M.Phil thesis on children with Borderline intelligence. She is a growing researcher with 3 published works, 1 submitted and 3 in preparation and co-resource person for a workshop on CBT with 14 invited lectures to her credit delivered at the National Institute of Public Cooperation & Child Development, Directorate of Prosecution, and Central Detective Training Institute.

Ambika Kathju is a licensed Clinical Psychologist from India. She completed her M.Phil. in Clinical Psychology from Gujarat Forensic Sciences University, Gandhinagar in 2018, and M.A in Psychology from the IIS University, Jaipur, in 2013. Apart from working as a clinician, she has also worked as an Assistant Professor at Mody University. She is passionate about her work and is working towards creating awareness and bringing quality services in the field of mental health. Currently, she is working as a freelance consultant in Melbourne, Australia.

Tanay Maiti (MBBS, DPM, DNB Psych) is a young enthusiastic psychiatrist and mental health professional from India, with more than half a decade experience as a trainee, learner and later as a full time professional in the field, though his inquisitive nature and exploring mind hasn't come to a pause ever! He has multiple national and international publications to his credits, and has won multiple awards for his paper/posters as well. He has also been chosen for the prestigious fellowship from 'Dr. Ramachandra N Moorthy Foundation' at 6th Leadership and Professional Skills course for Early Career Psychiatrist' at NIMHANS, Feb 2018 (one among the sixteen from the entire SAARC region) and also been recognized amongst the promising young psychiatrists and won a fellowship from World Psychiatric Association(one of the thirty seven winners from the entire globe)for the same at recently conducted 'World Congress of Psychiatry' September 2018 at Mexico City, Mexico. There, he participated in a 3-continent symposium and presented the scenario of of child psychiatry in India. He also had 2 brief presentations where he talked about public health perspectives in current Indian mental health scenario, and contribution of Indian philosophy and yoga in the mental health interventions. With direct experience to work and learn from the three of the premier institutes in country(VIMHANS, New Delhi; Christian Medical College, Vellore and AIIMS, Bhubaneswar) Dr. Tanay is currently focusing his work on extensive research and both undergraduate and post graduate training(writing books and book chapters for them), along with regular clinical works and managing difficult patients and clinical scenarios. Dr. Maiti's primary interest of work and research lies upon child and adolescent psychiatry, developmental psychology, adolescent substance abuse and stress, coping and personality factors.

Jahirul Mullick has more than fifteen years of research experience with a demonstrated history of working in higher education industry both in research and teaching capacity. He received his doctoral degree in leadership practice and inclusive education, and Master of Education degree in Applied Behaviour Analysis from Monash University. He works as Sessional Lecturer in Early Childhood Education Program at School of Education, RMIT University. As a behaviour science practitioner he provides early interventions to children (3 to 7) with autism or ADHD, and positive behaviour support to individuals with ASD or other intellectual disabilities. He has published several academic articles and book chapters that focus on leadership practice, inclusive and special education, applied behaviour analysis and teacher development.

Chirag Parmar has finished his postgraduate study in Psychiatry from Smt. NHL Municipal Medical college in 2014. He is working at Gujarat Institute of Mental Health as a Consultant Psychiatrist since 2015. His area of interest is Addiction Medicine.

Krunal Patel has done his MD in Psychiatry from PDU Medical College, Rajkot, India in 2018. After graduating from medical school he has joined Gujarat Institute of Mental Health as in capacity of Consultant Psychiatry. His work interest area are biological psychiatry and psycho-pharmacology.

Girija Patwardhan, a student of a unique school in Pune, namely 'Jnana Prabodhinee Prashala', has completed her masters degree in Clinical Psychology from Fergusson College Pune in 2014. After completing her Masters in Clinical Psychology she worked as a faculty for undergraduate students in the department of Psychology in Abasaheb Garware College, Pune for one academic year. Later she completed her RCI recognized M.Phil in Clinical Psychology, from Gujarat Forensic Sciences University, Gandhinagar, Gujarat in the year 2017. She has worked for Baya Karve Women's Study and Research Center of Maharshi Karve Stree Shikshan Samstha, Pune as a Clinical Psychologist during October 2017 to October 2018. During this, she played a vital role in a research study on Effects of Burnout on Health and Job Performance among Women which was funded and appreciated by the Maharashtra State Commission for Women. Currently she is practicing as Consulting Clinical Psychologist and one of the Directors at Dhruv Educational and Research Foundation, Pune. Besides this she is also associated with Prasanna Autism Centre, Pune where she has worked voluntarily with the autistic children in the centre, using dance as a therapeutic base.

Ann Paul is currently pursuing her M.Phil. in Clinical Psychology from SRM University, Chennai. She completed her MSc in psychology. After Completing her Postgraduation, she worked with children with learning disabilities. Her research interest lies in child and adolescent mental health, neuropsychology and positive psychology.

Pangajam Ponnuswamy is an Assistant professor of Clinical Psychology at the SRM Medical college Hospital & Research Centre. She has completed her master of Philosophy in Clinical Psychology at Sri Ramachandra University in the year 2002, Chennai, India. She has eleven years of teaching experience and 15 years of clinical experience in providing psychotherapy to students and patients. She is done research work on the women's problem of premenstrual syndrome and Poly Cystic Ovarian Disorder. Presented a Paper on Management of a Case of Depression with Marital and Cognitive Behavior Therapy. Published articles on the impact of stress in marital satisfaction and quality of life among primary infertile, secondary infertile and fertile women and Management of a Child with Generalized Anxiety Disorder using Play Therapy.

Kalpana Raman is currently pursuing her Doctoral degree at the Auckland University of Technology and also a practicing Clinical Psychologist at the Counties Manukau District Health Board. She is a registered practitioner by the New Zealand Psychology Board and the Rehabilitation Council of India. She has been the top scorer of her batch during her M.Phil Clinical Psychology at the Gujarat Forensic Sciences University and has completed her MSc from Durham University, UK with merit. She possesses excellent work experience at renowned and noticeable hospitals and clinical setups and has extensive background of dealing with psychiatric cases She has presented various research papers, and has been resource person at various corporate and professionals' workshops, talk-shows and documentary film at the national and international platforms.Passionate about making her voice being heard in the world of academia, she continues to publish research papers on distinguished journals, and presenting her research at nationwide and international conferences (ICM-Asia Pacific, Auckland, Stanford University, USA) and seminars. Her current research interests include understanding of meditation practices and neuropsychology, mindfulness and psychometrics.

Rajesh Sharma, BCBA, has an extensive professional experience in special education, psychology practice, and applied behaviour analysis (ABA) in a variety of setting including schools, psychiatric & drug addiction facilities, department of education, and NGO sector. Jay has keen interest in developing innovative interventions to treat maladaptive & problematic behaviours and help people improve their quality of life. He is a clinical director at Sunrise Behavioural Health Pty Ltd. Jay practises applied behaviour analysis (ABA) and teachs special education at Torrens University Australia in Melbourne.

Nikita Variyani is an RCI registered Clinical Psychologist. She has done M.Phil in Clinical Psychology from Gujarat Forensic Sciences University, Gandhinagar. She has also pursued Masters in Yoga. At present, she is working as a Clinical Psychologist at Hospital for Mental Health, Vadodara. She has been working in this field since last 6 years. She has worked with various types of population suffering from different mental ailments. Her interest lies in working with children with special needs and childhood disorders. She believes in combining the alternative therapies alongwith psychotherapies for intervention of the psychological disorders. Her research interest focused in examining the effect of different alternative therapies like Yoga, Pranayama on mental health.

Yesha A. Vyas is a Rehabilitation Counselor and a Psychotherapist. She has received advanced training in Rational Emotive Cognitive Behavior Therapy(RECBT) from the Albert Ellis Institute, New York. She has a Masters in Clinical Psychology and a Post Graduate Diploma in Rehabilitation Psychology. She has 12+ years of experience in working with parent-child issues, anxiety, depression, issues related to self and interpersonal relationships. She has worked with multiple premier institutes in the capacity of a Psychotherapist. She also works in the capacity of a Behavioral Trainer and conducts training programmes for teachers, parents, individuals and corporates.

York Williams, Ph.D., Associate Professor of Special Education at West Chester University, conducts research primarily in gifted and special education and urban school choice reform. Specifically, his work focuses on: (1) recruiting and retaining culturally diverse students in gifted education; (2) multicultural and urban education school choice; (3) minority student achievement and underachievement; and (4) family involvement. He consults with school districts and educational organizations in the areas of gifted education and multicultural/urban education. Additional interests include the intersection of urban school violence and achievement amongst African American males through the lens of social and juvenile justice. Dr. Williams has been a public school teacher for over fifteen years and has worked as an administrator and supervisor over special and gifted education programs. Dr. Williams is the founder of Children's Advocates for Social Justice (CASJ, 2003) and Young Urban Leaders Program (YULP, 2007) Dr. Williams' work has been recognized by various professional organizations: American Education Research Association (AERA); Family Involvement Network of Educators (FINE); Temple Education Research Award (TERA); The Temple University Benjamin Verdile Alumni Association Award; and Whose Who Amongst America's Teachers Recognition Award. As a scholar, Dr. Williams is the author of "Urban Charter Schools: African American Parents' School Choice Reform" (2013) and has written over two dozens of research papers and articles and presented them at numerous conferences and workshops nationwide.

Prateek Yadav is a Graduate from MLB Medical College Jhansi and has done his M.D. Psychiatry from AFMC Pune. He is an Assoc Prof and has over ten years of experience in Psychiatry working in various hospitals and teaching institutes and has various publications in national and international journals and is presently working in Guwahati.

Index

T

U

V

Y

www.ingramcontent.com/pod-product-compliance
Lightning Source LLC
LaVergne TN
LVHW080533300926
849162LV00007B/1600